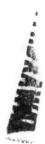

Glutamine, Glutamate, and GABA in the Central Nervous System

Neurology and Neurobiology

EDITORS
Victoria Chan-Palay and Sanford L. Palay
The Harvard Medical School

ADVISORY BOARD

Günter Baumgartner
University Hospital, Zurich

Gösta Jonnson
Karolinska Institute

Bruce McEwen
Rockefeller University

Masao Ito
Tokyo University

Glutamine, Glutamate, and GABA in the Central Nervous System

Proceedings of a Satellite Symposium of the 9th Meeting of the
International Society for Neurochemistry on the Metabolic Relationship
Between Glutamine, Glutamate and GABA in the Central Nervous System,
Held in Saskatoon, Saskatchewan, Canada, July 17–20, 1983

Editors

Leif Hertz

Department of Pharmacology
University of Saskatchewan
Saskatoon, Saskatchewan, Canada

Elling Kvamme

Neurochemical Laboratory
University of Oslo
Oslo, Norway

Edith G. McGeer

Kinsmen Laboratory of
Neurological Research
University of British Columbia
Vancouver, British Columbia, Canada

Arne Schousboe

Department of Biochemistry
The Panum Institute
University of Copenhagen
Copenhagen, Denmark

ALAN R. LISS, INC., NEW YORK

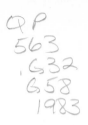

Address all Inquiries to the Publisher
Alan R. Liss, Inc., 150 Fifth Avenue, New York, NY 10011

Copyright © 1983 Alan R. Liss, Inc.

Printed in the United States of America.

Library of Congress Cataloging in Publication Data

Satellite Meeting on the Metabolic Relationship Between Glutamine, Glutamate, and GABA in the Central Nervous System (1983: Saskatoon, Sask.)
Glutamine, glutamate, and GABA in the central nervous system.

"Satellite Symposium of the 9th Meeting of the International Society for Neurochemistry in Vancouver."
Bibliography: p.
Includes index.
1. GABA—Metabolism—Congresses. 2. Glutamine—Metabolism—Congresses. 3. Glutamic acid—Metabolism—Congresses. 4. Brain chemistry—Congresses. I. Hertz, Leif, 1930–   . II. International Society for Neurochemistry. Meeting (19th: 1983: Vancouver, B.C.) III. Title.
[DNLM: 1. Brain-—Metabolism—Congresses. 2. GABA—Metabolism—Congresses. 3. Glutamates—Metabolism—Congresses. 4. Glutamine—Metabolism—Congresses. W1 NE 337B v.7/QU 60 S253g 1983]
QP563.G32S28   1983   599'.0188   83-25529
ISBN 0-8451-2706-3

Contents

METABOLISM OF GLUTAMINE, GLUTAMATE, AND GABA AT THE
CELLULAR AND SUBCELLULAR LEVEL

Contributors

Richard A. Altschuler, Laboratory of Neuro-Otolaryngology, National Institutes of Health, Bethesda, MD 20205 **[33]**

A.M. Benjamin, Department of Pharmacology, University of British Columbia, Vancouver, British Columbia, V6T 1W5, Canada **[399]**

Soll Berl, Department of Neurology, Mount Sinai School of Medicine, New York, NY 10029 **[205,233, 609]**

Claes-Henric Berthold,Department of Anatomy, University of Göteborg, S-400 33, Göteborg, Sweden **[473]**

J. Borg, Centre National de la Recherche Scientifique, Centre de Neurochimie, 67084 Strasbourg Cedex, France **[317]**

H.F. Bradford, Department of Biochemistry, Imperial College, London SW7 2AZ, England **[249,643]**

Edward A. Brunner, Department of Anesthesia, Northwestern University Medical School, Chicago, IL 60611 **[653]**

Roel Bruntink, Studygroup Inborn Errors and Brain, Department of Psychiatry, Faculty of Medicine, University of Groningen, Groningen, The Netherlands **[619]**

Steven P. Butcher, Department of Physiology and Pharmacology, University of Southampton, Southampton SO9 3TU, England **[517]**

Roger F. Butterworth, Laboratory of Neurochemistry, Clinical Research Center, Hôpital Saint-Luc (University of Montreal), Montreal, Quebec, H2X 3J4, Canada **[595]**

Graham LeM. Campbell, Department of Neurology, The Graduate Hospital, Philadelphia, PA 19146 **[343,355]**

Astrid G. Chapman, Department of Neurology, Raine Institute, King's College Hospital Medical School, London SE5 9NU, England **[625]**

Sze-Chuh Cheng, Department of Anesthesia, Northwestern University Medical School, Chicago, IL 60611 **[653]**

M. Teresa Ciotti, Istituto di Biologia Cellulare, Consiglio Nazionale delle Ricerche, 00196 Roma, Italy **[493]**

Donald D. Clarke, Department of Chemistry, Fordham University, Bronx, NY 10458 **[205,233]**

J.F. Collins, Department of Chemistry, City of London Polytechnic, London EC1, England **[643]**

Arthur J.L. Cooper, Department of Neurology, Cornell University Medical College, New York, NY 10021 **[77,371]**

Barrett R. Cooper, Department of Pharmacology, The Wellcome Research Laboratories, Burroughs Wellcome Co., Research Triangle Park, NC 27709 **[145]**

J.T. Cummins, Addiction Research Laboratory, VA Medical Center, Sepulveda, CA 91343 **[669]**

The number in brackets is the opening page number of the contributor's article.

Maria del Carmen Gutierrez, Department of Pharmacology, Southern Illinois University School of Medicine, Springfield, IL 62708 **[571]**

J. Drejer, Department of Biochemistry A, Panum Institute, University of Copenhagen, DK2200 Copenhagen, Denmark **[297,509]**

D.R. Dvorak, Department of Behavioral Biology, Research School of Biological Sciences, Australian National University, Canberra, ACT 2601, Australia **[287]**

Thomas E. Duffy, Department of Neurology, Cornell University Medical College, New York, NY 10021 **[77,371]**

Bernt Engelsen, Neurological Department, Haukeland Hospital, 5616 Haukeland Sykehus, Norway **[241]**

Thomas E. Fisher, Department of Pharmacology, University of Saskatchewan, Saskatoon, Saskatchewan, S7N OWO, Canada **[327]**

Frode Fonnum, Division of Environmental Toxicology, Norwegian Defence Research Establishment, N-2007 Kjeller, Norway **[241]**

M. Frolich, Addiction Research Laboratory, VA Medical Center, Sepulveda, CA 91343 **[669]**

Karen N. Gale, Department of Pharmacology, Georgetown University Schools of Medicine and Dentistry, Washington, DC 20007 **[177]**

J.W. Geddes, Department of Biochemistry, University of Saskatchewan, Saskatoon, Saskatchewan, S7N OWO, Canada **[675]**

Ezio Giacobini, Department of Pharmacology, Southern Illinois University School of Medicine, Springfield, IL 62708 **[571]**

Anders Hamberger, Institute of Neurobiology, University of Göteborg, S-400 33, Göteborg, Sweden **[473]**

G. Hamel, Centre National de la Recherche Scientifique, Centre de Neurochimie, 67084 Strasbourg Cedex, France **[317]**

Leif Hertz, Department of Pharmacology, University of Saskatchewan, Saskatoon, Saskatchewan, S7N OWO, Canada **[xiii,297,327,431]**

Elisabeth Hösli, Department of Physiology, University of Basel, CH-4051 Basel, Switzerland **[441]**

Leo Hösli, Department of Physiology, University of Basel, CH-4051 Basel, Switzerland **[441]**

James L. Howard, Department of Pharmacology, The Wellcome Research Laboratories, Burroughs Wellcome Co., Research Triangle Park, NC 27709 **[145]**

K. Hummeler, Joseph Stokes Research Institute, The Children's Hospital of Philadelphia, Philadelphia, PA 19104 **[389]**

Kouiji Kanmori, Department of Pharmacology, Kyoto Prefectural University of Medicine, Kawaramachi-Hirokoji, Kamikyo-ku, Kyoto 602, Japan **[559]**

Birgitta Karlsson, Institute of Neurobiology, University of Göteborg, S-400 33, Göteborg, Sweden **[473]**

E. Keller, Addiction Research Laboratory, VA Medical Center, Sepulveda, CA 91343 **[669]**

S. Kim, Department of Medicine, University of British Columbia, Vancouver, British Columbia, V6T 1W5, Canada **[389]**

Povl Krogsgaard-Larsen, Department of Chemistry BC, Royal Danish School of Pharmacy, 2100 Copenhagen, Denmark **[297,537]**

Kinya Kuriyama, Department of Pharmacology, Kyoto Prefectural University of Medicine, Kawaramachi-Hirokoji, Kamikyo-ku, Kyoto 602, Japan **[559]**

Elling Kvamme, Neurochemical Laboratory, University of Oslo, Blindern, Oslo 3, Norway [xiii,51]

O.M. Larsson, Department of Nuclear Medicine, The State University Hospital, DK-2100 Copenhagen, Denmark [297]

Anders Lehmann, Institute of Neurobiology, University of Göteborg, S-400 33, Göteborg, Sweden [473]

Giulio Levi, Istituto di Biologia Cellulare, Consiglio Nazionale delle Ricerche, 00196 Roma, Italy [493]

P. Madtes, Laboratory of Vision Research, National Eye Institute, Bethesda, MD 20205 [273]

J. Mark, Centre National de la Recherche Scientifique, Centre de Neurochimie, 67084 Strasbourg Cedex, France [317]

David L. Martin, Center for Laboratories and Research, New York State Department of Health, Albany, NY 12201 [129]

S.C. Massey, Department of Ophthalmology, Washington University School of Medicine, St. Louis, MO 63110 [273]

Alun D. McCarthy, Department of Biochemistry, University of Dundee, Medical Sciences Institute, Dundee DD1 4HN, Scotland [19]

Edith G. McGeer, Kinsmen Laboratory of Neurological Research, Department of Psychiatry, University of British Columbia, Vancouver, British Columbia, V6T 1W5, Canada [xiii,3]

P.L. McGeer, Kinsmen Laboratory of Neurological Research, Department of Psychiatry, University of British Columbia, Vancouver, British Columbia, V6T 1W5, Canada [3]

E. Meier, Department of Biochemistry A, Panum Institute, University of Copenhagen, DK2200 Copenhagen, Denmark [509]

Brian S. Meldrum, Department of Neurology, Institute of Psychiatry, London SE5 8AF, England [625]

Ian G. Morgan, Department of Behavioural Biology, Research School of Biological Sciences, Australian National University, Canberra, ACT 2601, Australia [287]

William J. Nicklas, Department of Neurology, UMDNJ-Rutgers Medical School, Piscataway, NJ 08854 [219]

I. Nissim, Isotope Department, Weizmann Institute, Rehovot, Israel [389]

Michael D. Norenberg, Department of Pathology-D-33, University of Miami School of Medicine, Miami, FL 33101 [95]

Britta Nyström, Institute of Neurobiology, University of Göteborg, S-400 33, Göteborg, Sweden [473]

O.P. Ottersen, Anatomical Institute, University of Oslo, Oslo 1, Norway [185]

Thomas L. Perry, Department of Pharmacology, University of British Columbia, Vancouver, British Columbia, V6T 1W5, Canada [581]

D.W. Peterson, Department of Biochemistry, Imperial College, London SW7 2AZ, England [643]

Andreas Plaitakis, Department of Neurology, Mount Sinai School of Medicine, New York, NY 10029 [609]

D. Pleasure, Division of Biochemical Development and Molecular Diseases, The Children's Hospital of Philadelphia, Philadelphia, PA 19104 [389]

Fred Plum, Department of Neurology, Cornell University Medical College, New York, NY 10021 [371]

Richard L. Potter, Department of Biology, California State University, Northridge, CA 91330 [327]

D.A. Redburn, Department of Neurobiology and Anatomy, University of Texas Medical School, Houston, TX 77025 [273]

Peter J. Roberts, Department of Physiology and Pharmacology, University of Southampton, Southampton SO9 3TU, England **[517]**

Arne Schousboe, Department of Biochemistry A, Panum Institute, University of Copenhagen, Copenhagen, Denmark **[xiii,297,327,509]**

S. Segal, Division of Biochemical Development and Molecular Diseases, The Children's Hospital of Philadelphia, Philadelphia, PA 19104 **[389]**

Richard P. Shank, Department of Biological Research, McNeil Phamaceutical, Spring House Lane, PA 19477 **[343,355]**

David C. Spink, Department of Chemistry, University of Maryland, College Park, MD 20742 **[129]**

B. Spitz, Centre National de la Recherche Scientifique, Centre de Neurochimie, 67084 Strasbourg Cedex, France **[317]**

Jon Storm-Mathisen, Anatomical Institute, University of Oslo, Oslo 1, Norway **[69,185]**

Gerd Svenneby, Neurochemical Laboratory, University of Oslo, Blindern, Oslo 3, Norway **[69]**

John C. Szerb, Department of Physiology and Biophysics, Dalhousie University, Halifax, Nova Scotia, B3H 4H7, Canada **[457]**

Ricardo Tapia, Departamento de Neurociencias, Centro de Investigaciones en Fisiología Celular, Universidad Nacional Autónoma de México, AP 70-600, 04510 México DF, México **[113]**

C.M. Thanki, Department of Biochemistry, Imperial College, London SW7 2AZ, England **[249]**

S. Thompson, Kinsmen Laboratory of Neurological Research, Department of Psychiatry, University of British Columbia, Vancouver, British Columbia, V6T 1W5, Canada **[3]**

J. Tyson Tildon, Department of Pediatrics, University of Maryland School of Medicine, Baltimore, MD 21201 **[415]**

Keith F. Tipton, Department of Biochemistry, Trinity College, University of Dublin, Dublin 2, Ireland **[19]**

Cees J. Van den Berg, Department of Biological Psychiatry, University Psychiatric Clinic, 9713 EZ Groningen, The Netherlands **[619]**

Fernando Vergara, Department of Neurology, Cornell University Medical College, New York, NY 10021 **[77]**

Mary J. Voaden, Department of Visual Science, Institute of Ophthalmology, London WC1H 9QS, England **[261]**

H.K. Ward, Department of Biochemistry, Imperial College, London SW7 2AZ, England **[249]**

Robert J. Wenthold, Department of Neurophysiology, University of Wisconsin Medical School, Madison, WI 53706 **[33]**

Helen L. White, Department of Pharmacology, The Wellcome Research Laboratories, Burroughs Wellcome Co., Research Triangle Park, NC 27709 **[145]**

J.D. Wood, Department of Biochemistry, University of Saskatchewan, Saskatoon, Saskatchewan, S7N OWO, Canada **[675]**

Jang-Yen Wu, Department of Cell Biology, Baylor College of Medicine, Texas Medical Center, Houston, TX 77030 **[161]**

Yukio Yoneda, Department of Pharmacology, Kyoto Prefectural University of Medicine, Kawaramachi-Hirokoji, Kamikyo-ku, Kyoto 602, Japan **[559]**

Albert C.H. Yu, Department of Pharmacology, University of Saskatchewan, Saskatoon, Saskatchewan, S7N OWO, Canada **[327,431]**

M. Yudkoff, Division of Biochemical Development and Molecular Diseases, The Children's Hospital of Philadelphia, Philadelphia, PA 19104 **[389]**

Preface

This book is one outcome of a meeting with 70 scientists participating from 16 countries, which was held in Saskatoon, Saskatchewan, Canada, July 17–20, 1983 as a satellite symposium of the 9th meeting of the International Society for Neurochemistry in Vancouver. The purpose of the satellite meeting—and thus of this book—has been to try to integrate observations from many different research areas into a unified concept of the role of glutamine, glutamate, and GABA in the function of the central nervous system. This has been done on many different organizational levels, ranging from studies on the whole brain or the histologically simpler retina, through whole cells or subcellular structures, to purified enzyme preparations. Many parameters were discussed not only under normal conditions but also in specific disease states or under the influence of external factors. The topics that were emphasized comprised metabolism, including regulatory mechanisms; transport processes, including cellular localizations and interactions; and receptors, including drug effects.

The meeting was generously supported by the Medical Research Council of Canada; by the University of Saskatchewan and its colleges of medicine and of graduate studies; by the Province of Saskatchewan and the city of Saskatoon; and by the Upjohn Medical Company (Don Mills, Ontario), Caltec Scientific (Edmonton, Alberta), and Amersham Radiochemicals (Oakville, Ontario). We have received invaluable assistance from many persons. Although we cannot thank all of them individually, we would like to extend a special thanks to Dr. J.S. Richardson, Department of Pharmacology, University of Saskatchewan, for his great help in arranging the meeting, and to Dr. R.G. Murray, Dean of Medicine, University of Saskatchewan, for his moral and financial support, without which this meeting, and thus this book, would not have been possible. We are also grateful to Mrs. Margaret Matheson, Miss Jackie Bitz, and Mrs. Rosemary Wallace for secretarial assistance in connection with the meeting and with the preparation of this book; and to the publishers, Alan R. Liss, Inc., New York, for their prompt and efficient handling of the manuscripts. Above all, however, we want to express our sincere appreciation and gratitude to all participants in the meeting. Thanks to them it was held in an atmosphere of cooperation and, occasionally, constructive criticism. Such personal interaction is a second, intangible outcome of the meeting, and is essential for arriving at any unified concept in this complex field. Although such a concept is still sketchy and incomplete, we hope it will be evident from this book that progress has been made toward that goal.

Leif Hertz
Elling Kvamme
Edith G. McGeer
Arne Schousboe

KEY ENZYMES OF GLUTAMINE, GLUTAMATE, AND GABA METABOLISM

Glutamine, Glutamate, and GABA
in the Central Nervous System, pages 3–17
© 1983 Alan R. Liss, Inc., 150 Fifth Avenue, New York, NY 10011

GABA AND GLUTAMATE ENZYMES

E.G. McGeer, P.L. McGeer and S. Thompson

Kinsmen Laboratory of Neurological Research
Department of Psychiatry, University of B.C.,
Vancouver, Canada

INTRODUCTION

Our laboratory has long been interested in defining the
neurotransmitters used by various pathways in brain and
changes in these neurotransmitter systems in human diseases.
We have studied enzymes concerned in neurotransmitter synthesis and catabolism as possible indicators of biochemical
neuroanatomy and pathology. The amino acid systems in brain
are extremely difficult because of an embarrassment of
riches. GABA and glutamate/aspartate (Glu/Asp) are, respectively, the probable inhibitory and excitatory "workhorses"
responsible for a majority of neurons in mammalian brains
(McGeer, McGeer 1981). Glu/Asp systems are particularly
difficult because of the lack of good chemical indices and
the occurrence of Glu/Asp in many compartments of brain.
Their diverse roles explain why the levels are not in themselves good indices to their neurotransmitter function.
Sodium dependent uptake or K^+-induced release has been used
but these almost certainly involve glia as well as neurons.
If an enzyme can be identified which is highly concentrated
in one amino acid neuron, such an enzyme would be useful,
not only in animal studies aimed at localization, but in
human pathological studies. The thrust of this chapter is a
consideration of various enzymes as possible indicators of
amino acid neurons.

Before an enzyme can be regarded as a specific indicator of a particular neuronal system, its localization to
such neuronal system must be established. There are three
general procedures commonly used to study the localization

of a particular enzyme. These are:
1. Histochemical methods
2. Biochemical measures in selectively lesioned animals
3. Biochemical studies on neuronal or glial cultures
There are difficulties with each method. The histochemical
procedures are often difficult to establish and may not reveal the proportion of enzyme in neurons vs glia if it is in
both compartments. Combinations of histochemical procedures
with lesion or pharmacological techniques may give further
information but offer their own complicating factors.

Interpretations of lesion data usually involve the
assumption that only neuronal components are affected but it
is by no means certain that the glia which normally exist in
close association with nerve endings still remain after
destruction of those nerve endings. The increasing evidence
that there is marked chemical specialization of glia (Currie
Kelly 1981; Drejer et al. 1982; Henn 1976; Schousboe, Divac
1979; Schrier, Thompson 1974) may mean that some of the
changes seen after brain lesions are due to glial rather than
neuronal components. This is particularly true in the case
of lesions induced by injections of kainic acid (KA) or
other excitotoxin which have been reported to destroy neurons
in a area without effect on glia, axons of passage or afferent nerve endings. Glia cultures derived from KA-injected
adult rat striata have characteristics akin to those of glia
cultures derived from fetal rather than adult brain (van
Alstyn, personal communication). The probability of chemical
specialization of glia, the difficulty of getting pure cultures and the possibility that cells in culture do not reflect
entirely the chemical characteristics of cells in vivo, all
provide difficulties in interpretation of tissue culture
studies. All three methods are, of course, very valuable
but it is difficulties such as these which probably underlie
the many controversies which exist in the literature.

In our work, we have used some histochemical procedures
but most of the data are derived from biochemical measurements on the neostriatum of rats with various types of lesions. The neostriatum is a convenient structure for studying
the localization of enzymes through lesion techniques because
at least some of the biochemical neuroanatomy is known (Figure 1). The long axoned corticostriatal glutamate tract can
be lesioned surgically without affecting GABAergic, dopaminergic or cholinergic indices in the striatum; the extent of
the lesion can be determined by measurement of glutamate

uptake in striatal synaptosomes although maximum decreases
in this non-specific index are of the order of 50%. Similarly the long axoned dopaminergic tract can be destroyed by 6-
hydroxydopamine (60HDA) injections without effect on the
other systems shown in Fig. 1; assays of tyrosine hydroxylase in the striatum provide a convenient index of the extent
of dopaminergic neuronal loss. On the other hand, injections

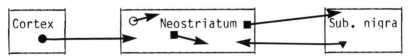

Fig. 1. Some tracts in the extrapyramidal system:
● glutamate; ○ acetylcholine; ■ GABA; ▼dopamine.

of KA or ibotenic acid into adult rat neostriatum produce
marked degeneration of local GABAergic, cholinergic and
other neuronal perikarya in the striatum with no significant
degeneration of afferent systems; measurements of glutamate
decarboxylase (GAD) and/or choline acetyltransferase (ChAT)
give a convenient measure of neuronal loss. In neonatal
rats, the GABAergic neurons are not affected by KA which
provides still another aspect of lesion specificity.

GABA ENZYMES

The routes of synthesis and metabolism of GABA through
the "GABA shunt" are well established (Equation 1) but there
are still some questions relating to enzyme localization.

Equation 1:

$$\text{Glutamine} \underset{5}{\overset{1}{\rightleftarrows}} \text{Glutamate} \quad \alpha\text{-Ketoglutarate}$$

Glutamine ⇌ Glutamate α-Ketoglutarate
            2↓   ✕ 3
              GABA   Succinic ──4──→ Succcinic
                      semialdehyde   acid

1. Glutaminase

It has long been believed that GABA neurons do not take
up glutamate but rather take up glutamine which is converted
in the nerve ending into glutamate by glutaminase (McGeer et
al. 1978). The evidence that glutamine is a better precursor

than glutamate for the GABA releasable by K^+-depolarization is consistent with such a picture (Tapia, Gonzalez 1978). Glutaminase is also found in glia and possibly in glutamate neurons (Wenthold 1980; Ward et al. 1983). Measurements of GAD, glutamate uptake and glutaminase in the neostriata of rats after lesions of the corticostriatal tract or intra-striatal injections of KA (Table 1) are consistent with the

TABLE 1 GLUTAMATE UPTAKE GAD AND GLUTAMINASE (AS PERCENT OF CONTROL) IN THE NEOSTRIATA OF RATS AFTER VARIOUS LESIONS

Lesion of:	Glutamate Uptake	GAD	Glutaminase
Corticostriatal tract	50±17%*	104±12%	91±12%
Kainic acid - 4 nm	119±11%	43±13%*	67±11%*
- 10 nm	112±14%	23±12%*	56±9%*

*Significantly different from control

belief that GABA neurons do not take up glutamate and indi-cate that significant amounts of glutaminase do not occur in glutamate nerve endings of the corticostriatal tract.

A comparison of GAD and glutaminase in the striatum of rats lesioned with varying amounts of KA (Figure 2) suggests that some 60% of the glutaminase activity in the neostriatum is located in GABAergic structures with about 40% in glia. Difficulties in interpretation of such data have already been described but the probable association of much of the glutaminase in the extrapyramidal system with GABAergic neurons was also indicated by the fact that it decreased in parallel with GAD in the substantia nigra of rats following these KA injections (McGeer, McGeer 1979). The decrease in GAD reflects degeneration of descending striatonigral GABAergic systems.

2. GAD

This synthetic enzyme, which takes glutamate to GABA, is specific to GABAergic neurons in the central nervous system and is probably the most widely used index of the

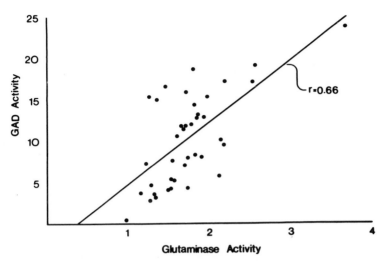

Fig. 2. GAD and glutaminase activities in the neostriata of rats lesioned with varying amounts of kainic acid

integrity of such neurons. GAD has been purified by several laboratories and immunohistochemical work with GAD antibodies is yielding valuable information on the anatomy and morphology of central GABAergic systems (for references see Nagai et al. 1983). One problem is that the enzyme is rapidly transported from the cell bodies with most of the total GAD activity being found in nerve terminals (Ribak et al. 1978). Immunohistochemical studies do not generally reveal the cell bodies except in colchicine-treated animals; hence this procedure cannot readily be combined with a retrograde tracer to establish the projections of GABAergic neurons. Thus there still appears to be some room for less definitive histochemical methods involving other enzymes, notably GABA transaminase (GABA-T).

3. GABA Transaminase

The key enzyme for metabolism of GABA is GABA-T. This enzyme, like acetylcholinesterase in cholinergic neurons, is not completely specific and may also occur in other non-GABAergic neurons as well as in glia. Nevertheless, some recent studies indicate that histochemical work with GABA-T may provide clues to the anatomy of GABA systems. This would make it analogous to acetylcholinesterase which has been a very valuable, although not definitive, tool in studying cholinergic systems. Both chemical (cf Table 2) and histochemical (Vincent et al. 1981) studies in lesioned rats indicate that much of the GABA-T is in GABAergic systems with no significant amounts in cholinergic cells (selectively destroyed by KA injections in neonates) or dopaminergic nerve endings (selectively destroyed by the 6-OHDA). In the latter case there was also no decrease in GABA-T activity in the substantia nigra, indicating that this enzyme does not occur in appreciable amounts in dopamine cells or dendrites even though these are strongly GABA receptive. It had previously been suggested that GABA released at synapses is taken up

TABLE 2.   SOME ENZYME ACTIVITIES AS PERCENT OF CONTROLS IN
           THE STRIATUM OF RATS AFTER VARIOUS LESIONS

| Enzyme | Intrastriatal Injections of KA | | 10-day-old | 6-OHDA |
| | Adult | | | |
	5 nm	10 nm	20 nm	Lesions
Tyrosine hydroxylase	112%	109%	--	48%**
ChAT	55%**	18%	43%**	101%
GAD	64%**	25%**	93%	113%
GABA-T	62%**	34%**	110%	101%

Significantly different from control, *p < 0.01, **p < 0.001
Data taken from Vincent et al. 1980b.

and catabolized in the post-synaptic neuron and in surrounding glial elements since these were the structures thought to contain most of the GABA-T (Baxter 1976). However, this experiment indicated that dopamine neurons of the substantia nigra do not contain much GABA-T, although they are thought to be postsynaptic to a major GABAergic system. Hence, it appears that neurons which receive GABAergic synapses do not necessarily contain GABA-T.

A surprising aspect of these data is the indication (from the parallel falls in GAD and GABA-T) that very little striatal GABA-T activity is in glial cells. As mentioned in the introduction, such an interpretation may be dangerous since KA may affect particular types of glia cells. Studies with the gliatoxic D,L-α-aminoadipic acid in the retina, however, have also been interpreted as indicating a neuronal localization for GABA-T in that region (Linser, Moscona 1981). Recently reported data on the postnatal increases in GABA-T in rat cerebral hemispheres and the higher levels in such tissue as compared with cortical cultures are also consistent with a predominantly neuronal localization (Hansson, Sellstrom 1983). However, histochemical studies clearly indicate the presence of GABA-T in some glia, particularly, for example, Bergmann glia of the cerebellum which can be doubly stained for both GABA-T and the glial marker, GFA.

A histochemical procedure for GABA-T was introduced by van Gelder in 1965 and improved by Hyde and Robinson (1976a, b). A problem with their procedure is that the intense and diffuse staining of the neuropile makes it difficult to differentiate between stained glia or neurons, and between cell bodies or nerve terminals in juxtaposition with them (Hyde, Robinson 1974). If the animal is treated 8-48 hours before sacrifice with an irreversible inhibitor of GABA-T, such as ethanolamine-O-sulfate or gabaculine, only those structures capable of rapid synthesis of new enzyme will be visualized (Fig. 3)(cf Vincent et al. 1980a,1982). Using this pharmacohistochemical technique we have mapped such GABA-T-intensive neurons in rat brain. The stained cells

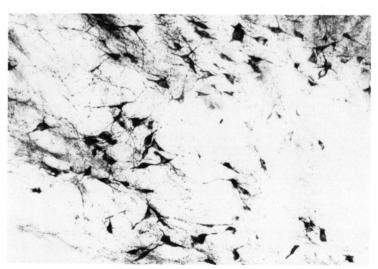

Fig. 3. Neurons stained for GABA-T in globus pallidus of a rat killed 17 hrs after treatment with gabaculine (Nagai et al. 1983)

include all neuronal groups previously reported to be GABA-ergic on the basis of other methods. Other cell groups, not yet identified by such techniques, also stain intensely for GABA-T and may be GABAergic. Known non-GABA neuronal groups are negative for GABA-T staining under these conditions, reinforcing the hypothesis that GABA neurons are far more GABA-T intensive than other neurons (Nagai et al. 1983). This technique can be combined with retrograde tracing methods and thus may be extremely useful in identifying the projections of presumptive GABAergic neurons.

4 and 5. Succinic Dehydrogenase and Glutamine Synthetase

The metabolism of GABA by GABA-T produces one molecule of succinic semialdehyde and one of glutamate. The succinic semialdehyde may be oxidized by succinic dehydrogenase (SSDH) to succinic acid which is returned to the Kreb's cycle. If the glutamate is formed from GABA-T within the GABA nerve ending, it may be decarboxylated by GABA. If, on the other hand, the glutamate is formed in glial cells, it is apparent-ly transformed by glutamine synthetase into glutamine before being returned to the GABAergic nerve ending. Glutamine synthetase has been reported to be restricted to glia (Norenberg, Martin-Hernandez 1979; Linser, Moscona 1981; Patel et al. 1983), while SSDH is in both neurons and glia. Neither of these enzymes appears of use in studying the anatomy of GABAergic systems and we have not ourselves worked with them.

GLUTAMATE ENZYMES

Glutamate plays many roles in the central nervous system and there are correspondingly many different enzymic reactions by which it can be formed or destroyed. We will limit our discussion to the few we have studied in a search for the source of neurotransmitter glutamate.

The synaptic pools of many neurotransmitters are regu-lated by feedback effects on a key synthetic enzyme. Since excess glutamate is itself neurotoxic (McGeer, McGeer 1976), it would seem that feedback control would be particularly necessary. Hence, we hypothesized some years ago that the neurotransmitter pool of glutamate should arise by some enzy-mic step specific to glutamate neurons which would allow for such control. Using the types of lesions already described, we attempted to determine whether aspartate transaminase or ornithine δ-transaminase in the rat neostriatum might be specific or highly localized to glutamate systems. We have also done some histochemical studies on 5-Δ¹-pyrrolidine-carboxylate dehydrogenase and proline oxidase since these offer a possible route to glutamate.

Aspartate Transaminase

This enzyme (Asp-T) catalyzes the reversible conversion shown in Equation 2. If it were responsible for the synthesis of the Glu/Asp, it might be possible for some neurons to secrete both amino acids since they might be freely interconvertible in the nerve terminals. Such a possibility would

Equation 2:

$$\text{Aspartate} + \alpha\text{-Ketoglutarate} \underset{}{\overset{\text{Asp-T}}{\rightleftharpoons}} \text{Oxaloacetate} + \text{Glutamate}$$

explain the frequent conflicts in the literature as to whether a particular path uses aspartate or glutamate and makes even more apropos the use of the term Glu/Asp to refer to neurons using glutamate and/or aspartate. Co-release of aspartate and glutamate has been reported from granule cells (Flint et al. 1981). Specific histochemical localizations of Asp-T in the granule cell areas of the rat olfactory bulb, in the nuclear layer of the retina (Recasens, Delaunoy 1981; Altschuler et al. 1982), and in the fiber endings of the basket cells in the chicken cerebellum (Martinez-Rodriguez et al. 1974) have been reported. Asp-T has also been localized in terminals of the auditory nerve (Altschuler et al. 1981; Fex et al 1982), which may utilize Glu/Asp as transmitter (Wenthold, Gulley 1978; Wenthold 1979; Martin, Adams 1979); it contains 2-5 times the Asp-T found in other nerves, and Asp-T decreases in the ventral cochlear nucleus after the auditory nerve is lesioned (Wenthold 1980). Asp-T could, therefore, have an intricate role to play in the regulation of the relative levels of glutamate and aspartate in nerve terminals.

As indicated in Table 3, however, lesioning the cortico-striatal tract, which markedly affected glutamate uptake, had no effect on striatal Asp-T activity. It is consistent with this finding that lesioning Glu/Asp afferents to the

TABLE 3. Glutamate uptake and some enzyme activities (as percent of control) in neostriatum of decorticated and KA-lesioned rats (Wong et al. 1982)

	Decorticated	Kainic acid
Glutamate uptake	64%*	92%
Orn-T	81%**	62%**
Asp-T	102%	80%**
GAD	101%	9%***
ChAT	97%	10%***

*P < 0.025; **P < 0.005; *** P < 0.0005

hippocampus (Nadler et al. 1978) did not cause decreases in hippocampal Asp-T. Kainic acid lesions of the striatum produced a small but significant loss in local Asp-T in our hands (Table 3), as well as in those of Nicklas et al. (1979) who reported almost identical data. The relatively small loss seen after KA suggests that much of the enzyme is in glia or other structures unaffected by the neurotoxin. Our findings that striatal Asp-T was not altered after cortical lesions argue against any significant localization of Asp-T in striatal Glu/Asp terminals.

Ornithine δ-Transaminase (Orn-T)

Another possible route to neurotransmitter glutamate might be from ornithine through transamination and subsequent oxidation of the intermediate Δ^1-pyrroline-5-carboxylic acid (P5C; Equation 3). The biochemistry of the interconversion

Equation 3:

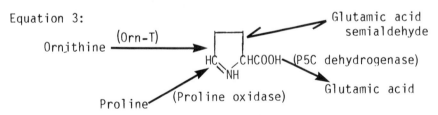

between glutamate and ornithine has been reviewed (Roberts 1981). This hypothesis gained some support from studies showing some parallelism between the regional distributions of Orn-T activity and glutamate uptake, localization of about 85% of the activity in the synaptosomal fraction and marked post-natal increases in activity (Wong et al. 1981; Wong, McGeer 1981). The losses in Orn-T found in the cortex and striatum in patients with Huntington's disease are also consistent with a neuronal localization (Wong et al. 1982b).

In animals with lesions of the corticostriatal tract, however, striatal Orn-T activity decreased very slightly, suggesting that only about 19% may be present in the Glu/Asp terminals (Table 3). The more marked reduction of Orn-T activity in the KA-lesioned striatum (Table 3) suggests that at least 38% of the total striatal Orn-T is present in intrinsic neurons or neuronal perikarya. The remaining 43% seems to be localized in elements other than the glutamate nerve endings but equally insensitive to KA, most probably in glia. The degree of specificity indicated by these results is not sufficient to allow the use of Orn-T as a reliable index for glutamate systems. But one cannot conclude that Orn-T is not involved in the synthesis of transmitter glutamate. Ornithine may well be one of several putative precursors for glutamate. Shank and Campbell (1983) have come to a similar conclusion from studies on uptake and metabolism of ornithine in various cerebellar fractions and Yoneda et al. (1982) reported the synaptosomal conversion of ornithine to glutamate and GABA.

P5C Dehydrogenase and Proline Oxidase

Another possible route to glutamate is from proline (Equation 3). Histochemical studies on P5C dehydrogenase, using a modification of van Gelder's method for GABA-T but with Δ^1-pyrrolidine-5-carboxylic acid (P5C; Strecker 1960) as substrate, show regionally specific staining of a few selected groups of glial cells. There is, for example, selective staining of Bergmann glial cells (Figure 4), of astrocytic-like cells in the hippocampal pyramidal layer and in fibrous astrocytes of the corpus callosum and white matter of the cerebral hemispheres. No staining was seen in neurons, nor were the glia stained in many regions of the brain. When proline was substituted for the P5C as a histochemical substrate for proline oxidase, the Bergmann glia were also stained; no other specific staining was seen. The evidence therefore is against these enzymes being neuronal in brain.

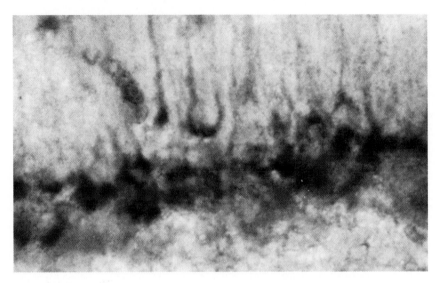

Fig. 4 Staining of Bergmann glia in cerebellum by the histo-chemical procedure for Δ^1-pyrrolidine-5-dehydrogenase

CONCLUSIONS

The enzymes connected with glutamate metabolism pose a fascinating challenge. It is clear that much remains to be learned but the importance of Glu/Asp neurons in brain suggests the needed efforts are worthwhile.

REFERENCES

Altschuler RA, Neises GR, Harmison GG, Wenthold RJ, Fex J (1981). Immunocytochemical localization of aspartate aminotransferase immunoreactivity in cochlear nucleus of the guinea pig. Proc Soc Natl Acad Sci USA 78:6553

Altschuler RA, Mosinger JL, Harmison G, Parakkal MH, Wenthold RJ (1982). Aspartate aminotransferase-like immunoreactivity as a marker for aspartate/glutamate in guinea pig photo-receptors. Nature 298:657.

Baxter CF (1976). Some recent advances in studies of GABA metabolism and compartmentation, in "GABA in Nervous System Function" (E Roberts, TN Chase, DB Tower, eds.), Raven Press, N.Y., p. 11

Bradford HF, HK Ward (1976): On glutaminase activity in mammalian synaptosomes. Brain Res 110: 115

Currie DN, Kelly JS (1981). Glial versus neuronal uptake of glutamate. J Exp Biol 95:181

Drejer J, Larsson OM, Schousboe A. (1982) Characterization of L-glutamate uptake into and release from astrocytes and neurons cultured from different brain regions. Exp Brain Res 47:259.

Fex J, Altschuler RA, Wenthold RJ, Parakkal MH (1982). Aspartate aminotransferase immunoreactivity in cochlea of guinea pig. Hearing Res 7:149

Flint RS, Rea MA, McBride WJ (1981). In vitro release of endogenous amino acids from granule cell-, stellate cell-, and climbing fiber-deficient cerebella. J Neurochem 37:1425

Hansson E, Sellstrom A (1983). MAO, COMT, and GABA-T activities in primary astroglial cultures. J Neurochem 40:220

Henn FA (1976). Neurotransmission and glial cells. A functional relationship? J Neurosci Res 2:271

Hyde JC, Robinson N (1974). Gamma-aminobutyrate transaminase activity in rat cerebellar cortex: a histochemical study. Brain Res 82:109

Hyde JC, Robinson N (1976a). Improved histological localization of GABA-transaminase in rat cerebellar cortex after aldehyde fixation. Histochem 46:261

Hyde JC, Robinson N (1976b). Electron cytochemical localization of gamma-aminobutyric acid in rat cerebellar cortex. Histochem 49:51

Linser PJ, Moscona AA (1981). Induction of glutamine synthetase in embryonic neural retina: Its suppression by the gliatoxic agent α-aminoadipic acid. Devel Brain Res 1:103

Martin MR, Adams JC (1979). Effects of DL-α-aminoadipate on synaptically and chemically evoked excitation of anteroventral cochlear nucleus neurons in the cat. Neuroscience 4:1097

Martinez-Rodriguez R, Fernandez B, Cevallos C, Gonzalez M (1974). Histochemical location of glutamic dehydrogenase and aspartate aminotransferase in chicken cerebellum. Brain Res 69:31

McGeer EG, McGeer PL (1976). Duplication of biochemical changes of Huntington's chorea by intrastriatal injections of glutamic and kainic acid. Nature 263: 517

McGeer EG McGeer PL (1978). Localization of glutaminase in the rat neostriatum. J Neurochem 32:1071

McGeer PL, McGeer EG (1981). Amino acid transmitters. In Siegel GJ, Alberts RW, Agranoff BW, Katzman R (eds): "Basic Neurochemistry", 3rd edition, Little, Brown & Co., p. 233

McGeer PL, Eccles JC, McGeer EG (1978). "Molecular Neurobiology of the Mammalian Brain", Plenum Press, New York.

Nadler JV, White WF, Vaca KW, Perry BW, Cotman CW (1978). Biochemical correlates of transmission mediated by glutamate and aspartate. J Neurochem 31:147

Nagai T, McGeer PL, McGeer EG (1983). Distribution of GABA-T-intensive neurons in the rat forebrain and midbrain. J Comp Neurol 218: (in press)

Nicklas WJ, Nunez R, Berl S, Duvoisin R (1979). Neuronal-glial contributions to transmitter amino acid metabolism: studies with kainic acid-induced lesions of rat striatum. J Neurochem 33:839

Norenberg MD, Martin-Hernandez A (1979). Fine structural localization of glutamine synthetase in astrocytes of rat brain. Brain Res 161:303

Patel AJ, Hunt A, Tahourdin CSM (1983). Regional development of glutamine synthetase activity in the rat brain and its association with the differentiation of astrocytes. Dev Brain Res 8:31.

Recasens M, Delaunoy JP (1981). Immunological properties and immunohistochemical localization of cysteine sulfinate or aspartate aminotransferase-isoenzyme in rat CNS. Brain Res 205:351

Ribak CE, Vaughn JE, Saito K (1978). Immunocytochemical localization of glutamic acid decarboxylase in neuronal somata following colchicine inhibition of axonal transport. Brain Res 140:315

Roberts E (1981). Strategies for identifying sources and sites of formation of GABA-precursor or transmitter glutamate in brain. Di Chiara G, GL Gessa (eds): "Glutamate as a neurotransmitter", Adv Biochem Psychopharm, Vol. 27, New York: Raven Press, pp 91-102.

Schousboe A, Divac I (1979). Differences in glutamate uptake in astrocyte cultures from different brain regions. Brain Res 177:407

Schrier BK, Thompson E (1974). On the role of glial cells in the mammalian nervous system. J Biol Chem 249:1769

Strecker HJ (1960). The interconversion of glutamic acid and proline. J Biol Chem 235:2045

Shank RP, Campbell GL-M (1983). Ornithine as a precursor of glutamate and GABA. J Neurosci Res 9:47

Tapia R, Gonzalez RM (1978). Glutamine and glutamate as precursors of the releasable pool of GABA in brain cortex slices. Neurosci Lett 10:165

van Gelder NM (1965). The histochemical demonstration of γ-aminobutyric acid metabolism by reduction of a tetrazolium salt. J Neurochem 12:231

Vincent SR, Kimura H, McGeer EG (1980a). The pharmacohistochemical demonstration of gaba-transaminase. Neurosci
Lett 16:345

Vincent SR, Lehmann J, McGeer EG (1980b). The localization
of GABA-transaminase in the striato-nigral system. Life
Sci 27:595

Vincent SR, Kimura H, McGeer EG (1981). The histochemical
localization of GABA transaminase in the efferents of the
striatum. Brain Res 222:198

Vincent SR, Kimura H, McGeer EG (1982) GABA-transaminase in
the basal ganglia: A pharmacohistochemical study. Brain
Res 251:104

Ward HK, Thanki CM, Bradford HF (1983). Glutamine and
glucose as precursors of transmitter amino acids: Ex vivo
studies. J Neurochem 40:855

Wenthold RJ (1979). Release of endogenous glutamic acid,
aspartic acid and GABA from cochlear nucleus slices.
Brain Res 162:338

Wenthold RJ (1980). Glutaminase and aspartate
aminotransferase decrease in the cochlear nucleus after
lesion of the auditory nerve. Brain Res 190:293

Wenthold RJ, Gulley RL (1978). Glutamic acid and aspartic
acid in the cochlear nucleus of the waltzing guinea pig.
Brain Res 158:279

Wong PTH, McGeer EG (1981). Postnatal changes of GABAergic
and glutamatergic parameters. Develop Brain Res 1:519

Wong PTH, McGeer EG, McGeer PL (1981). A sensitive
radiometric assay for ornithine aminotransferase:
Regional and subcellular distribution in rat brain. J
Neurochem 36:501

Wong PT-H, McGeer EG, McGeer PL (1982a). Effects of kainic
acid injections and cortical lesions on ornithine and
aspartate aminotransferases in rat striatum. J Neurosci
Res 8:643

Wong PTH, McGeer PL, Rossor M, McGeer EG (1982b). Ornithine
aminotransferase in Huntington's disease. Brain Res
231:466

Yoneda Y, Roberts E, Dietz GW Jr (1982). A new synaptosomal
biosynthetic pathway of glutamate and GABA from ornithine
and its negative feedback inhibition by GABA. J Neurochem
38:1694

**Glutamine, Glutamate, and GABA
in the Central Nervous System, pages 19–32
© 1983 Alan R. Liss, Inc., 150 Fifth Avenue, New York, NY 10011**

GLUTAMATE DEHYDROGENASE

Alun D McCarthy[1] & Keith F Tipton

Department of Biochemistry
Trinity College, Dublin 2,
Ireland.

The enzyme glutamate dehydrogenase (L-glutamate-NAD(P)$^+$ oxidoreductase (deaminating), EC 1.4.1.3) catalyses the reaction:

$$L\text{-Glutamate} + NAD(P)^+ + H_2O \rightleftharpoons 2\text{-Oxoglutarate} + NAD(P)H + H^+ + NH_4^+$$

The results of several studies on the metabolism of glutamate in liver have failed to yield any clear concensus on the role of this enzyme. Studies with isolated hepatocytes led Krebs et al. (1978) to conclude that the net flux through the reaction was in the direction of ammonia production for urea synthesis, a conclusion also supported by the results of Rognstad (1977). A similar function, of producing ammonia under conditions of metabolic acidosis, has also been suggested for the enzyme in kidney (Schoolwerth et al. 1978). In contrast McGivan and Chappell (1975) suggested that the activity of the purine nucleotide cycle (see Tornheim, Lowenstein, 1972) might be adequate to supply ammonia for urea production. They interpreted the results of Mendes-Mourao et al. (1975), that showed leucine (an activator of glutamate dehydrogenase) to inhibit urea production from alanine in isolated hepatocytes, as indicating that this enzyme operated in the direction of glutamate synthesis in vivo. A similar conclusion has also been reached from studies on the effects of ADP and pH on the activity of the enzyme (Bailey et al. 1982). These workers

[1] Present address: Department of Biochemistry, Medical Sciences Institute, The University, Dundee DD1 4HN, Scotland, U.K.

suggested that the main function of the enzyme was the rapid removal of ammonia, but that the glutamate formed could also result in increased concentrations of N-acetylglutamate that would activate the urea cycle by a direct effect on the activity of carbamoylphosphate synthase.

The role of the enzyme in brain is far from clear. Although isolated liver mitochondria will readily catalyse the oxidative deamination of glutamate (Mendes-Mourao et al. 1975; Krebs, Lund 1977), those from brain are apparently unable to do this (Dennis, Clark 1977). It appears that transamination, rather than deamination accounts for the metabolism of exogenous glutamate or that produced endogenously in brain mitochondria (Dennis, Clark 1978). These mitochondria do, however, readily catalyse the synthesis of glutamate from 2-oxoglutarate and ammonia, which might suggest the involvement of glutamate dehydrogenase in the detoxification of ammonia in brain. The suggestion that ammonia toxicity might result, in part, from the activity of glutamate dehydrogenase resulting in a depletion of citric acid cycle intermediates does not, however, appear to be valid since chronic ammonia administration was not found to deplete these intermediates (Hawkins et al. 1973).

In view of the importance of glutamate and γ-aminobutyrate as neurotransmitters in brain, it would be tempting to ascribe a major role in the metabolism of these compounds to glutamate dehydrogenase. Investigation of these processes are complicated by the existence of more than one metabolically distinct pool of glutamate in brain (van den Berg et al. 1970) but there is no convincing evidence to suggest that glutamate dehydrogenase plays a major part in the formation of these neurotransmitters (see van den Berg 1970). The observation that a number of psycho-active drugs, including chlorpromazine (Fahien, Shemisa 1969) and the phenothiazines and butyrophenones (Veronese et al. 1979) are powerful inhibitors of brain glutamate dehydrogenase raises the intriguing possibility that the effects of these drugs might be complicated by their interference with the function of this enzyme.

The complicated allosteric regulation of glutamate dehydrogenase activity has been the subject of many studies (for review see: Fisher 1973; Smith et al. 1975). Inhibitors of the enzyme include GTP, GDP and, to a lesser extent, ITP and IDP (see Yielding, Tompkins 1961; Fisher

1973). ADP generally acts as an activator of the enzyme. These regulatory effects, however, depend on the assay pH, the coenzyme used and its concentration (see Fisher 1973; Bailey et al. 1982). For example, at pH 6.0 GTP can act as an activator of the enzyme whereas ADP inhibits it (Di Prisco 1975).

The behaviour of the enzyme is further complicated by its polymerisation at higher protein concentrations. At low concentrations the enzyme exists as a hexamer but this associates to form higher aggregates as the concentration is increased; a process that is generally inhibited by allosteric inhibitors and promoted by allosteric activators (see e.g. Markau et al. 1971; Cohen et al. 1976). It has been argued that this aggregation phenomenon, which has no effect on the specific activity of the enzyme (Fisher et al. 1962), is important for the action of allosteric effectors in vivo (Cohen et al. 1976; Cohen, Benedek 1979; but see Thusius 1977; Zeiri, Reisler 1978). In addition to this self-association, the association of glutamate dehydrogenase with other cellular components, such as aspartate amino-transferase (see Churchich 1978; Fahien et al. 1978) or the mitochondrial inner membrane (Godinot 1974; Nemat-Gorgani, Dodd 1977a,b), may play a part in regulating its activity.

In order to investigate the roles of the enzyme in brain and the possible significance of its interactions with drugs we decided to study the properties of the enzyme from ox brain. However, in the course of this work we found that the commonly-used preparations of the enzyme had suffered limited proteolytic digestion during the purification (McCarthy et al. 1980). Because of this, it became necessary to compare the properties of the enzymes prepared from brain and liver by our procedure with those of the previously well-studied proteolysed preparations.

PURIFICATION PROCEDURES AND PROTEOLYSIS

The procedure that was initially adopted for the purif-ication of the enzyme from ox brain (McCarthy et al. 1980) involved ammonium sulphate precipitation, chromatography on DEAE-cellulose and affinity chromatography on GTP-Sepharose (see Godinot et al. 1974). This procedure, which yielded an apparently homogeneous preparation of the enzyme, was also found to give satisfactory results in the purification of glutamate dehydrogenase from ox liver (McCarthy et al. 1980). The method was less time-consuming than those that had previously been commonly used to purify the enzyme from liver (see e.g. Olson, Anfinsen 1952; Fahien et al. 1969) and these latter methods were found to be unsuitable for use with brain.

Studies of the behaviour of the enzyme preparations purified from liver and brain on polyacrylamide gel electrophoresis in the presence of sodium dodecyl sulphate revealed that they had slightly slower mobilities than were obtained when the ox liver enzyme preparations from a number of commercial suppliers (which have been used in almost all the more recent studies with this enzyme) were analysed in the same way (McCarthy et al. 1980). These results suggested that the enzymes prepared by our procedure were slightly larger than the preparations obtained from the commercial sources. When an ammonium sulphate precipitate from an ox liver homogenate was taken up in 20 mM sodium-potassium phosphate buffer, pH 7.4, dialysed and stored for 14 days before the purification procedure of McCarthy et al. (1980) was completed, the mobility of the purified enzyme on polyacrylamide gel electrophoresis was found to be the same as that of a commercially-supplied preparation, suggesting that the difference between the preparations resulted from a modification occurring during the purification of the commercially-obtained samples.

Amino-terminal analysis of the preparations obtained from ox liver and brain by the method of McCarthy et al. (1980) and that from a commercial source (Boehringer Corp.) revealed the sequences shown in Table 1.

Table 1. N-Terminal Sequences of Glutamate Dehydrogenase Preparations from Ox.

Source	Preparation	Sequence
Brain	McCarthy et al. (1980)	H_2N-X-Asp-(Ala)$_3$-Asp-Y-Glu-
Liver	" " " "	H_2N-X-Asp-(Ala)$_3$-Asp-Y-Glu-
Liver	Boehringer Corp.	H_2N-Ala-Asp-Y-Glu-

The unidentified terminal amino acid, X, may be cysteine or cysteic acid and Y may be arginine. The sequence of the preparation from the Boehringer Corp. is similar to that reported for the enzyme from ox liver by Moon et al. (1972). These results suggest that the N-terminal tetrapeptide has been lost during the procedure used in the preparation of the commercially-obtained sample. Since the C-terminal sequences of these preparations have not been determined, the possibility that proteolysis may also have occurred at this end of the polypeptide cannot be excluded.

Comparison of the peptides produced by tryptic digestion of the enzyme preparations using the method of Cleveland et al. (1977) showed some differences between the mobilities of the peptides liberated from the native and commercially-obtained preparation. There was, however, no difference between the preparations from ox brain and liver that had been prepared by the method of McCarthy et al. (1980). This result is consistent with earlier reports (Talal, Tompkins 1964; Fahien, Shemisa 1969) that the enzymes from these two sources are identical. This, however, may contrast with the situation in the rat where Chee et al (1979) have reported the brain and liver enzymes to have different properties.

Recently we have found that N_2,N_2-adipodihydrazido-bis (N^6-carbonylmethyl-NAD) (bis-NAD$^+$) can be used in the preparation of the enzymes from ox brain and liver and from rat liver (Beattie et al. 1983). This bifunctional reagent consisting of two NAD$^+$ molecules covalently linked by a "spacer" has been shown to be able to cross-link the active sites of some multimeric dehydrogenases under appropriate conditions causing precipitation. At low concentrations of bis-NAD$^+$ no appreciable cross-linking occurs, however, the addition of the substrate analogue glutaric acid displaces the enzyme binding equilibrium resulting in the formation of inter-molecular cross-links and precipitation of the enzyme. This procedure has been shown to be effective in replacing the affinity chromatography step in the purification procedure, further reducing the time taken to achieve complete purification.

PROPERTIES OF NATIVE AND PROTEOLYSED GLUTAMATE DEHYDROGENASE

The discovery that the commercially-available preparations of glutamate dehydrogenase, that had been used in the majority of studies on this enzyme, had suffered limited proteolytic digestion during their purification necessitated a re-evaluation of the kinetic properties. In the following sections some of the properties of the native (unproteolysed) preparations obtained by the method of McCarthy et al. (1980) are compared with those of commercially-obtained (proteolysed) preparations of the enzyme.

(a)   Behaviour at High Concentrations

The differences in the relative molecular masses of the native and proteolysed preparations of glutamate dehydrogenases were too small to be detectable by their sedimentation behaviour at low concentrations. As the protein concentration was increased analytical ultracentrifugation showed all preparations to form aggregates, but there was no significant differences between the native and proteolysed preparations in this respect. In the presence of 3 mM GTP plus 3 mM NADH, which have been reported to promote disaggregation (Markau et al. 1971), it was found that the native preparations depolymerised more readily than the commercially-obtained samples (McCarthy et al. 1981).

It is tempting to ascribe this difference in the aggregation behaviour of the enzyme preparations to differences between their affinities for the nucleotides since Hucho et al. (1975) have produced evidence implicating the N-terminal region of the molecule in the interactions with allosteric nucleotides. Such an explanation would be consistent with the data in Table 2 that indicate that increasing the concentrations of GTP and NADH tends to minimise the differences between the sedimentation behaviour of the native and proteolysed preparations. These results do not, however, exclude the possibility of some difference in the self-association constants of the enzyme-nucleotide complexes.

Table 2.   Sedimentation Coefficients of Ox Liver Glutamate Dehydrogenase Preparations (adapted from McCarthy et al. 1981).

Effector Concentration (mM)		Sedimentation Coefficient $(S_{20,w}.10^{-13}S)$	
GTP	NADH	Native Enzyme	Commercial (Boehringer) Enzyme
0.7	0.7	14.7	16.1
3.0	3.0	14.4	15.2
7.0	7.0	13.9	14.4

(b)   Behaviour at Low Concentrations

Despite the possibility that the use of higher protein concentrations may provide a truer reflection of the situation in vivo (see e.g. Tompkins et al. 1963), the majority of kinetic studies with glutamate dehydrogenase have been performed at much lower concentrations.   In order to investigate whether the proteolysis that had occurred during the purification of the enzyme had resulted in any significant changes in its kinetic properties, a series of comparisons were made at such low concentrations (0.12 μg.ml^{-1}), where the association phenomena discussed above do not occur. Because of the complexity of the reaction catalysed by glutamate dehydrogenase and its regulation, a complete kinetic analysis has not been carried out but a wide range of experiments have been performed to allow the apparent kinetic parameters to be determined.

Activity in the direction of reductive amination was assayed spectrophotometrically in a mixture containing, unless otherwise stated, 80 μM NAD(P)H, 5 μM 2-oxoglutarate, 100 mM NH$_4$Cl, enzyme and 50 mM sodium potassium phosphate buffer, pH 7.4.   The reaction in the direction of oxidative deamination was assayed fluorimetrically in a reaction mixture containing, unless otherwise stated, 1 mM NAD(P)$^+$, 40 mM L-glutamate, enzyme and the same buffer solution.

When the enzymes were assayed in the direction of oxidative deamination the dependence on NAD$^+$ concentration was found to be complex and similar to that reported by Engel

and Dalziel (1969).   The native and proteolysed preparations behaved similarly in this respect.   Neither were there
any major differences in the K_m values for the other substrates, assayed in either direction, or in the maximum
velocity values.   The dependence of the initial velocity on
pH, determined in a variety of buffers, was also similar
with the native and proteolysed preparations.

When the dependence of the initial rate of reductive
amination on the concentration of NH_4Cl was studied, there
was inhibition at high concentrations of this substrate
(> 600 μM) and the proteolysed preparation appeared to be
somewhat more sensitive than the native ox brain enzyme.
Further studies suggested that this inhibition was due to
Cl^- ions since similar inhibition was observed with KCl or
NaCl but not with Na_2SO_4.   In all cases the commercially-
obtained preparation was somewhat more sensitive to this
inhibition.   Although these results might suggest that the
proteolysis had affected anion binding sites on the enzyme,
the high concentrations involved make any physiological
significance doubtful.

With both the native and proteolysed preparations of
the enzyme the reaction in the direction of reductive amination was inhibited by high concentrations of NADH (> 32 μM).
This high-substrate inhibition was found to be partial in
nature and, as shown in Fig. 1, the native preparation was
found to be more sensitive to inhibition than the commercially
obtained preparation..   This difference may be related to
the more efficient depolymerization of the former enzyme
preparation by NADH and GTP that was discussed earlier.   No
significant inhibition of either preparation by NADPH could
be detected at concentrations of up to 80 μM.

Significant differences were also observed in the sensitivities of the preparations to nucleoside phosphates.   The
response of the reaction assayed in the direction of reductive amination were found to show marked differences when
determined at inhibitory concentrations (80 μM) and non-
inhibitory concentrations (16 μM) of NADH.   These data are
summarized in Table 3.

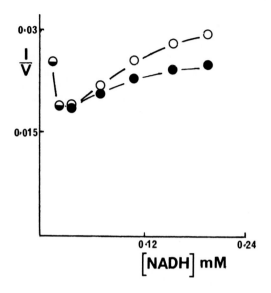

Fig. 1.   A Dixon (1953) plot for the inhibition of glutamate dehydrogenase preparations by NADH.   The reaction was
assayed in the direction of reductive amination as described
in the text.   Initial velocities are given in μmol product.
min^{-1}.mg $enzyme^{-1}$.   O Native (ox brain) enzyme; ● Ox liver
enzyme from Boehringer Corp.

Although the native enzyme preparation was somewhat
more sensitive to inhibition by GTP, the relative sensitivities were similar regardless of the coenzyme used or whether
the concentrations of NADH were inhibitory or not.   In
contrast, the two preparations only showed differences in
their sensitivities to activation by ADP at inhibitory concentrations of NADH.   Similarly a difference in the response to the weaker activation by ATP was observed at
inhibitory concentrations of NADH but not when NADPH was
used.   These differences might be related to the differences
in the affinities of the two forms for inhibitory concentrations of NADH.

There was no significant difference between the sensitivities of the two preparations to activation by ADP (K_a =
32 - 33 μM) when the reaction was assayed in the direction
of oxidative deamination with either NAD^+ or $NADP^+$ as the

coenzyme.   In contrast, when assayed with NAD^+, the native
enzyme preparation was somewhat more sensitive to activation
by ATP (K_a = 85 µM) than was the proteolysed preparation
(K_a = 130 µM).   The former preparation when assayed in this
direction with $NADP^+$ as the coenzyme, was somewhat more
sensitive to inhibition by GTP (K_i = 18 µM) than was the
commercially-obtained preparation (K_i = 30 µM).   When NAD^+
was used as the coenzyme, the difference between the sensitivities of the two preparations was even smaller although,
again the native preparation was the more sensitive.

Table 3.   The Effects of Allosteric Nucleotides on the
Reductive Amination of 2-Oxoglutarate.

Nucleotide	Coenzyme	Concentration (µM)	$K_i[K_a]$ (µM)	
			Native (Ox Brain Enzyme)	Commercial (Boehringer) Enzyme
GTP	NADH	16	12	18
"	NADH	80	6.5	9
"	NADPH	80	9	16
ADP	NADH	16	[18]	[16]
"	NADH	80	[154]	[85]
"	NADPH	80	[20]	[20]
ATP	NADH	80	[480]	[250]
"	NADPH	80	[130]	[130]

THE EFFECTS OF Mg^{2+} IONS

Previous studies on the effects of nucleoside triphos-
phates on the activity of glutamate dehydrogenase have used
the free, uncomplexed, forms of these nucleotides. However,
it is likely that these compounds will exist largely as their
metal ion complexes within the mitochondria.   Our own
studies (McCarthy, Tipton manuscript in preparation) have
shown that the magnesium complexes of ATP and GTP have no
effects on the activity assayed in the direction of NAD^+
reduction.   ADP, however, has a considerably lower affinity
for divalent cations and substantial amounts would be
expected to remain uncomplexed under physiological conditions.

In addition Bailey et al. (1982) have stated that Mg^{2+}, Mn^{2+} and Ca^{2+} have no effect on the activation of glutamate de-hydrogenase by ADP. These considerations suggest that within the cell the effects of GTP and ATP on the activity of glutamate dehydrogenase may be of considerably less importance than those of ADP.

CONCLUSIONS

The discovery that commonly used preparations of glut-amate dehydrogenase had undergone limited proteolysis during preparation (McCarthy et al. 1980) necessitated a re-eval-uation of the behaviour of the enzyme. The differences revealed in the present studies, while suggesting that the proteolytic digestion may have affected the nucleotide bind-ing sites, were small and their in vivo significance may be doubtful. Perhaps the most important differences revealed in these studies are those in the responses of the aggregat-ion-disaggregation behaviour at higher concentrations and further work will be required to assess their significance.

Limited proteolysis of commercially-prepared ox liver glutamate dehydrogenase by chymotrypsin has been shown to have a pronounced activatory effect (Place, Beynon 1982) but it is not known whether this behaviour has any physiological significance. In the case of the enzyme preparations studied here, the specific activities of the native prepar-ations and those from commercial sources were similar.

Mihara et al. (1982) have shown that glutamate dehydro-genase is synthesised outside the mitochondrion as a pre-cursor of higher molecular weight. It is unlikely, however, that the proteolysis discussed in the present work is related to the processing of the higher molecular weight material associated with its insertion into the mito-chondrion.

REFERENCES

Bailey J, Bell ET, Bell JE (1982). Regulation of bovine glutamate dehydrogenase. The effects of pH and ADP. J Biol Chem 257:5579.
Beattie RE, Graham LD, Griffin TO, Tipton KF (1983). Purification of NAD^+-dependent dehydrogenases by affinity

precipitation with N_2,N_2' adipodihydrazido-bis-(N^6-carboxy-methyl-NAD$^+$).

Chee PY, Dahl JL, Fahien LA (1979). The purification and properties of rat brain glutamate dehydrogenase. J Neurochem 35:52.

Churchich JE (1978). Interaction between brain enzymes glutamate dehydrogenase and aspartate aminotransferase. Biochem Biophys Res Commun 83:1105.

Cleveland DW, Frischer SG, Kuschner MW, Laemmli UK (1977). Peptide mapping by limited proteolysis in sodium dodecyl sulfate and analytical gel electrophoresis. J Biol Chem 252:1102.

Cohen RJ, Benedek GB (1979). The functional relationship between the polymerization and catalytic activity of beef liver glutamate dehydrogenase. III. Analysis of Thusius' critique. J Mol Biol 129:37.

Cohen RJ, Jedziniak JA, Benedek GB (1976). The functional relationship between polymerization and catalytic activity of beef liver glutamate dehydrogenase. II. Experiments. J Mol Biol 108:179.

Dennis SC, Clark JB (1977). Regulation of glutamate metabolism by TCA cycle activity in rat brain mitochondria. Biochem J 168:521.

Dennis SC, Clark JB (1978). The synthesis of glutamate by rat brain mitochondria. J Neurochem 31:673.

DiPrisco A (1975). Effect of pH and ionic strength on the catalytic and allosteric properties of native and chemically modified preparations of ox liver mitochondrial glutamate dehydrogenase. Arch Biochem Biophys 171:604.

Dixon M (1953). Determination of enzyme inhibitor constants. Biochem J 55:170.

Engel PC, Dalziel K (1969). Kinetic studies of glutamate dehydrogenase with glutamate and norvaline as substrates. Biochem J 115:621.

Fahien LA, Shemisa O (1969). Effects of chlorpromazine on glutamate dehydrogenase. Mol Pharmacol 6:156.

Fahien LA, Strmecki M, Smith S (1969). Studies on gluconeogenic mitochondrial enzymes. I. A new method of preparing beef liver glutamate dehydrogenase and effects of purification methods on the properties of the enzyme. Arch Biochem Biophys 130:449.

Fahien LA, Ruoho A, Kmiotek E (1978). A study of glutamate dehydrogenase-aminotransferase complexes with a bifunctional imidate. J Biol Chem 253:5745.

Fisher HF, Cross DG, McGregor LL (1962). Catalytic activity of subunits of glutamate dehydrogenase. Nature 196:895.

Fisher HF (1973).   Glutamate dehydrogenase-ligand complexes
   and their relationship to the mechanism of the reaction.
   Adv Enzymol 39:369.
Godinot C (1974).   Nature and possible functions of assoc-
   iation between glutamate dehydrogenase and cardiolipin.
   Biochemistry 12:4029.
Godinot C, Julliard JH, Gautheron DC (1974).   A rapid and
   efficient new method of purification of glutamate dehydrogenase by affinity chromatography on GTP-Sepharose. Anal
   Biochem 61:264.
Hawkins RA, Miller AL, Nielsen RC, Veech RL (1973).   The
   acute action of ammonia on rat brain metabolism in vivo.
   Biochem J 134:1001.
Hucho F, Rasched I, Sund H (1975).   Studies of glutamate
   dehydrogenase: analysis of functional areas and function-
   al groups.   Eur J Biochem 52:221.
Krebs HA, Lund P (1977).   Aspects of the regulation of the
   metabolism of branched-chain amino acids.   Adv Enz Reg
   15:375.
Krebs HA, Hems R, Lund P, Halliday D, Read WWC (1978).
   Sources of ammonia for mammalian urea synthesis. Biochem
   J 176:733.
McCarthy AD, Walker JM, Tipton KF (1980).   Purification of
   glutamate dehydrogenase from ox brain and liver. Biochem
   J 191:605.
McCarthy AD, Johnson P, Tipton KF (1981).   Sedimentation
   properties of native and proteolysed preparations of ox
   glutamate dehydrogenase.   Biochem J 199:235.
McGivan JD, Chappell JB (1975).   On the metabolic function
   of glutamate dehydrogenase in rat liver.   FEBS Lett 52:1.
Markau K, Schneider J, Sund H (1971).   Studies of glutamate
   dehydrogenase. The mechanism of the association-dissoc-
   iation equilibrium of beef liver glutamate dehydrogenase.
   Eur J Biochem 24:393.
Mendes-Mourao J, McGivan JD, Chappell JB (1975).   The
   effects of L-leucine on the synthesis of urea, glutamate
   and glutamine by isolated rat liver cells. Biochem J
   146:457.
Mihara K, Omura T, Harano T, Brenner S, Fleischer S, Rajag-
   opalan KV, Blobel G (1982). Rat liver L-glutamate
   dehydrogenase, D-β-hydroxybutyrate dehydrogenase, malate
   dehydrogenase and sulfite oxidase are each synthesised as
   larger precursors by cytoplasmic-free polysomes. J Biol
   Chem 257:3355.
Moon K, Piskiewicz D, Smith EL (1972). Glutamate dehydrog-
   enase:amino-acid sequence of the bovine enzyme and compar-

isons with that from chicken liver. Proc Nat Acad Sci USA 69:1380.

Nemat-Gorgani M, Dodd G (1977a). The interaction of phospholipid membranes and detergents with glutamate dehydrogenase. 1. Kinetic studies. Eur J Biochem 74:129.

Nemat-Gorgani M, Dodd G (1977b). The interaction of phospholipid membranes and detergents with glutamate dehydrogenase. 2. Fluorescence and stopped-flow studies. Eur.J Biochem 74:139.

Olson JA, Anfinsen CB (1952). Crystallization and characterization of L-glutamic acid dehydrogenase. J Biol Chem 197:67.

Place GA, Beynon RJ (1982). The chymotrypsin-catalysed activation of bovine liver glutamate dehydrogenase. Biochem J 205:75.

Rognstad R (1977). Sources of ammonia for urea synthesis in isolated rat liver cells. Biochim Biophys Acta 496:249.

Schoolwerth AC, Nazar BL, LaNoue KF (1978). Glutamate dehydrogenase activation and ammonia formation in rat kidney mitochondria. J Biol Chem 253:6177.

Smith EL, Austen BM, Blumenthal KM, Nyc JF (1975). Glutamate dehydrogenase. The Enzymes 11:293.

Talal N, Tompkins GM (1964). Allosteric properties of glutamate dehydrogenases from different sources. Science 146:1309.

Thusius D (1977). Does a functional relationship exist between the polymerization and catalytic activity of glutamate dehydrogenase. J Mol Biol 115:243.

Tompkins GM, Yielding KL, Talal N, Curran TF (1963). Protein structure and biological regulation. Cold Spring Harbor Symp Quant Biol 28:461.

Tornheim K, Lowenstein JM (1972). The purine nucleotide cycle. The production of ammonia from aspartate by extracts of rat skeletal muscle. J Biol Chem 247:162.

Van den Berg CJ (1970). Glutamate and glutamine. In Lajtha A (ed.): Handbook of Neurochemistry 3, New York: Plenum Press, p355.

Veronese FM, Bevilacqua R, Chaiken IM (1979). Drug-protein interactions: evaluation of the binding of antipsychotic drugs to glutamate dehydrogenase by quantitative affinity chromatography. Mol Pharmacol 15:313.

Yielding KL, Tompkins GM (1961). An effect of L-leucine and other essential amino acids on the structure and activity of glutamic dehydrogenase. Proc Nat Acad Sci USA 47:983.

Zeiri L, Reisler E (1978). Uncoupling of the catalytic activity and the polymerization of beef liver glutamate dehydrogenase. J Mol Biol 124:291.

**Glutamine, Glutamate, and GABA
in the Central Nervous System, pages 33–50**
© 1983 Alan R. Liss, Inc., 150 Fifth Avenue, New York, NY 10011

IMMUNOCYTOCHEMISTRY OF ASPARTATE AMINOTRANSFERASE AND
GLUTAMINASE

Robert J. Wenthold and Richard A. Altschuler

Department of Neurophysiology, University
of Wisconsin, Madison, Wisconsin, 53706
(RJW) and Laboratory of Neuro-otolaryngology,
NIH, Bethesda, Maryland 20205 (RAA)

There is strong evidence supporting a neurotransmitter
role for glutamate (glu) and aspartate (asp). Both amino
acids have been shown to be selectively enriched in populations of nerve fibers and terminals, calcium-dependent
release has been demonstrated in a number of systems, high
affinity uptake for glu and asp has been shown, and pharmacological studies have revealed receptors for glu and asp
which are characteristic of neurotransmitter receptors.
However, very little is known concerning the nature and
regulation of the synthesis and degradation of glu and asp
when they may be functioning as neurotransmitters, and
relationships between the pools of transmitter amino acid
and non-transmitter amino acid remain to be defined. It has
not been possible to distinguish neurons using glu as a
neurotransmitter from those using asp or a structurally or
metabolically related compound. Furthermore, no direct
method exists for the identification of neurons which use
glu or asp as neurotransmitters. To address such issues,
we have undertaken an immunocytochemical study of enzymes
involved in the metabolism of glu and asp. Determination
of the cellular and subcellular locations of enzymes associated with a neurotransmitter's synthesis and breakdown will
provide insights into the nature and regulation of these
events as well as a potential method for localizing neurons
using a particular neurotransmitter. However, because of
the many functions in which glu and asp are involved, in
addition to possible neurotransmitter roles, it cannot be
expected that localizations of glu or asp related enzymes
will be as straightforward as those for other neurotransmitters such as acetylcholine and the catecholamines. In

our studies, we hypothesized that neurons which use glu or
asp as a neurotransmitter would have a much greater capability
for the synthesis of these amino acids than those which use
a neurotransmitter such as acetylcholine. This difference
would be expected to be greatest in the presynaptic terminals
which are largely devoted to the production, storage and
release of neurotransmitter.

Our study of the immunocytochemistry of glu and asp-
related enzymes arose from our work on the auditory nerve
neurotransmitter. Extensive data suggest glu or asp as the
neurotransmitter of the auditory nerve, including high levels
of glu and asp in auditory nerve terminals and fibers,
release of glu and asp from auditory nerve terminals, the
presence of enzymes capable of synthesizing glu and asp in
auditory nerve terminals, retrograde transport of D-asp in
auditory nerve fibers and the presence of excitatory amino
acid receptors on neurons receiving auditory nerve input
in the cochlear nucleus (for reviews, see Wenthold, 1981;
Wenthold and Martin, 1983). In the course of the study on
this pathway, we found that we were unable to demonstrate
a high affinity uptake of glu or asp into terminals of the
auditory nerve. While slices and synaptosome preparations
from the cochlear nucleus took up both amino acids, the uptake was not reduced by prior lesion of the auditory nerve
and the release of the accumulated amino acids from the slices
was neither calcium-dependent nor changed by auditory nerve
lesion. On the other hand, the release of endogenous glu
and asp from cochlear nucleus slices was calcium-dependent
and this release was significantly reduced by lesion of the
auditory nerve (Wenthold, 1979). Thus, little uptake of
exogenous glu or asp was taking place into auditory nerve
terminals. Because of these results, we investigated possible
enzymatic routes for the production of glu and asp in auditory nerve terminals. Four enzymes were measured, aspartate
aminotransferase (AAT), glutaminase (GLNase), glutamate
dehydrogenase (GD), and glutamine synthetase (GS). Glutamate
decarboxylase (GAD), the enzyme catalyzing the synthesis
of GABA from glu, had been studied previously and found not
to be enriched in auditory nerve terminals and fibers (Fex
and Wenthold, 1976). After lesion of the auditory nerve,
it was found that GLNase and AAT decreased in the cochlear
nucleus, GD did not change and GS increased. These results
are consistent with GLNase and AAT being enriched in fibers
and terminals of the auditory nerve and GS being present
in glial cells which proliferate after the lesion. GS had

been studied immunocytochemically and shown to be present
in glial cells (Norenberg and Martinez-Hernandez, 1979).
These results raised the interesting possibility that GLNase
and AAT may be involved in the production of glu and asp
in terminals of the auditory nerve. Several studies have
implicated GLNase in the production of glutamate for release
as a neurotransmitter. GLNase is enriched in synaptosomes
(Bradford and Ward, 1976) and enriched in neurons relative
to astrocytes (Hamberger et al., 1978; Patel et al., 1982).
Radioactive glutamine is readily converted into releasable
glu in brain slices (Hamberger et al., 1979), in synaptosome
preparations (Bradford et al., 1978), and in slice preparations after in vivo labeling (Ward et al., 1983). Maintenance of the neurotransmitter pool of glu appears to require
glutamine since both release and tissue levels of glu are
decreased in slices in media lacking glutamine (Hamberger
et al., 1979). Based on these data, several models have
been proposed in which glutaminase plays a central role in
the production of glu in the presynaptic terminal. AAT has
been less directly implicated in the production of releasable glu or asp. Levels of AAT are higher in bulk prepared
neurons compared to bulk prepared astrocytes (Hertz, 1979)
and AAT is present in isolated synaptosomes (Fonnum, 1968).
Glu, glutamine and α-ketoglutarate can serve as precursors
for asp in synaptosome preparations (Hertz, 1979) and it
has been suggested that the conversion of α-ketoglutarate
to glutamate in presynaptic terminals may involve AAT (Shank
and Campbell, 1982). To further investigate the possibility
that GLNase and AAT may play a role in the synthesis of glu
and asp in the auditory nerve and to extend these studies
to other areas of the nervous system, antibodies were made
to allow immunocytochemical localization of these enzymes.

ANTIBODIES TO AAT AND GLNASE

Cytoplasmic AAT (obtained from Boehringer Mannheim)
was purified by gel filtration. This preparation was either
used directly for antibody production or was subjected to
SDS acrylamide gel electrophoresis and the band corresponding
to the AAT subunit was cut out and used for antibody production. Both antisera produced the same results in the immunocytochemical studies. Antibodies to AAT immunoprecipitated
a single polypeptide, corresponding to the subunit of AAT,
after labeling of auditory nerve proteins with ^{35}S-methionine
(Altschuler et al., 1981). The characterization of antibodies

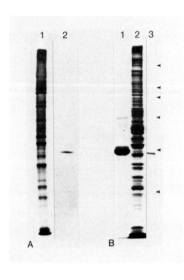

Figure 1. Immunoprecipitation (A) and immunoblotting (B) of the rat cerebellum using antibodies to AAT. For immunoprecipitation the cerebellum was injected with 250 µCi ^{35}S-methionine. The cerebellum was removed 3 h later and solubilized with 1% Triton and 1% deoxycholate and immunoprecipitated with antibodies against AAT (Altschuler et al., 1981). The precipitated proteins were analyzed by SDS gel electrophoresis and fluorography. Immunoblotting was done as described by Towbin (1979) using antibodies to AAT at 1/200 dilution. A.1. Total labeled cerebellar proteins after ^{35}S-methionine injection. 2. Immunoprecipitated cerebellar proteins using anti-AAT antibodies. B.1. Purified AAT (from pig heart, Coomassie blue stain). 2. Total cerebellar proteins (Coomassie blue stain). 3. Immunoblot of total cerebellar proteins using anti-AAT antibodies. Arrowheads indicate position of molecular weight standards of 200, 130, 94, 68, 45 and 29 kilodaltons.

to AAT has been extended to other brain regions using immunoprecipitation and electroblotting techniques. Data obtained using the cerebellum are shown in Figure 1. As with the auditory nerve, the major component recognized by the antibody preparation corresponds to the subunit of AAT. Antibodies to phosphate-dependent glutaminase were produced in the laboratory of Dr. N. Curthoys using enzyme purified from rat kidney. Antibodies to the kidney enzyme were previously shown to crossreact with GLNase from rat brain (Curthoys et al., 1976) and immunoprecipitation and peptide mapping studies show that the antibodies bind to the same protein species from brain and from kidney (Haser and Curthoys, 1983, in preparation). Antibodies to both AAT and GLNase were localized using either the indirect immunofluorescence technique or the peroxidase-antiperoxidase technique. Controls to establish the specificity of staining included absorption controls and substitution of normal serum for the primary antibody.

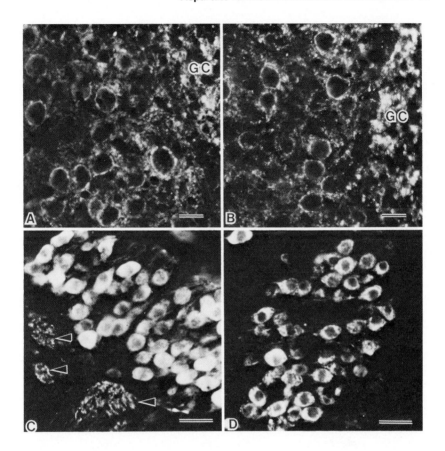

Figure 2. Fluorescence micrographs of the guinea pig
cochlear nucleus and spiral ganglion stained with antibodies
against AAT (A,C) and GLNase (B,D). Immunofluorescent rings
of AAT-IR (A) and GLNase-IR (B) around spherical cells of
the anteroventral cochlear nucleus and labeling of granule
cells (GC) are shown. The cell bodies of the auditory nerve,
the spiral ganglion cells, are also intensely labeled with
antibodies against AAT (C) or GLNase (D). In C, efferent
fibers are also labeled (arrowheads). Primary antisera
used at 1/1200 dilution. Bar = 25 μm.

COCHLEAR NUCLEUS

     As discussed above, biochemical studies showed that
GLNase and AAT were enriched in terminals and fibers of the

auditory nerve. Immunocytochemical studies using antibodies
to GLNase and to AAT show similar distributions for both
enzymes (Figure 2). Most apparent are rings of immunoreactivity in the ventral cochlear nucleus. Experiments involving lesion of the auditory nerve and electron microscopy
immunocytochemistry show these rings to correspond to the
large axosomatic terminals that the auditory nerve makes on
neurons in the cochlear nucleus (Altschuler et al., 1981).
At the electron microscopic level, AAT immunoreactivity was
most intense in terminals of the auditory nerve, but also
present at lower levels in postsynaptic cell bodies and glial
cells. Presynaptic terminals in this region not originating
from the auditory nerve were unlabeled (Altschuler et al.,
1981). Two populations of spiral ganglion cells have been
identified based on morphological criteria, a large population comprising 90-95% of the total, and a small population
made up of the remaining cells. Our studies show that the
small population of cells labels much less intensely using
antibodies to both enzymes than does the large population
(Fex et al., 1982; Altschuler et al., submitted for publication). This could be due to a difference in processing the
enzymes for axonal transport or may reflect different amounts
in the terminals, possibly suggesting that different neurotransmitters are used for these two populations of neurons.

We have identified another population of neurons in
the cochlear nucleus which contains high levels of AAT-like
immunoreactivity (AAT-IR) and GLNase-like immunoreactivity
(GLNase-IR), the granule cells of the ventral cochlear nucleus. The immunoreactivity of these cells is not affected
by auditory nerve lesion. Recently, it was shown that
cochlear nucleus granule cells can also take up and retro-
gradely transport D-asp (Oliver et al., 1983).

RETINA

A number of studies indicate that glu and asp function
as neurotransmitters in the retina. Pharmacology (Wu and
Dowling, 1978; Slaughter and Miller, 1981; Slaughter and
Miller, 1983), uptake (Marc and Lam, 1981; Ehinger, 1981)
and release studies (Neal and Massey, 1981) suggest that
photoreceptors use an excitatory amino acid neurotransmitter.
Recent physiological studies have suggested that an excitatory
amino acid may also be the neurotransmitter for a class of
amacrine cells (Ikeda and Sheardown, 1982) and uptake and

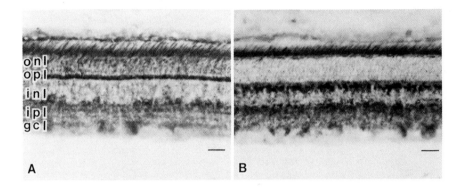

onl
opl
inl
ipl
gcl

A   B

Figure 3. AAT-IR (A) and GLNase-IR (B) in guinea pig retina
visualized with PAP technique. Primary antiserum used at
1/1200 dilution. Bar = 20 μm. onl = outer nuclear layer;
opl = outer plexiform layer; inl = inner nuclear layer;
ipl = inner plexiform layer; gcl = ganglion cell layer.

retrograde transport of D-asp has been reported for a population of retinal ganglion cells in the pigeon (Beaudet et
al., 1981).

When antisera to AAT is applied to the retina of the
rat or guinea pig, labeling is seen in photoreceptors and
their terminals in the outer plexiform layer (opl) as shown
in Figure 3A (Altschuler et al., 1982). At the ultrastructural level, AAT-IR is seen in cone pedicles in the guinea
pig retina (unpublished observation). AAT-IR is also seen
in a class of amacrine cells and their fibers in the inner
plexiform layer (ipl) and in a class of retinal ganglion
cells. Using antisera against GLNase labeling is also seen
in the opl, but with an appearance differing from that seen
with AAT antiserum (Figure 3B). It appears that GLNase-IR
is not associated with photoreceptors but rather with cells
in the inl. Ultrastructural studies will be necessary to
resolve this question. GLNase-IR is also seen in some
amacrine cells and their fibers in the ipl as well as in
some cells in the ganglion cell layer.

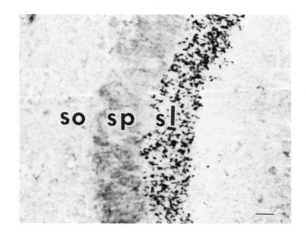

Figure 4. GLNase-IR in rat hippocampus demonstrated with
PAP technique. Intense labeling seen in mossy fiber terminals in sl and lighter labeling of pyramidal cells in sp.
Primary antiserum used at 1/2000 dilution. Bar = 20 µm.
so = stratum oriens; sp = stratum pyramidale; sl = stratum
lucidum.

HIPPOCAMPUS

There is evidence that a number of neurons within and
to the hippocampus use an excitatory amino acid neurotransmitter: the perforant pathway, the mossy fiber pathway and
Schaffer collaterals and commissural fibers of pyramidal
cells (see Cotman, 1981 and Storm-Mathisen, 1981 for review).
Our immunocytochemical studies on the hippocampus show GLNase-
like immunoreactive labeling of the mossy fiber system, with
label in granule cells, fibers and their terminals in stratum
lucidum in regio inferior in the guinea pig and rat hippocampus (Figure 4). GLNase-like immunoreactivity is also
seen in many, but not all, pyramidal cells. No AATase-like
immunoreactivity is seen in the mossy fiber system and only
very light labeling is seen in pyramidal cells. Neither
GLNase nor AATase-like immunoreactivities are seen in the
dentate gyrus where the perforant pathway terminates on
granule cells.

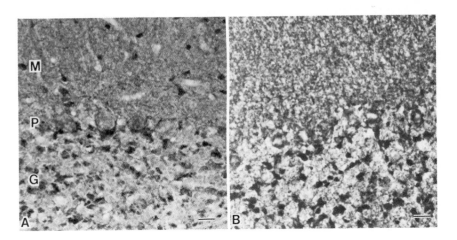

Figure 5. AAT-IR (A) and GLNase-IR (B) in rat cerebellum demonstrated with PAP technique. Primary antiserum used at 1/400 dilution. Bar = 20 μm. M = molecular layer; P = Purkinje cell layer; G = granule cell layer.

CEREBELLAR CORTEX

Neurotransmitters of the cerebellar cortex have been extensively studied and the major cell types have been assigned a putative neurotransmitter. GABA is believed to be a predominant neurotransmitter in the cerebellum, being associated with Purkinje, Golgi, stellate and basket cells. It has recently been suggested that GABA may not be the neurotransmitter of all Purkinje cells based on immunocyto-chemical studies (Chan-Palay et al., 1981, 1982), but these results may be due to the nature of the antibody against GAD used, since other studies reported that all Purkinje cells contain GAD (Oertel et al., 1981). Also, taurine has been suggested as the neurotransmitter of stellate cells (McBride and Frederickson, 1980; Chan-Palay et al, 1982; Okamoto et al., 1983). An excitatory amino acid has been suggested to be the neurotransmitter of the cerebellar gran-ule cells, based on biochemical (Rodhe et al., 1979; Gallo et al., 1982) and pharmacological (Stone, 1979; Crepel, 1982) evidence. The fact that some granule cells are labeled with antibodies against cysteine-sulfinic acid decarboxylase may suggest that taurine also plays a role in these neurons (Chan-Palay et al., 1982).

Our immunocytochemistry studies on the cerebellum show
marked differences in labeling patterns using antibodies
to AAT and antibodies to GLNase (Figure 5). Both antibodies
show labeling in the granule cell layer, with GLNase showing
a more intense reaction product. In the molecular layer,
antibodies to AAT label basket and stellate cells, while
those to GLNase do not show labeling of cell bodies in this
region. However, GLNase-IR appears to be associated with
nerve fibers and terminals in the molecular layer. In the
Purkinje cell layer, Purkinje cell bodies are unlabeled or
lightly labeled using both antisera while AAT antibodies
show labeling at the base of the Purkinje cells. While it
is clear at the light microscopic level that stellate and
basket cells are immunoreactive for AAT, the other reaction
product cannot be definitively assigned to a structure in
the absence of electron microscopy. Based on location and
structure, the immunoreactivity at the base of Purkinje cells
is likely to be associated with baskets formed by basket
cell axons. This would also be consistent with labeling
of basket cell bodies. In the granule cell layer, both AAT-
IR and GLNase-IR are associated with granule cell bodies.
Reaction product is also present which does not appear confined to granule cell bodies. This may represent clusters
of granule cells or could arise from damage due to fixation
or the immunocytochemistry procedure. It is also possible
that the reaction product is associated with granule cell
dendrites or axons and terminals from mossy fibers.

DISCUSSION

Our results show a specific enrichment in immunoreactivity of AAT and GLNase in several neuronal populations.
While in an immunocytochemical study we cannot definitively
conclude that the immunoreactivity corresponds to the particular enzyme, the immunoprecipitation and immunoblotting
studies on AAT and GLNase show that the major species recognized by the antibodies correspond to the subunits of the
respective enzymes. Measurement of enzymatic activities
of AAT and GLNase in the auditory nerve is consistent with
the immunocytochemical findings (Wenthold, 1980; Altschuler
et al., 1981). Since AAT and GLNase fulfill general metabolic roles and are widely distributed in both neuronal and
non-neuronal tissue, they are unlike enzymes involved in
the synthesis of acetylcholine, GABA, catecholamines and
serotonin, which are largely confined to neurons which

release the related neurotransmitter. However, our results
clearly show that specific populations of neurons are
enriched in AAT-IR and GLNase-IR. When these studies were
begun, we felt that the major difference between glu/asp
releasing neurons and non-glu/asp releasing neurons would
be in the presynaptic terminal, where enzymes involved in
the synthesis of glu and asp would be enriched in terminals
releasing these amino acids compared to those releasing a
neurotransmitter unrelated to these amino acids. However,
we have found in many cases that neuronal cell bodies are
also enriched in AAT-IR and GLNase-IR. This finding is
consistent with those on the immunocytochemistry of GAD
where it has been suggested that differences in cell body
immunoreactivity may be associated with variation in fixation
of different neuronal cell types or loss of antigen during
the immunocytochemistry procedure (Oertel et al., 1981).
Differential cell body labeling may also reflect different
processing of particular enzymes for axonal transport.

Results from a study of a number of putative glutamergic
and aspartergic neurons and other neurons are summarized in
Table 1. These results show that three types of labeling
are found: neurons containing AAT-IR alone, neurons containing GLNase-IR alone, and those containing both. There are
several possible explanations for the different labeling
patterns observed for putative glutamergic and aspartergic
neurons. These range from the possibility that some of these
neurons may not use an excitatory amino acid neurotransmitter
to the possibility that these enzymes play no role in the
production of the neurotransmitters, glu and asp, and are
present in those neurons for other reasons. Both explanations seem unlikely. There is strong evidence supporting
a neurotransmitter role for glu or asp for many of the
neurons in which we find AAT-IR or GLNase-IR. The presence
of GLNase and/or AAT in a large number of putative glu/asp
neurons and their absence from a number of other neurons,
would be difficult to reconcile on any basis other than a
link to the neurotransmitter. Our results showing GLNase
in mossy fiber terminals in the hippocampus are consistent
with recent results showing glu is present in these same
terminals as shown using an antibody against glu itself
(Storm-Mathiesen et al., 1983).

The different labeling patterns of putative excitatory
amino acid neurons that we find using antibodies against
AAT and GLNase may suggest that these neurons have varying

TABLE 1. IMMUNOCYTOCHEMICAL DISTRIBUTION OF AAT AND GLNASE

Neuron	Enzyme	Other Evidence[a]
Auditory Nerve	AAT, GLNase	Levels, Release, Pharmacology, D-asp
Granule Cells- Cochlear Nucleus	AAT, GLNase	D-asp
Cochlear Efferents	AAT, GLNase	Uptake
Photoreceptors	AAT	Uptake, Release, Pharmacology
Amacrine Cells	AAT, GLNase	Uptake, Pharmacology
Mossy Fibers- Hippocampus	GLNase	Levels, Uptake, Pharmacology
Pyramidal Cells- Hippocampus	GLNase	Levels, Uptake, Release, Pharmacology
Granule Cells- Cerebellum	AAT, GLNase	Levels, Release, Pharmacology
Stellate, Basket Cells-Cerebellum	AAT	
Neocortex Layers II, III	AAT	Levels, Uptake, Release, Pharmacology
Neocortex Layers V, VI	GLNase	Levels, Uptake, Release, Pharmacology

[a]Refers to other evidence supporting glu or asp as a neurotransmitter for these neurons.

capabilities and mechanisms for glu and asp production. While glutamine may be the major precursor of releasable glutamate, evidence suggests that glutamate in the presynaptic terminal can be obtained by other routes. Glucose can serve as a precursor for glu (Hamberger et al., 1978) and α-ketoglutarate can be taken up by presynaptic terminals and converted to releasable glu (Shank and Campbell, 1982). Another route, which has been studied in detail, is high affinity uptake of glu or asp into the presynaptic terminal. Since most studies investigating routes of glu and asp production have been done on heterogeneous preparations, it is impossible to conclude if different routes of labeling take place in different synaptic populations or if several routes occur simultaneously in a single population. However, high affinity uptake can be localized by autoradiography and several studies point to differences in the degree of high affinity uptake into presynaptic terminals of neurons believed to use glu or asp as a neurotransmitter. For example, it has been convincingly demonstrated that putative glutamergic terminals in the hippocampus acquire glu through a high affinity uptake mechanism (Storm-Mathisen and Iversen, 1979). On the other hand, it has been shown that granule cells of the cerebellum, which are also believed to use glu as a neurotransmitter, take up little or no glutamate (for example, De Barry et al., 1982; Wilkin et al., 1982). Uptake also appears to play a minor role in the supply of glu and asp in auditory nerve terminals (Wenthold, 1979; Oliver et al., 1983). It may be proposed, then, that there are several routes of production of presynaptic glu and asp, and the degree to which a particular route is used may vary from neuron to neuron. Such a mechanism may be advantageous since it would allow for differential regulation of neurotrans-mitter production at synapses based on availability of a particular precursor. Differential labeling of putative excitatory amino acid neurons with antibodies to GLNase and AAT may also suggest that different neurotransmitters are released from these synapses. Glu can be produced from glutamine by glutaminase while asp production would require AAT. Therefore, it may be suggested that neurons which only contain GLNase release glu, while those that contain both AAT and GLNase could release glu, asp or both. This reason-ing could also be extended to putative glutamergic and aspartergic neurons that are not enriched in AAT or GLNase. While glu and asp probably are neurotransmitters, it is thought that they are only two of several excitatory amino acid neurotransmitters that are structurally related and have similar postsynaptic receptors. For example, quinolinic acid, which is not synthesized from glu or asp, is present in brain and is an agonist for NMDA receptors (Perkins and Stone, 1983). Therefore, putative excitatory amino acid neurons which do not contain AAT or GLNase may be non-glu and non-asp excitatory amino acid pathways.

Glu, in addition to being a neurotransmitter, is also a precursor for GABA. Glutamine is readily converted to GABA in synaptosomes and brain slices, and it has therefore been suggested that GLNase plays a role in the production

of GABA (Hertz, 1979). Our results, however, do not show
an enrichment of GLNase in putative GABAergic neurons. Since
electron microscopy has not been carried out, it remains
possible that GLNase is selectively elevated only in the
presynaptic terminals of GABAergic neurons. Furthermore,
relatively low levels of GLNase may be sufficient for
production of glu in these neurons. AAT, however, is found
to be present in cerebellar stellate and basket cells,
neurons which are believed to release GABA. Since it appears
that most basket and stellate cells are labeled with antibodies against AAT, it is unlikely that the labeled neurons
represent only a subpopulation which uses an excitatory
amino acid neurotransmitter. Rather, these results suggest
that AAT may play a role in the production of GABA in these
neurons. On the other hand, we do not see labeling of other
putative GABAergic neurons such as Golgi and Purkinje cells
in the cerebellum as well as cells in the cortex and retina.
Furthermore, in the retina, the immunocytochemical distribution of AAT is reported to differ significantly from that
of GAD (Lin et al., 1983). Variations in levels of AAT
among putative GABAergic neurons may explain these results.
It has been suggested that GABA may not be the only neurotransmitter of stellate and basket cells, but rather that
some of these neurons use taurine as a neurotransmitter
(McBride and Frederickson, 1980; Chan-Palay et al., 1982;
Okamoto et al., 1983). It has also been suggested that AAT
and cysteine-sulfinic acid transaminase may be the same
protein (Recasens et al., 1980). If this is the case, the
presence of AAT (or cysteine-sulfinic acid transaminase)
in basket and stellate cells would be consistent with taurine
being present in these neurons. However, studies on the
retina show that AAT and cysteine-sulfinic acid decarboxylase,
which is believed to be a marker for taurine-containing
neurons (Wu, 1982), have different immunocytochemical distributions (Lin et al., 1983).

In summary, our results show that AAT and GLNase are
enriched in several populations of neurons which are believed
to use glu or asp as their neurotransmitter. However, not
all putative excitatory amino acid neurons contain both
enzymes and some may contain neither. This finding suggests
that different metabolic routes may be involved in the
production of the neurotransmitters, glu and asp, and that
these routes may be used to varying degrees in different
populations of neurons. One objective of our studies was
to determine if AAT, GLNase or both enzymes could serve as

immunocytochemical markers for glutamergic and aspartergic neurons. We find that AAT may be present in other neurons, perhaps some GABAergic neurons, while GLNase appears more likely to be enriched only in those neurons which are believed to release glu or asp. Certainly, these results are preliminary and a more extensive survey of the nervous system is required. Our findings also suggest that a study of additional enzymes involved in the production of glu and asp may be a fruitful approach to the further characterization of excitatory amino acid neurotransmitters.

REFERENCES

Altschuler RA, Mosinger JL, Harmison GG, Parakkal MH, Wenthold RJ (1982). Aspartate aminotransferase-like immunoreactivity as a marker for aspartate/glutamate in guinea pig photoreceptors. Nature 298:657.

Altschuler RA, Neises GR, Harmison GG, Wenthold RJ, Fex J (1981). Immunocytochemical localization of aspartate aminotransferase immunoreactivity in cochlear nucleus of the guinea pig. Proc Natl Acad Sci 78:6553.

Beaudet A, Burkhalter A, Reubi JC, Cuenod M (1981). Selective bidirectional transport of [^{3}H]D-aspartate in the pigeon retino-tectal pathway. Neurosci 6:2021.

Bradford HF, Ward HK (1976). On glutaminase activity in mammalian synaptosomes. Brain Res 110:115.

Bradford HF, Ward HK, Thomas AJ (1978). Glutamine as a substrate for nerve endings. J Neurochem 30:1453.

Chan-Palay V, Lin CT, Palay S, Yamamoto M, Wu JY (1982) Taurine in the mammalian cerebellum: Demonstration by autoradiography with [^{3}H]taurine and immunocytochemistry with antibodies against the taurine-synthesizing enzyme, cysteine-sulfinic acid decarboxylase. Proc Natl Acad Sci USA 79:2695.

Chan-Palay V, Nilaver G, Palay SL, Beinfeld MG, Zimmerman EA, Wu JY, O'Donohue TL (1981). Chemical heterogeneity in cerebellar Purkinje cells: Existence and coexistence of glutamic acid decarboxylase-like and motilin-like immunoreactivities. Proc Natl Acad Sci USA 78:7787.

Cotman CW, Foster A, Lanthorn T (1981). An overview of glutamate as a neurotransmitter. In Di Chiara G, Gessa GL (eds): "Glutamate as a Neurotransmitter," New York: Raven Press, pp 1.

Crepel F, Dhanjal SS, Sears TA (1982). Effect of glutamate, aspartate and related derivatives on cerebellar Purkinje cell dendrites in the rat: An in vitro study. J Physiol

329:297.

Curthoys NP, Kuhlenschmidt T, Godfrey SS, Weiss RF (1976). Phosphate-dependent glutaminase from rat kidney. Arch Biochem Biophys 172:162.

De Barry J, Langley OK, Vincendon G, Gombos G (1982). L-glutamate and L-glutamine uptake in adult cerebellum: An autoradiographic study. Neuroscience 7: 1289.

Ehinger B (1981). [H^3]-D-aspartate accumulation in the retina of pigeon, guinea pig and rabbit. Exptl Eye Res 33: 381.

Fex J, Altschuler RA, Wenthold RJ, Parakkal MH (1982). Aspartate aminotransferase immunoreactivity in cochlea of guinea pig. Hearing Res 7:149.

Fex J, Wenthold RJ (1976). Choline acetyltransferase, glutamate decarboxylase and tyrosine hydroxylase in the cochlea and cochlear nucleus of the guinea pig. Brain Res 109:575.

Fonnum F (1968). The distribution of glutamate decarboxylase and aspartate transaminase in subcellular fractions of rat and guinea pig brain. Biochem J 106:401.

Gallo V, Ciotti MT, Coletti A, Aloisi F, Levi G (1982). Selective release of glutamate from cerebellar granule cells differentiating in culture. Proc Natl Acad Sci 79: 7919.

Hamberger AC, Chiang CH, Nylen ES, Scheff SW, Cotman CW (1979). Glutamate as a CNS transmitter I. Evaluation of glucose and glutamine as precursors for the synthesis of preferentially released glutamate. Brain Res 168:513.

Hamberger A, Cotman CW, Sellstrom A, Weiler CT (1978). Glutamine, glial cells and their relationship to transmitter glutamate. In Franck G, Hertz L, Tower DB (eds): "Dynamic Properties of Glial Cells," New York: Plenum Press, p 163.

Hertz L (1979) Functional interactions between neurons and astrocytes I. Turnover and metabolism of putative amino acid transmitters. Prog Neurobiol 13:277.

Ikeda H, Sheardown MJ (1982). Asparate may be an excitatory transmitter mediating visual excitation of "sustained" but not "transient" cells in the cat retina: Iontophoretic studies in vivo. Neuroscience 7:25.

Lin CT, Li HZ, Wu JY (1983). Immunocytochemical localization of L-glutamate decarboxylase, gamma aminobutyric acid transaminase, cysteine-sulfinic acid decarboxylase, aspartate aminotransferase and somatostatin in rat retina. Brain Res In Press.

Marc RE, Lam DMK (1981). Uptake of aspartic and glutamic acid by photoreceptors in goldfish retina. Proc Natl Acad Sci 78:7185.

McBride WJ, Frederickson RCA (1980). Taurine as a possible inhibitory transmitter in the cerebellum. Fed Am Soc Exptl Biol 39:2701.

Neal MJ, Massey SC (1980). The release of acetylcholine and amino acids from the rabbit retina in vivo. Neurochem 1: 191.

Norenberg MD, Martinez-Hernandez A (1979). Fine structural location of glutamine synthetase in astrocytes of rat brain. Brain Res 161:303.

Oertel WH, Schmechel DE, Mugnaini E, Toppaz ML, Kopin IJ (1981). Immunocytochemical localization of glutamate decarboxylase in rat cerebellum with a new antiserum. Neuroscience 6:2715.

Okamoto K, Kimura H, Sakai Y (1983). Evidence for taurine as an inhibitory neurotransmitter in cerebellar stellate interneurons: Selective antagonism by TAG (6-aminomethyl-3-methyl-4H,1,2,4-benzothiadiazine-1,1-dioxide). Brain Res 265:163.

Oliver DL, Potashner SJ, Jones DR, Morest DK (1983). Selective labeling of spiral ganglion and granule cells with D-asparatate in the auditory system of cat and guinea pig. J Neurosci 3:455.

Patel AJ, Hunt A, Gordon RD, Balazs R (1982). The activities of different neural cell types of certain enzymes associated with the metabolic compartmentation of glutamate. Dev Brain Res 4:3.

Perkins MN, Stone TW (1983). Quinolinic acid: Regional variations in neuronal sensitivity. Brain Res 259:172.

Recasens M, Benezra R, Basset P, Mandel P (1980). Cysteine-sulfinate aminotransferase and aspartate aminotransferase isoenzymes of rat brain. Purification, characterization and further evidence for identity. Biochemistry 19:4583.

Rohde BH, Rea MA, Simon JR, McBride WJ (1979). Effects of x-irradiation induced loss of cerebellar granule cells on the synaptosomal levels and the high affinity uptake of amino acids. J Neurochem 32:1431.

Shank RP, Campbell GL (1982). Glutamine and alpha-ketoglutarate and metabolism by nerve terminal enriched material from mouse cerebellum. Neurochem Res 7:601.

Slaughter MM, Miller RF (1981). Two-amino-4-phosphorobutyric acid: A new pharmacological tool for retina research. Science 211:182.

Slaughter MM, Miller RF (1983). An excitatory amino acid antagonist blocks cone input to sign-conserving second order retina neurons. Science 219:1230.

Stone TW (1979). Glutamate as the neurotransmitter of cerebellar granule cells in the rat: Electrophysiological evidence. Br J Pharmacol 66:291.

Storm-Mathisen J (1981). Glutamate in hippocampal pathways. In DiChiara G, Gessa GL (eds): "Glutamate as a Neurotransmitter," New York: Raven Press, p 43.

Storm-Mathisen J, Iversen LL (1979). Uptake of 3H glutamic acid in excitatory nerve endings: Light and electronmicroscopic observation in the hippocampal formation of the rat. Neuroscience 4:1237.

Storm-Mathisen J, Leknes AK, Bore AJ, Vaaland JL, Edminson P, Haug FMS, Ottersen OP (1983). First visualization of glutamate and GABA in neurones by immunocytochemistry. Nature 301:517.

Towbin H, Staechelin T, Gordon J (1979). Electrophoretic transfer of proteins from polyacrylamide gels to nitrocellulose sheets: Procedure and some applications. Proc Natl Acad Sci 76:4350.

Ward HK, Thanki CM, Bradford HF (1983). Glutamine and glucose as precursors of transmitter amino acids: ex vivo studies. J Neurochem 40:855.

Wenthold RJ (1979). Release of endogenous glutamic acid, aspartic acid and GABA from cochlear nucleus slices. Brain Res 162:338.

Wenthold RJ (1980). Glutaminase and aspartate aminotransferase decrease in the cochlear nucleus after lesion of the auditory nerve. Brain Res 190:293.

Wenthold RJ (1981). Glutamate and aspartate as neurotransmitters for the auditory nerve. In DiChiara G, Gessa GL (eds): "Glutamate as a Neurotransmitter," New York: Raven Press, p 69.

Wenthold RJ, Martin MR (1983). Neurotransmitters of the auditory nerve and central auditory system. In Berlin C (ed): "Recent Advances: Hearing Sciences," College Hill Press, In Press.

Wilkin GP, Garthwaite J, Balazs R (1982). Putative acidic amino acid transmitters in the cerebellum II. Electron microscope localization of transport sites. Brain Res 244:69.

Wu SM, Dowling JE (1978). L-aspartate: Evidence for a role in cone photoreceptor synaptic transmission in the carp retina. Proc Natl Acad Sci 75:5205.

Wu JY (1982). Purification and characterization of cysteic acid and cysteine-sulfinic acid decarbolylase and L-glutamate decarboxylase from bovine brain. Proc Natl Acad Sci 79:4270.

Glutamine, Glutamate, and GABA
in the Central Nervous System, pages 51–67
© 1983 Alan R. Liss, Inc., 150 Fifth Avenue, New York, NY 10011

GLUTAMINASE (PAG)

Elling Kvamme

Neurochemical Laboratory
Preclinical Medicine, Oslo University
P.O.Box 1115 - Blindern, Oslo 3, Norway

Phosphate activated glutaminase (PAG) (EC 3.5.1.2)
appears to be a dominant Gln metabolizing enzyme in brain
(Review Kvamme 1983). We purified pig kidney PAG (Kvamme
et al. 1970) and pig brain PAG (Svenneby et al. 1973; Kvamme
and Svenneby 1975) to apparent homogeneity (10-15,000 fold),
making use of the property of the enzyme to solubilize and
polymerize in a reversible manner. PAG has also been purified from rat kidney by Curthoys et al. (1976), and from pig
brain by Nimmo and Tipton (1980) using modifications of our
method.

Pig brain PAG (as well as pig kidney PAG) exists in a
monomeric form (Tris-HCl enzyme, mol.wt. 120-135,000), but
at a protein concentration above 0.1 mg/ml it dimerizes on
addition of phosphate (phosphate form) and insoluble polymers are formed on addition of phosphate plus borate
(phosphate-borate enzyme, mol.wt. 1,5-2,0 mill.) (Kvamme et
al. 1970).

In addition, a membrane-bound insoluble form has been
suggested (Nimmo and Tipton 1981). Pig brain PAG contains
subunits with mol.wts. of 64,000 (Kvamme and Svenneby 1975).
However, Nimmo and Tipton (1980) report that the subunit of
pig brain PAG has a mol.wt. of 73,000. By electron microscopy pig kidney and brain PAG show similar pictures (Olsen
et al. 1970; 1973; Svenneby 1970).

GENERAL ACTIVATORS AND INHIBITORS OF PAG

Pig brain and kidney PAG have rather similar properties.
Phosphate is a potent activator of PAG, and the enzyme is
also stimulated by a variety of other compounds such as citrate, succinate (Greenstein and Leuthardt 1948; O'Donovan
and Lotspeich 1966; Katunuma et al. 1966; Kvamme et al.
1970; Svenneby et al. 1970), thyroxine (Hovhannesian et al.
1970; Badalian et al. 1975), various phosphorylated compounds (Weil-Malherbe and Beall 1970; Weil-Malherbe 1972),
acetyl-CoA (Kvamme and Torgner 1974), and acyl-CoA derivatives (Kvamme and Torgner 1975). The enzyme is therefore not
phosphate-dependent and for that reason the old term
phosphate-activated glutaminase is preferred. Anionic activation is apparently a general characteristic of PAG.

The activation by anions differs for the monomeric and
polymeric forms. We found that the polymeric form is more
susceptible than the Tris-HCl enzyme to activation by anions, such as succinate and citrate. Maleate also activates
the purified PAG to the same extent as do the above mentioned citric acid cycle intermediates. This activation disappears when PAG is inactivated by heat and is therefore not
caused by contamination of PAG with "maleate-activated glutaminase" (gamma-GT), which is resistant to heat treatment.
The citric acid cycle intermediates and acetyl-CoA produce
no additional activation to that of phosphate at high concentrations. Hence they appear to compete for the same anionic site (Weil-Malherbe 1969; Svenneby et al. 1970; Svenneby 1971; Kvamme and Torgner 1974). The specific activity
(units·mg protein^{-1}) of the dimeric and polymeric forms of
PAG is three times that of the monomeric form. Therefore,
the Tris-HCl form of purified PAG is characterized by time-
dependent activation followed by polymerization (hysteretic
effect) when incubated for varying length of time with anionic activators, such as phosphate, phosphate-borate or
acyl-CoA derivatives and at a protein concentration above
0.1 mg·ml^{-1} (Svenneby et al. 1970; Kvamme and Torgner 1974).
Dimerization does not appear to be a prerequisite for activation of the Tris-HCl form. Thus, when incubated with the
activators malonate or citrate, we found the same sedimentation coefficient as for the purified Tris-HCl form.

PAG is an allosteric enzyme (Kvamme et al. 1970; Kvamme
and Svenneby 1975). The kinetic behavior of the purified
enzyme is pH dependent and double reciprocal plots of acti-

vity against Gln give straight lines only at pH 8.

The most prominent inhibitor is the end-product of the PAG reaction, glutamate. The other reaction product, ammonia, as well as N-ethylmaleimide, inhibits only structural-bound PAG and not the purified enzyme (Kvamme et al. 1970; Svenneby 1971; Kvamme and Olsen 1981). PAG is also inhibited by cyclic AMP, cyclic GMP (Weil-Malherbe 1972), protons and long-chain acyl-CoA derivatives (Kvamme and Torgner 1975) in higher concentrations than those which activate the enzyme.

PAG IN INTACT SYNAPTOSOMES AND ASTROCYTES

Inhibition by Glu, 2-Oxoglutarate and Ammonia

The major findings from our laboratory discribed in this paper, have been confirmed using synaptosomes prepared both by the method of Whittaker and Barker (1972) and that of Booth and Clark (1982).

The PAG content of synaptosomes is very high, since they contain 40% of the total tissue PAG and only 10% of the protein (Bradford and Ward 1976).

Synaptosomes
Percent activity of PAG

Added (mM)	0	0.05	0.10	0.20	0.30	0.40	1.00	2.00
Glu	100	97	93	85	54	52	49	48
2-oxo	100		89		55			49
NH_4^+	100	88	78	72	69	65	60	58

Table 1. Percent activity of PAG following incubation for 2 min at 25°C at pH 7.4 with Glu, 2-oxoglutarate or ammonia in concentrations as indicated. Mean of 2 experiments, run in duplicate. Other additions: 2 mM L-[(U)-^{14}C] Gln, 5 mM Na-phosphate, 90 mM NaCl, 56 mM KCl, 4 mM Hepes, 5 mM $MgCl_2$, 10 mg/l oligomycin and 0.6 mg/l antimycin A. Experimental procedure as described by Kvamme and Lenda(1982).

Although synaptosomal PAG appears to have major properties in common with the purified enzyme, there are important differences. Table 1 demonstrates that synaptosomal PAG has

a great sensitivity to inhibition by its reaction products,
Glu and ammonia, in the low concentration range of 0-0.4 mM.
At 0.4 mM the PAG activity is 40-50% inhibited and the activity is little further reduced on increasing the inhibitor
concentration to 2 mM. As discussed above, purified PAG is
not inhibited by ammonia and less sensitive to inhibition by
Glu in this concentration range. It is noteworthy that Glu,
which has a restricted permeability to the inner mitochondrial membrane, appears to be just as easily available to
PAG as ammonia.

Synaptosomes
Percent activity of PAG

	No AOA	AOA
2-oxo	57 + 4	97
2-oxo + Asp	49 + 5	110 + 9
2-oxo + Ala	52 + 6	109

Table 2. The effect of aminooxyacetic acid (AOA) on the
inhibition of PAG by 2-oxoglutarate (2-oxo). Additions:
1 mM 2-oxo, 1 mM Asp, 1 mM Ala, 5 mM AOA. Otherwise, conditions as Table 1. Mean of 6 experiments + SEM or of 2
experiments, run i duplicate.

It is also of interest as shown in Table 1, that 2-oxo-
glutarate inhibits synaptosomal PAG, and that the extent of
inhibition is almost equal to Glu on a molar basis. Asp and
Ala may produce some additional inhibition to that of 2-oxo-
glutarate, but these amino acids do not inhibit PAG when
added without 2-oxoglutarate. However, the aminotransferase
inhibitor aminooxyacetic acid (AOA) completely abolishes the
inhibition exerted by 2-oxoglutarate alone, or combined with
Asp or Ala (Table 2).

As demonstrated in Table 3, a concentration-dependent relationship has been found between the 2-oxoglutarate added and
Glu formed at the end of incubation. In these experiments
the synaptosomes are incubated without Gln. The inhibition
of PAG by 2-oxoglutarate can therefore be explained by an
effect of aminotransferase reactions converting 2-oxo-
glutarate to Glu, and we have obtained no evidence that 2-
oxoglutarate as such has any effect on PAG. The Glu dehydrogenase reaction appears to be unimportant for the Glu formation in synaptosomes. Thus, ammonia 1-2 mM does not stimulate Glu formation from 2-oxoglutarate when omitting the inhi-

Synaptosomes
nmoles Glu·mg protein^{-1} at the end of incubation
(mM)

2-oxo	0.1	1.3
2-oxo	0.5	4.0
2-oxo	2.0	9.0 + 0.7
2-oxo	2.0 + Asp	12.5 + 0.7
2-oxo	2.0 + Ala	10.9
2-oxo	2.0 + AOA	0.1 + 0.01
2-oxo	2.0 + Asp + AOA	0.1 + 0.01

Table 3. The effect of aminooxyacetic acid (AOA) on Glu
formation. Additions: 5 mM Na-phosphate, 2-oxoglutarate
(2-oxo) as shown, 2 mM Asp, 2 mM Ala, 2 mM AOA, 90 mM NaCl,
56 mM KCl, 4 mM Hepes, 5 mM MgCl$_2$, 10 mg/l oligomycin, 0.6
mg/l antimycin A. The synaptosomes were incubated for 2 min
at 25°C and pH 7.4 (Kvamme and Lenda 1982). Mean of 6 experiments + SEM or mean of 2 experiments.

bitors antimycin A and oligomycin from the reaction mixture
and adding glucose and malate for energy generation. This is
in accordance with the low Glu dehydrogenase activity which
previously has been reported by Dienel et al. (1977). Since
we have been unable to detect any maleate activated glutaminase in synaptosomes (Kvamme and Olsen 1981), PAG appears
to be a dominant Gln metabolizing enzyme in this structure.

Synaptosomes
Percent activity of PAG

	pH 7.6	pH 7.0
	100	44 + 7
Glu	48 + 4	35 + 5
NH$_4^+$	53 + 8	30 + 6

Table 4. The effect of pH on the inhibition of PAG by ammonia and Glu. Additions: 1 mM Glu, 1 mM ammonia. Otherwise, conditions as Table 1. Mean of 5 experiments + SEM.

As shown in Table 4, PAG is markedly inhibited by lowering the pH from 7.6 to 7.0, and the effects of Glu and ammonia are greatly reduced by this change in pH. Thus, synaptosomal PAG may be regulated by pH, as well as by the Glu and
ammonia concentration in the extracellular space. However,

synaptosomal preparations contain a high concentration of endogenous Glu (4 mM) which, if not compartmentalized, would exert a constant inhibition of PAG (Kvamme and Lenda 1981). We tested this by comparing the susceptibility of PAG to activation by phosphate and inhibition by Glu in disrupted and intact synaptosomes. If inhibited by endogenous Glu, the susceptibility to addition of phosphate or Glu should be reduced in intact synaptosomes as compared to disrupted ones, where endogenous Glu presumably has leaked out. We found no difference between these two preparations, indicating that the endogenous Glu in intact synaptosomes is compartmentalized (Kvamme and Lenda 1981). Storm-Mathisen (1983) has recently obtained evidence using immunocytochemical methods, that the transmitter amino acids are concentrated in synaptic vesicles.

In astrocytes cultured from mouse brain, PAG is not inhibited by ammonia, similarly to purified PAG, whereas the inhibitory effect of Glu corresponds to that of PAG in synaptosomes (Kvamme et al. 1982). The physiological importance of this is unclear, but the result may suggest that synaptosomal PAG has a greater regulatory potential than glial PAG.

The Localization of PAG in Synaptosomal Mitochondria

PAG is known to be a mitochondrial enzyme (Errera and Greenstein 1949) and some workers report that renal PAG is localized to the matrix region (Kalra and Brosnan 1974), whereas others provide convincing evidence that the enzyme is bound to the inner mitochondrial membrane (Curthoys and Weiss 1974; Kovačević 1976; Kvamme 1982).

Using glutathione as a marker for the matrix region, it can be distinguished among two groups of sulfhydryl group reagents, those reacting with glutathione and thus permeable to the inner mitochondrial membrane, and those impermeable to this membrane (Tietze 1969). N-ethylmaleimide (NEM) belongs to the former group and mersalyl (Mers) and P-mercuribenzoate (PMB) to the latter. Furthermore, these inhibitors can be used to localize sulfhydryl group containing enzymes, also within the inner mitochondrial membrane. In this way beta-hydroxybutyrate dehydrogenase (BHBD) has been found to be bound to the inner face of the inner mitochondrial membrane (Gaudemer and Latruffe 1975; McIntyre et al. 1978), and the enzyme can be considered an inner face marker.

Percent inhibition

Inhibitor	Synaptosomes	Synaptosomal mitochondria	Sonicated synaptosomal mitochondria
NEM	81 + 10	94 + 4	63 + 3
Mersalyl	13 + 10	25 + 13	80 + 2
PMB	-	23 + 4	80 + 2

Table 5. Inhibition of beta-hydroxybutyrate dehydrogenase by sulfhydryl group reagents. Additions: 1 mM N-ethylmaleimide (NEM), 0.1 mM mersalyl, and 0.5 mM p-mercuribenzoate (PMB). The synaptosomal mitochondria were prepared according to Lai and Clark (1976).

By this technique we tested the permeability of synaptosomes to NEM, Mers and PMB. We found that BHBD in intact synaptosomes and synaptosomal mitochondria is strongly inhibited by NEM (80-90%) and relatively little affected by Mers and PMB. However, following sonication BHBD is inhibited about 80% by Mers and PMB, demonstrating that these inhibitors now are accessible to the enzyme (Table 5).

Percent inhibition

Inhibitor	Synaptosomes	Synaptosomal mitochondria	Disrupted synaptosomal mitochondria
NEM	50 + 4	53 + 8	60 + 13
Mersalyl	64 + 4		
PMB	72 + 2		

Table 6. Inhibition of PAG by sulfhydryl group reagents. Additions: 1 mM N-ethylmaleimide (NEM), 0.1 mM mersalyl (Mers), 0.5 mM p-mercuribenzoate (PMB), and 10 mM phosphate. The synaptosomes and mitochondria were disrupted by sonication. Otherwise, conditions as Table 1 and 5.

Since we have shown that the permeability characteristics of synaptosomes, synaptosomal mitochondria and rat liver mitochondria to sulfhydryl group reagents are similar, we can use these inhibitors to localize PAG. As shown in Table 6, synaptosomal PAG is inhibited 50% by NEM, and 64 and 72% respectively, by Mers and PMB. The inhibition by NEM of synaptosomal PAG is about the same as that of PAG in disrupted synaptosomes and disrupted synaptosomal mito-

chondria. These results demonstrate that Mers and PMB
either inhibit PAG itself or the sulfhydryl group reagent-
sensitive carrier of phosphate or Gln.

Synaptosomes
Percent activity of PAG

Additions	1 -	2 Ca^{2+}	3 NEM	4 Ca^{2+} + NEM
A	100 $\pm$ 4	175 $\pm$ 5	57 $\pm$ 12	170 $\pm$ 3
B	100 $\pm$ 13	172 $\pm$ 14	54 $\pm$ 3	154 $\pm$ 8

Table 7. Effect of preincubation of the synaptosomes with
phosphate (10 mM) (A 1, 3), or calcium (1 mM) and phosphate
(A 2, 4) before addition of NEM (1 mM) (A 3, 4) and Gln, as
compared to preincubation with phosphate (B 1, 2), or NEM
and phosphate (B 3, 4), before the addition of calcium (B 2,
4) and Gln. The preincubation was performed for 5 min at
25°C. Mean of 4 experiments $\pm$ SEM.

However, preloading the synaptosomes with phosphate has no
influence on the inhibition of PAG by NEM (Table 7), and
sonication of the synaptosomes or synaptosomal mitochondria
is also without appreciable effect (Table 6). Therefore, an
inhibition of PAG mediated by an effect on the phosphate or
Gln carrier is rendered unlikely. PAG itself appears to be
inhibited, similar to what has been found in rat liver mitochondria (Josef and Meijer 1981), and our results support
the conclusion that PAG is localized, at least in part, to
the outer face of the inner mitochondrial membrane.

Making use of the same sulfhydryl group reagents, we
have produced evidence to show that also in pig renal mitochondria PAG is localized externally in the inner mitochondrial membrane.

The maximal inhibition of PAG by NEM is only about 50%,
and this inhibition is reached at a NEM concentration of 0.5
mM (Kvamme and Olsen 1979; Kvamme and Olsen 1981). Thus,
some Mers and PMB sensitive sulfhydryl groups on PAG may not
be accessible to NEM.

It is of interest to note that the sulfhydryl group
reagents produce similar pattern of inhibition of PAG in
astrocytes cultured from mouse brain, as in synaptosomes
(Kvamme et al. 1982).

Synaptosomes
Percent activity of PAG

Added [Pi](mM)	No NEM		NEM	
	pH 7.0	pH 7.6	pH 7.0	pH 7.6
0	82 + 4	100 + 3	60 + 4	37 + 2
5	92 + 7	137 + 4	51 + 7	59 + 4
10	118 + 7	192 + 3	44 + 7	41 + 4

Table 8. The counteraction by N-ethylmaleimide (NEM) of the activation of PAG by phosphate (Pi) and effect of pH. The synaptosomes were preincubated with 1 mM NEM (when indicated) for 5 min at 25°C, before the addition of Gln. Otherwise, conditions as Table 1. Mean of 6 experiments + SEM.

As demonstrated in Table 8, the phosphate activation of synaptosomal PAG as well as the effect of pH in the presence of phosphate is almost abolished by NEM. The sensitivity of PAG to pH, phosphate and Glu in the surrounding medium, is in accord with external localization of PAG in the inner mitochondrial membrane, and supports the view that these compounds together with ammonia and calcium (see below), may be important regulators of synaptosomal PAG in vivo.

The Calcium Activation of Synaptosomal PAG

Calcium (0-1 mM) activates structural-bound PAG, but has no effect on purified PAG. The calcium activation is dependent on phosphate (Table 9) and promotes phosphate activation, similarly to the dye Bromothymol Blue, and several acyl-CoA derivatives (Kvamme and Torgner 1974; 1975). However, the latter compounds also activate purified PAG. To our knowledge calcium is the only cationic compound activating PAG with exception of ammonia which in high concentrations (10-20 mM) may activate purified PAG (Kvamme et al. 1970; Svenneby 1971).

Synaptosomes
Specific acitivity of PAG
(nmoles $Glu \cdot min^{-1} \cdot mg$ protein^{-1})

[Pi](mM)	0	10
-	2.3 + 0.1	6.1 + 0.4
Ca^{2+}	1.2 + 0.1	10.7 + 0.4

Table 9. Calcium acitivation as affected by phosphate. Addition: 1 mM calcium. Otherwise, conditions as Fig. 1.

The calcium activation of PAG was first observed in synaptosomes and renal mitochondria (Kvamme 1979; Kvamme and Olsen 1979; Kvamme 1982; Kvamme et al. 1983), later in brain slices, brain homogenates (Benjamin 1981) and in astrocytes cultured from mouse brain (Kvamme et al. 1982).

	Synaptosomes Percent activity of PAG	
	No Ca^{2+}	Ca^{2+}
–	100 + 2	160 + 10
Glu	55 + 3 a)	36 + 4 a)
NH$_4{}^+$	52 + 4	50 + 5

Table 10. The counteraction by Glu and ammonia of the calcium activation. Additions: 0.8 mM Glu, 0.8 mM ammonia, 10 mM phosphate, and 0.5 mM calcium. Otherwise, conditions as Table 1. Mean of 6 experiments + SEM. a) Significant difference (p < 0.001. Student's test).

It should be noted that potassium in depolarizing concentrations (56 mM) does not by itself affect calcium activation (Kvamme et al. 1983). The calcium activation of PAG in synaptosomes and synaptosomal mitochondria is unrelated to energy requiring transport mechanisms, because it is not affected by the uncoupler 2,4 dinitrophenol which inhibits the mitochondrial proton pump (Mitchell 1967). As shown in Table 10 the calcium activation of PAG is however, abolished by the product inhibitors Glu and ammonia.

	Synaptosomes Percent activity of PAG	
	No NEM	NEM
No calcium	100 + 8	34 + 8
Calcium	184 + 18	132 + 12

Table 11. The counteraction by calcium of the N-ethylmaleimide (NEM) inhibition. Additions: 0.5 mM calcium and 10 mM phosphate. The synaptosomes were preincubated for 5 min at 25°C with NEM before the addition of Gln or Gln and calcium. Otherwise, conditions as Table 1. Mean of 6 experiments + SEM.

Calcium counteracts the inhibition by NEM, Mers and PMB as shown (with NEM) in Table 11.

Disrupted synaptosomal mitochondria
Specific acitivity of PAG
(nmol Glu·min^{-1}·mg protein^{-1})

[Pi](mM)	0		10	
-	5.6 + 2.0		15.9 + 2.3	
Ca^{2+}	4.3 + 1.4		32.7 + 5.5	
NEM	2.2 + 0.7		6.3 + 2.1	
Ca^{2+} + NEM	2.3 + 0.8		29.2 + 5.0	

Table 12. Additions: 1 mM calcium, 1 mM N-ethylmaleimide (NEM) and 1 mM calcium. The synatosomal mitochondria were prepared according to Lai and Clark (1976). The mitochondria were disrupted by freezing and thawing. The preparation was preincubated for 5 min at 25°C with NEM (when added) before the addition of Gln or Gln and calcium. Otherwise, conditions as Table 1. Mean of 5 experiemnts + SEM.

Since the calcium activation of PAG is dependent on phosphate, and calcium is known to affect the phosphate transport into mitochondria (Fiskum and Lehninger 1980), an indirect effect of calcium on the phosphate transport should be expected. This is unlikely, because as shown in Table 7, preincubation of phosphate together with calcium does not enhance the calcium activation, as compared to preincubation with phosphate alone (compare A$_2$ with B$_2$). Moreover, preincubation with NEM does not reduce the calcium effect appreciably (compare A$_4$ with B$_4$). On the contrary, calcium counteracts the NEM effect in either case. A decisive argument against any effect of calcium on phosphate transport is provided by the experiment shown in Table 12. Thus, the calcium activation of PAG as well as the phosphate dependence of calcium activation can be demonstrated to occur to the same extent in disrupted synaptosomal mitochondria as in intact synaptosomes. The NEM effect is also simmilar and so is the abolition by calcium of the NEM effect. This indicates that calcium affects PAG by causing a conformational change, which makes the enzyme more sensitive to phosphate. Since NEM binds sulfhydryl groups covalently and calcium counteracts the NEM-inhibition of PAG, the NEM-sensitive sulfhydryl group may not be essential for the activity of PAG. These groups may be of importance for the accessibility of phosphate to its activator site and masked by the calcium induced conformational change of PAG.

PERSPECTIVES

Being a mitochondrial-bound enzyme, PAG is present in all brain areas. It has however, been suggested that 60% of PAG in neostriatum is located in GABA-ergic structures (McGeer and McGeer 1979). This is of interest in view of the findings by Bradford et al. (1978), Hamberger et al. (1978) and Reubi et al. (1978) that Gln is a likely precursor for the transmitter Glu and GABA.

Since PAG is susceptible to a variety of activators and inhibitors, it has a great regulatory potential, which may explain why brain and renal PAG that have almost the same properties, can serve different functions. Thus, the set of regulatory ligands available to brain PAG may be different from that of renal PAG, making the enzyme functionally different in the two organs. However, another important factor is probably the variation in concentration which a regulatory ligand can undergo in a particular organ.

Since PAG appears to be bound to the outer face of the inner mitochondrial membrane, it has a far greater regulatory potential than if it were localized on the inside of the inner membrane. The enzyme may thus be regulated by compounds in the extramitochondrial and extracellular space, such as Glu, ammonia, calcium and acyl-CoA derivatives, which may undergo considerable variation in their concentrations. In this way the PAG activity may be adjusted according to the physiological needs.

The PAG activity has been reported to be higher in nerve endings than in glial cells (Salganicoff and De Robertis 1965); Bradford and Ward 1976), and this has been used as an argument in support of the hypothetical Gln cycle. However, the maximal activity of PAG may be unrelated to its functional activity. Since the extracellular Gln concentration is assumed to be 0.5 mM (Gjessing et al 1972; Johnson 1978), and the mitochondrial phosphate concentration is 5-8 mM, the activity of pig brain PAG is at most 5-10% of that obtained at maximal activity in the presence of 20 mM Gln and 100 mM phosphate. Therefore, from a functional perspective the availability and variability of regulatory ligands are likely to be considerably more important than differences in maximal activity.

Calcium activation of PAG may not be directly involved

in neurotransmission, because this activation is unaffected by potassium in depolarizing concentrations. In the recovery phase, however, replenishing of depleted stores of Glu (or GABA) may be triggered by calcium activating the PAG.

SUMMARY

Phosphate activated glutaminase appears to be a dominant glutamine metabolizing enzyme in brain. The pig brain enzyme has been purified to homogeneity and it has similar properties as renal glutaminase. The purified enzyme may exist in a monomeric, dimeric and polymeric form, and the specific activity increases three fold by conversion of the monomeric form to one of the others. Phosphate activated glutaminase is susceptible to a large number of activators and inhibitors.

Purified glutaminase has somewhat different properties than the synaptosomal enzyme, which is more susceptible to inhibition by Glu than the purified enzyme. Furthermore, it is inhibited by ammonia and activated by calcium in contrast to this enzyme. Calcium is a cationic activator, which is unusual, and it acts by promoting phosphate activation. Making use of the differential permeability of the mitochondrial inner membrane to sulfhydryl group reagents, evidence has been produced to show that phosphate activated glutaminase is localized to the outer face of the inner mitochondrial membrane.

Phosphate activated glutaminase in astrocytes cultured from mouse brain is not inhibited by ammonia, but it appears otherwise to have similar properties as the synaptosomal enzyme.

Phosphate activated glutaminase in nerve endings may function at less than 5-10% of its maximal activity in vivo, and is likely to be predominantly regulated by extramitochondrial (and extracellular) changes in the concentration of protons, Glu, ammonia and compounds which promote phosphate activation, such as acyl-CoA derivatives and calcium. In addition, since 2-oxoglutarate is a strong inhibitor (by Glu formation), the enzyme may in vivo be controlled by the operation of the citric acid cycle. It is suggested that phosphate activated glutaminase may be important in the recovery phase following neurotransmission by replenishing de-

pleted stores of Glu and possibly other amino acid neurotransmitters, in response to calcium activation of the enzyme.

If the lack of ammonia inhibition of phosphate activated
glutaminase in cultured astrocytes reflects a general glial
property, the enzyme may have a greater regulatory potential
in nerve endings than in glial cells.

REFERENCES

Badalian LL, Buniatian HC, Hovhannissian VS (1975). Effect
of glutamic acid in the interaction of various activators
of brain glutaminase. Voprosy Biochimii Mozga Akad Nauk
Armjan SSR 10:40.
Benjamin AM (1981). Control of glutaminase activity in rat
brain cortex in vitro: Influence of glutamate, phosphate,
ammonium, calcium and hydrogen ions. Brain Res 208:363.
Booth RF, Clark JB (1978). A rapid method for the preparation of relatively pure metabolically competent synaptosomes from rat brain. Biochem J 176:365.
Bradford HF, Ward HK (1976). On glutaminase activity in
mammalian synaptosomes. Brain Res 110:115.
Bradford HF, Ward KH, Thomas AJ (1978). Glutamine - a major
substrate for nerve endings. J. Neurochem 30:1453.
Curthoys NP and Weiss R (1974). Regulation of renal ammoniagenesis. Subcellular localization of rat kidney glutaminase isoenzymes. J Biol Chem 249:3261.
Curthoys NP, Kuhlenschmidt T, Godfrey SS (1976). Regulation
of renal ammoniagenesis. Purification and characterization of phosphate-dependent glutaminase from rat
kidney. Arch Biochem Biophys 174:82.
Dienel G, Ryder E, Greengard O (1977). Distribution of
mitochondrial enzymes between the perikaryal and synaptic
fractions of immature and adult rat brain. Biochem
Biophys Acta 496:484.
Errera M, Greenstein JP (1949). Phosphate-activated glutaminase in kidney and other tissues. J Biol Chem 178:495.
Fiskum and Lehninger (1980). The mechanisms and regulation
of mitochondrial Ca^{2+} transport. Fed Proc 39:2432.
Gaudemer Y, Latruffe N (1975). Evidence for penetrant and
non-penetrant thiol reagents and their use in the location
of rat liver mitochondrial D(-)-beta-hydroxybutyrate
dehydrogenase. FEBS Lett 54:30.
Gjessing LR, Gjesdahl P, Sjaastad O (1972). The free amino
acid in human cerebrospinal fluid. J Neurochem 19:1807.

Greenstein JP, Leuthardt FM (1948). Effect of phosphate and other anions on the enzymatic desamidation of various amides. Arch Biochem Biophys 17:105.

Hamberger A, Chiang G, Nylén ES, Scheff SW, Cotman CW (1978). Stimulus-evoked increase in the biosynthesis of the putative neurotransmitter glutamate in the hippocampus. Brain Res 143:549.

Hovhannissian VS, Buniatian HC, Ukrdumova GS, Badalian LL (1970). The participation of thyroxine in the interaction of the isoenzymes of brain glutaminase and certain features of its action. Voprosy Biochimii Mozga Akad Nauk Armjan SSR 6:5.

Johnson JL (1978). The excitant amino acids glutamic and aspartic acid as transmitter candidates in the vertebrate central nervous system. Prog Neurobiol 10:155.

Josef SK, Meijer AJ (1981). The inhibitory effects of sulphydryl reagents on the transport and hydrolysis of glutamine in rat-liver mitochondria. Eur J Biochem 119:523.

Kalra J and Brosnan JT (1974). The subcellular localization of glutaminase isoenzymes in rat kidney cortex. J Biol Chem 249:3255.

Katunuma N, Tomino L, Nishino H (1966). Glutaminase isoenzymes in rat kidney. Biochem Biophys Res Commun 22:321.

Kovačević Z (1976). Importance of the flux of phosphate across the inner membrane of kidney mitochondria for the activation of glutaminase and the transport of glutamine. Biochem Biophys Acta 430:399.

Kvamme E, Tveit B, Svenneby G (1970). Glutaminase from pig renal cortex. I. Purification and general properties. J Biol Chem 245:1871.

Kvamme E, Torgner I (1974). The effect of acetyl-coenzyme A on phosphate-activated glutaminase from pig kidney and brain. Biochem J 137:525.

Kvamme E, Svenneby G (1975). Phosphate activated glutaminase in brain. In Marks N, Rodnight T (eds): "Research Methods in Neurochemistry", Vol 3, New York: Plenum Press, p 277.

Kvamme E, Torgner I (1975). Regulatory effect of fatty acyl-coenzyme A derivatives on phosphate-activated pig brain and kidney glutaminase in vitro. Biochem J 149:83.

Kvamme E (1979). Regulation of glutaminase and its possible implication for GABA metabolism. In Mandel P, DeFeudis FV (eds): "GABA-Biochemistry and CNS Functions", New York: Plenum Publ Corp, p 111.

Kvamme E, Olsen BE (1979). Evidence for two species of mammalian phosphate-activated glutaminase having different regulatory properties. FEBS Lett 107:33.

Kvamme E, Lenda K (1981). Evidence for compartmentalization of glutamate in rat brain synaptosomes using the glutamate sensitivity of phosphate activated glutaminase as a functional test. Neurosci Lett 25:193.

Kvamme E, Olsen BE (1981). Evidence for compartmentation of synaptosomal phosphate-activated glutaminase. J Neurochem 36:1916.

Kvamme E (1982). Regulation of pig kidney phosphate-activated glutaminase. In Tannen RL, Goldstein L, Lemieux G, Simpson D, Vinay P (eds): "Renal Ammonia Metabolism". In Berlyne GM, Giovannetti S, Thomas S (eds): "Contributions to Nephrology ", Vol 31, Basel: Karger, p 60.

Kvamme E, Lenda K (1982). Regulation of glutaminase by exogenous glutamate, ammonia and 2-oxoglutarate in synaptosomal enriched preparation from rat brain. Neurochem Res 7:667.

Kvamme E, Svenneby G, Hertz L, Schousboe A (1982). Properties of phosphate activated glutaminase in astrocytes cultured from mouse brain. Neurochem Res 7:761.

Kvamme E (1983). Deaminases and amidases. In Lajtha A (ed): "Handbook of Neurochemistry", Vol 4, New York: Academic Press, p 85.

Kvamme E, Svenneby G, Torgner IAa (1983). Calcium stimulation of glutamine hydrolysis in synaptosomes from rat brain. Neurochem Res 8:23.

Lai JCK, Clark JB (1976). Preparation and properties of mitochondria derived from synaptosomes. Biochem J 154:423.

McGeer EC, McGeer PL (1979). Localization of glutaminase in the rat neostriatum. J Neurochem 32:1071.

McIntyre JO, Bock H-GO, Fleischer S (1978). The orientation of D-beta-hydroxybutyrate dehydrogenase in the mitochondrial inner membrane. BBA 513:255.

Mitchell P (1967). Proton-translocation phosphorylation in mitochondria, chloroplasts and bacteria: natural fuel cells and solar cells. Fed Proc 26:1370.

Nimmo GA, Tipton KF (1980). Purification of soluble glutaminase from pig brain. Biochem Pharmacol 29:359.

Nimmo GA, Tipton KF (1981). Kinetic comparisons between soluble and membrane-bound glutaminase preparations from pig brain. Eur J Biochem 11:57.

O'Donovan J, Lotspeich WD (1966). Activation of kidney mitochondrial glutaminase by inorganic phosphate and organic acids. Nature (Lond) 212:930.

Olsen BR, Svenneby G, Kvamme E, Tveit B, Eskeland T (1970). Formation and ultrastructure of enzymically active polymers of pig renal glutaminase. J. Mol Biol 52:239.

Olsen BR, Torgner I, Christensen TB, Kvamme E (1973). Ultrastructure of pig renal glutaminase. Evidence for conformational changes during polymer formation. J Mol Biol 74:239.

Reubi JC, Van den Berg CJ, Cuénod M (1978). Glutamine as precursor for the GABA and glutamate transmitter pools. Neurosci Lett 10:171.

Salganicoff L, De Robertis E (1965). Subcellular distribution of the enzymes of the glutamic acid, glutamine and gamma-aminobutyric acid cycles in rat brain. J Neurochem 12:287.

Storm-Mathisen J, Leknes AK, Bore AT, Vaaland JL, Edminson P, Haug F-MS, Ottersen OP (1983). First visualization of glutamate and GABA in neurones by immunocytochemistry. Nature 301:517.

Svenneby G (1970). Pig brain glutaminase. Purification and identification of different enzyme forms. J Neurochem 19:1591.

Svenneby G, Tveit B, Kvamme E (1970). Glutaminase from pig renal cortex. II. Activation by inorganic and organic anions. J Biol Chem 245:1878.

Svenneby G (1971). Activation of pig brain glutaminase. J Neurochem 18:2201.

Svenneby G, Torgner I, Kvamme E (1973). Purification of phosphate-dependent pig brain glutaminase. J Neurochem 20:1217.

Tietze F (1969). Enzymic method for quantitative determinations of nanogram amounts of total and oxidized glutathione: Applications to mammalian blood and other tissues. Anal Biochem 27:502.

Weil-Malherbe H (1969). Activators and inhibitors of brain glutaminase. J Neurochem 16:855.

Weil-Malherbe H (1972). Modulators of glutaminase activity. J Neurochem 19:2257.

Weil-Malherbe H, Beall GD (1970). Riboflavin 5'-phosphate: a potent activator of brain glutaminase. J Neurochem 17:1101.

Whittaker VP, Barker LA (1972). The subcellular fractionation of brain tissue with special reference to the preparation of synaptosomes and their component organelles. In Rainer F (ed): "Methods of Neurochemistry", Vol 2, New York: Marcel Dekker, p 1.

**Glutamine, Glutamate, and GABA
in the Central Nervous System, pages 69-76**
© 1983 Alan R. Liss, Inc., 150 Fifth Avenue, New York, NY 10011

IMMUNOLOGICAL STUDIES ON PHOSPHATE ACTIVATED GLUTAMINASE

Gerd Svenneby and Jon Storm-Mathisen*

Neurochemical Laboratory
Preclinical Medicine, Oslo University
P.O.Box 1115 - Blindern, Oslo 3, Norway

Phosphate activated glutaminase (PAG) (EC 3.5.1.2) from both pig brain and pig kidney (Kvamme, Svenneby 1975; Kvamme, these Proceedings) has for many years been studied at the Neurochemical Laboratory. In an early attempt to establish the purity of our pig brain preparation of PAG, we raised an antiserum in rabbit (Svenneby, Torgner 1982). In double immunodiffusion experiments (Ouchterlony) this serum gave only one precipitin line, indicating a homogenous enzyme preparation. In this report we describe some recent immunochemical work using more sensitive immunoassay systems, and applying a characterized antibody preparation to demonstrate PAG immunocytochemically in brain tissue.

METHODS

PAG from pig brain and pig kidney was purified as described (Kvamme, Svenneby 1975; Kvamme et al. 1984). Rabbits were immunized with 200 ug of partly purified PAG (approx. 50% pure), in an equal volume of Freund's complete adjuvant. The rabbits were boosted every month with 100 ug of the same preparation in Freund's incomplete adjuvant. Blood samples were taken before and at several intervals during the course of immunization. The sera obtained were pooled, and the immunoglobulins were isolated (Harboe, Ingild 1973). The final immunoglobulin fraction was 30% reduced in volume compared with the starting material.

*Anatomical Institute, University of Oslo, Karl Johansgt. 47, Oslo 1, Norway.

The presence of antibodies was tested by double immunodiffusion (Ouchterlony double gel diffusion) technique using
different dilutions of antibodies against antigens in tris-
HCl buffer. Crossed immunoelectrophoresis (CIE) was done
according to Weeke (1973). Identification of the precipitates was carried out by visualization of PAG by a histochemical method (Davis, Prusiner 1973).

Immunoblotting was performed following separation of
antigen preparations on SDS-polyacrylamide-slab gel
electrophoresis by the method of Towbin et al. (1979),
slightly modified. The blots were usually stained reversibly with toluidine blue (Towbin et al. 1982). The proteins were marked on the nitrocellulose (NC) sheet with a
soft pencil. To test the possible use of the antibodies in
immunocytochemistry, the NC sheets in some experiments were
treated for 30 min with 5% glutaraldehyde followed by 1 M
aminoethanol-HCl for 30 min, both in 0.1 M sodium phosphate
buffer at pH 7.4. To block unspecific binding sites the NC
sheets were soaked in tris-NaCl containing 0.5 % Tween 20,
pH 10.2, (blocking buffer) (Batteiger et al. 1982) for 2 hrs
and incubated overnight with our immunoglobulin preparation
diluted 1:1000 with the blocking buffer. Bound antibodies
were visualized by peroxidase labelled swine anti-rabbit IgG
(Dakopatts, 1:1000) (Ørstavik 1981). Alternatively, immu-
noblots not stained with toluidine blue were processed
exactly as the immunocytochemical sections.

Vibratome sections (10 um) were cut from the hippocampus
of a mouse perfusion fixed with 5% glutaraldehyde in
phosphate buffer (0.1 M, pH 7.4). The sections were treated
with aminoethanol and alcohols, incubated free floating with
the immunoglobulins at 4°C overnight, and processed with the
peroxidase-antiperoxidase method as previously described
(Storm-Mathisen et al. 1983). Qualitatively similar results
were obtained whether the immunoglobulins were diluted 1:500
or 1:1000.

RESULTS AND DISCUSSION

In double immunodiffusion, immunoglobulins from rabbits
immunized with brain PAG (approx. 50% pure) gave a single
precipitin line against the enzyme from pig brain. This
precipitin showed confluence with a precipitin line against
crude mitochondria preparations from human brain and the

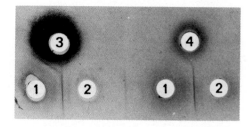

Fig. 1. Double immunodiffusion. 1: antibodies, 2: partly
purified pig brain PAG, 3: purified pig kidney PAG, 4:
extract from human brain mitochondria. Note the confluence
between the precipitin lines against antigens from pig brain
(2) and human brain (4). A spur is seen indicating immunological differences between PAG from pig kidney (3) and pig
brain (2).

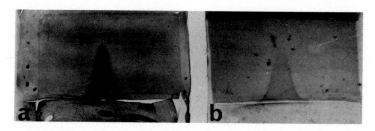

Fig. 2. Crossed immunoelectrophoresis. The antigen is 5 ug
partly purified PAG (approx. 50% pure). The upper gel contains 0.2 ml antibody preparation ml gel^{-1}. a: stained for
PAG activity, b: stained with Coomassie brilliant blue R
250. Note the similar pattern using either staining method.

enzyme purified from pig kidney (Fig. 1). A spur can be
seen between the precipitin lines against pig brain and pig
kidney, indicating partial immunological identity.

When the brain enzyme was incubated overnight on ice
with the antibody preparation, the enzymatic activity did
not decrease in the incubation mixture. Following centrifugation, however, the activity decreased in the supernatant
with increasing amount of antibody. No inhibition of enzyme
activity therefore occurred when antigen-antibody complexes
were formed. This can be further demonstrated using CIE.

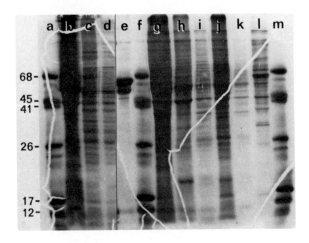

Fig. 3. SDS-gel electrophoresis. a, f, m: standard proteins
(bovine serum albumin mol.wt. 68 K, ovalbumin 45 K, alcohol
dehydrogenase 41 K, alpha-chymotrypsinogen A 25.7 K, myoglo-
bin 17 K, cytochrome C 11.9 K). Crude extract from b: monkey brain; c, d, j: rat brain; g: pig kidney; h: pig brain;
i: pig brain mitochondria; k: human brain mitochondria; e:
highly purified pig kidney PAG; l: partially purified (50%
pure approx.) pig brain PAG. 1-5 ug prot. per lane.

Following two identical runs of CIE, one was stained with
Coomassie brilliant blue, whereas the other one was stained
for enzymatic activity. Fig. 2 shows that similar precipitin patterns were obtained using either method, although
some extra minor precipitin lines can be seen in Fig. 2 b.
When the gel was stained with Coomassie brilliant blue
following the staining for enzymatic activity, the main precipitin coincided with that showing PAG activity. We therefore conclude that, although our antibody preparation is not
completely monospecific, it precipitates mainly PAG.
Production of antibody secreting hybridomas and their
subcloning to get monoclonal antibodies is in progress
(colaboration with Ulf Johnsen, M.D., Rikshopitalet, Oslo).

    To investigate the possible use of our rabbit antibodies
in immunocytochemistry, we have used immunoblotting
following SDS electrophoresis. When we treated the NC-blot
with glutaraldehyde prior to the incubation with antibodies,
the immunostaining was somewhat fainter, indicating a

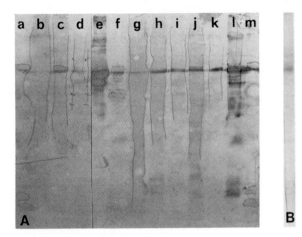

Fig. 4 A. Immunoblot of a duplicate gel to the one presented in Fig. 3. Note one main immunoreactive band with
mol.wt. 64 K. (There is some PAG-immunoreactivity in the
standard protein preparation).
B. Similar immunoblot of crude mouse brain extract, not
stained with toluidine blue, but fixed in glutaraldehyde and
precessed to show PAGimmunoreactivity in the same conditons
as the sections (Fig. 5).

decrease in avidity. The purified PAG preparations from
both pig brain and pig kidney gave several immunoreactive
bands, in addition to the main band, whereas the crude preparations from pig brain, rat brain or human brain gave rise
to mainly a single band with mol.wt. 64 kilo Daltons (K)
(Fig. 4). The pig brain PAG consists of only one subunit of
64 K (Svenneby et al. 1973). It was surprising that the pig
kidney preparation, containing 2 subunits of 64 K and 57 K,
which was almost homogenous according to the staining with
Commassie brilliant blue (row e in Fig. 3), gave rise to so
many proteins reacting with our antibodies (Fig. 4 A, row
e). However, these proteins are apparently not present to
any significant extent in human, rat or pig brain, since
essentially one protein band of mol.wt. 64 K was observed
using the sensitive immunoblotting procedure on crude
extracts from these species (rows c, d, h, j in Fig. 4 A).
The same holds true for mouse brain, processed as the immunostained sections (Fig. 4 B). Our antibodies should thus
be suitable for immunocytochemical studies on PAG.

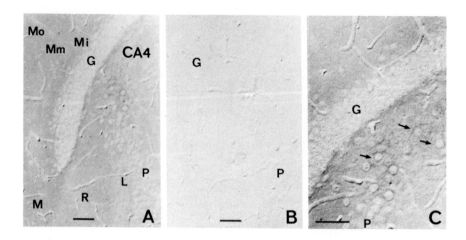

Fig. 5. Immunocytochemistry of PAG in mouse hippocampus.
Interference contrast (Leitz). A and C, rabbit immunoglobulin fraction (1:500). B, pre-immune serum (1:500). Note
that PAG-like immunoreactivity is present everywhere, except
in cell nuclei and capillaries. M, R, L, and O, strata moleculare, radiatum, lucidum, pyramidale and oriens of hippocampus CA3; Mo, Mm, and Mi, outer, middle and inner zones
of stratum moleculare of area dentata; G, stratum granulosum
of area dendata; arrows, CA4 cells. Perforant path fibres
terminate in M, Mo and Mm; mossy fibres in L and CA4; CA3
pyramidal cell fibres in R and O; CA4 derived fibres in Mi.
Scale bars 50 um.

Preliminary immunocytochemical studies on mouse hippocampus showed a rather diffuse distribution of staining
(Fig. 5). Thus there was some immunoreactivity in all
layers, except alveus (white matter). Cell nuclei were
unstained. In the neuropil the strongest intensity occurred
infragranularly and in the molecular layers, particularly in
CA3, and in the inner zone of the dentate molecular layer.
The mossy fibre layer had the lowest immunoreactivity among
the neuropil layers. The cytoplasm of cell bodies had about
the same staining intensity as the adjoining neuropil,
except in CA4, where some large multipolar cells were
conspicuously immunoreactive. These cells seemed to be different from the GABA-containing cells, and probably belongs
to the population of cells that project to the inner zone of
the dentate molecular layer (Laurberg, Sørensen 1981). Exa-

mination at high magnification suggested that in the neuropil boutons as well as dendrites were stained. Thus, the picture is somewhat similar to that obtained with an anti-glutamate antibody in perfusion fixed tissue (Storm-Mathisen et al. 1983, and these Proceedings), except that, with the PAG antibody, dendrites and cell bodies were less strongly stained and no weakly stained interneurones were seen. The low contrast between the layers is also reminescent of the rather uniform distribution of endogenous glutamate in dissected freeze-dried sections (Berger et al. 1977; Nitsch et al. 1979). The fact that glial cells were not easily identified, suggests that they contain about average PAG immunoreactivity.

These preliminary immunocytochemical results are compatible with the interpretation that PAG could be present in all the links in the excitatory chain of neurones, neurones that are likely to be glutamatergic (see Storm-Mathisen et al. 1983 for references), as well as in the GABA-containing interneurones, in the hippocampal formation. The relatively low staining in the mossy fibre layer is at variance with the reports by Altschuler et al. (1982 and Wenthold, Altschuler, these Proceedings), who found PAG-like immunoreactivity in the mossy fibres in rat and guinea pig using an antiserum raised against PAG prepared from rat kidney. Our finding of a wide distribution of PAG-like immunoreactivity is consistent with the notion that PAG has a role in the metabolism of cells in general.

REFERENCES:

Altschuler RA, Wenthold RJ, Haser WG, Monaghan DT, Cotman CW, Fox J (1982). Glutaminase-like immunoreactivity in the hippocampus of the rat and guinea pig. Soc Neurosci Abs 8:663.
Batteiger B, Newhall VWJ, Jones RB (1982). The use of Tween 20 as a blocking agent in the immunological detection of proteins transfered to nitrocellulose membranes. J Immunol Meth 55:297.
Berger SJ, Carter JG, Lowry OH (1977). The distribution of glycine, GABA, glutamate and aspartate in rabbit spinal cord, cerebellum and hippocampus. J Neurochem 28:149.
Davis JN, Prusiner S (1973). Stain for glutaminase activity. Anal Biochem 54:272.
Harboe N, Ingild A (1973). Immunization, isolation of immu-

noglobulins, estimation of antibody titre. In Axelsen NH, Krøll J, Weeke B (eds): "A Manual of Quantitative Immunoelectrophoresis", Oslo: Universitetsforlaget, p 161.

Kvamme E, Svenneby G (1975). Phosphate activated glutaminase in brain. In Marks N, Rodnight T (eds): "Research Methods in Neurochemistry", Vol 3, New York: Plenum Press, p 277.

Kvamme E, Torgner I Aa, Svenneby G (1984) L-glutaminase (mammalian). In Colowick SP, Kapaln NO (eds): "Methods in Enzymology", New York: Academic Press (in press).

Laurberg S, Sørensen KE (1981). Associational and commissural collaterals of neurons in the hippocampal formation (hilus fascia dentatae and subfield CA3). Brain Res 212:287.

Nitsch C, Kim J-K, Shimada C (1979). The commissural fibres in rabbit hippocampus: synapses and their transmitter. Progr Brain Res 51:193.

Storm-Mathisen J, Leknes AK, Bore AT, Vaaland JL, Edminson P, Haug F-MS, Ottersen OP (1983). First visualization of glutamate and GABA in neurones by immunocytochemistry. Nature 301:517.

Svenneby G, Torgner I Aa, Kvamme E (1973). Purification of phosphate-activated glutaminase. J Neurochem 20:1217.

Svenneby G, Torgner I Aa (1982). Immunological studies of phosphate activated glutaminase from brain. In Stella AMG, Gombos G, Benzi G, Bachelard HS (eds): "Basic and Clinical Aspects of Molecular Neurobiology", Milano: Fondazione Internazionale Menarini, p 447.

Towbin H, Staehelin T, Gordon J (1979). Electrophoretic transfer of proteins from polyacrylamide gels to nitrocellulose sheets. Procedure and some applications. Proc Natl Acad Sci USA 76:4350.

Towbin H, Ramjoue H-P, Kuster H, Liverani D, Gordon J (1982). Monoclonal antibodies against Eucaryotic ribosomes. J Biol Chem 257:12709.

Weeke B (1973). Crossed immunoelectrophoresis. In Axelsen NH, Krøll J, Weeke B (eds): "A Manual of Quantitative Immunoelectrophoresis", Oslo: Universitetsforlaget, p 47.

Ørstavik KH (1981). Alloantibodies to factor IX in Haemophilia B characterized by crossed immunoelectrophoresis and enzyme-conjugated antisera to human immunoglobulins. Brit J Haematol 48:15.

**Glutamine, Glutamate, and GABA
in the Central Nervous System, pages 77–93**
© 1983 Alan R. Liss, Inc., 150 Fifth Avenue, New York, NY 10011

CEREBRAL GLUTAMINE SYNTHETASE

Arthur J.L. Cooper, Fernando Vergara and
Thomas E. Duffy

Departments of Neurology and Biochemistry
Cornell University Medical College
1300 York Avenue, New York, New York   10021

Glutamine synthetase is a crucial enzyme for the maintenance of nitrogen homeostasis because it replenishes L-
glutamine, an amino acid which is a constituent of most
proteins and which serves as a nitrogen source for a variety of important metabolites (Fig. 1). The amide nitrogen
of glutamine is used for the synthesis of nitrogen 3 and 9
of the purine ring, the amide of NAD^+, asparagine amide,
nitrogen 1 of the imidazole ring of histidine, the pyrrole
nitrogen of tryptophan, the amino groups of glucosamine-6-
phosphate, guanine, cytidine and p-aminobenzoate, and carbamyl phosphate. Carbamyl phosphate is in turn used for
the synthesis of urea, arginine and nitrogen 1 of the pyri-
midine ring (see Meister, 1980). In the abovementioned
reactions glutamine seems to play a role that could conceivably have been fulfilled by ammonia[1] (Tate and Meister,
1973). However, ammonia is toxic to many animal tissues,
particularly the central nervous system, and it may be that
for thermodynamic reasons, ammonia cannot bind easily to
most enzymes catalyzing nitrogen incorporation reactions
except at high, toxic concentrations. Glutamine, on the
other hand, has a carbon skeleton "handle" which allows its
binding to glutamine amidotransferases. Glutamine thus
serves as a non-toxic store of easily transferable nitrogen
and of glutamate. Glutamine also participates as α-amino
group donor in a number of transamination reactions (Cooper
and Meister, 1981, 1983).[2] The product, α-ketoglutaramic

---

[1]For convenience, ammonia refers to the sum of ammonium ion
(NH_4^+) and ammonia free base (NH_3). At physiological pH,
~99% of total ammonia exists as NH_4^+.

acid, is hydrolyzed by ω-amidase to α-ketoglutaric acid and
ammonia. Glutamine is utilized in man (and probably in
higher apes) for a unique detoxication reaction: phenyl-
acetic acid, derived from phenylalanine, is coupled with
glutamine (via phenylacetyl adenylate and phenylacetyl coenzyme A) to form phenylacetylglutamine; daily urinary output of phenylacetylglutamine in man is about 300 mg (Moldave and Meister, 1957; Meister, 1980). Recently, glutamine has been recognized to be a major fuel of the small
intestine (Windmueller and Spaeth, 1980), bone (Biltz et
al., 1982), human diploid fibroblasts (Zielke et al., 1980)
and HeLa cells (Reitzer et al., 1979). Glutamine amide is
a major source of urinary ammonia; the carbon skeleton of
glutamine is utilized as an energy source in the kidney
(Pitts, 1975).

Despite this multitude of enzymatic reactions that can
potentially deplete glutamine, glutamine is generally present in high concentration in most cells and body fluids.
For example, glutamine is the amino acid of highest concentration in mammalian blood and cerebrospinal fluid (CSF).
In man, glutamine accounts for ∿20% and ∿67% of the plasma
and CSF amino acid content, respectively (Record et al.,
1976). In rats, glutamine occurs in millimolar concentrations in brain, heart, liver, small intestine, and sketetal
muscle (Herbert et al., 1966). The widespread occurrence
and high activity of glutamine synthetase largely accounts
for the high concentrations of glutamine in most body
tissues. Glutamine synthetase plays a particularly important role in the central nervous system (CNS) for the
removal of ammonia (a neurotoxin) and of glutamate (a
putative neurotransmitter), as well as for the generation
of glutamine as a source of carbon and nitrogen to replace
glutamate and GABA released from neurons (Hertz, 1979,
1982).

---

[2]Transfer of the amide nitrogen of glutamine to α-ketoglutarate to yield glutamate in a reaction catalyzed by glutamate synthase occurs in microorganisms and in plants (Miflin and Lea, 1977; Tempest et al., 1970). Glutamate synthase has not been detected in mammalian tissues, but
O'Donovan and Lotspeich (1968) have presented evidence from
studies with L-[^{15}N-amide]glutamine suggesting that kidney
cortex homogenates can transfer the amide nitrogen of
glutamine directly to pyruvate, α-ketoglutarate and oxaloacetate. However, the mechanism remains to be elucidated.

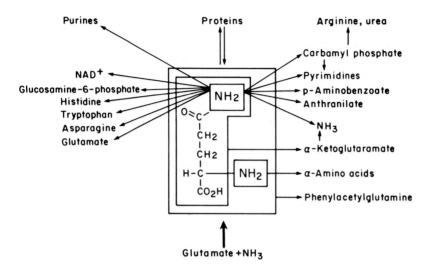

Fig. 1. Central role of glutamine in nitrogen homeostasis. The bold arrow emphasizes the fact that only one route for glutamine formation is known (the glutamine synthetase reaction), whereas glutamine breakdown is catalyzed by many enzymes. Adapted from Tate and Meister (1973).

STRUCTURE AND CATALYTIC FUNCTIONS OF SHEEP BRAIN GLUTAMINE SYNTHETASE.

Glutamine synthetase catalyzes the reversible formation of glutamine from glutamate, ammonia and ATP (Eq. 1) (Levintow and Meister, 1954). A divalent cation (Mg^{2+}, Mn^{2+} or Co^{2+}) is required for activity.

$$\text{L-Glutamate} + \text{ATP} + \text{NH}_3 \overset{\rightarrow}{\underset{\leftarrow}{}} \text{L-glutamine} + \text{ADP} + \text{P}_i \quad (1)$$

Glutamine synthetases have been purified from a number of sources, including rat liver, rat and sheep brain, pea, E. coli and B. subtilis (see refs. quoted by Meister, 1980). The first essentially homogeneous preparation of glutamine synthetase was obtained from sheep brain (Pamiljans et al., 1962). The sheep brain enzyme has an apparent molecular weight of 392,000 and is composed of eight identical subunits arranged as a cube (Haschemeyer, 1970). The specificity of the sheep brain enzyme toward nucleotides is narrow. In addition to ATP, only dATP is appreciably active; low activity occurs with adenosine tetraphosphate,

ITP, GTP and UTP (Wellner and Meister, 1966). In contrast, ammonia can be replaced by a number of nucleophiles, including hydroxylamine, hydrazine, monomethylhydrazine, methylamine, ethylamine and glycine ethyl ester, to yield the corresponding γ-glutamyl compound (Meister, 1974). With glutamate as acceptor, hydroxylamine is as effective as ammonia. The specificity of glutamine synthetase toward amino dicarboxylic acid substrates is curious. The enzyme is active toward both D- and L-glutamate but is active only toward the L-isomer of α-methylglutamate. L-Aspartate is neither a substrate nor an effective inhibitor, whereas both D- and L-α-aminoadipate are substrates. Furthermore, the rigid glutamate analog, cis-L-1-amino-1,3-dicarboxycyclohexane (cis-L-cycloglutamate) is a good substrate of glutamine synthetase. These considerations suggest that glutamate binds to glutamine synthetase in a fully (or almost fully) extended configuration.

The overall mechanism of the glutamine synthetase reaction is complex. An important component of the mechanism appears to be the formation of an acyl phosphate intermediate; nucleophilic displacement of P_i by NH_3 leads to glutamine formation. In support of this hypothesis is the finding that L-methionine-SR-sulfoximine (MSO), an analog of the tetrahedral transition state intermediate, is phosphorylated to MSO-phosphate which binds tightly to the active site and renders glutamine synthetase inactive. Glutamate provides some protection against MSO inactivation, but ammonia does not. On the other hand, glutamate plus ammonia affords complete protection. Glutamine synthetase also catalyzes the direct phosphorylation of cycloglutamate in the absence of ammonia to yield an enzyme-[cycloglutamyl phosphate][ADP] complex. A listing of the partial reactions catalyzed by sheep brain glutamine synthetase is given below (Meister, 1980).

$$\text{L-Glutamine} + \text{NH}_2\text{OH} \xrightarrow[\text{P}_i(\text{As}_i)]{\text{ADP (ATP), M}^{2+}} \text{γ-glutamylhydroxamate} + \text{NH}_3 \qquad (2)$$

$$\text{L-Glutamine} + \text{H}_2\text{O} \xrightarrow[\text{As}_i]{\text{ADP, M}^{2+}} \text{L-glutamate} + \text{NH}_3 \qquad (3)$$

$$\text{L-(or D-)Glutamate} + \text{ATP} \xrightarrow{\text{M}^{2+}} \text{2-L-(or D-)pyrrolidone-5-carboxylate} + \text{ADP} + \text{P}_i \qquad (4)$$

$$\beta\text{-Glutamyl phosphate} + ADP \xrightarrow{M^{2+}} \beta\text{-glutamate} + ATP \quad (5)$$

$$\text{Acetyl phosphate} + ADP \xrightarrow{M^{2+}} \text{acetate} + ATP \quad (6)$$

$$\text{Carbamyl phosphate} + ADP \xrightarrow{M^{2+}} CO_2 + NH_3 + ATP \quad (7)$$

$$ENZYME + \text{cycloglutamate} + ATP \xrightarrow{M^{2+}} ENZYME[\text{cycloglutamyl phosphate}][ADP] \quad (8)$$

$$ENZYME + \text{L-methionine-S-sulfoximine} + ATP \xrightarrow{M^{2+}}$$
$$ENZYME[\text{L-methionine-S-sulfoximine phosphate}][ADP] \quad (9)$$

An investigation of the glutamine synthesis reaction (Eq. 1) and the partial reactions (Eq. 2-9) has led to a detailed knowledge of the reaction characteristics (Meister, 1980). A summary is as follows: (1) The enzyme possesses separate binding sites for glutamate, ATP and ammonia, but the substrates do not bind covalently to these sites. (2) Ammonia binding requires prior binding of glutamate. (3) MSO binds to both the glutamate and ammonia sites. (4) Formation of an acyl phosphate intermediate is likely; the slow rate of 2-pyrrolidone-5-carboxylate formation in the presence of glutamate, ATP and M^{2+} (in the absence of ammonia) suggests that the enzyme stabilizes this acyl phosphate intermediate.

DISTRIBUTION OF BRAIN GLUTAMINE SYNTHETASE

The activity of brain glutamine synthetase, when measured under optimal conditions (γ-glutamylhydroxamate assay), is quite similar among different mammalian species. For example, the activity ($\mu mol/hr/g$ wet weight, 37°C) has been reported as follows: whole rat brain (76), (Vogel et al., 1975), (54) (Cooper et al., 1979); cat brain (34-123) (Berl, 1966); human brain (17-96) (Vogel et al., 1975). Glutamine synthetase activity has been detected in every structure examined in human brain (Vogel et al., 1975) and in adult cat brain (Berl, 1966). Activity is highest in the grey matter of the cerebral cortex, with smaller amounts in the brain stem (20-50% of that in cortex). The low activity of glutamine synthetase in brain stem may account, in part, for the findings that acute hyperammonemia, of a degree sufficient to cause coma, has little or no effect on forebrain concentrations of ATP but causes a marked decline in brain stem ATP (Schenker et al., 1967; Hindfelt and Siesjö, 1971; Hindfelt et al., 1977; McCandless and Schenker, 1981). Ultrastructural immunocytochemical techniques strongly suggest that astrocytes contain most, if not all, of the brain glutamine synthetase activity (Martinez-Hernandez et al., 1976; Norenberg and Martinez-Hernandez, 1979). In the retina, glutamine synthetase is localized in the Müller (glial) cells (Riepe and Norenberg, 1977).

In the cat, glutamine synthetase activity is low in cerebral cortex, cerebellum and brain stem at birth, but activity increases 3- to 8-fold in cortex and cerebellum with age and reaches a plateau at about 6 weeks of age. In the brain stem, activity barely doubles between birth and adulthood (Berl, 1966). The specific activity of glutamine synthetase in cultures of rat C-6 glioma cells is 2% of that in whole adult rat brain (Nicklas and Browning, 1978), but on passage of the cells, the specific activity rises markedly to near adult brain levels (Parker et al., 1980). The specific activity of glutamine synthetase in primary rat and mouse astrocytic cultures shows a slow increase in parallel with the increase in activity of the developing whole brain (Hertz et al., 1978; Hallermayer et al., 1981; Juurlink et al., 1981; Potter et al., 1982). The maximum specific activity attained in cultured glial cells is twice that of brain as a whole (Juurlink et al., 1981).

Studies with a variety of nitrogen- and carbon-labeled precursors suggest that glutamate/ammonia metabolism is compartmented in brain (Berl et al., 1961; 1962a; Cooper et al., 1979). That is, cerebral glutamine is synthesized in a small, metabolically active pool of glutamate that does not readily exchange with a large pool of glutamate that turns over more slowly. The evidence favors the astrocytes as the small compartment (see Duffy et al. and other chapters in this volume). Cerebral metabolic compartmentation of glutamate/ammonia metabolism is not present at birth in a number of species but develops postnatally (Berl, 1965; Patel and Balázs, 1970; Van den Berg, 1970). In rat brain, compartmentation is evident at 15 days of age and is fully developed at 30 days of age (Patel and Balázs, 1970), the period over which glial proliferation and maturation is most pronounced (e.g., Bignami and Dahl, 1973; Skoff et al., 1976).

INHIBITION OF BRAIN GLUTAMINE SYNTHETASE BY L-METHIONINE-SR-SULFOXIMINE (MSO) AND RELATED COMPOUNDS

MSO is a strong irreversible inhibitor of sheep brain glutamine synthetase and it has been known for many years that administration of MSO to animals produces generalized convulsions. A subconvulsive dose of MSO in mice rapidly (< 1 hr) inactivates liver glutamine synthetase (> 95%) but protein synthesis rapidly replenishes most (> 80%) of the activity within a few days (Rao and Meister, 1972). In the brain, activity is decreased to about 15% of control within 10 h, but activity recovers only to about 40% of control within 8-15 days; thereafter, activity continues to increase but never reaches control values even after 3 months (see also data of Sellinger et al., 1968). These data suggest two loci in brain for the synthesis of glutamine synthetase with different turnover times. After MSO treatment, the residual glutamine synthetase activity of the brain is apparently insufficient to remove excess brain ammonia, and brain ammonia concentrations rise. This rise of brain ammonia has been implicated as the cause of the astrocytic proliferation and appearance of Alzheimer type II astrocytes in brain within 8 h of the administration of a convulsive dose of MSO to rats (Gutierrez and Norenberg, 1975).

The concept that the convulsant activity of MSO is directly related to inhibition of glutamine synthetase is, however, controversial. Warren and Schenker (1964) and Folbergrová et al. (1969) noted that brain ammonia in mice administered MSO reaches a maximum several hours before the onset of seizures. Sellinger and colleagues have pointed out that MSO alters cerebral methylation reactions, disrupts serotonin metabolism, and may interfere with cell membrane function and protein synthesis (Sellinger et al., 1968; Ghittoni et al., 1970; Schatz and Sellinger, 1975; Sellinger and Dietz, 1981). Following administration of [3H]MSO to rats or [35S]MSO to mice, considerable label is recovered in particulate fractions of brain homogenates (Ghittoni et al., 1970; Rao and Meister, 1972). Warren and Schenker (1964) found that MSO treatment protects mice against a potentially lethal dose of ammonia. This observation was confirmed by Hindfelt and Plum (1975) in rats and was extended to show that the protective effect is not due to specific influences on respiration, circulation, acid-base homeostasis or body temperature. The protective effect of MSO was found to be limited to the prevention of ammonia-induced tonic convulsions, which usually terminate in death, but otherwise the toxic manifestations of ammonia were the same.

Although MSO is a novel substrate for a number of enzymes (Cooper et al., 1976), it seems unlikely that a metabolite of MSO is the convulsant or that the convulsant activity is due to inhibition of enzymes other than glutamine synthetase. Labeled MSO, added to brain homogenates, may be quantitatively extracted unchanged (Ghittoni et al., 1970). The S-isomer of MSO which inhibits glutamine synthetase is also the convulsant isomer (Rowe and Meister, 1970). MSO reversibly inhibits γ-glutamylcysteine synthetase (Richman et al., 1973); however, α-ethyl MSO, which is a convulsant, inhibits glutamine synthetase but not γ-glutamylcysteine synthetase. α-Ethyl MSO is unlikely to be metabolized since it does not possess an α-C-H bond. Conversely, buthionine sulfoximine (BSO), which is not a convulsant, inhibits γ-glutamylcysteine synthetase but not glutamine synthetase (Griffith and Meister, 1978, 1979;

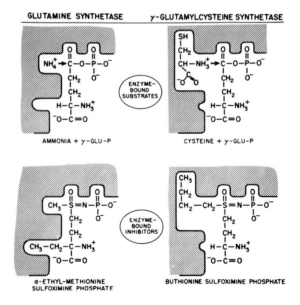

Fig. 2. Analogues of MSO as selective inhibitors of glutamine synthetase and γ-glutamylcysteine synthetase. The conformation of the active site of glutamine synthetase permits binding of an α-ethyl group but not an S-butyl group. The active site of γ-glutamylcysteine synthetase accommodates the S-butyl group but not the α-ethyl group. γ-Glu-P, γ-glutamyl phosphate. (Meister, 1980).

Griffith et al., 1979). The selective binding of α-ethyl MSO to glutamine synthetase and of BSO to γ-glutamylcysteine synthetase are in accord with the known topography of the active sites of these two enzymes (Fig. 2). The finding that α-ethyl MSO is both a selective inhibitor of glutamine synthetase and a convulsant would seem to rule out (a) inhibition of enzymes other than glutamine synthetase, and (b) appearance of secondary enzymatic breakdown products as causes of the MSO-induced convulsions.

Warren and Schenker (1964) postulated that the protective effect of MSO against ammonia intoxication was related to its interference with ammonia removal, decreasing the cerebral energy demands. However, Hindfelt (1973) has argued that glutamine synthetase is of minor importance for maintaining the cerebral energy balance and its inhibition probably could not entirely account for the protective effect of MSO against ammonia intoxication. In order to investigate the mechanism of protection afforded by MSO, we studied the effect of MSO treatment and ammonia infusion on ammonia, glutamine, glutamate and α-ketoglutarate levels in the cerebral cortex of paralyzed, anesthetized and artificially respirated rats (Table 1).

Infusion of ammonium acetate into rats greatly elevated blood and brain ammonia levels and gave rise to a large increase in brain glutamine compared to values obtained in sodium acetate-infused controls (Table 1); brain glutamate levels declined by a small but significant amount. Despite a net increase in 5-carbon amino acids (glutamate + glutamine), the concentration of α-ketoglutarate was not altered. The mechanism for this increase in 5-carbon units is unknown but may reflect ammonia-stimulated CO_2 fixation (cf Berl et al., 1962b) or impaired glutamine breakdown (Matheson and Van den Berg, 1975; Tyce et al., 1981).

MSO treatment increased cerebral ammonia concentrations and decreased glutamine (Table 1); brain glutamate levels also fell following MSO administration, as has been reported by others (Tews and Stone, 1964; Folbergrová et al., 1969; Van den Berg and Van den Velden, 1970; Hindfelt, 1973). Interestingly, the reduction of brain glutamate occurred in the face of elevated α-ketoglutarate and ammonia concentrations (Table 1) which would be expected to promote glutamate formation via the glutamate dehydrogenase reaction. Furthermore, the decrease in glutamate concentration occurred under conditions in which the incorpora-

TABLE 1

METABOLITE CONCENTRATIONS (mmol/kg wet wt ± S.E.) IN RAT CEREBRAL CORTEX DURING AMMONIA-INDUCED AND L-METHIONINE-SR-SULFOXIMINE-INDUCED INTOXICATION

Metabolite	NaAc-infused (control) (N = 4)	NH4Ac-infused (N = 5)	MSO-treated + NaAc-infused (N = 3)	MSO-treated + NH4Ac-infused (N = 4)
Ammonia	0.326 ± 0.063	0.985 ± 0.084*	0.855 ± 0.031*	2.48 ± 0.06*
α-Ketoglutarate	0.096 ± 0.011	0.112 ± 0.011	0.157 ± 0.006*	0.141 ± 0.018*
Glutamate	12.87 ± 0.43	11.07 ± 0.26*	10.07 ± 0.32*	11.58 ± 0.44*†
Glutamine	8.04 ± 0.32	18.48 ± 0.81*	3.79 ± 0.54*	6.97 ± 1.00
Ammonia (arterial blood)(mmol/l)	0.191 ± 0.019	0.710 ± 0.150*	0.432 ± 0.089*	1.02 ± 0.07*

Adult male Wistar rats (242-325 g) were anesthetized with divinyl ether and catheters were inserted into the tail artery and one femoral vein. The rats were then tracheotomized, curarized, and passively ventilated with 30% O_2-70% N_2O. Rectal temperature was maintained at 37 ± 1°C, and respiratory rate and depth were adjusted to maintain arterial blood acid-base balance [PaO_2 = 111 ± 5 mm Hg; $PaCO_2$ = 37.3 ± 0.9 mm Hg; pH = 7.390 ± 0.005 (mean ± S.E., n = 16)]. Animals that received MSO were injected i.p. with 150 mg/kg of the compound [a dose that prevents ammonia-induced tonic convulsions in rats (Hindfelt and Plum, 1975)], 2-2.5 h before the infusions were begun. The rats were infused i.v. with either 3.0 M sodium acetate (NaAc) or 3.0 M ammonium acetate (NH4Ac) for 2 h at a rate of 6.2 μl/min, after which they were killed by freezing their brains in situ with liquid nitrogen (Pontén et al., 1973). Cortical tissue was dissected from the frozen brains, pulverized under liquid nitrogen, weighed at -20°C, and extracted with 3 M perchloric acid. Metabolite concentrations were determined on neutralized perchloric acid extracts by enzymatic, fluorometric methods (Hindfelt et al., 1977).

*Different from control values with p < 0.01 by Dunnett's test for multiple comparisons.
†Different from value in MSO-treated, NaAc-infused animals with p < 0.05 by Student's t-test.

tion of blood-borne [^{13}N]ammonia (Cooper et al., 1979) and [^{14}C]acetate (Van den Berg and Van den Velden, 1970) into brain glutamate is enhanced. These labeling data can best be explained by assuming that in the presence of MSO, metabolic compartmentation of glutamate/ammonia is disrupted, i.e., the precursors enter the large compartment from which they are largely excluded under normal conditions.

If the effects of MSO treatment and ammonia infusion on brain glutamate concentrations were additive, a large fall in glutamate would have been expected in animals that received both of these treatments. However, this was not the case (Table 1); glutamate levels were still significantly decreased in animals that received both MSO and ammonia, but they were closer to normal in this group compared with animals that received MSO, and tended to be higher than those that received only ammonium acetate.

Although the reductions of brain glutamate in the MSO-treated or ammonium acetate-infused rats are small (22% and 14%, respectively), the changes may not be uniformly distributed throughout the brain but confined to a single compartment, perhaps the small (astrocytic) compartment. If so, the decrease of glutamate in that compartment would be much greater than that measured in the brain as a whole and could be critical for the functioning of the compartment. The origins of small-compartment glutamate appear to be (1) entry from the large compartment, (2) reductive amination of small-compartment α-ketoglutarate, and (3) transamination of small-compartment α-ketoglutarate with amino acids, notably branched-chain amino acids, that enter from the large compartment and from the blood. The relative importance of uptake of glutamate from the large compartment in MSO-treated or ammonia-treated animals is not known, although uptake is thought to be dependent upon neuronal activity and release of glutamate from nerve terminals (Hertz, 1979, 1982). Under normal circumstances, reductive amination of α-ketoglutarate seems to play a minor role in the synthesis of glutamate in the small compartment, based upon data derived from [^{13}N]ammonia incorporation studies (Cooper et al., 1979), and Yu et al. (1982) have shown that the glutamate dehydrogenase reaction is active in the oxidative direction in cultured astrocytes. We suggest that transamination of small-pool α-ketoglutarate with branched-chain amino acids may represent an important source of small-pool glutamate (Cooper et al., 1979; Duffy et al., this volume). The brain contains branched-chain amino acid transaminase activity (Benuck et al., 1971); the branched chain amino acids (valine and leucine) are readily taken up by the brain (Oldendorf, 1971); and the intermediary metabolism of these amino acids provides a source of glutamate carbon (cf Patel and Balázs, 1970) as well as glutamate nitrogen.

If the cerebral concentrations of the branched-chain amino acids are indeed important for the maintenance of small-compartment glutamate, then it is noteworthy that in dogs infused with ammonium chloride, brain valine is lowered (Tews et al., 1963), and in dogs treated with MSO, both valine and leucine concentrations in brain are depressed (Tews and Stone, 1964). Whatever factors tend to decrease small-compartment glutamate formation after ammonia or MSO treatment, they are apparently offset by the increase in synthesis of glutamate (presumably by the glutamate dehydrogenase reaction) due to the extraordinarily high concentration of ammonia in animals treated with MSO and ammonium acetate (Table 1). This glutamate may be important for maintaining energy metabolism of the astrocytes (Hindfelt et al., 1977; Yu et al., 1982), both as a key component of the malate-aspartate shuttle of intracellular hydrogen transport and as oxidizable substrate.

CONCLUDING REMARKS

Glutamine synthetase is crucial in regulating the concentration of glutamate in brain and in maintaining the concentration of ammonia at low levels. However, the system appears to operate normally at near maximum efficiency since the enzyme cannot maintain low brain ammonia levels in the face of continuous high concentrations of ammonia in blood or following reduction of the enzyme activity by inhibitors. Decreased glutamate in a small critical compartment (astrocytes, nerve endings) may contribute to the neurotoxicity of elevated ammonia and MSO poisoning.

ACKNOWLEDGMENTS

We thank Dr. Alton Meister for his helpful suggestions. Part of the work mentioned from the authors' laboratory was supported by U.S. Public Health Service Grant AM-16739.

Benuck M, Stern F, Lajtha A (1971). Transamination of amino acids in homogenates of rat brain. J Neurochem 18:1555.

Berl S (1965). Compartmentation of glutamic acid metabolism in developing cerebral cortex. J Biol Chem 240:2047.

Berl S (1966). Glutamine synthetase. Determination of its distribution in brain during development. Biochemistry 5:916.

Berl S, Lajtha A, Waelsch H (1961). Amino acid and protein metabolism. VI. Cerebral compartments of glutamic acid metabolism. J Neurochem 7:186.

Berl S, Takagaki G, Clarke DD, Waelsch H (1962a). Metabolic compartments in vivo. Ammonia and glutamic acid metabolism in brain and liver. J Biol Chem 237:2562.

Berl S, Takagaki G, Clarke DD, Waelsch H (1962b). Carbon dioxide fixation in the brain. J Biol Chem 237:2570.

Bignami A, Dahl D (1973). Differentiation of astrocytes in the cerebellar cortex and pyramidal tracts of the newborn rat. An immunofluorescence study with antibodies to a protein specific to astrocytes. Brain Res 49:393.

Biltz RM, Letteri JM, Pellegrino ED, Pinkus L (1982). Glutamine: a new metabolic substrate. In Massry SG, Letteri JM, Ritz E (eds): "Regulation of Phosphate and Mineral Metabolism." Advances in Exp Med Biology, vol. 151. New York: Plenum Press, p. 423.

Cooper AJL, McDonald JM, Gelbard AS, Gledhill RF, Duffy TE (1979). The metabolic fate of ^{13}N-labeled ammonia in rat brain. J Biol Chem 254:4982.

Cooper AJL, Meister A (1981). Comparative studies of glutamine transaminases from rat tissues. Comp Biochem Biophys 69B:137.

Cooper AJL, Meister A (1983). Glutamine and asparagine transaminases. In Metzler DE, Christen P (eds): "The Transaminases." New York: Academic Press. In press.

Cooper AJL, Stephani RA, Meister A (1976). Enzymatic reactions of methionine sulfoximine. Conversion to the corresponding α-imino and α-keto acids, and to α-ketobutyrate and methane sulfinimide. J Biol Chem 251:6674.

Folbergrová J, Passonneau JV, Lowry OH, Schulz DW (1969). Glycogen, ammonia and related metabolites in the brain during seizures evoked by methionine sulphoximine. J Neurochem 16:191.

Ghittoni NE, Ohlsson WG, Sellinger OZ (1970). The effect of methionine on the regional and intracellular disposition of [3H]methionine sulfoximine in rat brain. J Neurochem 17:1057.

Griffith OW, Anderson ME, Meister A (1979). Inhibition of glutathione biosynthesis by prothionine sulfoximine (S-n-propylhomocysteine sulfoximine), a selective inhibitor of γ-glutamylcysteine synthetase. J Biol Chem 254:1205.

Griffith OW, Meister A (1978). Differential inhibition of glutamine and γ-glutamylcysteine synthetases by α-alkyl analogs of methionine sulfoximine that induce convulsions. J Biol Chem 253:2333.

Griffith OW, Meister A (1979). Potent and specific inhibition of glutathione synthesis by buthionine sulfoximine (S-n-butyl homocysteine sulfoximine). J Biol Chem 254:7558.

Gutierrez JA, Norenberg MD (1975). Alzheimer II astrocytosis following methionine sulfoximine. Arch Neurol 32:123.

Hallermayer K, Harmening C, Hamprecht B (1981). Cellular localization and regulation of glutamine synthetase in primary cultures of brain cells from newborn mice. J Neurochem 37:43.

Haschemeyer RH (1970): Electron microscopy of enzymes. Adv Enzymol 33:71.

Herbert JD, Coulson RA, Hernandez T (1966). Free amino acids in the caiman and rat. Comp Biochem Physiol 17:583.

Hertz L (1979). Functional interactions between neurons and astrocytes. I. Turnover and metabolism of putative amino acid transmitters. Prog Neurobiol 13:277.

Hertz L (1982). Astrocytes. In Lajtha A (ed) "Handbook of Neurochemistry," vol. 1, 2nd edition. Plenum: New York, p. 319.

Hertz L, Bock E, Schousboe A (1978). GFA content, glutamate uptake and activity of glutamate metabolizing enzymes in differentiating mouse astrocytes in primary cultures. Dev Neurosci 1:226.

Hindfelt B (1973). The effect of acute ammonia intoxication upon the brain energy state in rats pretreated with L-methionine D-L-sulphoximine. Scand J Clin Lab Invest 31:289.

Hindfelt B, Plum F (1975). L-Methionine-DL-sulphoximine and acute ammonia toxicity. J Pharm Pharmac 27:456.

Hindfelt B, Siesjö BK (1971). Cerebral effects of acute ammonia intoxication. II. The effect upon energy metabolism. Scand J Clin Lab Invest 28:365.

Hindfelt B, Plum F, Duffy TE (1977). Effect of acute ammonia intoxication on cerebral metabolism in rats with portacaval shunts. J Clin Invest 59:386.

Juurlink BHJ, Schousboe A, Jørgensen OS, Hertz L (1981). Induction by hydrocortisone of glutamine synthetase in mouse primary astrocyte cultures. J Neurochem 36:136.

Levintow L, Meister A (1954): Reversibility of the enzymatic synthesis of glutamine. J Biol Chem 209:265.

Martinez-Hernandez A, Bell KP, Norenberg MD (1976). Glutamine synthetase: glial localization in brain. Science 195:1356.

Matheson DF, Van den Berg CJ (1975). Ammonia and brain glutamine: Inhibition of glutamine degradation by ammonia. Biochem Soc Trans 3:525.

McCandless DW, Schenker S (1981). Effect of acute ammonia intoxication on energy stores in the cerebral reticular activating system. Exp Brain Res 44:325.

Meister A (1974): Glutamine synthetase of mammals. In Boyer PD (ed.): "The Enzymes," vol. 10, 3rd edition. New York: Academic Press, p. 699.

Meister A (1980): Catalytic mechanism of glutamine synthetase; overview of glutamine metabolism. In "Glutamine: Metabolism, Enzymology and Regulation." New York: Academic Press, p. 1.

Miflin BJ, Lea PJ (1977). Amino acid metabolism. Ann Rev Plant Physiol 28:299.

Moldave K, Meister A (1957). Synthesis of phenylacetylglutamine by human tissue. J Biol Chem 229:463.

Nicklas WJ, Browning ET (1978). Amino acid metabolism in glial cells: homeostatic regulation of intra- and extracellular milieu by C-6 glioma cells. J Neurochem 30:955.

Norenberg MD, Martinez-Hernandez A (1979). Fine structural localization of glutamine synthetase in astrocytes in brain. Brain Res 161:303.

O'Donovan DJ, Lotspeich WD (1969). The role of the amide group of glutamine in renal biosynthesis of amino acids. Enzymologia 36:301.

Oldendorf WH (1971). Brain uptake of radiolabeled amino acids, amines and hexoses after arterial injection. Am J Physiol 221:1629.

Pamiljans V, Krishnaswamy PR, Dumville G, Meister A (1962). Studies on the mechanism of glutamine synthesis; isolation and properties of the enzyme from sheep brain. Biochemistry 1:153.

Parker KK, Norenberg MD, Vernadakis A (1980). "Transdifferentiation" of C6 glial cells in culture. Science 208:179.

Patel AJ, Balázs R (1970). Manifestation of metabolic compartmentation during the maturation of the rat brain. J Neurochem 17:955.

Pitts RF (1975). Production of CO_2 by the intact function-
ing kidney of the dog. In Baruch S (ed): "The Medical
Clinics of North America". Vol. 59:3. Symposium on
Renal Metabolism. Philadelphia: Saunders, p. 507.

Pontén U, Ratcheson RA, Salford LG, Siesjö BK (1973).
Optimal freezing conditions for cerebral metabolites in
rats. J Neurochem 21:1127.

Potter RL, Yu AC, Schousboe A, Hertz L (1982). Metabolic
fate of [U-^{14}C]-labeled glutamate in primary cultures of
mouse astrocytes as a function of development. Dev
Neurosci 5:278.

Rao SLN, Meister A (1972). In vivo formation of methionine
sulfoximine phosphate, a protein-bound metabolite of
methionine sulfoximine. Biochemistry 11:1123.

Record CO, Buxton B, Chase RA, Curzon G, Murray-Lyon IM,
Williams R (1976). Plasma and brain amino acids in
fulminant hepatic failure and their relationship to
hepatic encephalopathy. Eur J Clin Invest 6:387.

Reitzer LJ, Wice BM, Kennell D (1979). Evidence that glutamine, not sugar, is the major energy source for cultured HeLa cells. J Biol Chem 254:2669.

Richman PG, Orlowski M, Meister A (1973). Inhibition of
γ-glutamylcysteine synthetase by L-methionine-S-sulfoximine. J Biol Chem 248:6684.

Riepe RE, Norenberg MD (1977). Müller cell localization of
glutamine synthetase in rat retina. Nature 268:654.

Rowe WB, Meister A (1970). Identification of L-methionine-S-sulfoximine as the convulsant isomer of methionine sulfoximine. Proc Natl Acad Sci USA 66:500.

Schatz RA, Sellinger OZ (1975). Effect of methionine and
methionine sulfoximine on rat brain S-adenosylmethionine
levels. J Neurochem 24:63.

Schenker S, McCandless DW, Brophy E, Lewis MS (1967).
Studies on the intracerebral toxicity of ammonia. J
Clin Invest 46:838.

Sellinger OZ, Azcurra JM, Ohlsson WG (1968). Methionine
sulfoximine seizures. VIII. The dissociation of the
convulsant and glutamine synthetase inhibitory effects.
J Pharmacol Exp Ther 164:212.

Sellinger OZ, Dietz DD (1981). The metabolism of 5-hy-
droxytryptamine in the methionine sulfoximine epileptogenic rat brain. J Pharmacol Exp Ther 216:77.

Skoff RP, Price DL, Stocks A (1976). Electron microscopic
autoradiographic studies of gliogenesis in rat optic
nerve. II. Time of origin. J Comp Neurol 169:313.

Tate SS, Meister A. (1973). Glutamine synthetases of mammalian liver and brain. In Prusiner S, Stadtman ER (eds): "The Enzymes of Glutamine Metabolism." New York: Academic Press, p. 77.

Tempest DW, Meers JL, Brown CM (1970): Synthesis of glutamate in Aerobacter aerogenes by a hitherto unknown route. Biochem J 117:405.

Tews JK, Carter SH, Roa PD, Stone WE (1963). Free amino acids and related compounds in dog brain; post-mortem and anoxic changes, effects of ammonium chloride infusion, and levels during seizures induced by picrotoxin and by pentylenetetrazol. J Neurochem 10:641.

Tews JK, Stone WE (1964). Effects of methionine sulfoximine on levels of free amino acids and related substances in brain. Biochem Pharmacol 13:543.

Tyce GM, Ogg J, Owen Jr CA (1981). Metabolism of acetate to amino acids in brains of rats after complete hepatectomy. J Neurochem 36:640.

Van den Berg CJ (1970). Compartmentation of glutamate metabolism in the developing brain: Experiments with labelled glucose, acetate, phenylalanine, tyrosine, and proline. J Neurochem 17:973.

Van den Berg CJ, Van den Velden J (1970). The effect of methionine sulfoximine on the incorporation of labelled glucose, acetate, phenylalanine and proline into glutamate and related amino acids in the brains of mice. J Neurochem 17:985.

Vogel WH, Heginbothom SD, Boehme DH (1975). Glutamic acid decarboxylase, glutamine synthetase and glutamic acid dehydrogenase in various areas of human brain. Brain Res 88:131.

Warren KS, Schenker S (1964). Effect of an inhibitor of glutamine synthesis (methionine sulfoximine) on ammonia toxicity and metabolism. J Lab Clin Med 64:442.

Wellner VP, Meister A (1966). Binding of adenosine triphosphate and adenosine diphosphate by glutamine synthetase. Biochemistry 5:872.

Windmueller HG, Spaeth AE (1980). Respiratory fuels and nitrogen metabolism in vivo in small intestine of fed rats. J Biol Chem 255:107.

Yu AC, Schousboe A, Hertz L (1982). Metabolic fate of ^{14}C-labeled glutamate in astrocytes in primary cultures. J Neurochem 39:954.

Zielke HR, Ozand PT, Tildon JT, Sevdalian DA, Cornblath M (1980). Reciprocal regulation of glucose and glutamine utilization by cultured human diploid fibroblasts. J Cell Physiol 95:41.

**Glutamine, Glutamate, and GABA
in the Central Nervous System, pages 95–111**

IMMUNOHISTOCHEMISTRY OF GLUTAMINE SYNTHETASE

Michael D. Norenberg

Laboratory Service, Veterans Administration
Medical Center and Depts. of Pathology and
Neurology, Univ. of Miami Med. Ctr, Miami, FL

Glutamine synthetase (GS) is involved in a number of important metabolic functions in brain (Van den Berg, 1970; Meister, 1974). Of particular relevance with the theme of this conference is its involvement in ammonia detoxification and glutamate and GABA metabolism. Due to its crucial role in key areas of metabolism, the precise localization of GS in brain was deemed essential.

The evolution of the concept of different metabolic pools of glutamate (Balázs and Cremer, 1972; Berl et al., 1975) led to the proposal of a glutamate-glutamine cycle (Van den Berg and Garfinkel, 1971; Benjamin and Quastel, 1975) whereby released glutamate and GABA are taken up by glial cells and subsequently converted to glutamine through the action of GS. Glutamine then diffuses out of glia into neurons where it replenishes the transmitter pools of glutamate and GABA. Immunohistochemical studies in our laboratory have lent strong support to these concepts by demonstrating that glia are the only cellular elements in brain that contain GS and that more specifically this enzyme is localized in astrocytes.

It is the purpose of this article to briefly review our immunohistochemical findings of GS in the rat as well as to present more recent material regarding its distribution in other species, to discuss developmental aspects of this enzyme, and to summarize observations in tissue culture and its status in certain pathological conditions.

DISTRIBUTION OF GS IN THE RAT

The distribution of GS as evaluated by immunohistochemistry has been most extensively studied in the rat
(Norenberg, 1979). In general, the pattern of staining was
almost identical to that obtained with metallic impregnation methods used for the demonstration of astrocytes, as
well as that observed with GFAP immunohistochemistry
(Ludwin et al, 1976). Except for a trace amount in
ependymal cells, GS was confined to astrocytes and was not
encountered in any other cell of the nervous system. The
perikaryon and processes stained very well as did the peri-
vascular end-feet (Fig. 1), the glia limitans adjacent to
the pia and the astrocytic processes which terminated
beneath the ependymal surface (Fig. 2). This distribution
of GS-containing astrocyte processes appears to serve as a
barrier against ammonia and explains the extraordinarily
rapid conversion of ammonia to glutamine in brain (Cooper
et al., 1979).

The cerebellum showed intense staining of the Bergmann
glial cells (Fig. 3) while in the retina, GS was localized
in the Müller (glial) cells (Riepe and Norenberg, 1977).

Ultrastructural immunohistochemical studies have
served to pinpoint the localization of GS to the astrocyte
(Norenberg and Martinez-Hernandez, 1979) (Figs. 4,5).
Specifically, no other neuronal, glial or mesenchymal elements contained reaction product. In addition to confirming the distribution of GS as revealed by light microscopy,
EM findings emphasized the intimate association of GS-
containing glial processes with synaptic endings (Fig. 5B).

PHYLOGENETIC ASPECTS

Using the same antibody prepared in rabbit against
sheep GS, the staining pattern in human and chick brains
was similar to that observed in the rat. The Bergmann
glial cells in the chick stained well in contrast to the
lack of GFAP immuno-reactivity reported by Dahl and
Bignami (1973). More primitive vertebrates such as the
goldfish and toad do not have astrocytes but instead have
ependymoglial cells whose cell bodies are located on the
ventricular surface and possess cytoplasmic processes that
reach the pial surface. In these species GS was localized

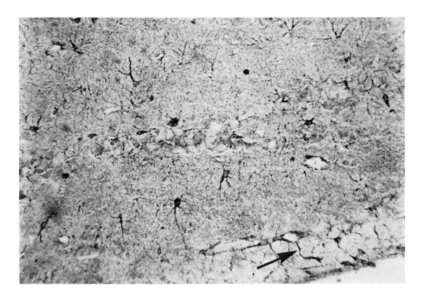

Fig. 1. Section of rat hippocampus stained for GS by the indirect immunoperoxidase method. Many prominently stained astrocytes are evident. There is intense staining around blood vessels. Note astrocyte process ending on blood vessel (arrow). 150X.

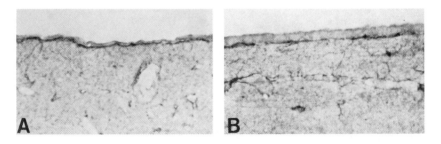

Fig. 2. A. Rat cerebral cortex demonstrates a well-stained glia limitans. 150X. B. Conspicuous subependymal staining is shown in this micrograph. 150X.

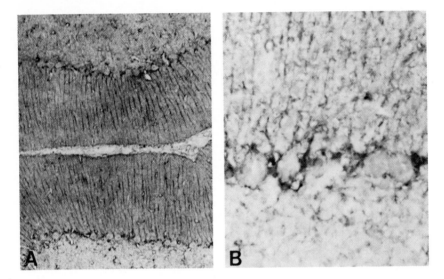

Fig. 3. A. Radial processes of Bergmann glial cells are
well illustrated. 75X. B. Higher magnification shows
absence of stain in the Purkinje cells. 300X.

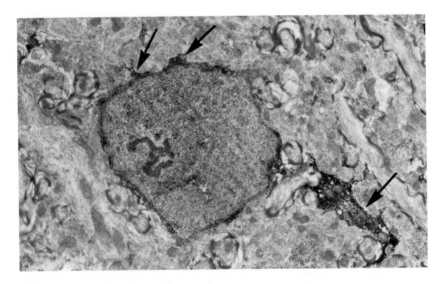

Fig. 4. Immunoperoxidase demonstration of GS at the
ultrastructural level. Note dense granules in the
cytoplasm and processes of an astrocyte (arrows). 10,500X.

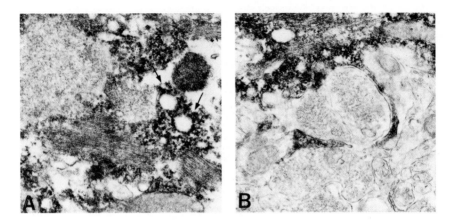

Fig. 5. A. Electronmicrograph of astrocyte showing glial filaments and dense reaction product in the cytoplasm especially in relation to cisternae of endoplasmic reticulum (arrows). 23,400X. B. Synaptic ending is outlined by GS-containing glial processes. 23,400X.

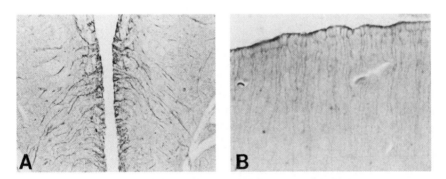

Fig. 6. A. Third ventricle of goldfish stained for GS. Note prominently stained fibers radiating from the ventricular surface. 250X. B. Optic lobe of toad with positively-staining ependymal cells. Cell bodies are on the luminal surface while their cytoplasmic processes extend into the brain parenchyma. 625X.

to these ependymoglial cells (Fig. 6). These cells apparently also do not possess GFAP. It would thus appear that GS may be a more fundamental marker of glial cells in general than GFAP.

Preliminary studies carried out in collaboration with Dr. Betty I. Roots have shown that GS in the cattle tick, earthworm and aplysia is also localized to glial cells.

DEVELOPMENTAL ASPECTS

The developmental pattern of GS in the rat was studied from embryonic day 15 (E15) through the 60th postnatal day (P60). In the neocortex positively stained cells were first seen on the day of birth (P0) but were localized only in the deeper portions (Fig. 7A). By contrast, the entorhinal cortex (a phylogenetically older area), basal ganglia and brain stem contained many positive cells throughout. Over the next few days more positive staining cells were observed in more superficial areas of the neocortex so that by P10 all areas had positive cells (Fig. 7B).

The cerebellar cortex at P0 did not show any GS activity whereas positive cells were identified in the deep cerebellar nuclei. Perikaryal staining of the Bergmann glial cells was initially observed on P1 and by P2 early radial fibers could be identified. By P4 a few of these radial fibers had extended to the pial surface. Intense staining was observed in the cerebellar cortex by P7-10 (Fig. 8).

The spinal cord at E17 showed pronounced staining around the central canal as well as within the parenchyma. Prominent radial fibers could be identified reaching the pia particularly in the anterolateral zone (Fig. 9A).

As early as E15 GS activity was observed in the ventricular zone. GS development in the ventricular zone and in its associated radial fibers (Fig. 9B) proceeded pari passu with its subsequent development in the adjacent portion of the brain parenchyma. Thus, in the lateral ventricles GS activity was initially seen ventrally and medially corresponding to the subsequent appearance of positive staining glial cells in the entorhinal cortex and septal area respectively. Later on, staining appeared in the lateral and dorsal walls of the ventricles anticipating

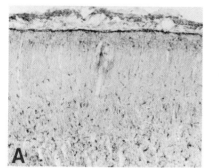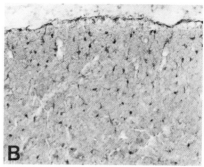

Fig. 7. A. Cerebral cortex of postnatal day 1 rat shows positively staining cells chiefly in the deeper layers. The glia limitans is well-stained. B. Astrocytes of post-natal day 10 rat cortex stain well throughout. Both 250X.

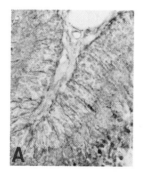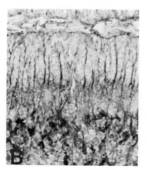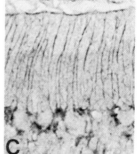

Fig. 8. Cerebellar cortex of postnatal day 2, 4 and 10 rats (A, B, C respectively). Note the progressive development of the Bergmann glial cells. All 625X.

the development of positive staining cells in the lateral
and dorsal portions of the neocortex. Thus we observed a
ventro-medial to dorso-lateral gradient along the
ventricular surface.

With further development of GS in brain parenchyma,
there was a progressive diminution of staining from the
ependymal surface which presumably resulted from the migra-
tion of the cell body into the subependymal zone while its
positively stained process remained extended to the luminal
surface (Fig. 10). Eventually that process was retracted
so that by P31 there was only minimal ependymal staining
left. By P60 little to no ependymal staining remained
which is similar to the pattern observed in the adult.

It thus appears that in the embryo GS-requiring functions are assumed by ependymal cells. This ontogenetic
scheme is apparently a throw-back to the early phylogenetic
pattern observed in more primitive species as noted above.
When brain matures, GS-requiring functions then seem to be
taken over by astrocytes. A similar pattern was observed
in the development of GS in rat retina where the earliest
staining was noted in the pigment epithelium, an ependymal
derived-structure (Riepe and Norenberg, 1978). While GS
increased in the Müller cells a corresponding reduction in
the pigment epithelium occurred so that in the adult that
layer no longer contained any GS.

Our histochemical findings correlate very well with
the biochemical developmental pattern of GS which is characterized by low activity at birth and a gradual progressive rise to reach adult levels by 1 month postnatally (Wu,
1964; Bayer and McMurray, 1967; Ozand et al., 1975). A
more important observation of this study is that the pattern of GS development almost precisely coincides with the
development of astrocytes as determined by autoradiographic
methods (Das, 1979).

In sum, the developmental pattern of GS is characterized by its initial appearance in older phylogenetic areas
followed by its development in newer ones. Within these
zones, GS appears initially in the ventricular zone and
then later in the adjacent parenchyma. Moreover, it
appears that the presence of GS may be one of the earliest,
if not the earliest, evidence of differentiation of gli-
oblasts into an astrocyte lineage. In this regard it may

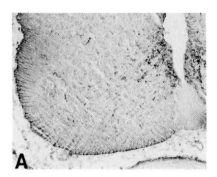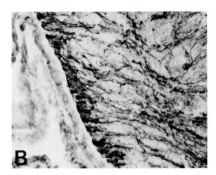

Fig. 9. A. Embryonic day 17 rat spinal cord shows staining in the ventricular zone and adjacent parenchyma. Conspicuous radial processes terminate on the pia. 250X. B. Postnatal day 1 rat lateral ventricle displays prominent ependymal and radial fiber staining. Note similarity to the pattern in adult goldfish and toad. 625X.

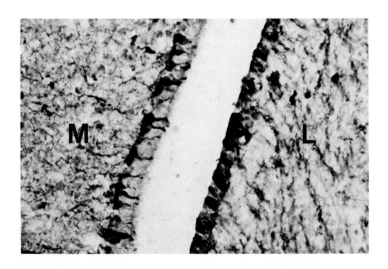

Fig. 10. Postnatal day 2 rat lateral ventricle. The ependyma on the lateral (L) surface contains more stain than the medial (M) side. Medial surface staining is found principally in processes extending to the luminal surface whose cell bodies are located in the subependymal zone. 940X.

be noted that glial fibrillary acidic protein (GFAP), the most widely used astrocyte marker, is not detected until several days after the appearance of GS (Bignami and Dahl, 1973, 1974).

TISSUE CULTURE AND INDUCTION STUDIES

High concentration of GS in primary astrocyte cultures was first reported by Schousboe et al (1977) and its identification immunohistochemically has been demonstrated by Juurlink et al. (1981). Dr. Lee Mozes and I have also carried out immunohistochemical studies in primary astrocyte cultures and found similar results (Fig. 11). Recently, Raff and co-workers (1983) have reported the immunohistochemical presence of GS in astrocytes in culture and its absence in oligodendrocytes. Pilkington et al. (1982) have shown immunoreactive GS in astrocyte tumor lines.

GS induction by cortisol in chick retina by immunohistochemical means has been shown by Linser and Moscona (1979) as well as by Norenberg and co-workers (1980). Additionally, Dutt and co-workers (1981) have reported that with both biochemical and immunohistochemical methods, cyclic and non-cyclic derivatives of adenosine and guanosine in vitro show similar induction of GS. Hallermayer et al. (1981) demonstrated GS induction immunohistochemically in primary astrocyte cultures.

PATHOLOGICAL ASPECTS

The most common response to destructive injury in the CNS is the hypertrophy and apparent proliferation of astrocytes commonly referred to as reactive fibrous astrocytosis or fibrous gliosis. This phenomenon has generally been viewed as a reparative process to isolate the injured area from the more viable regions of the CNS.

To evaluate the status of GS in these reactive astrocytes, destructive lesions were produced in the parietal lobes of rats and immunoperoxidase procedures were carried out at intervals from 7 minutes to 5 months after lesion formation (Fig. 12) (Norenberg, 1982). As early as 15 minutes following injury increased amounts of immunoreactive GS could be identified in astrocytes. There

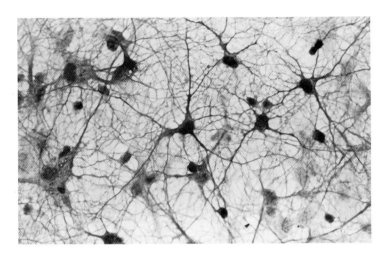

Fig. 11. Two-week old primary astrocyte culture from 2-day-old rat brain treated with dibutyryl cAMP for the last 2 days and stained for GS. 940X.

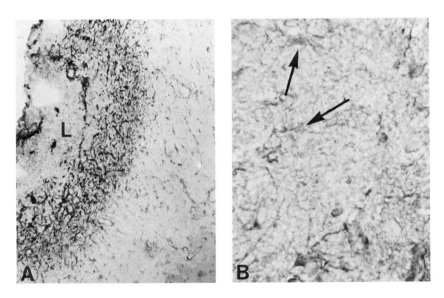

Fig. 12. A. Striking astrocytic GS staining is observed 3 weeks after the production of a lesion (L) in rat brain. GS forms a "wall" around the lesion. 75X. B. At 5 months some astrocytes possess little to no GS (arrows). 300X.

was a progressively marked increase in GS which reached a peak of activity at about 3 weeks followed by a gradual return to normal levels over the next few months.

This marked and early activity in GS suggests that following injury astrocytes may be more concerned with the elimination of ammonia resulting from the trauma as well as be involved in the uptake of a number of amino acid neurotransmitters and perhaps other potentially deleterious substances released from their normal intracellular location. It would thus appear that these reactive astrocytes may be more engaged with the correction of the metabolic derangement resulting from the traumatic injury rather than just the simple laying down of an inert scar tissue. The finding of increased GS activity is in keeping with the observation of increased labeling of the acetate-derived glutamate pool (a measure of the "small" or glial pool) following destructive lesions (Hamberger et al. 1980).

Of possible relevance was that at 5 months following trauma, numerous astrocytes around these lesions possessed little to no GS (Fig. 12B). This decrease in GS may perhaps create a critical rise in ammonia and glutamate thereby leading to seizures since both agents are potentially epileptogenic. It is possible that this apparent GS deficiency in these older reactive astrocytes may be one mechanism whereby the "glial scar" may contribute to the pathogenesis of post-traumatic epilepsy.

Methionine sulfoximine (MSO) is a potent convulsant agent with epileptogenic properties which appear to be related to the inhibition of GS (Lamar and Sellinger, 1965; Rowe and Meister, 1970). Morphologically, MSO acts principally on astrocytes resulting in degenerative changes in these cells (Gutierrez and Norenberg, 1977). The relationship between GS inhibition and such morphological changes in astrocytes, however, remains to be elucidated. Possibly the increased brain ammonia resulting from GS inhibition may be responsible for these astrocytic changes as similar changes are observed in ammonia intoxication (Norenberg, 1981). Since these degenerative changes in astrocytes appear during the pre-ictal period we have speculated that deranged astroglial function may perhaps contribute to the subsequent development of seizures.

Immunohistochemical study of rats treated with MSO

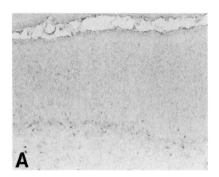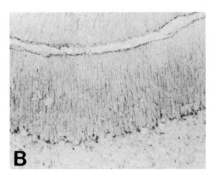

Fig. 13. A. Cerebellar cortex stained for GS from rat
treated with methionine sulfoximine (MSO). Note almost
total absence of staining. B. Normal control. Both 250X.

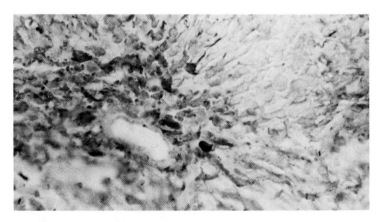

Fig. 14. Glioblastoma multiforme showing tumor
cells oriented about a blood vessel. Note the
variation in GS-staining. 940X.

(150-200 mg/kg) resulted in an almost complete absence of staining in gray matter astrocytes in all areas of brain (Fig. 13). Surprisingly, astrocytes of the white matter showed no significant reduction in stain. The sparing of white matter astrocytes may perhaps explain the small amount of residual GS activity found after MSO treatment. GS in astrocytes first disappeared from the processes which appeared to be undergoing fragmentation (clasmatodendrosis) and then was lost from the perikaryon as well. This decrease in GS immunoreactivity was seen pre- as well as post-ictally.

Immunohistochemical studies in an experimental model of hepatic encephalopathy associated with hyperammonemia have shown no significant change except for a slight increase in staining in astrocytes of the hippocampus and the Bergmann glia of the cerebellum (unpublished observation). This apparent lack of alteration in GS activity is in keeping with biochemical findings (Colombo et al., 1977; Sadasivudu, 1977). This would suggest that the GS content normally present is sufficient to keep up with the demands of excessive ammonia.

The identification of immuno-reactive GS has become a useful adjunct in the diagnosis of human brain tumors. Pilkington and Lantos (1982) in a detailed study found positive staining in all astrocytic tumors with the intensity of staining correlating very well with the degree of differentiation in these neoplasms. We have observed similar findings (Fig. 14). Pilkington and Lantos further noted that GS was not found in other primary brain tumors except for a slight amount in ependymomas. As noted previously, a trace amount of GS appears to be present in normal ependymal cells.

CONCLUDING REMARKS

The precise localization of GS in astrocytes has substantially aided our understanding of the role of these cells in the nervous system. It has clearly established these cells as foremost in the detoxification of ammonia as well as clarified its participation in the neurotransmitter actions of glutamate and GABA. GS localization in astrocytes in all species thus far studied along with its early ontogenetic appearance makes its presence one of the most fundamental characteristics of astrocytes. Furthermore, GS has shown its usefulness in the biological and pathological study of astrocytes. Finally, these observations serve to dispel the impression that astrocytes are mere bystanders and instead confer on these cells a uniquely crucial role in the efficient operation of the nervous system.

ACKNOWLEDGMENTS: The skilled and patient typing of Linda Williams and the photographic assistance of Greg Castiglione are greatly appreciated.

REFERENCES

Balá" zs R, Cremer JE (eds) (1972). "Metabolic Compartmentation in the Brain." New York: Wiley.

Bayer SM, McMurray WC (1967). The metabolism of amino acids in developing rat brain. J Neurochem 14:695.

Benjamin AM, Quastel JH (1975). Metabolism of amino acids and ammonia in rat brain cortex slices in vitro: a possible role of ammonia in brain function. J Neurochem 25:197.

Berl S, Clarke DD, Schneider D (eds) (1975). "Metabolic Compartmentation and Neurotransmission." New York: Plenum Press.

Bignami A, Dahl D (1973). Differentiation of astrocytes in the cerebellar cortex and the pyramidal tracts of the newborn rat. An immunofluorescence study with antibodies to a protein specific to astrocytes. Brain Res 49:393.

Bignami A, Dahl D (1974). Astrocyte-specific protein and neuroglial differentiation. An immunofluorescence study with antibodies to the glial fibrillary acidic protein. J Comp Neurol 153:27.

Colombo JP, Bachman C, Peheim E, Berüter J (1977). Enzymes of ammonia detoxification after portocaval shunt in the rat. II. Enzymes of glutamate metabolism. Enzyme 22:399.

Cooper AJL, McDonald JM, Gelbard AS, Gledhill RF, Duffy TE (1979). The metabolic fate of ^{13}N-labeled ammonia in rat brain. J Biol Chem 254:4982.

Dahl D, Bignami A (1973). Immunochemical and immunofluorescence studies of the glial fibrillary acidic protein in vertebrates. Brain Res 61:279.

Das GP (1979). Gliogenesis and ependymogenesis during embryonic development of the rat: an autoradiographic study. J Neurol Sci 43:193.

Dutt K, Norenberg MD, Reif-Lehrer L (1981). Effect of nucleotides and related compounds on glutamine synthetase activity in chick embryo retina: a biochemical and immunohistochemical study. J Neurochem 36:1239.

Gutierrez JA, Norenberg MD (1977). Ultrastructural study of methionine sulfoximine induced Alzheimer type II astrocytosis. Amer J Pathol 86:285.

Hallermayer K, Harmening C, Hamprecht B (1981). Cellular localization and regulation of glutamine synthetase in primary cultures of brain cells from newborn mice. J Neurochem 37:43.

Hamberger A, Jacobson I, Lindroth P, Mopper K, Nyström B, Sandberg M (1980). Neuron-glia interactions in the biosynthesis and release of transmitter amino acids. In Mandel P, Defeudis FV (eds) "Amino Acid Neurotransmitters," New York: Raven Press.

Juurlink BHJ, Schousboe A, Jørgensen OS, Hertz L (1981). Induction by hydrocortisone of glutamine synthetase in mouse primary astrocyte cultures. J Neurochem 36:136.

Lamar C Jr, Sellinger OZ (1965). The inhibition in vivo of cerebral glutamine synthetase and glutamine transferase by the convulsant methionine sulfoximine. Biochem Pharmacol 14:489.

Linser P, Moscona AA (1979). Induction of glutamine synthetase in embryonic neural retina: localization in Müller fibers and dependence on cell interactions. Proc Nat Acad Sci (USA) 76:6476.

Ludwin SK, Kosek JC, Eng LF (1976). The topographical distribution of S-100 and GFA proteins in the adult rat brain: an immunohistochemical study using horseradish peroxidase-labeled antibodies. J Comp Neurol 165:197.

Meister A (1974). Glutamine synthetase of mammals. In Boyer PD (ed) "The Enzymes," vol 10, New York: Academic Press, p 699.

Norenberg MD (1979). The distribution of glutamine synthetase in the rat central nervous system. J Histochem Cytochem 27:756.

Norenberg MD (1981). The astrocyte in liver disease. In Fedoroff S, Hertz L (eds). "Advances in Cellular Neurobiology," Vol 2. New York: Academic Press, p 303.

Norenberg MD (1982). Immunohistochemical study of glutamine synthetase in brain trauma. J Neuropathol Exp Neurol 41:347.

Norenberg MD, Dutt K, Reif-Lehrer L (1980). Glutamine synthetase localization in cortisol-induced chick embryo retinas. J Cell Biol 84:803.

Norenberg MD, Martinez-Hernandez A (1979). Fine structural localization of glutamine synthetase in astrocytes of rat brain. Brain Res 161:303.

Ozand PT, Stevenson JH, Tildon JT, Cornblath M (1975). The effects of hyperketonemia on glutamate and glutamine metabolism in developing rat brain. J Neurochem 25:67.

Pilkington GJ, Lantos PL (1982). The role of glutamine synthetase in the diagnosis of cerebral tumors. Neuropath Appl Neurobiol 8:227.

Pilkington GJ, Lantos PL, Darling JL, Thomas DGT (1982). Three cell lines from a spontaneous murine astrocytoma show variation in astrocytic differentiation. Neurosci Lett 34:315.

Raff MC, Miller RH, Noble M (1983). A glial progenitor cell that develops in vitro into an astrocyte or an oligodendrocyte depending on culture medium. Nature 303:390.

Riepe RE, Norenberg MD (1977). Müller cell localization of glutamine synthetase in rat retina. Nature 268:654.

Riepe RE, Norenberg MD (1978). Glutamine synthetase in the developing rat retina: an immunohistochemical study. Exp Eye Res 27:435.

Rowe WB, Meister A (1970). Identification of L-methionine-S-sulfoximine as the convulsant isomer of methionine sulfoximine. Proc Natl Acad Sci (USA) 66:500.

Sadasivudu B, Rao TI, Radhakrishna C, Murthy CR (1977). Acute metabolic effects of ammonia in mouse brain. Neurochem Res 2:639-655.

Schousboe A, Svenneby G, Hertz L (1977). Uptake and metabolism of glutamate in astrocytes cultured from dissociated mouse brain hemispheres. J Neurochem 29:999.

Van den Berg CJ (1970). Glutamate and glutamine. In Lajtha A (ed) "Handbook of Neurochemistry," vol 3, New York: Plenum Press, p 355.

Van den Berg CJ, Garfinkel D (1971). A simulation study of brain compartments: metabolism of glutamate and related substances in mouse brain. Biochem J 123:211.

Wu C (1964). Glutamine synthetase. III. Factors controlling its activity in the developing rat. Arch Biochem Biophys 106:394.

**Glutamine, Glutamate, and GABA
in the Central Nervous System, pages 113–128**
© 1983 Alan R. Liss, Inc., 150 Fifth Avenue, New York, NY 10011

REGULATION OF GLUTAMATE DECARBOXYLASE ACTIVITY

Ricardo Tapia

Departamento de Neurociencias
Centro de Investigaciones en Fisiología Celular
Universidad Nacional Autónoma de México
04510-México D.F., México

The synthesis of GABA in brain depends mainly, if not only, on the activity of glutamate decarboxylase (GAD). Because of the importance of GABA as the most widely distributed inhibitory transmitter in the brain, the regulation of GAD activity is closely linked to the physiological inhibitory mechanisms of the CNS. In fact, soon after the initial studies on the activity of GAD had indicated its notable dependence on the availability of pyridoxal 5'-phosphate (PLP) (Roberts 1960), experiments in vivo using some hydrazides as carbonyl-trapping agents beautifully demonstrated that these compounds produced convulsions and inhibited GAD activity in vivo, these effects being reversed by the injection of pyridoxine or by the addition of PLP in vitro to GAD incubation media (Killam et al. 1960).

Some years later, in several studies (Minard 1967; Tapia, Awapara 1969; Tapia et al. 1969; Dakshinamurti, Stephens 1969; Tapia, Pasantes 1971; Bayoumi, Smith 1972) a decrease of brain PLP levels was demonstrated to occur after dietary pyridoxine deficiency or after the administration of certain drugs, and it was observed that the PLP-deficient animals had convulsions and a diminished activity of GAD, which was returned to normal either by the addition of PLP in vitro or by a single injection of pyridoxine. In the latter case the neurological symptoms disappeared.

Many subsequent studies, both in vitro and in vivo, have produced overwhelming evidence in favor of the view

that PLP plays a fundamental role in the regulation of GAD
activity, and that such regulation is directly related to
the role of GABA as a transmitter at inhibitory synapses
(see Meldrum 1975; Tapia 1975, 1983; Tower 1976). Although
PLP is also a cofactor of GABA-transaminase and of course
of other amino acid transaminases and decarboxylases
present in brain, there is evidence that GAD is comparatively
considerably more labile than other B_6-enzymes, with the
exception of DOPA-decarboxylase, to a decrease of brain
PLP in vivo (Fig. 1). In the present chapter I try to
present in an integrated manner some of the main findings
of our laboratory, obtained both in vitro and in vivo,
on the mechanisms underlying PLP function as the main
single factor responsible for the regulation of GAD
activity.

STUDIES IN VITRO ON GAD MECHANISMS

Clearly, any compound normally present in brain and
capable of inhibiting GAD is a potential physiological
regulator of its activity, whatever its mechanism of
action may be. On the other hand, the use of certain
inhibitors designed specifically to study GAD mechanisms
provide a better tool to obtain information on such
mechanisms and consequently on the regulation of the enzyme
activity. For our kinetic studies on GAD inhibition we
have synthesized several derivatives of PLP, in which the
carbonyl group of this molecule has reacted with the amino
group of hydrazides, hydrazines or amino acids. The
resulting derivatives -hydrazones, oximes or Schiff bases-
were used as such or after stabilization by reduction of
the carbon-nitrogen double bond (Table 1). The unstability
of the double bond in the presence of GAD was clearly
demonstrated by the finding that the PLP-hydrazones I, II,
IV and V, when added in vitro, produced an activation of
GAD similar to that observed with PLP, whereas the
corresponding reduced hydrazines had no effect on GAD
activity (Table 2). This indicates not only that PLP is
somehow released from the PLP-hydrazone molecule and made
available to the apoGAD, but also that the reduced
hydrazones do not fit the active site of GAD, in spite of
their structural similarities with the natural PLP-substrate
Schiff base. In contrast, the PLP-oxime-O-acetic acid
(compound VI, Table 1), either reduced or not, inhibited

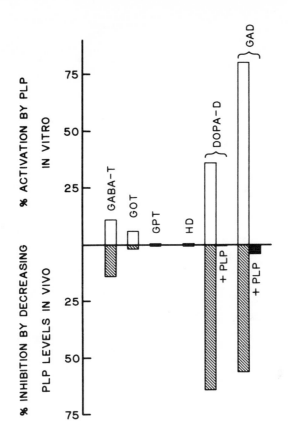

Fig. 1. Differences in the sensitivity to PLP availability
of several brain enzymes in vitro and in vivo. The upper
part shows the activation by 0.1 mM PLP in vitro as
compared to the activity in the absence of added coenzyme.
The lower part shows the inhibition after decreasing PLP
levels in vivo through the injection of PLP-ɣ-glutamyl
hydrazone (compound I, Table 1), which blocks pyridoxal
kinase activity; except when indicated (+PLP), activities
were measured in the absence of added PLP. GABA (GABA-T),
glutamic-oxalacetic (GOT) and glutamic-pyruvic (GPT)
transaminases, and histidine (HD), DOPA (DOPA-D) and
glutamic (GAD) decarboxylases, were measured. Data from
Tapia, Pasantes (1971).

Table 1. Derivatives of PLP synthesized and used to study GAD mechanisms

PLP	Hydrazide, hydrazine or amino acid	Hydrazone, oxime of Schiff base	Reduced derivative

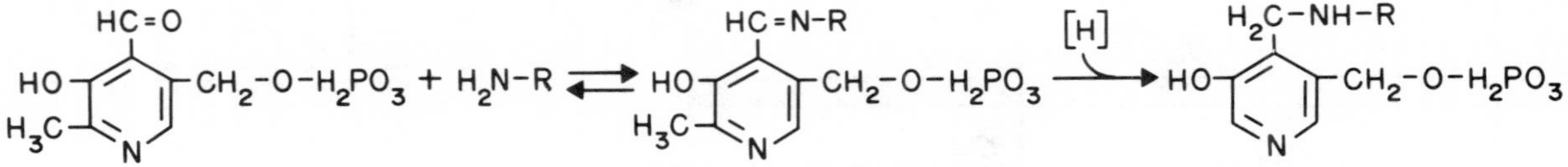

$$\text{PLP} + H_2N-R \rightleftharpoons \text{Hydrazone} \xrightarrow{[H]} \text{Reduced derivative}$$

R:

I $-NH-C(=O)-CH_2-CH_2-CH(NH_2)-COOH$

II $-NH_2$

III $-NH-CH_3$

IV $-NH-C(=O)-$ (pyridin-4-yl)

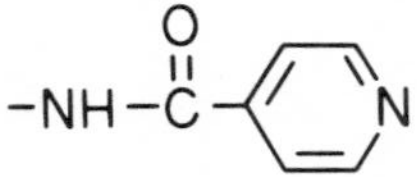

V $-NH-C(=S)-NH_2$

VI $-O-CH_2-COOH$

VII $-CH(COOH)-CH_2-CH_2-COOH$

VIII $-CH_2-CH_2-CH_2-COOH$

IX $-CH(COOH)-CH_2-SO_3H$

Table 2. Effect on GAD activity in vitro of some
of the compounds shown in Table 1

Compound (0.1 mM)	Per cent change
PLP	+ 93
I	+ 73
Reduced	+ 6
II	+ 66
Reduced	+ 5
IV	+ 81
Reduced	+ 3
V	+ 57
Reduced	+ 1
VI	− 49
Reduced	− 51

The roman numbers refer to the compounds listed in Table 1.
Data from Tapia, Awapara (1969).

GAD by about 50% (Table 2), suggesting that the unreduced
compound is more stable than the hydrazones and that both
forms of the oxime fit the active site of GAD. Interestingly
enough, this PLP-oxime had no effect at all on the activity
of brain GABA-transaminase and DOPA-decarboxylase, neither
on the activity of GAD from E. coli (Tapia, Sandoval 1971).

On the basis of the above results, we carried out more
detailed studies on the mechanism of the inhibitory effect
of PLP-oxime-O-acetic acid, and we also tested the action
of the reduced amino acid-Schiff bases VII-IX (phospho-
pyridoxyl-amino acids) (Table 1). The results of these
kinetic experiments indicated that compounds VI-IX behaved
as mixed function inhibitors with respect to glutamate and
as competitive inhibitors with respect to PLP (Bayón et al.
1977a). However, relatively high concentrations of the
inhibitors, even at very low PLP concentrations, cannot
decrease the enzyme activity to zero but only to a fixed
limit velocity. These studies suggested to us the existence
of two forms of GAD activity: one that is dependent on the
availability of free PLP, which is inhibited by the stable

PLP-derivatives fitting into the active site, and competing
with PLP, and the other possessing tightly bound PLP and
therefore independent of the free coenzyme (Tapia, Sandoval
1971; Bayón et al. 1977a).

The above postulation was strongly supported by kinetic
studies carried out in the absence of inhibitors (Bayón et
al. 1977b). In these experiments the dissociation constant
of the glutamate-PLP Schiff base was determined under the
experimental conditions to be used, and GAD activity was
measured in a wide range of glutamate and PLP concentrations,
in such a way that three limit situations were approached:
1) absence of glutamate-PLP Schiff base; 2) when all glutamate
was trapped in the form of Schiff base; 3) when all PLP was
trapped in the form of Schiff base.

The results of these kinetic experiments in the absence
of inhibitors were fully consistent with the existence of
the free PLP-dependent and the free PLP-independent forms of
GAD activity. Furthermore, they permitted the mathematical
analysis of each separate enzyme activity, thus allowing
the following conclusions (Tapia, Sandoval 1971; Bayón et
al. 1977a 1977b, 1978): a) the Km for glutamate was identical
for the two forms of GAD; b) the free PLP-independent GAD
activity possesses tightly bound coenzyme, which cannot be
displaced by PLP analogs or by dialysis; c) the ratio free
PLP-dependent/free PLP-independent GAD is close to 2.8,
which means that 25-30% of the total GAD corresponds to the
enzyme possessing tightly bound PLP and 70-75% to the enzyme
requiring free PLP; d) the glutamate-PLP Schiff base cannot
be a substrate for either form of GAD activity; e) the two
forms of the enzyme are independent and cannot be
interconverted by changes in the availability of substrate
or coenzyme; f) the free-PLP dependent GAD seems to follow
a random bireactant mechanism with regard to the coenzyme
and the substrate.

The mechanistic model of GAD activity, taking into
account all the considerations mentioned above, is the
following:

$$Ea \underset{\xleftarrow{\hspace{2.5cm}}}{\xrightarrow{Ks_1 = Ks_2}} EaS \xrightarrow{Kp_1} Ea + P$$

$$E \underset{\xleftarrow{\hspace{2.5cm}}}{\xrightarrow{Ks_2 = Ks_1}} ES \qquad\qquad A \underset{\xleftarrow{\hspace{1cm}}}{\xrightarrow{Ko}} SA$$

$$Ka \updownarrow \qquad\qquad Ka \updownarrow \qquad\qquad Koi \updownarrow$$

$$AE \underset{\xleftarrow{\hspace{2.5cm}}}{\xrightarrow{Ks_1 = Ks_2}} AES \xrightarrow{Kp_2} E + P \qquad AI$$

where Ea is the free PLP-independent GAD ('a' represents the tightly bound coenzyme); E is the free PLP-dependent GAD; S is glutamate; A is PLP; P represents the reaction products; SA is the glutamate-PLP Schiff base; and I is any compound capable of forming a Schiff base with PLP. The equilibrium constants, as well as the rate constant for product formation, are indicated. All the kinetic observations leading to postulate this mechanistic model were reproduced by a computer using the experimentally determined kinetic constants (Bayón et al. 1977b).

An important consequence of the above conclusions is that only the free PLP-dependent activity is susceptible to regulation by the available PLP. In addition, any endogenous compound capable of reacting with PLP in the form of a Schiff base, including glutamate and GABA, would be potential regulators of this form of GAD activity, providing that their concentration at the subcellular GAD location is higher than the dissociation constant of the corresponding Schiff base. Any other endogenous compound capable of somehow displacing or interfering with the binding of PLP to the enzyme could also function as a GAD regulator.

Regulation by PLP of Different GAD Populations

The studies described above do not give information on the physical relationship between the two GAD activities: the two corresponding catalytic sites might be in the same molecule, in different subunits or in different populations of the enzyme. In one of their studies on the glutamate-promoted inactivation of a partially purified GAD preparation,

Martin et al. (1980) suggested that the two types of GAD activity might be located in one molecular species.

In our experiments on the Ca^{2+}-promoted binding of GAD to phospholipid vesicles (liposomes), we found that only a fixed percentage of total GAD activity was susceptible to be bound, in spite of increasing the proportion of liposomes present in the mixture to a large excess with respect to the protein (Covarrubias, Tapia 1978). In order to investigate the possibility that the populations of bound and soluble GAD activities might represent the two forms of GAD described above, in a subsequent work (Covarrubias, Tapia 1980) we studied comparatively some kinetic properties of the GAD bound to the liposomes and the GAD which remained soluble. We found that the activation by PLP of the bound GAD was more than double as compared to the soluble GAD, and that the inhibition of the bound GAD by the PLP-oxime-O-acetic acid (compound VI) was half that of the soluble GAD in the absence of PLP, whereas the inhibition was similar when PLP was added to the incubation medium (Fig. 2). Since we also measured the binding of PLP to the liposomes, and found that none of the PLP present in the incubation mixtures was bound, we concluded that the GAD capable of binding was a population of enzyme deficient in PLP as compared to the GAD which remained soluble (Covarrubias, Tapia 1980), and therefore much more susceptible to regulation by the availability of free PLP. The possible physiological importance of this interpretation will be analyzed in the next section.

STUDIES IN VIVO ON GAD REGULATION

The main interest for a neurobiologist concerns the physiological mechanisms that maintain the functions of the nervous system in the living animal, and the regulation of GAD is no exception. Some of the early studies indicating the dependence of GAD activity on the availability of PLP in brain, in vivo, have been already mentioned at the beginning of this chapter. Again some of the drugs listed in Table 1 have been extremely useful for this kind of studies. When the PLP-hydrazones I-III were injected to mice, they produced four parallel effects in brain: a) inhibition of pyridoxal kinase activity; b) a decrease in PLP concentration; c) a decrease in GAD activity and d) a decrease in GABA levels. All these changes were coincident with the

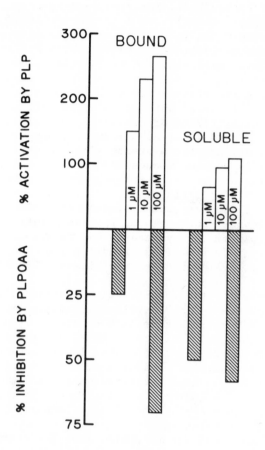

Fig. 2. Activation by PLP and inhibition by PLP-oxime-0-acetic acid (PLPOAA, compound VI, Table 1) of soluble GAD and GAD bound to phosphatidylcholine-phosphatidylserine vesicles. The concentrations of PLP are shown on each bar. The inhibition by PLPOAA (1 mM) in the absence (first bar) and in the presence of 0.1 mM PLP (second bar) is shown. Data from Covarrubias, Tapia (1980).

appearance of convulsions (Tapia et al. 1969; Tapia, Awapara 1969; Tapia, Pasantes 1971; Pérez de la Mora et al. 1973; Tapia et al. 1975a, 1975b), and a good correlation could be established between the inhibition of pyridoxal kinase activity and the diminution of PLP levels, and also between this decrease and the inhibition of GAD (Tapia et al. 1969).

Excellent correlations between PLP concentration and GAD activity in vivo were obtained also in animals treated with 1,1-dimethylhydrazine or subjected to a dietary vitamin B_6 deficiency (Minard 1967; Dakshinamurti, Stephens 1969). Interestingly, neither the hydrazones or the oxime of PLP (compounds IV-VI) nor the reduced hydrazines I-III, had any effect on pyridoxal kinase, PLP levels or GAD activity (Tapia, Awapara 1969; Tapia et al. 1969; Tapia 1974), in spite of their close structural similarities with the unreduced compounds. Furthermore, in these studies the inhibition of GAD by the hydrazones was reversed by the addition of PLP in vitro. These findings are consistent with the existence of a link between the kinase, PLP and GAD.

On the basis of the results discussed above, and since the parallel changes of PLP levels and GAD activity occur in the nerve endings (Pérez de la Mora et al. 1973), we have proposed that GAD activity in the GABAergic terminals is regulated to a great extent by PLP levels, which in turn depend on the activity of pyridoxal kinase (Tapia 1974). Furthermore, this chain of events seems to be closely linked to the physiological inhibitory role of GABA in the motor system, since disruption of the chain at any level results in seizures. Many of the findings discussed above have been confirmed and extended more recently (see for example Sawaya et al. 1978; Matsuda et al. 1979; Nitsch 1980).

GAD REGULATION AT THE PRESYNAPTIC ENDING

The revised findings in vitro and in vivo on the regulation of GAD activity in brain can be integrated at the subcellular level as shown in Fig. 3. This scheme represents an attempt to consider the pertinent data as related to the physiological aspects of the GABAergic terminal.

The two non-interconvertible forms of GAD activity are separated. The free PLP-independent activity is mainly

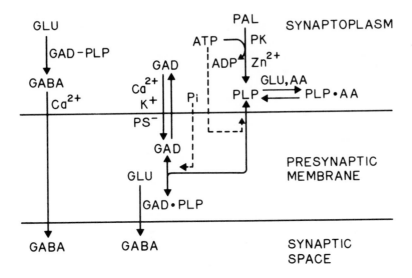

Fig. 3. Integrative view of the regulation of GAD activity
by PLP at the presynaptic level. GAD possessing tightly
bound PLP is mainly soluble (GAD–PLP, left part of the
figure) and the GABA synthesized by this form of GAD is
released upon depolarization in a calcium-dependent manner.
The free PLP-dependent GAD is preferentially bound to the
presynaptic membrane by electrostatic interactions mediated
by Ca^{2+} and/or K^+, which act as a cationic bridge between
GAD and the phosphatidylserine (PS$^-$) of the membrane. This
GAD population bound to the membrane is deficient in PLP and
can therefore be activated by the cofactor, which attaches
loosely to the active site (GAD·PLP). The availability of
free PLP is largely dependent upon the activity of the
Zn^{2+}-requiring pyridoxal kinase, and can be diminished by
the formation of Schiff bases (PLP·AA) with glutamate (GLU)
or other amino acids or amines (AA) present in sufficient
concentrations. Inorganic phosphate (Pi) may antagonize the
dissociation of GAD·PLP promoted by glutamate and stimulated
by ATP (discontinuous lines). The GABA produced by this form
of GAD will be immediately released into the synaptic cleft.
Further explanation in the text.

soluble and would synthesize GABA in the synaptoplasm, from
which the amino acid would be released by depolarization
in a Ca^{2+}-dependent manner. The free PLP-dependent enzyme
is shown preferentially bound to the presynaptic membrane
by an electrostatic mechanism involving the high intracellular K^+ concentrations and/or Ca^{2+} (Salganicoff, De
Robertis, 1965; Fonnum, 1968; Covarrubias, Tapia 1978, 1980).
Since this GAD is not soluble, the GABA produced by its
catalytic action will not be stored but released immediately
(tonic release), in such a way that the inhibition of this
GAD activity will result in seizures as a consequence of the
diminished GABAergic inhibition. Since this is the form of
GAD with absolute requirements for free PLP, any procedure
or alteration resulting in a decrease of PLP availability
(such as its chemical trapping, inhibition of its synthesis
or dietary pyridoxine deficiency), will necessarily lead to
its inhibition and therefore to convulsions (Tapia 1974,
1975; Tapia et al. 1975). The GAD that has been visualized
by electron microscopic immunocytochemistry in association
with the presynaptic membrane (Wood et al. 1976) might
correspond to this form of GAD.

The synthesis of PLP depends mainly on the activity of
pyridoxal kinase, an enzyme located in the synaptoplasm
(Loo, Whittaker 1967) and possibly regulated by Zn^{2+}
(McCormick et al. 1961; Loo, Whittaker 1967). The
phosphorylation of pyridoxal catalyzed by this enzyme
requires ATP as the donor of phosphate, and this creates
an interesting situation in the light of the studies carried
out by the group of Martin and Miller. These authors have
shown that glutamate promotes the dissociation of PLP from
GAD, and that this event is stimulated by ATP and other
nucleotides, whereas Pi antagonizes this stimulation (Miller
et al. 1978; Seligmann et al. 1978; Martin, Martin 1979;
Martin et al. 1980, 1982). Thus, as schematized in Fig. 3,
it seems possible that there is a balance between the
synthesis of PLP and the inhibition of GAD by ATP, which
can be also modified by Pi in such a way that when there
is an excess of PLP synthesis, ATP will dissociate it from
GAD, unless a sufficient concentration of Pi is present
to antagonize the latter action.

In Fig. 3 no consideration is made of the physical
identities of the two forms of GAD activity. The possibility
that the two active sites are located in the same molecule

has been already mentioned (Martin et al. 1980). However, other authors have observed that the inhibitory effect of ATP was greater on a low molecular weight GAD than on a high molecular weight enzyme (Tursky, Lassanová 1978). Furthermore, very recently Martin et al. (1983) have separated from porcine brain three molecular forms of GAD, apparently not interconvertible and with the same molecular weight, and one of them was in higher proportion in synaptosomal extracts than in whole brain extracts.

There seems to be little doubt that PLP is the most important physiological compound involved in the regulation of GAD activity in brain. This role of PLP is in my opinion one of the best examples in biochemistry for demonstrating not only the beautiful role of vitamins and coenzymes in enzymatic mechanisms, but also, in elegant neurobiological terms, the intimate relationships between neurochemical and neurophysiological events in the mammalian central nervous system. Future investigations undoubtedly will teach us many new and exciting facts regarding the molecular species of GAD, their location in the GABAergic endings, their relations with molecules of the presynaptic membrane and their implications in the neurobiology of GABAergic neurons.

Acknowledgements: Part of the work of the author, and travelling expenses, were supported by the Consejo Nacional de Ciencia y Tecnología, México, D.F. (grants PCCBNAL-800798 and ICCBXNA-720145).

Bayón A, Possani LD, Rode G, Tapia R (1978). Kinetics of brain glutamate decarboxylase. Dead-end and product inhibition studies. J. Neurochem 30:1629.
Bayón A, Possani LD, Tapia R (1977a). Kinetics of brain glutamate decarboxylase. Inhibition studies with N-(5'-phosphopyridoxyl)amino acids. J Neurochem 29:513.
Bayón A, Possani LD, Tapia M, Tapia R (1977b). Kinetics of brain glutamate decarboxylase. Interactions with glutamate, pyridoxal 5'-phosphate and glutamate-pyridoxal 5'-phosphate Schiff base. J Neurochem 29:519.
Bayoumi RA, Smith WRD (1972). Some effects of dietary vitamin B_6 deficiency on γ-aminobutyric acid metabolism in developing rat brain, J Neurochem 19:1883.
Covarrubias M, Tapia R (1978). Calcium-dependent binding of glutamate decarboxylase to phospholipid vesicles. J Neurochem 31:1209

Covarrubias M, Tapia R (1980). Brain glutamate decarboxylase: properties of its calcium-dependent binding to liposomes and kinetics of the bound and the free enzyme. J Neurochem 34:1682.

Dakshinamurti K, Stephens MC (1969). Pyridoxine deficiency in the neonatal rat. J Neurochem 16:1515.

Fonnum F (1968). The distribution of glutamate decarboxylase and aspartate transaminase in subcellular fractions of rat and guinea pig brain. Biochem J 106:401.

Killam KF, Dasgupta SR, Killam EK (1960). Studies on the action of convulsant hydrazides as vitamin B_6 antagonists in the central nervous system. In Roberts E, Baxter CF, van Harreveld A, Wiersma CAG, Adey WR, Killam KF (eds) "Inhibition in the Nervous System and Gamma-Aminobutyric Acid," New York: Pergamon, p 302.

Loo YH, Whittaker VP (1967). Pyridoxal kinase in brain and its inhibition by pyridoxylidene-β-phenylethylamine. J Neurochem 14:997.

Martin DL, Martin SB (1982). Effect of nucleotides and other inhibitors on the inactivation of glutamate decarboxylase. J Neurochem 39:1001.

Martin SB, Martin DL (1979). Stimulation by phosphate of the activation of glutamate apodecarboxylase by pyridoxal-5'-phosphate and its implications for the control of GABA synthesis. J Neurochem 33:1275.

Martin LD, Meeley MP, Martin SB, Pedersen S (1980). Factors influencing the activation and inactivation of glutamate decarboxylase. Brain Res Bull 5(Suppl 2):57.

Matsuda M, Abe M, Hoshino M, Sakurai T (1979). γ-Aminobutyric acid in subcellular fractions of mouse brain and its relation to convulsions. Biochem Pharmacol 28:2785.

McCormick DB, Gregory ME, Snell EE (1961). Pyridoxal phosphokinases-I. Assay, distribution, purification and properties. J Biol Chem 236:2076.

Meldrum BS (1975). Epilepsy and γ-aminobutyric acid. Internat Rev Neurobiol 17:1.

Miller LP, Martin DL, Mazumder A, Walters JR (1978). Studies on the regulation of GABA synthesis: substrate-promoted dissociation of pyridoxal-5'-phosphate from GAD. J Neurochem 30:361.

Minard FN (1967). Relationships among pyridoxal phosphate, vitamin B_6 deficiency, and convulsions induced by 1,1-dimethylhydrazine. J Neurochem 14:681.

Nitsch C (1980). Regulation of GABA metabolism in discrete rabbit brain regions under methoxypyridoxine- Regional differences in cofactor saturation and the preictal activation of glutamate decarboxylase activity. J Neurochem 34:822.

Pérez de la Mora, Feria-Velasco A, Tapia R (1973). Pyridoxal phosphate and glutamate decarboxylase in subcellular particles of mouse brain and their relationship to convulsions. J Neurochem 20:1575.

Roberts E (1960). Free amino acids of nervous tissue: some aspects of metabolism of gamma-aminobutyric acid. In Roberts E, Baxter CF, van Harreveld A, Wiersma CAG, Adey WR, Killam KF (eds) "Inhibition in the Nervous System and Gamma-Aminobutyric Acid, "New York: Pergamon, p 144.

Salganicoff L, De Robertis E (1965). Subcellular distribution of the enzymes of the glutamic acid, glutamine and γ-aminobutyric acid cycles in rat brain. J Neurochem 12:287.

Sawaya C, Horton R, Meldrum B (1978). Transmitter synthesis and convulsant drugs: effect of pyridoxal phosphate antagonists and allylglycine. Biochem Pharmacol 27:475.

Seligmann B, Miller LP, Brockman DE, Martin DL (1978). Studies on the regulation of GABA synthesis: The interaction of adenine nucleotides and glutamate with brain glutamate decarboxylase. J Neurochem 30:371.

Spink DC, Wu SJ, Martin DL (1983). Multiple forms of glutamate decarboxylase in porcine brain. J Neurochem 40:1113.

Tapia R (1974). The role of γ-aminobutyric acid metabolism in the regulation of cerebral excitability. In Myers RD, Drucker-Colín RR (eds) "Neurohumoral Coding of Brain Function," New York: Plenum, p 3.

Tapia R (1975). Biochemical pharmacology of GABA in CNS. In Iversen LL, Iversen SD, Snyder SH (eds) "Handbook of Psychopharmacology," New York: Plenum, Vol 4, p 1.

Tapia R (1983). γ-Aminobutyric acid: metabolism and biochemistry of synaptic transmission. In Lajtha A (ed) "Handbook of Neurochemistry" 2nd Ed, New York: Plenum Vol 3, p 423.

Tapia R, Awapara J (1969). Effects of various substituted hydrazones and hydrazines of pyridoxal-5'-phosphate on brain glutamate decarboxylase. Biochem Pharmacol 18:145.

Tapia R, Pasantes H (1971). Relationships between pyridoxal phosphate availability, activity of vitamin B_6-dependent enzymes and convulsions. Brain Res 29:111.

Tapia R, Pasantes H, Taborda E, Pérez de la Mora M (1975) Seizure susceptibility in the developing mouse and its relationship to glutamate decarboxylase and pyridoxal phosphate in brain. J Neurobiol 6:159.

Tapia R, Pérez de la Mora M, Massieu G (1969). Correlative changes of pyridoxal kinase, pyridoxal-5'-phosphate and glutamate decarboxylase in brain, during drug-induced convulsions. Ann NY Acad Sci 166:257.

Tapia R, Sandoval ME (1971). Study on the inhibition of brain glutamate decarboxylase by pyridoxal phosphate oxime-O-acetic acid. J Neurochem 18:2051.

Tapia R, Sandoval ME, Contreras P (1975). Evidence for a role of glutamate decarboxylase activity as a regulatory mechanism of cerebral excitability. J Neurochem 24:1283.

Tower DB (1976). GABA and seizures: clinical correlates in man. In Roberts E, Chase TN, Tower DB (eds) "GABA in Nervous System Function," New York: Raven, p 461.

Tursky T, Lassánová M (1978). Inhibition of different molecular forms of brain glutamate decarboxylase (GAD) with ATP. J Neurochem 30:903.

Wood JG, McLaughlin BJ, Vaughn JE (1976). Immunocyto-chemical localization of GAD in electron microscopic preparations of rodent CNS. In Roberts E, Chase TN Tower DB (eds) "GABA in Nervous System Function", New York: Raven, p 133.

**Glutamine, Glutamate, and GABA
in the Central Nervous System, pages 129–143**
© 1983 Alan R. Liss, Inc., 150 Fifth Avenue, New York, NY 10011

MULTIPLE FORMS OF GLUTAMATE DECARBOXYLASE IN HOG, RAT, AND HUMAN BRAIN

David C. Spink[*+] and David L. Martin[*]

[+]Department of Chemistry, University of Maryland, College Park, MD 20742, and [*]Center for Laboratories and Research, New York State Department of Health, Albany, NY 12201

The rate-limiting step in the synthesis of γ-aminobutyric acid (GABA) is catalyzed by glutamate decarboxylase (GAD; EC 4.1.1.15). Most studies of this enzyme have been in two basic areas, one focusing on the utility of GAD as a marker for GABAergic neurons in the CNS (discussed elsewhere in this volume), the second on the mechanisms controlling the rate of GABA synthesis in vivo. A number of low-molecular-weight species have been proposed as physiologic effectors of GAD activity, including chloride and other anions (Susz et al. 1966), adenine nucleotides (Turský 1970; Seligmann et al. 1978), inorganic phosphate (Martin, Martin 1979), and divalent cations (Wu, Roberts 1974). In vivo experiments showed that GAD is present in the brain predominantly as the apoenzyme (without bound cofactor), indicating that GAD may function much below its potential catalytic rate (Miller et al. 1977). A cycle of apoenzyme formation and reactivation of apoGAD by pyridoxal 5'-phosphate (pyridoxal-P) has been proposed as one of the mechanisms involved in the regulation of GABA synthesis (Martin et al. 1980; Meeley, Martin 1983a,b). It is also possible that multiple forms of GAD are important in regulating GABA synthesis (Wu et al. 1976, 1980; Bayón et al. 1977; Spink et al. 1983).

Brain GAD has been purified from several mammalian species, including the mouse (Wu et al. 1973), rat (Maitre et al. 1978), and human (Blindermann et al. 1978). These preparations have been well characterized, and many of the physical and kinetic properties of the purified enzymes have been described. However, kinetic studies of impure

preparations of brain GAD have been quite difficult to interpret in terms of a single form of the enzyme. A number of
peculiar results have been reported, including changes in
the kinetic parameters of GAD during purification (Susz et
al. 1966), the observation of two pH optima for the enzyme
(Miller et al. 1978), nonuniform dependence of GAD activity
on pyridoxal-P concentration (Tapia, Sandoval 1971; Bayón
et al. 1977), and biphasic kinetics of the substrate-
promoted inactivation of GAD (Meeley, Martin 1983a).

Physical analyses have also suggested that there are
multiple forms of GAD in mammalian brain. The apparent
molecular weight of mouse-brain GAD purified from the synaptosomal fraction was determined by gel filtration on Sephadex G-200 and by analytical ultracentrifugation. Each
method indicated a molecular weight of about 85,000 (Wu et
al. 1973). Similar molecular weight analyses of extracts of
whole brain by Sephadex G-200 chromatography showed GAD
activity at an elution volume corresponding to 85,000 and a
second peak of GAD activity in the void volume, indicating a
molecular weight of over 200,000 (Wu et al. 1976). The proposed subunit structure for brain GAD is a dimer of indistinguishable subunits (Wu et al. 1973; Blindermann et al.
1978; Maitre et al. 1978), yet [2-^{3}H]γ-acetylenic GABA, an
enzyme-activated, irreversible inhibitor of GAD, labeled two
polypeptides of differing molecular weight when allowed to
react with a partially purified preparation of GAD from rat
brain (Oertel et al. 1980). Also, experiments on the interaction of crude mouse-brain GAD with phospholipid vesicles
indicated that only a certain fraction (65%) of GAD would
bind to these vesicles, even when the lipid-to-protein ratio
was increased (Covarrubias, Tapia 1978). These and other
results have led investigators in a number of laboratories
to propose that there are multiple forms of GAD in mammalian
brain.

Among the major goals of the recent efforts in this laboratory have been the purification and physical and kinetic
characterization of GAD from hog brain. Initial attempts to
purify GAD from this source were carried out by the procedures developed for the purification of GAD from human brain
(Blindermann et al. 1978). Results comparable to those
previously reported (Blindermann et al. 1978; Maitre et al.
1978) were obtained during the initial stages of purification, although a portion of the GAD applied to the phenyl-
Sepharose column eluted before the displacing front of the

eluting agent, Triton X-100. In later preparations the column was eluted with an increasing glycerol gradient and a simultaneously decreasing sodium phosphate gradient to gradually decrease the dielectric constant of the eluant. Three distinct peaks of hog-brain GAD were resolved by this procedure (Fig. 1). The total yield of GAD from phenyl-Sepharose chromatography generally ranged from 60 to 80% of the enzyme activity applied to the column, indicating that these are not minor forms of the enzyme.

Isoelectric focusing was also investigated as a potential method for purifying GAD from hog brain. Experiments employing the sucrose gradient technique achieved substantial purification, but the enzyme generally focused over a rather wide pH range. Preparative isoelectric focusing of partially purified hog-brain GAD in a flat bed of granulated gel, using a pH gradient designed to be shallow over the range of the approximate isoelectric point (pI) as determined in earlier experiments (pH 5 to 6), resulted in three peaks of GAD activity. To determine whether the three components separated by phenyl-Sepharose chromatography were the same as those resolved by flat bed isoelectric focusing, samples from each phenyl-Sepharose peak were subjected to analytical isoelectric focusing in agarose gels (Fig. 2). The three components had different pI, and the three pI were virtually identical to those observed in the flat bed focusing experiments. Partially purified hog-brain GAD was also resolved into three components by nondenaturing polyacrylamide gel electrophoresis using the Ornstein and Davis procedure (Ornstein 1964; Davis 1964).

These results led us to conclude that there are multiple forms of GAD in hog brain (Spink et al. 1982, 1983). The three forms were referred to as α-GAD (pI 5.3), β-GAD (pI 5.5), and γ-GAD (pI 5.8) in the order of their elution from phenyl-Sepharose (Fig. 1.). All were low-molecular-weight forms, since each eluted from Sephadex G-200 at an elution volume corresponding to a molecular weight of 100,000. These forms were also observed when crude extracts of hog-brain synaptosomes prepared by hypotonic lysis of the P_2 fraction (Wu et al. 1973) were analyzed by phenyl-Sepharose chromatography. β-GAD was the major form in these preparations (66% of the total enzyme activity), and γ-GAD was the least abundant (16%).

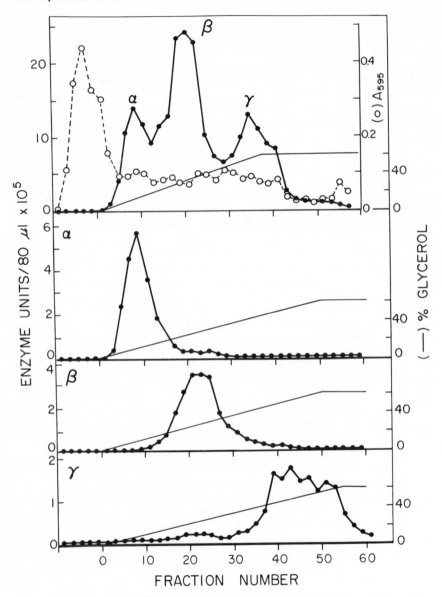

Fig. 1. Resolution and rechromatography of α-, ß-, and γ-GAD from hog brain on phenyl-Sepharose. Reprinted from Spink DC, Wu SJ, Martin DL (1983) J Neurochem 40:1113, with permission of Raven Press, NY.

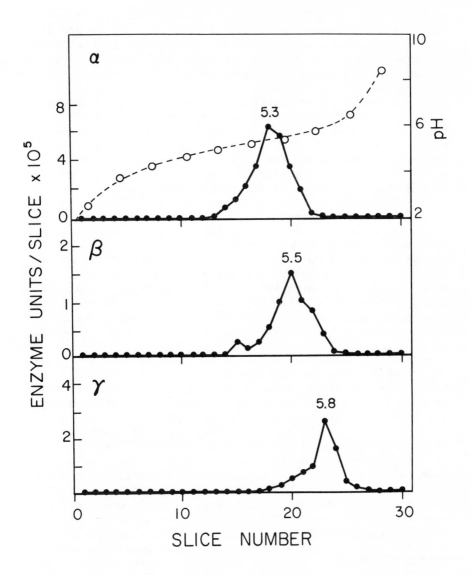

Fig. 2. Agarose gel isoelectric focusing of α-, ß-, and γ-
GAD from hog brain. Reprinted from Spink DC, Wu SJ, Martin
DL (1983) J Neurochem 40:1113, with permission of Raven
Press, NY.

We have recently investigated whether multiple forms of low-molecular-weight GAD are peculiar to the hog or are also found in other mammalian species. Wistar rats were killed by decapitation, and their brains were rapidly removed and frozen on solid CO_2 to eliminate postmortem changes. Extracts of rat brain were subjected to the same purification procedures as the hog-brain enzyme, including chromatography on DEAE-Sephacel, hydroxylapatite, Sephadex G-200, and phenyl-Sepharose. Only two peaks of rat-brain GAD were eluted from the phenyl-Sepharose in the glycerol gradient; however, a subsequent wash with buffer containing Triton X-100 eluted a third peak of enzyme activity (Spink, Porter, Wu, and Martin, submitted for publication).

Human-brain GAD was also purified by these methods. Chromatography on DEAE-Sephacel and hydroxylapatite resulted in single peaks of GAD activity, but subsequent chromatography on phenyl-Sepharose resolved two peaks of the enzyme (Fig. 3). In contrast to the purification of rat GAD, washing the column with buffer containing Triton X-100 did not elute more GAD. Thus only two forms of human-brain GAD were resolved by phenyl-Sepharose chromatography, whereas this procedure resolved three forms from rat and hog brain.

Species differences between the multiple forms of hog- and rat-brain GAD include differences in the relative amounts of the forms (ß-GAD is predominant in hog-brain preparations but appears to be the least abundant form in rat brain), differences in their hydrophobicity (rat γ-GAD requires Triton X-100 for elution from phenyl-Sepharose, while hog γ-GAD is eluted at a high glycerol concentration), and differences in the kinetic constants of the corresponding forms. The fact that only two forms of human-brain GAD were resolved by phenyl-Sepharose chromatography could be a species difference. There are, however, other possible reasons for this result. Human brain tissue cannot be obtained within minutes after death, as has been the case with rat and hog brain. Consequently the possibility of postmortem changes cannot be ruled out. Alternatively the procedures employed may not be sufficient to separate some forms of human-brain GAD.

Since multiple forms of brain GAD had now been resolved from three mammalian species, the possibility was intriguing that these forms might be responsible for the previously

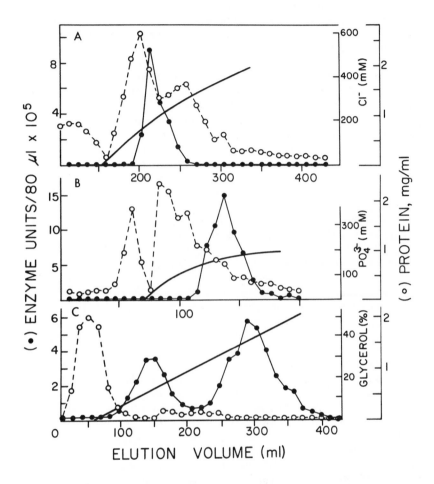

Fig. 3. Sequential chromatography of human brain GAD on (A) DEAE-Sephacel, (B) hydroxylapatite, and (C) phenyl-Sepharose.

observed kinetic oddities that have led others to hypothesize multiple forms of GAD in mammalian brain. Our results show that the multiple forms of hog-brain GAD do in fact differ significantly in their kinetic properties. The K_m

for glutamate was lowest for α-GAD (0.5 mM) and highest for
γ-GAD (1.3 mM) at pH 7.2 (Spink, Martin 1983). At pH 6.5
the differences were even more pronounced: the K_m were
0.5, 1.4 and 2.6 for the α, β and γ forms respectively
(Fig. 4).

The effects of varying pH on the activity of the multiple forms of GAD were investigated under two different assay
conditions: one in which substrate was highly saturating
for all forms (15 mM glutamate) and one in which glutamate
was not saturating (0.5 mM). At saturating glutamate each
form showed an apparent optimum at pH 6.5 to 6.8, which is
consistent with previous studies of brain GAD (Roberts,
Simonsen 1963; Wu et al. 1976; Blindermann et al. 1978).
However, at subsaturating glutamate concentrations varying
pH had significantly different effects: the α form of hog-
brain (Spink, Martin 1983) and rat-brain GAD showed maximal
activity at pH 6.5, while human α-GAD had an optimum at pH
6.8 (Fig. 5). The β and γ forms of GAD from these species
showed broader optima at pH 7.0 to 7.4.

The apparent reason for the observation of different pH
optima at different substrate concentrations is that K_m
and V_{max} for the various forms of GAD are affected differently by changing pH. Blindermann and co-workers found that
the K_m for glutamate of human-brain GAD was highly pH-
dependent, decreasing from 1.7 mM at pH 5.8 to 0.5 mM at pH
7.8, while V_{max} was highest at pH 6.8 (Blindermann et al.
1978). We have observed similar pH dependencies of the kinetic parameters of individual forms of hog- and rat-brain
GAD. As previously noted, the K_m of hog γ-GAD was 2.6 mM
at pH 6.5 and 1.3 mM at pH 7.2. In contrast, the K_m of
hog α-GAD was 0.5 mM at both pH 6.5 and 7.2. Further study
will be required to achieve a clear understanding of the
effects of pH on the kinetic constants of the individual
forms of GAD.

The presence of multiple forms of the enzyme could also
be responsible for some unexplained results, such as the
double pH optima observed for rat-brain GAD (Miller et al.
1978). Susz et al. (1966) observed a shift in the pH
optimum from 6.5 to 7.2 and a concomitant increase in K_m
for glutamate during the purification of mouse-brain GAD. A
possible explanation for this result could be selective loss

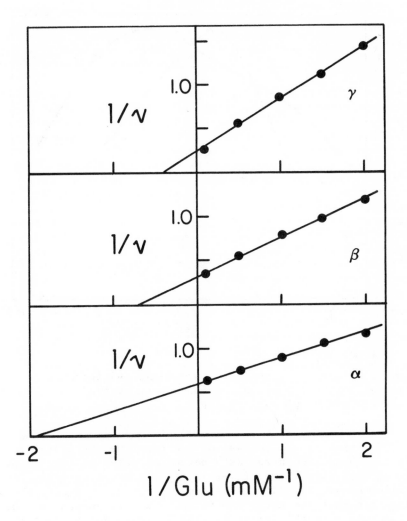

Fig. 4. Determination of K_m for glutamate of α-, ß-, and γ-GAD from hog brain at pH 6.5. Velocities are in nmol/min.

during this purification of a form of mouse-brain GAD similar to α-GAD of hog, rat, and human brain.

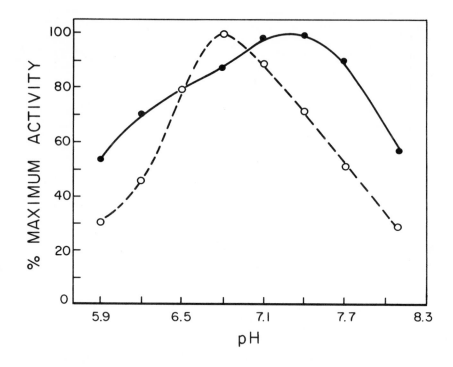

Fig. 5. Activity of α-GAD (o) and ß-GAD (●) from human brain as a function of pH. Samples were assayed with 0.5 mM glutamate and 20 μM pyridoxal-P.

The binding and release of the coenzyme, pyridoxal-P, has long been recognized as a potential point of regulation of GAD activity. Pyridoxal-P is tightly bound to brain GAD (Miller et al. 1978), yet in vivo experiments indicate that less than half the total GAD in rat brain is present in the holoenzyme form (Miller et al. 1977). HoloGAD is inactivated (converted to apoGAD) in the presence of saturating glutamate when pyridoxal-P is omitted from the medium (Miller et al. 1978; Meeley, Martin 1983a). This inactivation of brain GAD appears to be analogous to the inactivation of other amino acid decarboxylases by their substrates, including GAD from Escherichia coli (Sukhareva, Braunstein 1971) and the aromatic amino acid decarboxylase from hog kidney (O'Leary, Baughn 1977). Decarboxylation-dependent transamination, in which an aberrant protonation of a reaction intermediate causes the release of an aldehyde rather than an amine as product and converts enzyme-bound pyridoxal-P to pyridoxamine 5'-phosphate (an inactive form of the coenzyme), has been proposed as the mechanism of enzyme inactivation (Sukhareva, Braunstein 1971; O'Leary, Baughn 1977).

The initial studies of the substrate-promoted inactivation of partially purified hog-brain GAD were conducted at 30°C with 10 mM glutamate. In those experiments the inactivation did not conform to first-order kinetics, suggesting that there were two or more types of active sites undergoing inactivation at different rates (Meeley, Martin 1983a). When the kinetics of the individual α, β, and γ forms of hog-brain GAD were analyzed in similar experiments, each form was inactivated by an apparent first-order process. The half-times for inactivation were 8, 18, and 36 min for γ, β, and α respectively (Spink, Martin 1983). The multiple forms of GAD from rat brain also differed in their rates of substrate-promoted inactivation. As seen in Fig. 6, after a 20-min incubation in the presence of 10 mM glutamate without exogenous pyridoxal-P rat α-GAD had over 50% of its initial activity, while the β and γ forms had only about 30%. This inactivation was entirely dependent on the presence of glutamate for each form of GAD.

At present only two kinetic parameters, K_m for glutamate and the rate constant for glutamate-promoted inactivation, have been examined with respect to possible differences among the multiple forms of GAD. The differences observed in these two parameters suggest that the multiple forms of the enzyme could have substantially different catalytic rates in situ. In all of the species examined, α-GAD has a lower K_m for substrate and is inactivated more slowly by substrate than the β and γ forms. Depending on physiologic conditions, α-GAD could catalyze a significantly higher rate of GABA synthesis than β- or γ-GAD.

The multiple forms of hog-brain GAD differ in their pI and electrophoretic mobilities, indicating differences in surface charge (Spink et al. 1983). They also differ in hydrophobicity, as judged by their different affinities for phenyl-Sepharose. Currently it is not known whether these physical and kinetic differences among the forms of GAD are the result of posttranslational modifications of a single gene product or whether the α, β, and γ forms arise from

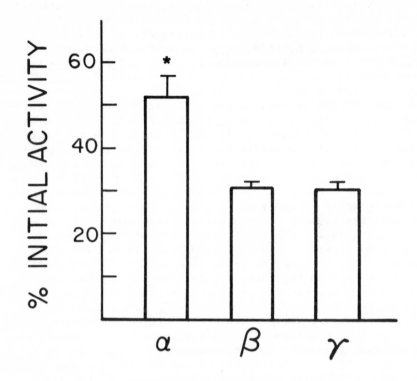

Fig. 6. Substrate-promoted inactivation of α-, ß-, and γ-GAD from rat brain. Samples were preincubated at 30°C for 20 min in the presence of 10 mM glutamate. * indicates significantly different from the other two forms of GAD (p <0.02) by Student's t-test.

distinct genes. The initial stages of purification are routinely carried out in the presence of a cocktail of protease inhibitors, yet the possibility that some of these forms result from partial degradation of GAD cannot be ruled out. Since gel filtration chromatography on Sephadex G-200 was not capable of separating the three forms of hog-brain GAD (each form had an apparent molecular weight of 100,000), proteolysis would have to be limited in extent (Spink et al. 1983).

It is not clear how the multiple forms of GAD discussed here are related to the high- and low-molecular-weight forms of the enzyme reported by Wu et al. (1976, 1980). The latter forms were indistinguishable by immunochemical methods, and it was suggested that high-molecular-weight GAD might be a polymeric form of the enzyme. As a result of subcellular fractionation experiments it was also postulated that high-molecular-weight GAD is a precursor to the low-molecular-weight form. The α, β, and γ forms also differ in subcellular distribution (Spink et al. 1983). Both of these results raise the possibility of posttranslational modification of GAD.

Since the GAD forms separated by phenyl-Sepharose chromatography and isoelectric focusing are low-molecular-weight forms, there is no obvious relationship between the α, β, and γ forms and the high-molecular-weight form of the enzyme. However, one or more of the forms of GAD separated by phenyl-Sepharose could be components of high-molecular-weight form. Many proteins, such as ornithine decarboxylase from rat liver (Kitani, Fujisawa 1983), show different apparent molecular weights depending on the ionic strength of the medium. Use of ammonium sulfate precipitation as a step in the purification procedure appears to increase the percentage of high-molecular-weight GAD in the initial stages of purification of the hog-brain enzyme (Meeley and Martin, unpublished observation).

The α, β, and γ forms of GAD differ from each other in surface charge and hydrophobicity. It is possible that certain domains of one or more of these forms participate in specific protein-protein interactions. The physical and kinetic characteristics of the various forms of mammalian-brain GAD, as well as the possible metabolic relationships among them, will be the focal points of further research.

Acknowledgements: This work was supported in part by grant MH-35664 from the National Institute of Mental Health, PHS/DHHS. Human cerebral and cerebellar cortex samples were obtained from E. D. Bird, M.D., Brain Tissue Resource Center, McLean Hospital, Belmont, MA. We greatly appreciate Susan J. Wu's contributions to this project.

Bayón A, Possani LD, Tapia M, Tapia R (1977). Kinetics of brain glutamate decarboxylase. Interactions with glutamate, pyridoxal 5'-phosphate and glutamate-pyridoxal 5'-phosphate Schiff base. J Neurochem 29:519.

Blindermann JM, Maitre M, Ossola L, Mandel P (1978). Purification and some properties of L-glutamate decarboxylase from human brain. Eur J Biochem 86:143.

Covarrubias M, Tapia R (1978). Calcium-dependent binding of brain glutamate decarboxylase to phospholipid vesicles. J Neurochem 31:1209.

Davis BJ (1964). Disc electrophoresis II. Method and application to human serum proteins. Ann NY Acad Sci 121:404.

Kitani T, Fujisawa H (1983). Purification and properties of ornithine decarboxylase from rat liver. J Biol Chem 258:235.

Maitre M, Blindermann JM, Ossola L, Mandel P (1978). Comparison of the structures of L-glutamate decarboxylases from human and rat brains. Biochem Biophys Res Commun 85:885.

Martin SB, Martin DL (1979). Stimulation by phosphate of the activation of glutamate apodecarboxylase by pyridoxal 5'-phosphate and its implications for the control of GABA synthesis. J Neurochem 33:1275.

Martin DL, Meeley MP, Martin SB, Pedersen S (1980). Factors influencing the activation and inactivation of glutamate decarboxylase. Brain Res Bull 5(Suppl 2):57.

Meeley MP, Martin DL (1983a). Inactivation of brain glutamate decarboxylase and the effects of adenosine 5'-triphosphate and inorganic phosphate. Cell Mol Neurobiol 3:39.

Meeley MP, Martin DL (1983b). Reactivation of substrate-inactivated brain glutamate decarboxylase. Cell Mol Neurobiol 3:55.

Miller LP, Walters JR, Martin DL (1977). Postmortem changes implicate adenine nucleotides and pyridoxal 5'-phosphate in regulation of glutamate decarboxylase. Nature 266:847.

Miller LP, Martin DL, Mazumder A, Walters JR (1978). Studies on the regulation of GABA synthesis: Substrate-promoted dissociation of pyridoxal 5'-phosphate from GAD. J Neurochem 30:361.

Oertel WH, Schmechel DE, Daly JW, Tappaz ML, Kopin IJ (1980). Localization of glutamate decarboxylase on line-immunoelectrophoresis and two-dimensional electrophoresis by use of the radioactive suicide substrate [2-^{3}H] - acetylenic GABA. Life Sci 27:2133.

O'Leary MH, Baughn RL (1977). Decarboxylation-dependent transamination catalyzed by mammalian 3,4-dihydroxyphenyl-alanine decarboxylase. J Biol Chem 252:7168.

Ornstein L (1964). Disc electrophoresis-I. Background and theory. Ann NY Acad Sci 121:321.

Roberts E, Simonsen DG (1963). Some properties of L-glutamic decarboxylase in mouse brain. Biochem Pharmacol 12:113.

Seligmann B, Miller LP, Brockman DE, Martin DL (1978). Studies on the regulation of GABA synthesis: The interaction of adenine nucleotides and glutamate with brain glutamate decarboxylase. J Neurochem 30:371.

Spink DC, Wu SJ, Martin DL (1982). Multiple forms of porcine brain glutamate decarboxylase. Trans Am Soc Neurochem 13:123.

Spink DC, Wu SJ, Martin DL (1983). Multiple forms of glutamate decarboxylase in porcine brain. J Neurochem 40:1113.

Spink DC, Martin DL (1983). Kinetic characterization of the multiple forms of glutamate decarboxylase. Trans Am Soc Neurochem 14:132.

Sukhareva BS, Braunstein AE (1971). Investigation of the nature of the interactions of glutamate decarboxylase from Escherichia coli with the substrate and its analogs. Mol Biol (Moscow) 5:302.

Susz JP, Haber B, Roberts E (1966). Purification and some properties of mouse brain L-glutamic decarboxylase. Biochemistry 5:2870.

Tapia R, Sandoval ME (1971). Study on the inhibition of brain glutamate decarboxylase by pyridoxal phosphate oxime-O-acetic acid. J Neurochem 18:2051.

Turský T (1970). Inhibition of brain glutamate decarboxylase by adenosine triphosphate. Eur J Biochem 12:544.

Wu J-Y, Matsuda T, Roberts E (1973). Purification and characterization of glutamate decarboxylase from mouse brain. J Biol Chem 248:3029.

Wu J-Y, Roberts E (1974). Properties of brain L-glutamate decarboxylase: Inhibition Studies. J Neurochem 23:759.

Wu J-Y, Wong E, Saito K, Roberts E, Schousboe A (1976). Properties of L-glutamate decarboxylase from brains of adult and newborn mice. J Neurochem 27:653.

Wu J-Y, Su YTT, Lam DMK, Brandon C, Denner L (1980). Purification and regulation of L-glutamate decarboxylase. Brain Res Bull 5(Suppl 2):63.

Glutamine, Glutamate, and GABA
in the Central Nervous System, pages 145–159
© 1983 Alan R. Liss, Inc., 150 Fifth Avenue, New York, NY 10011

REGULATION OF GABA-T: INHIBITION of GABA-T BY BW 357U

Helen L. White, Barrett R. Cooper, and James L. Howard

GABA-T (4-aminobutyrate-2-ketoglutarate transaminase; EC 2.6.1.19) is the enzyme principally responsible for catabolism of GABA, the major inhibitory neurotransmitter in mammalian brain (Baxter, 1976). A similar or perhaps identical enzyme is also found in some peripheral tissues including kidney and liver (Vasilev et al., 1973; Lancaster et al., 1973; White and Sato, 1978) and blood platelets (White, 1979). The importance of GABA-T in maintaining the concentration of brain GABA has been demonstrated by numerous investigators who have observed marked elevations of GABA after pretreatment of animals with inhibitors of the enzyme (Palfreyman, et al., 1981).

Following a brief discussion of possible endogenous regulation mechanisms and some known inhibitors of GABA-T, this presentation will focus on the properties of a newer inhibitor, BW 357U [1-(N-decyl)-3-pyrazolidinone], a compound synthesized by Dr. K. J. Ingold of the Wellcome Research Laboratories.

ENDOGENOUS REGULATION OF GABA-T

A Ping-Pong type of enzyme mechanism for GABA-T has been indicated by a kinetic analysis of the enzyme of mouse brain (Schousboe et al., 1973), rat brain (Maitre et al., 1975), lobster nerves (Hall and Kravitz, 1967), human brain, liver, and kidney (White and Sato, 1978), and platelets (White and Faison, 1980). This reaction is diagrammed in Fig. 1, with arrows indicating the forward reaction.

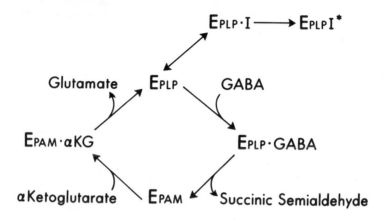

Fig. 1. <u>Ping-Pong mechanism for GABA-T</u>. E·PLP represents the enzyme bound to pyridoxal phosphate; E·PAM, the enzyme bound to pyridoxamine phosphate. E·PLP·I, a complex of enzyme with reversibly bound inhibitor; E·PLP·I*, an irreversibly bound enzyme-inhibitor complex.

Cofactor Availability

A Ping-Pong mechanism implies that the enzyme oscillates between two relatively stable forms, E·PLP and E·PAM, depending on whether the cofactor is bound to the enzyme as pyridoxal phosphate (PLP) or as pyridoxamine phosphate (PAM). The availability of this cofactor, which is derived from Vitamin B6, could be important for endogenous regulation of GABA-T activity. Very likely there are two cofactor binding sites on each enzyme molecule, with dissociation constants in the nM and μM ranges, respectively (Churchich and Moses, 1981). Only the more weakly bound cofactor can be removed by dialysis. When PLP is added back to dialyzed human brain enzyme, full activity is restored in a time-dependent manner at 37°C (White and Sato, 1978), suggesting that either a covalent interaction or conformational change is induced by cofactor binding. A variety of agents that can bind directly with PLP, such as phenelzine, Tris, cadmium and cupric ions, as well as other compounds that can interact with aldehydes, may inhibit GABA-T (Ho <u>et al</u>., 1975; White and Sato, 1978; Rej and Vanderlinde, 1975; Gallais <u>et al</u>., 1977). Such compounds may also affect many other transaminases or decarboxylases that require PLP. On the other hand, it is quite possible that PLP availability to GABA-T in vivo might be controlled by endogenous substances released in specific regions, or by competition among PLP-requiring enzymes for weakly-bound cofactor.

Substrate and Product Concentrations

Synthesis and catabolism of GABA in vivo in the central nervous system is dependent on glucose availability and its metabolism to glutamate via tricarboxylic acid cycles in at least two metabolic compartments. Thus, hypoglycemia and hypoxia can markedly influence endogenous GABA-T activity (Baxter, 1976). The conversion of the product succinic semialdehyde to succinate also depends on NAD+ availability; rapid metabolism of the semialdehyde helps drive the reaction in the forward direction. Glutamate can also inhibit the forward reaction, since it competes with GABA for the E-PLP form of the enzyme (Fig. 1) and, if succinic semialdehyde is also available, will favor the reverse reaction. With human brain GABA-T, the Ki for glutamate inhibition is 0.5 mM, competitive with GABA, which has a Km = 0.3 mM (White and Sato, 1978). Thus GABA-T, like other transaminases, may function in either direction depending on relative concentrations of participating substrates and products or alternate substrates. The reverse reaction will catalyze synthesis of GABA from succinic semialdehyde. This reaction forms part of a significant pathway for GABA synthesis in some peripheral tissues (Seiler and Wagner, 1976; White, 1981).

Halide Ions

Inhibition of GABA-T by halide ions has also been observed (Hall and Kravitz, 1967; Ho et al., 1975; White and Sato, 1978). For example, in the latter study, human brain GABA-T was inhibited by chloride ion with Ki = 0.13 M, a concentration that may have physiological relevance.

REGULATION OF GABA-T BY EXOGENOUS INHIBITORS

When GABA-T is inhibited in brain, the concentration of GABA increases dramatically. The pharmacological consequences of such GABA elevations have stimulated a continuing search for potent, selective, and safe inhibitors that may eventually have important clinical applications, for example in the treatment of convulsive illnesses, anxiety states, pain, circulatory problems, or problems associated with appetite regulation. Several inhibitors have been described in recent reviews (Metcalf, 1979; Ciesielski et al., 1980; Palfreyman et al., 1981), although none has yet fulfilled all requirements for safety and utility as a therapeutic agent. Examples of the most effective in laboratory studies are shown in Fig. 2. With the exception of BW 357U, these compounds are drawn to resemble an extended GABA structure, mimicking the more restricted structure of gabaculine. They have been shown to interact with GABA-T as substrate analogs that subsequently become irreversibly bound to the enzyme, thus inactivating it. This type of catalytic or "suicide enzyme" inhibition mechanism has been reviewed in detail by Metcalf (1979).

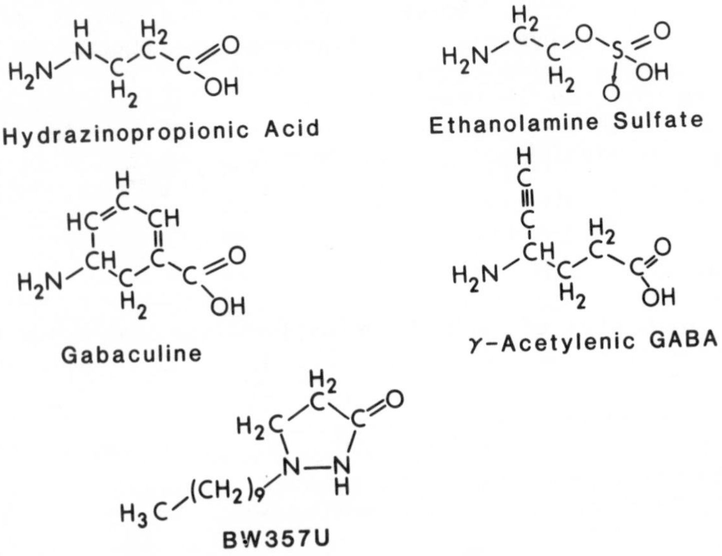

Hydrazinopropionic Acid

Ethanolamine Sulfate

Gabaculine

γ-Acetylenic GABA

BW357U

Fig. 2. Examples of GABA-T inhibitors.

In Vitro Inhibition by BW 357U

As seen in Table 1, BW 357U inhibits GABA-T of partially purified human brain (extracts prepared as by White and Sato, 1978) with an I_{50} of 0.02 µM. This inhibition was obtained in the presence of 20 µM pyridoxal phosphate and thus cannot be due to a removal of this cofactor from the enzyme. Rat brain GABA-T was also inhibited by BW 357U at a similar concentration. Other enzymes requiring pyridoxal phosphate as cofactor, including glutamate decarboxylase, were affected only at concentrations of inhibitor at least 1000-fold higher.

An indication that BW 357U became activated in aqueous solution before it was added to enzyme extracts was revealed in experiments such as that shown in Fig. 3. In distilled water solutions, having a pH of about 6, the inhibitor was positively charged, but could be titrated to the free base (by adding dilute aqueous NaOH) to pH 7-8. Even though the pH of the final enzyme assay was always controlled at pH 8.0 by 25 mM potassium phosphate buffer,

Table 1. In Vitro enzyme inhibition by BW 357U

Enzyme	Source	I_{50} or % Inhibition (Conc)
GABA-T	Human brain	2×10^{-8}M
ALA-AT	Rat liver	2.5×10^{-5}M
TYRO-AT	Rat liver	20% (0.1 mM)
GAD	Rat brain	35% (0.1 mM)
MAO-A	Rat brain	6% (10^{-5}M)
MAO-B	Rat brain	22% (10^{-5}M)
ChAc	Human brain	0% (0.1 mM)

GABA-T, γ-aminobutyrate aminotransferase; ALA-AT, alanine aminotransferase; TYRO-AT, tyrosine aminotransferase; GAD, glutamate decarboxylase; MAO-A and B, monoamine oxidase A and B; ChAc, choline acetyltransferase.

the inhibition obtained with the neutralized form of the inhibitor was much greater than when the inhibitor stock solution in distilled water was added directly to the buffered enzyme mixture (compare B with A in Fig. 3). Moreover, if the aqueous inhibitor solution, after titration to pH 7 or above, was further incubated in air at 37°C for an hour before addition to enzyme, the inhibition profile C in Fig. 3 was obtained.

In another experiment, outlined in Table 2, an inhibitor solution was prepared in deoxygenated glass-distilled water, and portions were titrated to pH 8 and incubated at 37°C for 1 hour before being added to the buffered enzyme. When the inhibitor was kept under nitrogen at pH 6, only 6% inhibition resulted (Table 2,A). Incubating the pH 6 solution in air tended to give slightly increased inhibition (data not shown), but raising the pH to 8 before this incubation gave maximum inhibition (Table 2,B). Preincubation of the enzyme with inhibitor decreased the reversibility of the inhibition on dialysis (Table 2,B compared with C). The presence of 1 mM GABA apparently prevented tight binding of BW 357U to the enzyme, since in this case no inhibition was observed after dialysis. This suggests that BW 357U binds only to the E·PLP form of GABA-T, because in the presence of GABA the enzyme will be converted to the E·PAM form (Fig. 1).

The above experiments demonstrated that the conversion of BW 357U to a more active inhibitor was favored by a pH of 7 or above and prolonged incubation at 37°C in water, conditions that could be expected to induce hydrolysis or oxidation of the compound. Hydrolysis of the pyrazolidinone ring of BW 357U would produce an open-ring compound having a net ionic charge of zero at neutral pH. Evidence for the formation of such a compound is given in Fig. 4, where [^{14}C]labeled BW 357U (carboxyl-labeled) was passed through a cation exchange resin before and after incubation. Initially the pyrazolidinone bears a positive ionic charge and was retained by the resin. However, after incubation at pH 8, at least half the compound was not retained and was apparently hydrolyzed. An equilibrium between open and closed-ring structures may be indicated, since a complete conversion was not achieved.

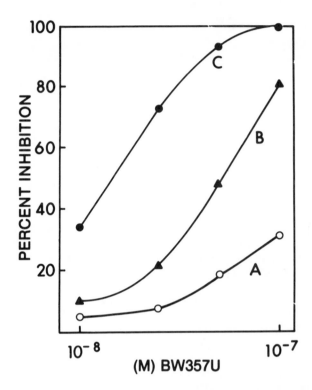

Fig. 3. <u>Inhibition of human brain GABA-T by BW 357U</u>. Inhibitor was dissolved in distilled water (pH ~ 6) under nitrogen and (A) added directly to GABA-T assay mixtures; (B) titrated to pH 7 in air before addition to enzyme; or (C) titrated and incubated at 37°C for 1 hr before addition to enzyme. For enzyme assays, human brain GABA-T was incubated in 50 mM potassium phosphate buffer, which also contained 20 μM pyridoxal phosphate, 50 μM EDTA, 25 μM dithiothreitol, 0.2 mM α-ketoglutarate, and 0.2 mM γ-aminobutyrate (2 Ci/mol) in a total volume of 0.10 ml. After incubation at 37°C for 30 min, mixtures were acidified with 10 μl of 2 N HCl and applied to 0.5 x 3 cm columns of Biorad AG50X8 cation exchange resin. Products (succinic acid or semialdehyde) were eluted into scintillation vials with 3 x 0.5 ml portions of distilled water and counted by scintillation techniques after the addition of 15 ml of Aquasol-2.

Table 2. <u>Factors that influence inhibition by BW 357U.</u>

Conditions	Percent Inhibition	
	(before dialysis)	(after dialysis)*
A. Inhibitor sol'n in O2-free water, pH 6	6.0	
B. Inhibitor sol'n at pH 8 incubated alone in air 1 hr at 37°C before adding to enzyme	98.7	69.7
GABA (1 mM) added to enzyme-inhibitor mixture in B before dialysis		4.8
C. Inhibitor sol'n incubated alone as above; then incubated with enzyme 15 min at 37°C before adding substrates	99.2	90.5
GABA (1 mM) added to C mixture before preinc. with enzyme		9.4

Inhibitor conc. = $4 \times 10^{-7}M$ in all experiments. GABA-T assays as in Legend of Fig. 3.

*Portions of each buffered enzyme + inhibitor mixture were dialyzed against buffer in order to determine reversibility of the inhibition. Dialysis was for 20 hr at 4°C vs 3 changes of 80-fold vol of 50 mM potassium phosphate, 0.5 mM dithiothreitol, 0.1 mM EDTA, 40 µM pyridoxal phosphate, pH 8.0.

Thin-layer chromatography of this preparation served
to distinguish the first two structures in Fig. 5 from
3-pyrazolidinone and hydrazinopropionic acid. Although a
trace of the latter compounds was detected in initial solutions of BW 357U, this did not increase during incubation
at 37°C. In addition, the I_{50} of preincubated BW 357U as
an inhibitor of GABA-T was similar to that obtained with
the ring-opened structure (Fig. 5). Thus the 10-carbon
alkyl substituent was probably not removed from BW 357U
during the activation step.

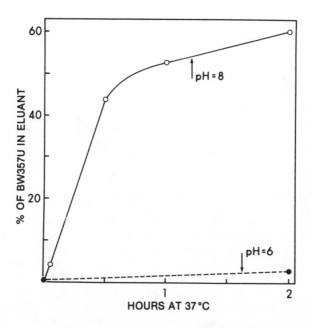

Fig. 4. <u>Evidence for ring opening of BW 357U in aqueous
solution</u>. A 50 µM aqueous solution of [3-^{14}C] BW 357U under
nitrogen was incubated at either pH 6 or pH 8 for up to 2
hours. At times indicated above, 1 ml aliquots (30540 dpm)
were applied to a 3 x 0.5 cm column of AG50X8 cation
exchange resin (hydrogen form; Bio-Rad Laboratories)
immediately followed by 1 ml of 50 mM potassium phosphate,
pH 8.0. The eluant was collected in a scintillation vial
and counted after adding 10 ml Aquasol-2. Percent in the
eluant represents percent of BW 357U that no longer bears a
net positive charge.

On the basis of these experiments, it appears most likely that hydrolysis of the pyrazolidinone ring of BW 357U must first occur in aqueous solution to produce the potent inhibition seen in Fig. 3,C. Like the other potent inhibitors shown in Fig. 1, BW 357U may then assume an extended conformational structure that may favor GABA-T inhibition. Although the hydrolyzed form of BW 357U resembles hydrazinopropionic acid, it differs from this latter compound in that it is much less toxic and is more selective as a GABA-T inhibitor.

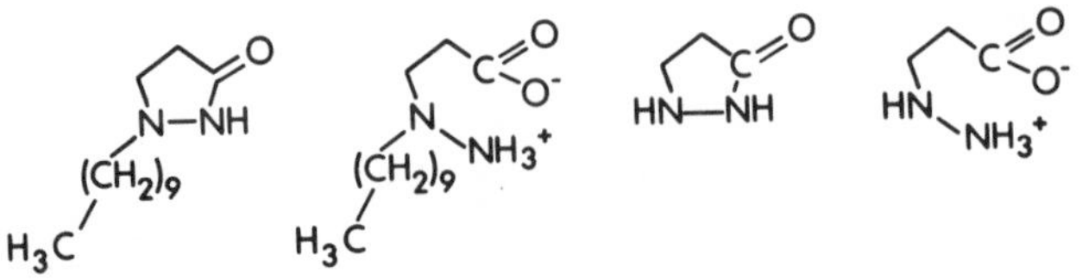

R_f =	0.83	0.80	0.40	<0.4 streaked
I_{50} (μM) =	0.2 (N$_2$) 0.015 (air)	0.02	5 (N$_2$) 0.012 (air)	0.003

Fig. 5. **Properties of BW 357U and possible hydrolysis or oxidation products.** R_f values were obtained by thin-layer chromatography on silica gel (Whatman LK5D) plates developed with n-butyl alcohol/water (100/72.5, top layer). I_{50} values (μM) were determined using partially purified human brain GABA-T, as in legend of Fig. 3. Compounds were dissolved in nitrogen-gassed distilled water and then either added directly to assay mixtures or adjusted to pH 8 and incubated in air for 1 hr at 37°C before addition to enzyme. All enzyme assays were performed at pH 8.0 in air.

In Vivo Regulation of GABA-T by BW 357U

When administered intraperitoneally or orally to rats, BW 357U produced a decrease in GABA-T activity that became maximal at 4 to 24 hours after dosing. This inhibition was accompanied by elevations in brain GABA levels as shown in Fig. 6. In this experiment rats were dosed once each day for 4 days and allowed to recover. Glutamate decarboxylase (GAD) in brain also decreased to some extent during the treatment period, but this did not seem to be caused by a direct inhibition of GAD or by a depletion of cofactor, since excess pyridoxal phosphate was added to all enzyme assays. Moreover, dialysis of brain homogenates did not significantly alter the inhibitions of either enzyme. A similar relatively weak inhibition of GAD has been observed after administration of other GABA-T inhibitors, including γ-acetylenic GABA (Jung et al., 1977) and ethanolamine O-sulfate (Fletcher and Fowler, 1980). It may reflect the action of a feedback mechanism whereby elevated GABA can inhibit synthesis of the enzyme responsible for GABA synthesis.

As seen in Fig. 6, after dosing was terminated, the return of GABA to normal levels proceeded more rapidly than might be expected from the rate of enzyme recovery. For example, on day 12 GABA levels were normal at a time when GABA-T was only 55% of normal value. This implies that new enzyme synthesized after cessation of treatment was probably fully functional.

With daily oral administration of BW 357U, a dose-dependent inhibition of GABA-T and consequent elevation of GABA levels could be maintained in rats for periods of several weeks at doses of 12.5 to 50 mg/kg per day. As seen in Fig. 7, a marked anorectic effect and decrease in body weights correlated with elevations of GABA achieved with BW 357U. Similar effects have been observed with another GABA-T inhibitor, ethanolamine O-sulfate (Howard et al., 1980; Cooper et al., 1980; White et al., 1982).

Although toxic effects developed after long-term chronic administration of BW 357U to laboratory animals, thus precluding a therapeutic use, this compound may find application in a variety of studies relating to the function of GABA in mammalian systems.

ACKNOWLEDGEMENTS

BW 357U [1-(N-decyl)-3-pyrazolidinone hydrochloride] and analogs were designed and synthesized by Dr. K. J. Ingold of the Organic Chemistry Dept., and the [^{14}C] labeled compounds, 3-[3-^{14}C]-pyrazolidinone hydrochloride and 1-(N-decyl)-3-[3-^{14}C]-pyrazolidinone hydrochloride, were synthesized by Dr. John A. Hill of Chemical Development Labs, Wellcome Research Laboratories, Research Triangle Park, North Carolina.

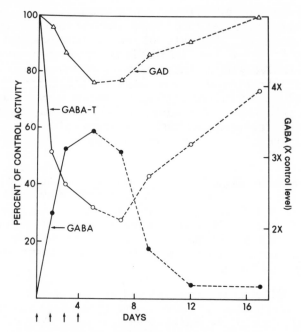

Fig. 6. Male Sprague-Dawley rats (Charles River; n = 5 rats/group) were treated orally with BW 357U at 30 mg/kg per day for 4 days indicated by arrows. GABA-T and GAD were determined during treatment (before each dose) and during recovery (dashed lines). For GABA-T, brain halves, cut along the sagital plane, were homogenized (1:10 tissue wt/buffer vol) in a buffer consisting of 50 mM potassium phosphate, 40 μM pyridoxal phosphate, 0.1 mM EDTA, 0.5 mM dithiothreitol, pH 8.0. Portions (10 μl) of this homogenate were incubated, for 30 min at 37°C, in a total volume of 75 μl of the above buffer with 5 mM α-keto-glutarate and 0.2 mM ^{14}C-GABA (New England Nuclear Corp., mixed with unlabeled GABA to give a specific radioactivity of 1 μCi/μmol). Products were separated by cation exchange as in the legend of Fig. 3. GABA was extracted from the other half of each brain by preparing 10% (tissue wt/solvent vol) homogenates in 80% ethanol, keeping these at 0°C for at least 15 min, centrifuging at 3000 x g for 10 min at 4°C, resuspending pellets in 75% ethanol, re-centrifuging, and combining supernatants from the 2 centrifugations. Aliquots of 5 or 10 μl were assayed for GABA using the fluorometric method of Graham and Aprison (1966). Control GABA levels = 2.04 ± 0.04 nmol/mg wet tissue.

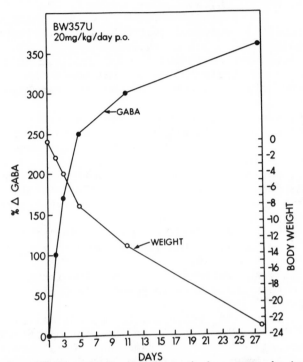

Fig. 7. <u>Correlation between percent increase in brain GABA and percent decrease in body weight</u>. Rats were treated orally once daily with 20 mg/kg of BW 357U. At various times following the onset of treatment, animals were sacrificed and their brains assayed for GABA content as in legend of Fig. 6.

REFERENCES

Baxter CF (1976). Some recent advances in studies of GABA metabolism and compartmentation. In Roberts E, Chase TN, Tower DB (eds): "GABA in Nervous System Function," New York: Raven Press, p 61.

Churchich JE and Moses U (1981). 4-Aminobutyrate aminotransferase. The presence of nonequivalent binding sites. J Biol Chem 256:1101-1104.

Ciesielski L, Simler S, Gensburger C, Mandel P, Taillandier G, Benoit-Guyod JL, Boucherle A, Cohen-Addad C, Lajzerowicz J (1979). GABA transaminase inhibitors. Adv Exp Med & Biol 123:21-41.

Cooper BR, Howard JL, White HL, Soroko F, Ingold K, Maxwell RA (1980). Anorexic effects of ethanolamine O-sulfate in the rat: evidence that GABA inhibits ingestive behavior. Life Sci 26:1997-2002.

Fletcher A, Fowler LJ (1980). γ-Aminobutyric acid metabolism in rat brain following oral administration of ethanolamine O-sulfate. Biochem Pharmacol 29:1451-1454.

Gallais F, Haran R, Laurent J-P, Nepveu-Juras F (1977). Complexation de la vitamine B_6 (pyridoxol) par le cation Cd^{++}: Étude par résonance magnétique du noyau ^{13}C. CR Acad Sc Paris 284:29-32.

Graham LT, Aprison MH (1966). Fluorometric determination of aspartate, glutamate, and γ-aminobutyrate in nerve tissue using enzymatic methods. Analyt Biochem 15:487-497.

Hall ZW, Kravitz EA (1967). The metabolism of γ-aminobutyric acid (GABA) in the lobster nervous system. J Neurochem 14:45-54.

Ho PPK, Young AL, Walters PC (1975). Two forms of 4-aminobutyrate transaminase in guinea pig brain. Enzyme 19:244-255.

Howard JL, Cooper BR, White HL, Soroko FE, Maxwell RA (1980). A role for GABA in the control of ingestive behavior: effects of ethanolamine O-sulfate and muscimol in rats. Brain Res Bull 5, Suppl 2:595-599.

Jung MJ, Lippert B, Metcalf BW, Schechter PJ, Böhlen P, Sjoerdsma A (1977). The effect of 4-amino hex-5-ynoic acid (γ-acetylenic GABA, γ-ethynyl GABA) a catalytic inhibitor of GABA transaminase, on brain GABA metabolism in vivo. J Neurochem 28:717-723.

Lancaster G, Mohyuddin F, Scrivner CR, Whelan DT (1973). A γ-aminobutyrate pathway in mammalian kidney cortex. Biochim Biophys Acta 297:229-240.

Maitre M, Ciesielski L, Cash C, Mandel P (1975). Purification and some properties of the 4-aminobutyrate: 2-oxoglutarate transaminase. Euro J Biochem 52:157-169.

Metcalf BW (1979). Inhibitors of GABA metabolism. Biochem Pharmacol 28:1705-1712.

Palfreyman MG, Schechter PJ, Buckett WR, Tell GP, Koch-Weser J (1981). The pharmacology of GABA-transaminase inhibitors. Biochem Pharmacol 30:817-824.

Rej R and Vanderlinde RE (1975). Effects of buffers on aspartate aminotransferase activity and association of the enzyme with pyridoxal phosphate. Clin Chem 21:1585-1591.

Schousboe A, Wu J-Y, Roberts E (1973). Purification and characterization of the 4-aminobutyrate-2-ketoglutarate transaminase from mouse brain. Biochemistry 12:2868-2873.

Seiler N, Wagner G (1976). NAD$^+$-Dependent formation of γ-aminobutyrate (GABA) from glutamate. Neurochem Res 1:113-131.

Vasilév VY, Eremin VP, Severin ES, Sytinskii IA (1973). Comparative characterization of porcine kidney and liver γ-aminobutyrate-glutamate-transaminases. Biokhimiya 38:355-364.

White HL (1979). 4-Aminobutyrate:2-oxoglutarate aminotransferase in blood platelets. Science 205:696-698.

White HL (1981). Glutamate as a precursor of GABA in rat brain and peripheral tissues. Molec & Cellular Biochem 39:253-259.

White HL, Faison LD (1980). GABA-T in blood platelets: Comparison with GABA-T of other tissues. Brain Res Bull 5, Suppl 2:115-119.

White HL, Howard JL, Cooper BR, Soroko FE, McDermed JD, Ingold KJ, Maxwell RA (1982). A novel inhibitor of gamma-aminobutyrate aminotransferase with anorectic activity. J. Neurochem 39:271-273.

White HL, Sato TL (1978). GABA-transaminases of human brain and peripheral tissues -- kinetic and molecular properties. J Neurochem 31:41-47.

**Glutamine, Glutamate, and GABA
in the Central Nervous System, pages 161–176
© 1983 Alan R. Liss, Inc., 150 Fifth Avenue, New York, NY 10011**

IMMUNOCYTOCHEMICAL IDENTIFICATION OF GABAERGIC
NEURONS AND PATHWAYS

Jang-Yen Wu

Department of Cell Biology and Program
in Neuroscience, Baylor College of Medicine
Texas Medical Center, Houston, Texas 77030

INTRODUCTION

GABA and taurine are two structurally related amino
acids and both have been proposed as inhibitory neurotransmitters or modulators in the mammalian central nervous system (for review, see Krnjevic 1976; Wu 1982a;
Rassin, Gaull 1978). The GABA-synthesizing enzyme, L-
glutamate decarboxylase (EC 4.1.1.15) (GAD) and the GABA-
degradative enzyme GABA-transaminase (EC 2.6.1.19) (GABA-
T) have been purified to homogeneity (Wu et al. 1973;
Schousboe et al. 1973; Wu 1976; Wu et al. 1981b). In
addition, specific antibodies to GAD and GABA-T have also
been obtained which made it possible to identify the GAD-
containing neurons and the GABAergic pathways by immunocytochemical methods (Saito et al. 1974b,c; Wu et al.
1981a, 1982b; Wu 1983). Unlike the GABA system, the biosynthetic pathways for taurine in the mammalian brain are
not clear. It has been postulated that the major route
for taurine synthesis in brain is through the decarboxylation of cysteinesulfinic acid to hypotaurine by cysteinesulfinic acid decarboxylase (EC 4.1.1.29) (CSAD) and
the subsequent oxidation of hypotaurine to taurine
(Jacobsen, Smith 1968). An alternative pathway is the
oxidation of cysteinesulfinic acid to cysteic acid,
followed by the decarboxylation of cysteic acid to taurine by cysteic acid decarboxylase (CAD) (Jacobsen, Smith
1968). Although the nature of the enzyme(s) decarboxyla-
ting cysteinesulfinic and cysteic acids is still disputed
(Sorbo, Heyman 1957; Lin et al. 1971), the balance of the
evidence indicates that the decarboxylation of cysteine-

sulfinic and cysteic acids is catalyzed by the same enzyme (Jacobsen, Smith 1968; Guion-Rain et al. 1975; Hope
1955; Blaschko, Hope 1954). Recently, a controversy arose
as to whether the same enzyme may catalyze the decarboxylation of L-glutamate and L-cysteinesulfinate in rat
brain (Blindermann et al. 1978; Urban et al. 1981). Since
GAD is the rate-limiting enzyme for GABA biosynthesis,
its presence in certain types of neurons, particularly at
the nerve terminal, has been regarded as evidence to
support the notion that these neurons use GABA as their
neurotransmitter. Should GAD and CSAD/CAD be the same
enzyme entity, the GABA neurons identified by the
presence of GAD will actually include the taurine-containing neurons and vice-versa. This communication is
intended to cover the following points: First of all to
present evidence to show that different enzyme entities
are responsible for the biosynthesis of GABA and taurine.
Secondly, to describe the procedures used in the author's
laboratory for the production and characterization of
both polyclonal and monoclonal antibodies. Thirdly, to
demonstrate the GABAergic neurons and their neuronal
connectivity by immunocytochemical localization of GAD.

NON IDENTITY OF GAD AND CSAD/CAD

In order to establish the identity or non-identity of
GAD and CSAD/CAD, these two enzymes have been purified to
homogeneity from bovine brain. The purification procedures involved various column chromatographies, e.g., gel
filtration, hydroxyapatite and DEAE-cellulose and preparative polyacrylamide gel electrophoresis. The following observations (Wu 1982a) obtained with the purified
enzyme preparations support the conclusion that CSAD/CAD
is the enzyme responsible for the biosynthesis of taurine
and GAD is responsible for GABA biosynthesis. First of
all, CSAD/CAD has a much higher affinity for cysteic and
cysteinesulfinic acids than GAD does (K_m values for
CSAD/CAD and GAD with cysteic and cysteinesulfinic acids
as substrate are 0.22 and 0.28 mM vs. 5.4 and 7.2 mM,
respectively). Secondly, although GAD can also use cysteic and cysteinesulfinic acids as substrates in addition
to glutamate, the affinity for cysteic and cysteinesulfinic acids is much lower than the affinity for L-glutamic acid as reflected in their K_m values (K_m for cysteic, cysteinesulfinic and L-glutamic acids is 5.4, 7.2

and 1.6 mM, respectively). Thirdly, GAD activity is strongly inhibited by L-glutamate (K_i = 0.45 mM) with L-cysteic acid as substrate. Furthermore, the concentration of L-glutamate in brain tissue is approximately 8-12 μmole/g fresh weight which is much higher than that of L-cysteic or cysteinesulfinic acids (Bachelard 1981). The high affinity of GAD for L-glutamate, the high concentration of L-glutamate in brain tissue and the strong inhibition of decarboxylation of L-cysteic acid by L-glutamate make it convincing that GAD is involved exclusively for GABA biosynthesis and not involved in the biosynthesis of taurine. On the other hand, CSAD/CAD which can use only L-cysteic and L-cysteinesulfinic acids, but not L-glutamate as substrates is the enzyme responsible for taurine biosynthesis. Immunodiffusion tests show that anti-GAD does not crossreact with CSAD/CAD and vice versa (Wu 1982a). The lack of cross-reactivity between anti-GAD and CSAD/CAD and vice versa definitely clears doubts about the validity of immunocytochemical results which we, as well as others, have used extensively for the identification of GAD-containing neurons and GABAergic pathways (for review, see Wu et al. 1981a, Wu et al. 1982a).

PRODUCTION OF ANTIBODIES AND IMMUNOCHEMICAL CHARACTERIZATIONS

In the past, we were able to obtain high titer antibodies with microgram quantities of antigens. In general, rabbits were injected biweekly with 3-180 μg of antigen in complete Freund's adjuvant into subscapular muscles. Animals were bled after the fifth injection. This technique has been successfully used in our laboratory for the production of antibodies against various proteins purified from the nervous system. For instance, a total of 15, 50, 50, 7 and 75 μg of purified GABA-T and GAD from mouse brain (Saito et al. 1974b,c; Wu et al. 1982a; Wu 1982b, 1983), choline acetyl transferase from electric organ of Torpedo (Brandon, Wu 1977), neurofilament protein from Myxicola (Lasek, Wu 1976), and GAD and CSAD from bovine brain (Wu 1982a), respectively, were able to evoke production of specific antibodies in rabbits. In addition to the conventional method, recently we have also employed the hybridoma technique (Kohler, Milstein 1975, 1976) for the production of monoclonal antibody against GAD (Wu et al. 1982b; Denner et al.

1983).

Briefly, the hybridoma was prepared according to the method of Kennett (1979) with some modifications. Each of two mice were immunized with purified rat brain GAD intraperitoneally for 6 weeks. The sera from the immunized mice had been shown to contain a high titer of antibody against rat brain GAD. The spleens were removed from the immunized mice and perfused with culture medium at several sites, thereby forcing the spleen cells into the culture medium. The erythrocytes were lysed with NH₄Cl, and the spleen cells were fused with plasmacytoma cell line (P3 x 63AG8) with a ratio of 10:1 in 50% polyethylene glycol for 5 min.

The hybrids were evenly suspended and gently distributed into 10 microplates (1 drop per well). The next day, an additional drop of the 2 x HAT medium (hypoxanthine, thymidine, and aminopterin) was added. The wells were fed two additional drops of HT medium (without aminopterin) 6-7 days later. Clones appeared 17 days later.

The positive wells were identified by screening the supernatant liquid for production of the antibody against GAD by ELISA test (enzyme-linked immunosorbent assay) using peroxidase-labeled goat anti-mouse IgG as second antibody and pure rat brain GAD as antigen. The anti-GAD producing clones were recloned until a single clone was obtained. The anti-GAD positive single clone was then injected into mice to produce ascites fluid. The culture medium and the ascites fluids were further screened by ELISA test or immunodot test using pure GAD as antigen. The anti-GAD producing clones appear to be stable upon storage in liquid nitrogen for several months.

The polyclonal antibodies were characterized by four immunochemical methods, namely, immunodiffusion and immunoelectrophoresis, neutralization of enzyme activities by antibodies, microcomplement fixation tests, and enzyme immunoassay (Saito et al. 1974b,c; Wong et al. 1974; Wu et al. 1982a, Wu 1982b, 1983). For monoclonal antibodies, they were characterized by ELISA and immunodot tests using pure rat brain GAD as antigen (Wu et al. 1982b; Denner et al. 1983).

IMMUNOCYTOCHEMICAL LOCALIZATION OF L-GLUTAMATE
DECARBOXYLASE

Some examples of immunocytochemical identification of
GABAergic neurons and their projections obtained in the
author's laboratory as well as from other laboratories
are summarized as follows:

a.   In rabbit retina

A combination of autoradiography and immunocytochemistry was used to identify GABAergic neurons in
rabbit retina. In the presence of Triton X-100, reaction
product was found in four broad, evenly spaced laminae
within the inner plexiform layer. In the absence of the
detergent, these laminae were seen to be composed of
small, punctate deposits. When colchicine was injected
intravitreally before GAD staining, cell bodies with the
characteristic shape and location of amacrine cells were
found to be immunochemically labeled. Electron microscopic examination showed that these processes were presynaptic to ganglion cell dendrites (infrequently),
amacrine cell telodendrons, and bipolar cell terminals.
Often, bipolar cell terminals were found which were
densely innervated by several GAD-positive processes. No
definite synapses were observed in which a GAD-positive
process represented the postsynaptic element. In autoradiographic studies by intravitreal injection of
[^{3}H]GABA, a diffuse labeling of the inner plexiform layer
and a dense labeling of certain amacrine cell bodies in
the inner nuclear layer was observed. Both immunocytochemical and autoradiographic results support the notion
that certain, if not all, amacrine cells use GABA as
their neurotransmitter (Brandon et al. 1979, 1980; Wu et
al. 1981a).

b.   In Goldfish and Frog Retina

Antibodies against purified catfish GAD were used in
this study. Immunocytochemical results revealed that GAD
was localized in some horizontal cells (H1 type), a few
amacrine cells in sublamina b of the inner plexiform
layer. Results from immunocytochemical studies of GAD-
containing neurons and autoradiographic studies of GABA

uptake revealed a marked similarity in the labeling
pattern suggesting that in goldfish retina, H1 type
horizontal cell and at least one type of amacrine cell
may use GABA as their neurotransmitter (Lam et al. 1979;
Wu et al. 1981a). Since GAD from frog brain crossreacted
with both antibodies against mouse brain GAD and catfish
GAD, either GAD antibodies could be used in the study of
frog retina. In the frog retina, dense GAD immunoreactivity was observed in the inner plexiform layer, both as
punctate deposits and as filled processes of stratified
and diffuse amacrine cells; in the inner nuclear layer,
where many cell bodies were labeled, including those of
some horizontal cells; and diffusely in the outer plexiform layer. These results suggest that at least some
types of amacrine cells and horizontal cells in frog
retina use GABA as their transmitter (Brandon et al.
1980).

c.   In Rat Habenula

    Biochemical and immunocytochemical methods have been
used to study GABA system in the rat habenula in both
normal and lesioned animals. GAD was found to be more
concentrated in the lateral (LH) than in the medial (MH)
habenula. A marked loss of GAD as well as a comparable
reduction in GABA uptake in the LH was observed following
stria medullaris (SM) lesions. The MH was not affected by
these lesions. Immunocytochemical results agreed well
with the biochemical findings, suggesting that SM contains GABAergic projections to the LH (Gottesfeld et al.
1980, 1981).

d.   In Monkey Striate Cortex and Geniculate Complex

    Neuronal cell bodies and synaptic terminals positive
for GAD have been located by immunocytochemical staining
in all layers of the macaque monkey cortex. In layers II
and III, the staining pattern of periodic dots is identical with that seen in sections stained for cytochrome
oxidase. The rows of dots run parallel with the ocular
dominance columns, suggesting that the labeled neurons
are preferentially related to each eye (Hendrickson et
al. 1981). In monkey geniculate complex, GAD-positive
cell bodies are found in all layers and in the interlami-

nar zones in the dorsal lateral geniculate nucleus (dLGN). The neuropil is more heavily labeled in the laminar than the interlaminar zones, with the magnocellular layers being most densely labeled. In the ventral lateral geniculate nucleus (vLGN), no stained cell bodies are seen, but the neuropil is intensely labeled, especially in the retinal input layer. The reticular nucleus of the thalamus (RNT) is just the opposite, with many GAD-positive neurons but sparsely labeled neuropil. The GAD-positive neurons in dLGN have small cell bodies with a large infolded, unlabeled nucleus. GAD reactivity is found in the thin rim of cytoplasm and in the two to four thick, straight dendrites, and on the cytoplasmic surfaces of mitochondria, Golgi and membraneous cisternae, and vesicles. GAD-positive synaptic profiles are found in both pre- and postsynaptic relationships in the dLGN. Some GAD-positive profiles are both pre- and postsynaptic in the same section, suggesting that these are presynaptic dendrites. In the laminae, GAD-positive presynaptic profiles are very commonly found within synaptic glomeruli where they lie postsynaptic to a retinal axon terminal and presynaptic to an unlabeled dendrite, which also receives input from the retinal terminal. Outside of glomeruli, individual GAD-positive profiles are presynaptic to either labeled or unlabeled cell bodies and dendrites. These data suggest that GAD-positive glomerular profiles are the presynaptic dendrites of the dLGN interneuron, whereas the individual GAD-positive contacts arise from axons of RNT neurons (Hendrickson et al. 1983).

e.   In Rat Hypothalamus and Pituitary Gland

A dense network of GAD-positive nerve fibers was observed to be essentially evenly distributed throughout the hypothalamus. A plexus of GABA terminals was also demonstrated both in the median eminence and within the posterior and intermediate lobes of the pituitary. Three distinct clusters of magnocellular GABA neurons were discovered in the posterior hypothalamus. In addition, GAD immunoreactive cell bodies were observed in many other hypothalamic nuclei, such as the arcuate nucleus and in the perifornical region. These results provide a morphological basis by which GABA of hypothalamic origin may regulate the neuroendocrine system (Vincent et al. 1982).

f.   In Rat Cerebellum

At least some populations of stellate, basket, Purkinje and Golgi cells in cerebellum have been identified
as GABAergic neurons by immunocytochemical localization
of GAD (Saito et al. 1974a; McLaughlin et al. 1974,
1975). GABAergic pathways in the cerebellum have also
been elucidated by retrograde and anterograde transport
of GAD antibody after in vivo injections (Chan-Palay et
al. 1979). In addition to GAD, some population of
Purkinje neurons have been shown to contain motilin, a
22-amino acid polypeptide (Chan-Palay et al. 1981), CSAD,
the taurine-synthesizing enzyme (Chan-Palay et al.
1982c,d) and some even contain both GAD and motilin as
demonstrated by double-staining procedures performed on
single sections of the cerebellum (Chan-Palay et al.
1981). The presence of motilin, GAD, and CSAD in the
Purkinje neurons calls for evaluation of the role of
motilin, GABA and taurine in cerebellar function.

g.   In Rat Pancreas

Both the GABA-synthesizing and degradative enzymes,
namely GAD and GABA-T, respectively, were found to occur
only in the β-cells of the islets of Langerhans. The
other endocrine cell types, the exocrine tissue and the
nervous elements in the pancreas did not contain either
enzyme. Animals treated with the β-cell toxins strepto-
zotocin or alloxan showed a loss of immunoreactive cells
in the islets. The results provide morphological evidence
of the coexistence of GABA and insulin in the β-cells of
the endocrine pancreas (Vincent et al. 1983b).

h.   In Cat Hippocampus

Several different types of GAD-positive cell bodies
were found in all layers in regions CA1 to CA3 in cat
hippocampus, suggesting that many kinds of GABAergic
interneurons are present in the hippocampus. Fibers and
varicosities that were immunoreactive for GAD were also
found in all layers. The most conspicuous patterns formed
by GAD-positive varicosities were in the pyramidal cell
layer, where they occurred as pericellular nets around
all pyramidal neurons. GAD-positive varicosities also

followed both apical and basal dendrites, but a very high density of GAD-positive varicosities was seen around fine (diameter 2 to 4 μm) tube-like structures that could sometimes be seen to lie at the base of pyramidal neurons. Electron microscopic analysis of GAD-positive structures that had first been identified in the light microscope established that the varicosities outlining such tube-like structures were boutons in symmetrical synaptic contact with the axon initial segments of pyramidal neurons; the other GAD-positive varicosities were boutons in symmetrical contact with cell bodies and apical and basal dendrites of pyramidal neurons. Detailed study of 19 axon initial segments showed that immunoreactive boutons occur most commonly along more distal parts of the initial segment, where they almost completely surround the axon and form symmetrical synapses not only along the main axon, but also with its spines. Since the GAD-positive boutons comprised 92% of all symmetrical synaptic boutons along the initial segments, it was concluded that the axoaxonic cell uses GABA as its transmitter (Somogy et al. 1983b).

i.   In Rat Dentate Gyrus

The distribution of GABA fibers within the dentate gyrus was immunohistochemically examined following lesions of the entorhinal cortex in the adult rat. A major change in the pattern of the GAD-positive fibers within the molecular layer was characterized by a marked increase in the density of fibers in the outer molecular layer. This change in the lamination of the dentate GABA fibers following entorhinal lesions appeared very similar to the changes which occur in acetylcholinesterase staining following entorhinal denervation of the dentate. These results provide morphological support for the sprouting of GABA fibers in the dentate gyrus in response to perforant path destruction (Goldowitz et al. 1982).

j.   In Tissue Cultures

GAD was immunohistochemically demonstrated in dissociated cultures from newborn rat neostriatum and substantia nigra. The size and shape of the enkephalin-immunoreactive cells varied, but they were generally larger

than substance P- and GAD-positive cells, which formed
relatively uniform cell populations. Cells of apparently
non-neuronal origin did not show any immunoreactivity. It
is unlikely that enkephalin is present in the same cells
that contain substance P or GAD because of morphological
differences between these cells. The possible coexistence
of substance P and GAD in the same cells, however, could
not be excluded (Panula et al. 1980, 1981a,b).

k. Others

GABAergic neurons and pathways have also been identified in many other regions of the mammalian central nervous system such as rat retina (Lin et al. 1983), dorsal
lateral geniculate nucleus (O'Hara et al. 1983), hypothalamic projection to the neocortex (Vincent et al.
1983a), rubrospinal neurons (Murakami et al. 1983), and
cat visual cortex (Somogyi et al. 1983a).

CONCLUDING REMARKS

It is the author's intention to choose GAD as an
example to show the approaches that have been taken in
the author's laboratory in the identification of GAD-containing neurons and their neuronal connectivity or GABA-
ergic pathways in various parts of the vertebrate central
nervous system, starting with the purification of GAD to
homogeneity, followed by production and characterization
of polyclonal and monoclonal GAD antibodies and finally
the visualization of GAD at cellular and subcellular
levels by immunocytochemical techniques. This approach
has proved to be very fruitful and should be applied to
other systems, e.g., taurine, aspartate and glutamate.
Indeed, the taurine synthesizing enzyme, CSAD, has been
localized in cerebellum (Chan-Palay et al. 1982c,d),
retina (Lin et al. 1983) and neuromuscular junction
(Chan-Palay et al. 1982a,b). Enzymes involved in the
metabolism of aspartate and glutamate, e.g., aspartate
amino transferase and glutaminase have also been localized in various parts of the mammalian central nervous
system (Altschuler et al. 1981; Lin et al. 1983; also see
Wenthold "Immunohistochemistry of Glutamate Amino Transferase and Glutaminase" in this volume). Since both aspartate and glutamate are ubiquitous and present in vir-

tually all cell types, it is expected that their synthetic enzymes, presumably aspartate aminotransferase and glutaminase, respectively, are also present in all cell types. Hence, aspartate aminotransferase and glutaminase may not be a good marker for aspartatergic and glutamatergic neurons, respectively. However, if the aspartatergic and glutamatergic neurons do have a substantially higher level of aspartate aminotransferase and glutaminase than the other cell types, then the immunocytochemical techniques which have been applied so successfully for the identification of GABAergic neurons and processes may prove to be still quite powerful for the identification of neurons or neuronal pathways using aspartate or glutamate as transmitter.

ACKNOWLEDGEMENT

Support by the National Institutes of Health, grants NS-17038, NS-13224, and EY-03909, is gratefully acknowledged.

REFERENCES

Altschuler RA, Neises GR, Harmison GG, Wenthold RJ, Fex J (1981). Immunocytochemical localization of aspartate amino transferase immunoreactivity in cochlear nucleus of the guinea pig. Proc Natl Acad Sci USA 78:6553.

Bachelard HS (1981). Biochemistry of centrally active amino acids. In DeFeudis FV, Mandel P (eds): "Amino Acid Neurotransmitters," New York: Raven Press, p 475.

Blaschko H, Hope DB (1954). Enzymatic decarboxylation of cysteic and cysteine sulfinic acid. J Physiol (London) 126:52P.

Blindermann JM, Maitre M, Ossola L, Mandel P (1978). Purification and some properties of L-glutamate decarboxylase from human brain. Eur J Biochem 86: 143.

Brandon C, Lam DMK, Su YYT, Wu J-Y (1980). Immunocytochemical localization of GABA neurons in the rabbit and frog retina. Brain Res Bull 5 (Suppl 2), 21.

Brandon C, Lam DMK, Wu J-Y (1979). The γ-aminobutyric acid system in rabbit retina: Localization by immunocytochemistry and autoradiography. Proc Natl Acad Sci USA 76:3557.

Brandon C, Wu J-Y (1977). Electrophoretic and immunochemical characterization of choline acetyltransferase from Torpedo. Soc Neurosci Abstr 3:404.

Chan-Palay V, Engel AG, Palay SL, Wu J-Y (1982a). Synthesizing enzymes for four neuroactive substances in motor neurons and neuromuscular junctions: Light and electron microscopic immunocytochemistry. Proc Natl Acad Sci USA 79:6717.

Chan-Palay V, Engel AG, Wu J-Y, Palay SL (1982b). Coexistence in human and primate neuromuscular junctions of enzymes synthesizing acetylcholine, catecholamine, taurine, and γ-aminobutyric acid. Proc Natl Acad Sci USA 79:7027.

Chan-Palay V, Lin CT, Palay S, Yamamoto M, Wu J-Y (1982c). Taurine in the mammalian cerebellum: Demonstration by autoradiography with [^{3}H]taurine and immunocytochemistry with antibodies against the taurine-synthesizing enzyme, cysteine-sulfinic acid decarboxylase. Proc Natl Acad Sci USA 79:2695.

Chan-Palay V, Nilaver G, Palay SL, Beinfeld MC, Zimmerman EE, Wu J-Y, O'Donohue TL (1981). Chemical heterogeneity in cerebellar Purkinje cells: existence and coexistence of glutamic acid decarboxylase-like and motilin-like immunoreactivities. Proc Natl Acad Sci USA 78:7787.

Chan-Palay V, Palay SL, Li C, Wu J-Y (1982d). Sagittal cerebellar microbands of taurine neurons: Immunocytochemical demonstration by using antibodies against the taurine synthesizing enzyme cysteine sulfinic acid decarboxylase. Proc Natl Acad Sci USA 79:4221.

Chan-Palay V, Palay SL, Wu J-Y (1979). Gamma-aminobutyric acid pathways in the cerebellum studied by retrograde and anterograde transport of glutamic acid decarboxylase antibody after in vivo injections. Anat Embryol 157:1.

Denner LA, Lin CT, Song GX, Wu J-Y (1983). Multiple forms of rat brain L-glutamate decarboxylase: Purification and immunochemical characterization. ASBC Abstract 42(7):2008.

Gottesfeld Z, Brandon C, Jacobowitz DM, Wu J-Y (1980). The GABA system in the mammalian habenula. Brain Res Bull 5:(Suppl 2)1.

Gottesfeld Z, Brandon C, Wu J-Y (1981). Immunochemistry of glutamate decarboxylase in the deafferented habenula. Brain Research 208:181.

Goldowitz D, Vincent SR, Wu J-Y, Hökfelt T (1982). Immunohistochemical demonstration of plasticity in GABA neurons of the adult rat dentate gyrus. Brain Res

238:413.

Guion-Rain M, Portemer C, Chateganer F (1975). Rat liver cysteine sulfinate decarboxylase: Purification, new appraisal of the molecular weight and determination of catalytic properties. Biochim Biophys Acta 384: 265.

Hendrickson AE, Hunt S, Wu J-Y (1981). Immunocytochemical localization of glutamic acid decarboxylase in monkey striate cortex. Nature 292:605.

Hendrickson AE, Ogren MP, Vaughn JE, Barber RP, Wu J-Y (1983). Light and electron microscopic immunocytochemical localization of the glutamic acid decarboxylase in monkey geniculate complex: Evidence for GABAergic neurons and synapses. J Neuroscience 3:1245.

Hope DB (1955). Pyridoxal phosphate as the co-enzyme of the mammalian decarboxylase for L-cysteine sulfinic and L-cysteic acids. Biochem J 59:497.

Jacobsen JB, Smith LH Jr. (1968). Biochemistry and physiology of taurine and taurine derivatives. Physiol Rev 48:424.

Kennett RH (1979). Cell fusion. In Jacoby W, Pastan J (eds): "Methods in Enzymology," New York: Academic Press, p 345.

Köhler G, Milstein C (1975). Continuous cultures of fused cells secreting antibody of predefined specificity. Nature 256:495.

Köhler G, Milstein C (1976). Derivation of specific antibody-producing tissue culture and tumor lines by cell fusion. Eur J Immunol 6:514.

Krnjevic K (1976). Inhibitory action of GABA and GABA-mimetics on vertebrate neurons. In Roberts E, Chase TN, Tower DB (eds): "GABA in Nervous System Function," New York: Raven Press, p 269.

Lam DMK, Su YYT, Swain L, Marc RE, Brandon C, Wu J-Y (1979). Immunocytochemical localization of glutamic acid decarboxylase in goldfish retina. Nature 278:565.

Lasek RJ, Wu J-Y (1976). Immunochemical analysis of the proteins comprising Myxicola (10 nm) neurofilaments. Soc Neurosci Abstr 2:40.

Lin CT, Li HZ, Wu J-Y (1983). Immunocytochemical localization of L-glutamate decarboxylase, γ-aminobutyric acid transaminase, cysteine-sulfinic acid decarboxylase, aspartate aminotransferase and somatostatin in rat retina. Brain Res 270:273.

Lin YC, Demeio RH, Metrione RM (1971). Purification and properties of rat liver cysteine sulfinate decarboxylase. Biochim Biophys Acta 250:558.

McLaughlin BJ, Wood JG, Saito K, Barber R, Vaughn JE, Roberts E, Wu J-Y (1974). The fine structural localization of glutamate decarboxylase in synaptic terminals of rodent cerebellum. Brain Res 76:377.

McLaughlin BJ, Wood JG, Saito K, Roberts E, Wu J-Y (1975). The fine structural localization of glutamate decarboxylase in developing axonal processes and presynaptic terminals of rodent cerebellum. Brain Res 85:355.

Murakami F, Katsumaru H, Wu J-Y, Matsuda T, Tsukahara N (1983). Immunocytochemical demonstration of GABAergic synapses on identified rubrospinal neurons. Brain Res 267:357.

O'Hara PT, Lieberman AR, Hunt SP, Wu J-Y (1983). Neural elements containing glutamic acid decarboxylase (GAD) in the dorsal lateral geniculate nucleus of the rat: Immunohistochemical studies by light and electron microscope. Neuroscience 8(2):189.

Panula P, Emson P, Wu J-Y (1980). Demonstration of enkephalin-, substance P-, and glutamate decarboxylase-like immunoreactivity in cultured cells derived from newborn rat neostriatum. Histochemistry 69:169.

Panula P, Wu J-Y, Emson P (1981a). Ultrastructure of GABA-neurons in culture of rat neostriatum. Brain Res 219:202.

Panula P, Wu J-Y, Emson P, Rechardt L (1981b). Demonstration of GABA-neurons in cultures of rat substantia nigra. Neuroscience Letters 22:303.

Rassin DK, Gaull GE (1978). Taurine and other sulphur-containing amino acids: Their function in the central nervous system. In Fonnum F (ed): "Amino Acids as Chemical Transmitters," New York: Plenum Press, p 571.

Saito K, Barber R, Wu J-Y, Matsuda T, Roberts E, Vaughn JE (1974a). Immunohistochemical localization of glutamic acid decarboxylase in rat cerebellum. Proc Natl Acad Sci USA 71:269.

Saito K, Schousboe A, Wu J-Y, Roberts E (1974b). Some immunochemical properties and species specificity of GABA-α-ketoglutarate transaminase from mouse brain. Brain Res 65:287.

Saito K, Wu J-Y, Roberts E (1974c). Immunochemical comparisons of vertebrate glutamic acid decarboxylase. Brain Res 65:277.

Schousboe A, Wu J-Y, Roberts E (1973). Purification and characterization of the 4-aminobutyrate-2-ketoglutarate transaminase from mouse brain. Biochemistry 12:2868.

Somogyi P, Freund T, Wu J-Y, Smith AD (1983a). The section Golgi impregnation procedure. II Immunocytochemical demonstration of glutamate decarboxylase in Golgi-impregnated neurons in their afferent and efferent synaptic boutons in the visual cortex of the cat. Neuroscience 9:475.

Somogyi P, Smith AD, Nunzi GA, Takagi H, Wu J-Y (1983b). Glutamate decarboxylase immunoreactive neurons and distribution of their synaptic terminals on pyramidal neurons in the hippocampus of the cat, with special reference to the axon initial segment. J Neuroscience 3:1450.

Sörbo B, Heyman T (1957). On the purification of cysteinesulfinic acid decarboxylase and its substrate specificity. Biochim Biophys Acta 23:624.

Urban PF, Reichert P, Mandel P (1981). Taurine metabolism and function. In DeFeudis FV, Mandel P (eds): "Amino Acid Neurotransmitters," New York: Raven Press, p 537.

Vincent SR, Hökfelt T, Skirboll LR, Wu J-Y (1983a). Hypothalamic GABA neurons project to the neocortex. Science 220:1309.

Vincent SR, Hökfelt T, Wu J-Y (1982). GABA neuron systems in hypothalamus and the pituitary gland: Immunohistochemical demonstration using antibodies against glutamate decarboxylase. Neuroendocrinology 34:117.

Vincent SR, Hökfelt T, Wu J-Y, Elde RP, Morgan LM, Kimmel JR (1983b). Immunohistochemical studies of the GABA system in the pancreas. Neuroendocrinology 36:197.

Wong E, Schousboe A, Saito K, Wu J-Y, Roberts E (1974). Glutamate decarboxylase and GABA-transaminase from six mouse strains. Brain Res 68:133.

Wu J-Y (1976). Purification and properties of L-glutamate decarboxylase (GAD) and GABA-aminotransferase (GABA-T). In Roberts E, Chase TN, Tower DB (eds): "GABA in Nervous System Function," New York: Raven Press, p 7.

Wu J-Y (1982a). Purification and characterization of cysteic/cysteine sulfinic acids decarboxylase and L-glutamate decarboxylase in bovine brain. Proc Natl Acad Sci USA 79:4270.

Wu J-Y (1982b). Decarboxylases: brain glutamate decarboxylase as a model. In Lajtha A (ed): "Handbook of Neurochemistry," New York: Plenum Press, 4:111.

Wu J-Y (1983). Preparation of glutamic acid decarboxylase as immunogen for immunocytochemistry. In Cuello AC (ed): "Neuroimmunocytochemistry," Sussex: IBRO Handbook Series: Methods in Neurosciences, in press.

Wu J-Y, Brandon C, Su YYT, Lam DMK (1981a). Immunocytochemical and autoradiographic localization of GABA system in the vertebrate retina. Molecular and Cellular
Biochem 39:229.

Wu J-Y, Lin CT, Brandon C, Chan DS, Mohler H, Richards JG
(1982a). Regulation and immunocytochemical characterization of GAD. In Palay S, Chan-Palay V (eds): "Cytochemical Methods in Neuroanatomy," New York: Alan R
Liss Inc, p 279.

Wu J-Y, Lin CT, Denner L, Su YYT, Chan DS (1982b). Monoclonal antibodies of GABA- and acetylcholine-synthesi-
zing enzymes. Amer Soc Neurochem Abstract 13(1):92.

Wu J-Y, Matsuda T, Roberts E (1973). Purification and
characterization of glutamate decarboxylase from mouse
brain. J Biol Chem 248:3029.

Wu J-Y, Su YYT, Lam DMK, Schousboe A, Chude O (1981b)
Assay methods, purification and characterization of L-
glutamate decarboxylase and GABA-transaminase," In
Marks N, Rodnight R (eds): New York: Plenum Publishing
Co 5:129.

**Glutamine, Glutamate, and GABA
in the Central Nervous System, pages 177–183
© 1983 Alan R. Liss, Inc., 150 Fifth Avenue, New York, NY 10011**

RADIOLABELLING OF GABA-TRANSAMINASE IN BRAIN HOMOGENATES
USING [^{3}H]GAMMA-VINYL-GABA

Karen Gale

Department of Pharmacology,
Georgetown University Schools of Medicine and Dentistry,
Washington, D.C., 20007

Gamma-vinyl-GABA (GVG) is thought to irreversibly inhibit
GABA-transaminase (GABA-T) by covalently binding to the active
site of the enzyme as it undergoes catalytic conversion by
GABA-T (1). An examination of the binding of radiolabelled
GVG should allow the further characterization of the interaction between GABA-T and GVG and potentially provide a method
for the isotopic labelling of the enzyme in vitro and in vivo.
Moreover, binding of labelled GVG may be used to estimate the
number of active enzyme molecules of GABA-T in a tissue homogenate. In the present report we describe a procedure for
the determination of [^{3}H]GVG binding to homogenates of tissue
from various brain regions, and characterize the specificity
of this interaction. In addition, we have used [^{3}H]GVG
binding to calculate the number of enzyme molecules of GABA-T
present in homogenates of striatal tissue.

MATERIALS and METHODS

Tissue from rat brain was homogenized in 20 volumes of 50mM
TRIS buffer (pH 8.4) containing 0.2% TRITON X-100, 2mM alpha-
ketoglutarate and 20mM mercaptoethanol. Binding was done in
1.5ml microcentrifuge tubes containing 40ul of tissue homogenate (200-300 ug protein), 5ul of [^{3}H]GVG (5pmoles), and 5ul of
buffer with or without 100 mM nonradioactive GVG. The tubes
were then placed in a shaking water bath at 37°C for 20min.
Following incubation, the reaction was stopped by the addition
of 950 ul of 85% ethanol. The ethanol-precipitated proteins
were then centrifuged at 20,000 x g for 20min, and free [^{3}H]GVG
was removed by aspirating the supernatant. The pellet was
washed by resuspending in ethanol and recentrifuging; the

supernatant was again removed by aspiration. The pellet was solubilized in 1 ml of a 1% solution of sodium dodecyl sulfate (SDS) and the radioactivity was determined by liquid scintillaation counting.

Assay of GABA-T was performed according to the method of DeBoer and Bruinvels (2). [³H]GVG (34 Ci/mmol) was prepared by New Engand Nuclear. The radiolabelled material was 97% pure as determined by HPLC analysis. Nonradioactive GVG was provided through the courtesy of Centre de Recherche, Merrell International, Strasbourg, France.

RESULTS

Amount of [³H]GVG bound:

Under the assay conditions used, less than 1% of the radioactivity used per assay tube was found to be bound to the ethanol-precipitated protein. Typically, 100,000 cpm were used per tube, of which 500-1000 cpm were recovered from the washed protein pellet.

Maximum inhibition of [³H]GVG binding was obtained when 10mM nonradioactive GVG was included in the reaction mixture. The binding remaining under these conditions is considered to be background or "nonspecific" binding and was found to represent approximately 30-40% of the total binding. Prior boiling of the homogenate did not alter the background [³H]GVG binding but did eliminate all binding above background, indicating that background binding was nonenzymatic. In addition, it was found that at least 50% of the background binding was still present in the absence of tissue, indicating that much of the background was due to binding of [³H]GVG to the reaction tube. Values for "specific" binding represent the difference between total binding and background.

Specificity:

Previous studies have demonstrated that amino-oxyacetic acid (AOAA) and 3-mercaptopropionic acid (3-MP) are capable of inhibiting GABA-T activity (3). We therefore examined the effect of these agents on the binding of [³H]GVG to tissue homogenates. Homogenates of striatum were assayed for [³H]GVG binding in the presence of various concentrations of AOAA or 3-MP. As shown in Table 1, complete inhibition of specific [³H]GVG binding was obtained in the presence of 100uM AOAA or 1mM 3MP. In the presence of 10uM AOAA, specific [³H]GVG binding binding was inhibited by greater than 90%, and with 100uM 3MP, the specific binding was inhibited by 50%. Neither AOAA nor 3MP altered the nonspecific binding.

TABLE 1.   Inhibition of [³H]GVG binding by AOAA and 3MPA.

Inhibitor	Conc.	Binding of ³H-GVG, CPM			
		TOTAL	NONSPECIFIC	SPECIFIC	% INHIBITION
Control		884	266	618	
AOAA	10^{-5}	306	253	53	91
	10^{-4}	264	269	0	100
3MPA	10^{-5}	771	317	454	27
	10^{-4}	549	268	281	55
	10^{-3}	297	287	10	98

Linearity with tissue concentration and comparison across different brain areas:

For determining whether the specific binding of [³H]GVG was linear as a function of tissue concentration, homogenates of striatum were prepared (800 ug prot/40 ul) and diluted with the incubation buffer to yield concentrations ranging from 75 ug/40 ul to 800 ug/40 ul. Both total and nonspecific binding were determined for each concentration of tissue used; tissue concentration was verified by protein determination. Fig. 1 shows specific binding as a function of tissue concentration. It can be seen that this function is linear up to 400ug/assay tube (8ug/ul). Note that nonspecific binding did not increase in proportion to protein, since a large portion of nonspecific binding was associated with the reaction tube and was independent of protein (see above).

Figure 1.   [³H]GVG binding to homogenates of rat striatum as a function of protein concentration.

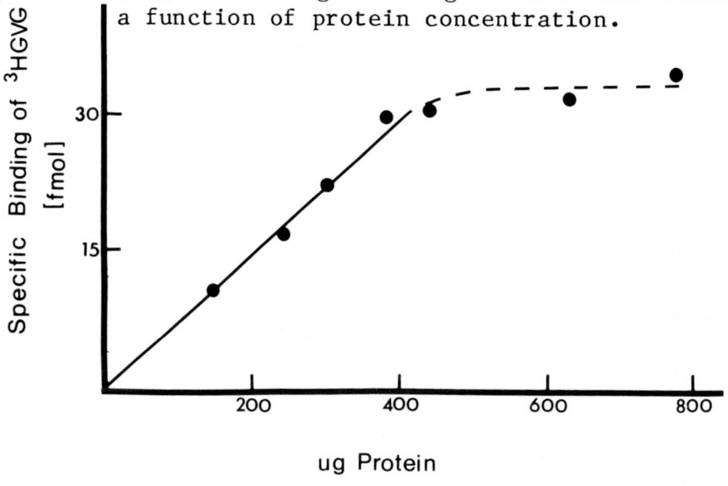

Table 2 shows the specific binding at different concentrations of tissue; 200-300 ug/ assay tube appears to be an optimal amount of tissue under our assay conditions. Table 2 also shows results from five other brain regions. Although the absolute binding activity per mg protein differs across brain areas, all areas examined show linearity with tissue concentrations up to at least 300 ug/assay tube.

TABLE 2
[3H]GVG Binding in various regions of rat brain

region	ug prot	CPM Total	CPM Nonspecific	CPM Specific	Specific/ug prot
Caudate	145	510	250	260	1.8
	240	663	253	410	1.7
	380	1005	275	730	1.9
Superior	120	568	258	310	2.6
colliculus	225	763	298	465	2.1
	244	817	272	545	2.2
	285	922	267	655	2.3
Substantia	248	518	252	266	1.1
nigra	285	619	266	353	1.2
	355	656	318	338	1.0
Cerebral	260	546	292	254	1.0
cortex	290	522	259	263	0.9
	375	660	270	390	1.0
Inferior	145	426	264	162	1.1
colliculus	240	500	262	238	1.0
	330	657	305	352	1.1
Cerebellar	170	365	257	108	0.64
cortex	230	420	282	138	0.60

Determination of amount of GABA-T enzyme molecules present in striatal tissue:

Nonradioactive GVG was mixed with [3H]GVG in varying proportions in order to prepare a series of GVG concentrations in a range (10^{-6} to 10^{-4}M) that is appropriate for producing measureable inhibition of GABA-T activity within a short incubation time. Following incubation, one aliquot of the incubation mixture was taken to measure amount of GVG bound, and another was taken for measurement of GABA-T activity.

The aliquots assayed for GABA-T activity were diluted at least 20-fold, so that the concentration of GVG in the assay tube was below that able to influence GABA-T measurement during the assay procedure. Thus, the calculations of inactivated enzyme are related solely to inactivation which occurred during the initial binding incubation. Fig. 2 shows the results of this experiment.

Figure 2. Relationship between inactivation of GABA-T and binding of GVG in a homogenate of rat striatum.

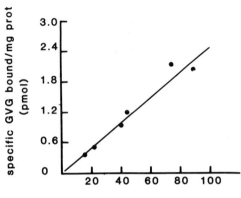

% inhibition of GABA-T activity

Amount of specific binding of GVG was calculated from the specific binding of [³H]GVG divided by the specific activity of [³H]GVG (radioactivity/moles GVG). The estimate of the number of enzyme molecules is based on the assumption that for every molecule of GVG bound, one molecule of enzyme has been inactivated. Thus, when the function is extrapolated to 100% enzyme inactivation, the amount of GVG bound is 2.6 pmol/mg protein, which corresponds to 1.6×10^{12} molecules of the enzyme present/mg protein of striatal tissue.

DISCUSSION

We have demonstrated the utility of [³H]GVG for measuring specific binding to GABA-T in brain homogenates. The procedure that we have developed appears specific for GABA-T and results in a relatively high percentage of specific binding. The resulting specific binding of [³H]GVG is linear with tissue obtained from several different brain regions up to concentrations of 8 ug protein/ul incubation mixture.

Our analysis of the binding of [³H]GVG in different regions of rat brain indicates a close correlation between [³H]GVG binding and GABA-T activity. Areas with highest [³H]GVG binding (superior colliculus, caudate putamen) also contain high GABA-T activity, while regions with lower [3H]GVG binding (cerebral cortex, cerebellar cortex) are also relatively low with respect to GABA-T activity. This observation is consistent with the mechanism of action of GVG being dependent upon the catalytic activity of GABA-T, an assumption supported by the fact that GABA-T inhibitors such as AOAA and 3-mercaptopropionic acid inhibit the binding of [3H]GVG. It is noteworthy that the concentrations of AOAA and 3MP that resulted in partial or complete inhibition of specific [3H]GVG binding correspond to those found to produce equivalent inhibition of the activity of the purified GABA-T (3,4). Since AOAA and 3MP at these concentrations are relatively selective inhibitors of GABA-T (3), it is likely that all of the specific binding of GVG is associated with GABA-T under the conditions of our assay. Furthermore, we have found that the pH optimum for [3H]GVG binding is 8.4 and the pH dependency of the binding (data not shown) corresponds precisely with that demonstrated for the activity of the purified enzyme (3,4).

Since there is a stoichiometric relationship between the number of [3H]GVG molecules bound and the number of GABA-T molecules inactivated, the labelled inhibitor affords us the possibility of calculating the number of enzyme molecules in a tissue homogenate. Previously, such calculations have been done for GABA-T with radioimmunoassay using an antibody to the enzyme (5). These calculations were based on competition with 125I-labelled purified GABA-T and assumed a molecular weight of 105,000. The problems inherent in such a procedure are typical of radioimmunoassay methods in general; the most outstanding concern is whether the crude GABA-T molecules in homogenates of various brain regions behave comparably to each other and to the purified GABA-T with respect to antibody binding. Whereas the procedure of Ossola et al. depends upon antigenicity, our procedure depends upon enzyme activity. Nevertheless, the value that we have obtained for the GABA-T concentration in homogenates of rat striatum using [3H]GVG (2.6 pmol/mg prot) are within an order of magnitude of the value reported by Ossola et al. (5) in rat striatum using the radioimmunoassay procedure (24 pmol/mg prot). It will be interesting to see whether the relative concentration of enzyme molecules across tissue from various brain regions derived from future studies with [3H]GVG will follow the same pattern observed using antibodies to GABA-T.

Radiolabelled GVG, in view of its ability to bind irreversibly to GABA-T, may now allow the characterization of the enzyme under conditions that have previously been inaccessible to experimental monitoring. In particular, since [^{3}H]GVG is readily taken up into brain tissue after either local micro-injection in vivo or perfusion of brain slices in vitro (Tavalalli and Gale, unpublished), [^{3}H]GVG may be used to probe ongoing GABA-T activity in intact animals or cellular elements. As Ossola et al (5) have commented with respect to measurements of GABA-T "ex vivo", "we cannot eliminate the possibility of an inactivating enzymatic process, ... in certain regions of the brain that is activated by tissue homogenization." Comparing the rates of in vivo labelling of GABA-T with [^{3}H]GVG in various brain areas may allow us to directly examine this possibility. Furthermore, [^{3}H]GVG may allow us to study changes in GABA-T activity in vivo as a function of development, drug treatments and other experimental variables.

[^{3}H]GVG may also prove useful for the direct autoradiographic localization of GABA-T. Again, the possibilities of irreversible labelling of the enzyme in vivo may afford a unique tracing procedure whereby labelled enzyme may be followed from its origin in GABAergic cell bodies to the axon terminals of these neurons.

In summary, [^{3}H]GVG was used to irreversibly label GABA-T in homogenates of rat brain. The binding procedure was specific for GABA-T and linear with tissue up to 8ug protein/ul. The specific binding was directly proportional to the enzyme activity in vitro and was completely inhibited by AOAA (100uM) and 3-MP (1.0mM). The binding procedure was used to estimate the amount of active enzyme in a homogenate of striatum.

1. Lippert B, Metcalf BW, Jung MJ and Casara P (1977). 4-amino-hex-5-enoic acid, a selective catalytic inhibitor of 4-aminobutyric acid amino transferase in mammalian brain. Eur J Biochem 74: 441
2. DeBoer TH, and Bruinvels J (1977). Assay and properties of 4-aminobutyric-2-oxoglutaric acid transaminase and succinic semialdehyde dehydrogenase in rat brain. J Neurochem 28: 471
3. Wu J-Y (1976). Purification, characterization and kinetic studies of GAD and GABA-T from mouse brain. in Roberts E, Chase TN and Tower DB (eds): "GABA in Nervous System Function", Raven Press, N.Y., p 7
4. Schousboe A, Wu J-Y and Roberts E (1973). Purification and characterization of the 4-aminobutyrate-2-ketoglutarate transaminase from mouse brain. Biochemistry 12: 2868
5. Ossola L, Maitre M, Blinderman J-M and Mandel P (1980). Turnover numbers of γ-aminobutyrate aminotransferase in some regions of rat brain. J Neurochem 34: 293

Glutamine, Glutamate, and GABA
in the Central Nervous System, pages 185–201
© 1983 Alan R. Liss, Inc., 150 Fifth Avenue, New York, NY 10011

IMMUNOHISTOCHEMISTRY OF GLUTAMATE AND GABA

J. Storm-Mathisen and O. P. Ottersen

Anatomical Institute, University of Oslo
Karl Johansgt. 47, Oslo 1, Norway

In contrast to the situation with amines and peptides,
there has been no satisfactory method for visualizing the
localization of amino acids in tissues. The success of
the immunocytochemical method for serotonin (Steinbusch et
al. 1978) encouraged us to try a similar approach for amino
acid transmitters (Storm-Mathisen et al. 1983). This should
be feasable because 1) free amino acids can be fixed in the
tissue by means of cross-linking agents such as glutaraldehyde, and 2) the fixation products thus formed are alien to
immunocompetent cells.

SERA AND SPECIFICITY

We crosslinked GABA or glutamate (Glu) with bovine serum
albumin (BSA) by means of distilled glutaraldehyde (G). The
dialysed conjugates, containing about 0.4umol of amino acid
bound pr. mg protein, were used to immunize rabbits. An
assay system was devised that allowed the specificities of
the sera to be evaluated in conditions similar to the ones
that tissue sections are exposed to when processed for
immunocytochemistry. Thus we extracted protein from rat
brain cortical tissue, dialysed it thoroughly against water
and coupling buffer till endogenous amino acids were no
longer detectable, and coupled the extract to cyanogen bromide activated Sepharose beads. Various amino acids and peptides were then bound to these beads by distilled G. For
processing, the beads were distributed in flat bottom wells
of microtiterplates which had been coated with
gelatin/chromalum to cause the beads to stick. The beads

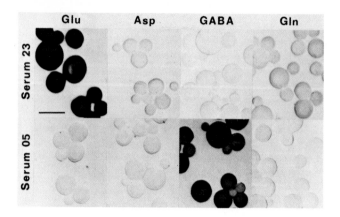

Fig. 1. Specificities of anti-Glu (upper row) and anti-GABA (lower row) sera after removing most of the crossreacting antibodies. Sepharose beads carrying brain protein were coupled to various amino acids by means of distilled glutaraldehyde, then processed with antisera in the same way as the tissue sections. Scale bar, 100um. (From Storm-Mathisen et al. 1983).

were preincubated with normal sheep serum, then incubated with antisera, and further processed according to the peroxidase-antiperoxidase method of Sternberger (1979). The beads were evaluated visually (Fig.1) or microdensitometrically (Table 1).

It proved necessary to remove undesired antibodies from the antisera in order to obtain the high specificities shown in Fig. 1 and Table 1. This was done by passing the sera through columns of Sepharose beads (S) to which were bound protein, and then an amino acid by means of G. The steps giving significant purification were for the anti-Glu sera: S-BSA, S-BSA-G-GABA (Fig. 1), S-BSA-G-Gln (Table 1); for the anti-GABA sera: S-BSA, S-BSA-G-Glu (Fig. 1), S-BSA-G-Tau (Table 1). Further passage of the sera through columns of beads carrying various polypeptides (native or treated with G), or of a Glu antiserum through S-BSA-G-Asp, had no discernible effect. The products showed high specificity, as the staining intensity was low with all amino acids tested other than the one against which the serum was

Compound fixed to brain protein	umol per ml gel	Glu antiserum 13 (1:200)	GABA antiserum 05 (1:80)
Glu	.32	100 ± 4	9 ± 1
Asp	.20	3 ± 1	5 ± 1
GABA	.53	5 ± 1	100 ± 7
Gln	.42	5 ± 1	12 ± 1
Gly	.49	2 ± 1	4 ± 1
Leu	.55	2 ± 1	11 ± 1
Pro	.84	5 ± 1	5 ± 1
Tau	.54	4 ± 1	6 ± 1
Ala	nd	1 ± 1	7 ± 1
Leu-Enk.	.62	5 ± 1	7 ± 1
Met-Enk.	nd	3 ± 1	8 ± 1
None	.00	7 ± 1	4 ± 1
Preimmune serum (Glu beads)		7 ± 1	4 ± 0.3

Table 1. Specificities of antisera demonstrated by microdensitometry of immuno-stained antigen-bearing Sepharose gel
beads. Absorbance (OD) is given as per cent of the maximum
for each serum (.189 ± .007 and .351 ± .024 for sera 13 and
05) and presented as mean ± s.e.m. of readings over 10-50
beads. (Data in part from Storm-Mathisen et al. 1983.)

raised. Similar low background staining was produced by a
preimmune serum (Table 1). The relatively low titres were
probably caused by the fact that the sera were frozen
and thawed repeatedly. Subsequent purified batches are
currently used at dilutions of 1:500 to 1:1500, and stored
at 4° with NaN_3.

Admittedly, the collection of amino acids and peptides
against which the sera have so far been tested (Table 1), is
relatively restricted. It does, however, comprise all the
free amino acids present at concentrations higher than
1umol/g in brain, and we feel the selectivity of the
staining is so good that the sera should be able to
visualize the tissue localizations of Glu and GABA.

TISSUE DISTRIBUTION, QUANTITATIVE ASPECTS

The tissue distributions of GABA-like and Glu-like immunoreactivities (GABA-LI and Glu-LI) suggest that this notion
is generally correct. We have used mice or rats fixed with
5% G in 0.1M sodium phosphate buffer pH 7.4 by perfusion
through the heart under pentobarbital anaesthesia after
briefly rinsing the vasculature with 2% dextran in buffer.
To minimize post mortem changes efforts were made to fix the
animals as rapidly as possible. Thus mice were becoming
stiff within one minute after opening the thorax. In model
experiments in slices we have found 5% G to cause retention
of about 50% of accumulated ^{3}H-labelled Glu or Asp, and
about 65% of GABA (Taxt, Storm-Mathisen 1979). Vibratome
sections (10-100um) were used and processed free-floating,
as already described (Storm-Mathisen et al. 1983). Control
sera (preimmune, immunized against wheat germ agglutinin, or
anti-Glu serum absorbed with S-BSA-G-Glu) produced weak and
diffuse staining (Fig. 3B). The very different staining
obtained by the anti-Glu and anti-GABA sera further emphasize the specificity.

In all parts of the CNS (see Ottersen, Storm-Mathisen
1984) there was a close similarity of the distribution of
GABA-LI to that of GAD, as visualized by immunocytochemistry
(Barber, Saito 1976; Barber et al. 1982; Goldowitz et al.
1982; Houser et al. 1980; Oertel et al. 1981; Perez de la
Mora et al. 1981; Ribak et al. 1977, 1978, 1979, 1980).
Regions known as rich in GAD, such as substantia nigra, globus pallidus, hypothalamus, preoptic region, and substantia
gelatinosa, were strongly stained.

The distribution of Glu-LI showed less dramatic differences between regions, as expected from the biochemically
determined distribution of endogenous Glu (Balcom et al.
1976). Particularly intense staining was found in the septal area, the periaqueductal grey and the interpeduncular
nucleus.

To obtain a more objective assessment of the relation
between staining intensity and endogenous contents of GABA
and Glu, microdensitometric measurements were taken over
stained sections and compared with biochemical data from the
literature (Fig. 2). To allow such a comparison, regions
were selected that are easily defined and relatively large and
homogeneous. The data of Balcom et al. (1975, 1976) were

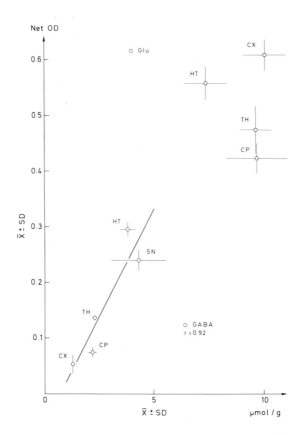

Fig. 2. Comparison of staining intensity (OD) for GABA-LI
and Glu-LI in immunocytochemical sections of perfusion fixed
mouse brains with biochemically determined tissue concentrations of GABA (Balcom et al. 1975) and Glu (Balcom et
al. 1976) in microwave fixed rat brains. The OD was determined microdensitometrically (Storm-Mathisen et al. 1983)
using a circular measuring spot of 60um diameter. Readings
(11-15 pr. section) were taken systematically to cover each
region and averaged. For each immunostained section a net OD
was obtained by subtracting the mean value of corresponding
averaged readings from 2-4 sections stained by control sera.
Mean net OD ($\overline{X}$) is based on 4 sections pr. region. Note
small interregional differences for Glu and Glu-LI and good
correlation between GABA and GABA-LI.

chosen because they are based on detailed dissection and on microwave killing, which may correspond more closely than conventional killing to our fast perfusion fixation. The correlation between microdensitometry and biochemistry is quite good for GABA, but not for Glu (Fig. 2). This is probably due in part to the relatively small interregional differences in Glu concentration, which are easily offset by uncertainties inherent in the different techniques. Thus one source of discrepancy is that the cytochemical reaction product is distributed differently between cell bodies, neuropil and fibres in the different regions, because the optical density (OD) underestimates the average concentration of a coloured product that is enriched in small areas (Ornstein 1952). This may explain the relatively low OD of Glu-LI in thalamus, where stained cells appeared to contribute particularly strongly to the total staining intensity, and in caudatoputamen, which contains myelinated fibre bundles with relatively low staining. Other obvious sources of differences are sampling (dissection/scanning with a 60um spot) and species (rat/mouse).

Further experiments should assess more directly the relation between staining intensity and amino acid content, and should also attempt to evaluate the possible influence of the microenvironment at the site of fixation. As the cross-linking by G is believed to occur largely with the E-amino groups of Lys, the protein composition may possibly affect the proportion of amino acid fixed. The relatively strong staining of nucleoplasm (rich in histones) and weak staining of nucleolus for both Glu-LI and GABA-LI (Fig. 3C, 5B,C) suggest that this factor has to be considered.

However, in spite of the necessary reservations, the presented data suggest that the staining intensities obtained by the immunocytochemical method may indeed be used as estimates of the endogenous contents of the amino acids.

CELLULAR LOCALIZATION

GABA-LI

The close similarity of GABA-LI and GAD immunocytochemistry (see above for refs.) was most striking at the cellular level. Stained bouton-like structures were seen in all regions, often in contact with cell bodies or dendrites (Fig. 3). Stained cell bodies generally appeared to be interneurones. In several cases, such as in the hippocampus (Fig. 3) and in the cerebellum, recognized GABA-ergic neurones contained GABA-LI. The great majority of thalamic cells with GABA-LI were located in the nucleus reticularis. The staining intensity in cell bodies appeared somewhat lower than in nerve terminals and axons. We have not tried colchicine pretreatment to augment perikaryal GABA-LI. Unlike GAD, GABA-LI was present even in the nucleus, which is to be expected as the nuclear pores should be penetrable to amino acids. Excitatory neurones, such as pyramidal cells of the cerebral neocortex and hippocampus, were not stained. An exception was the mossy fibres from area dentata to hippocampus CA3 and CA4 (Fig. 3A,C). The staining intensity in mossy fibre boutons was, however, much lower than in other GABA-LI positive boutons and is of unknown nature. It was not reduced following reduction of crossactivity to Tau after passage of the serum through S-BSA-G-Tau. Glial cells were usually not identifiable.

Axons with GABA-LI were abundant in capsula interna/crus cerebri rostral to the substantia nigra. As expected, they were also seen in cerebellar white matter and in the fasciculus longitudinalis medialis. It was somewhat unexpected to find such axons even in subcortical white matter and in fimbria hippocampi, as GABA in neocortex and hippocampus is mainly of intrinsic origin. This finding is, however, in line with recent evidence for GAD-containing afferents to neocortex (Vincent et al. 1983) and hippocampus (Seress, Ribak 1983), and with the observation that transection of the fimbria (Storm-Mathisen 1972) or cortical undercutting (Ulmar et al. 1975) lead to a small, but consistent reduction in hippocampal and cortical GAD.

Preliminary electronmicroscopic investigation in the hippocampus demonstrated GABA-LI in a subpopulation of nerve endings, often juxtaposed to dendritic shafts (Fig. 4). Nerve endings forming asymmetric contacts with spines were not seen to contain GABA-LI. The reaction product appeared concentrated to the core of synaptic vesicles. Mitochondria were relatively low in GABA-LI.

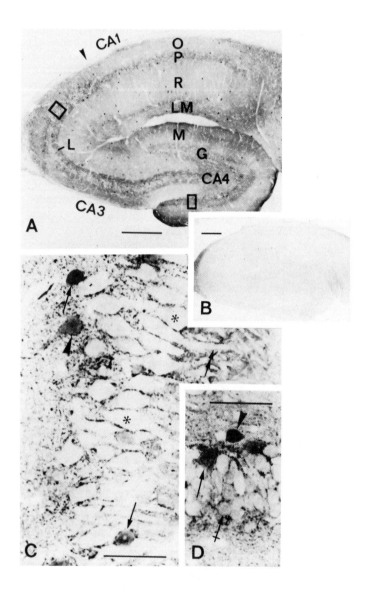

Fig. 3. (Facing page) Photomicrographs showing highly selective pattern of immunoreactivity in the perfusion fixed rat
hippocampal formation after incubation with an anti-GABA
serum (A,C,D), and absence of immunoreactivity after incubation with a preimmune serum (B). A: Neurones with GABA-LI
are scattered throughout the hippocampal formation. The
arrowhead is placed between CA1 and CA3; the upper and lower
frames indicate areas shown in C and D. Abbreviations in
this and other figures: G, stratum granulare; L, stratum
lucidum; LM, stratum lacunosum-moleculare; M, stratum moleculare fasciae dentatae, with zones Mo, Mm, and Mi; O, stratum oriens; P, stratum pyramidale; R, stratum radiatum; S,
subiculum. C: GABA-LI positive cells (arrows) are close to
the unstained pyramidal cells (asterisks). Arrowhead, GABA-
LI positive cell contacted by bouton-like stained dots;
double arrow, unstained pyramidal cell dendrite. Note weak,
diffuse staining in the stratum lucidum. D: GABA-LI positive
cells wedged between (arrow) or situated basal to
(arrowhead) the unlabelled granular cells (crossed arrow).
Scale: A,B: 0.5mm, C,D: 50um.

Glu-LI

In the perfusion fixed material Glu-LI was almost ubiquitous (see above). In grey matter the most conspicuous
feature was the strong staining of neuronal perikarya and
main dendrites (Fig. 5B,C). Like for GABA-LI, the nuclei
were stained, suggesting that Glu penetrates the nuclear
pores. The neuropil between large dendrites was relatively
diffusely stained, but bouton-like stained structures were
discernible in some preparations. Fibre tracts contained
numerous stained axons. In myelinated fibres the staining
was clearly restricted to the axis cylinder. Small glial-
like cell bodies could sometimes be identified as having a
low staining compared to the neuropil. The stained neuronal
perikarya included ones which are believed to use Glu or Asp
as transmitter, such as pyramidal cells in the cerebral cortex (Fig. 5C), but also ones not thought to be Glu-ergic.
The latter included cells in motor nuclei, locus coeruleus,
raphe, substantia nigra pars compacta, and the medial septal
area. At present we cannot say whether the concentration of
Glu-LI in these perikarya is different from that in putative
Glu-ergic cells. Some cells were, however, conspicuously
low in Glu-LI (Fig. 5B). These apparently included those

high in GABA-LI (Fig. 3C), suggesting that in these cells GAD has access to at least most of the Glu and converts the greater part of it to GABA.

The characteristic laminar distribution seen in regions such as the hippocampus for acidic amino acid uptake (Taxt, Storm-Mathisen 1979, 1983) was not reproduced for Glu-LI

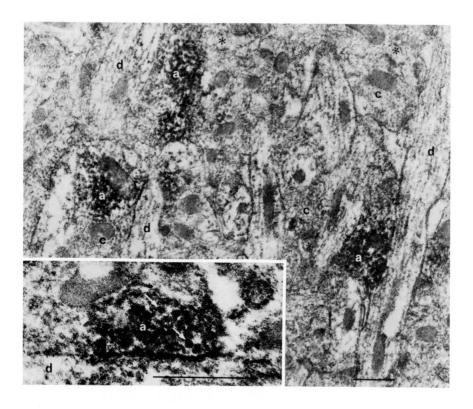

Fig. 4. Electronmicrographs from stratum radiatum of CA1 showing close relationship between GABA-LI positive boutons (a) and dendritic shafts (d). Unlabelled clear vesicle boutons (c) contact dendritic spines (asterisks) with dense postsynaptic specializations. Inset shows a GABA-LI positive bouton (a) at higher magnification. Note staining of vesicular structures (arrows) and at the zone of contact with the dendritic shaft (d). Material as in Fig. 3A, but osmicated and embedded in Araldite. Contrast staining with lead and uranyl salts. Scale: 0.5um.

in perfusion fixed material (Fig. 5A). The microscopic picture suggested that this could be due to the masking effect
of Glu-LI in dendrites and perikarya, structures that are
not labelled in the autoradiographic uptake experiments. In
agreement, slices (200um) cut from fresh hippocampus and
fixed in 5% G after incubation in Krebs solution at 25°,
exactly as for autoradiography after uptake of $[^3H]$Glu (or
$[^3H]$Asp), showed the distribution of Glu-LI to be the same
as that of Glu uptake sites. Microscopically the staining
was localized in bouton-like structures, while cell bodies
and larger dendrites were negative. In slices fixed
directly after cutting into cold sucrose (without incubation
in Krebs) the picture was similar, except that there was a
relatively stronger staining of bouton-like structures in
the area of termination of the lateral perforant path (Mo)
and of the mossy fibre boutons (L) (Fig. 6).

It seems that the in vitro treatment removes Glu from
the cell bodies and dendrites that are cut open in the
superficial parts of the slices accessible to immunochemistry and autoradiography, whereas the contents of the
boutons are left relatively intact. The ability of nerve
endings to retain endogeneous Glu in the Krebs medium may be
related to their ability to accumulate exogenous Glu. Glu
is known to be retained relatively well in synaptosomes
suspended in cold sucrose solution low in sodium and other
ions (Geddes et al. 1980; Nadler, Smith 1981). We would
like to suggest that the distribution of Glu-LI seen in slices treated with the sucrose medium may represent the in
vivo distribution of nerve terminal Glu (Fig. 6).

In one mouse the perfusion was inadequate in parts of the
brain, as evidenced by the presence of erythrocytes in
capillaries. Peripherally in the poorly perfused area the
distribution of Glu-LI was similar to that in slices cut into
cold sucrose before fixation, while centrally essentially all
Glu-LI was lost. GABA-LI was less affected. The lack of
Glu-LI in perikarya and dendrites in slices fixed in vitro may
therefore depend in part on factors other than the mechanical
damage, perhaps anoxia.

In electronmicroscopic preparations of sucrose treated
material mossy fibre boutons containing Glu-LI could be identified (Fig. 6C). As for GABA-LI, Glu-LI appeared to be concentrated in synaptic vesicles. Glu-LI in perfusion fixed
material has not yet been examined in the electronmicroscope.

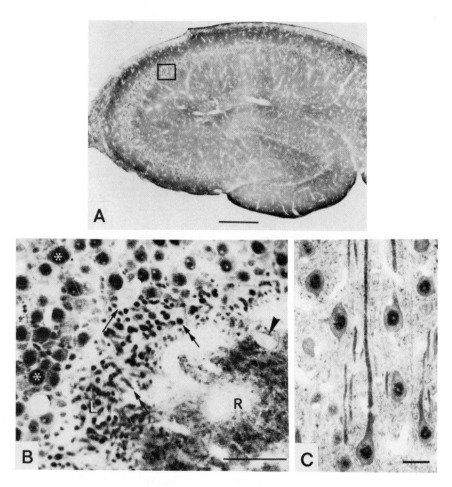

Fig. 5. Photomicrographs showing distribution of Glu-LI in the perfusion fixed rat (A) and mouse (B) hippocampus, and rat cerebral neocortex (C). Under low power the hippocampus appears rather uniformly stained (A), in striking contrast to immersion fixed hippocampi (Fig. 6A; see this for labelling of regions and zones). A part of CA3 (frame) of similar mouse material is enlarged in B. The pyramidal cell somata (asterisks) and dendrites (double arrows) are intensely labelled. Unstained, non-pyramidal cells occur e.g. in stratum radiatum (arrowhead) and pyramidale (arrow). Abbreviations in Fig. 3. C: Glu-LI positive pyramidal cells in the deep layers of the cortical barrel field (area 3). Scale: A: 0.5mm, B: 50um, C: 25um.

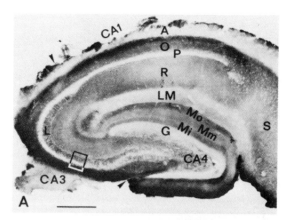

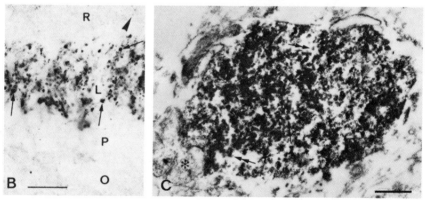

Fig. 6. Glu-LI in slices of rat hippocampal formation cut
into cold sucrose and immersion fixed. There is a highly
differential staining pattern (A; cf. Fig. 5A). Note that
the cell body layers (G,P) are unlabelled. The increased
staining intensity along the margins of the sections in this
and other figures is artifactual. Arrowheads indicate extent
of CA3; frame indicates area enlarged in B (adjacent slice).
B: Glu-LI is found in large dots, probably representing
mossy fibre terminals, in stratum lucidum (arrows), and in
smaller bouton-like dots (arrowhead) in stratum radiatum and
oriens. C: Electronmicrograph of same material, thin sectioned after embedding in Araldite, showing mossy fibre
bouton with Glu-LI in structures suggestive of vesicles
(double arrows). The bouton contacts an intraterminal spine
(asterisk). Abbreviations in Fig. 3. Scale: A: 0.5mm, B:
50um, C: 0.5um. (Adapted from Storm-Mathisen et al. 1983.)

CONCLUSIONS

The results show that GABA and Glu can be visualized immunocytochemically. The specificity appears very good, but further work is required to check all possible interfering substances, and to establish the quantitative relationship between endogeneous content and staining intensity, and the dependence of the latter on the local conditions during fixation.

The most important finding with the method so far is the apparent concentration of Glu-LI as well as GABA-LI in synaptic vesicles. Although better preparations must be awaited before firm conclusions can be drawn, this represents the first direct piece of evidence that amino acid transmitters are localized in synaptic vesicles. The observations are in line with biochemical data indicating that Glu is compartmentalized within nerve terminals (Kvamme, Lenda 1981) and accumulated by synaptic vesicles in vitro (Naito, Ueda 1983).

Another new finding is that tissue elements high in GABA-LI are generally low in Glu-LI, suggesting that in GABA-ergic neurones GAD is able to turn most of the Glu into GABA. In addition to confirming data known from GAD immunocytochemistry on the anatomy of GABA neurones, the results suggest that there are considerable amounts of GABA in the axons and perikarya of these neurones. The modest levels of Glu-LI as well as of GABA-LI in glia are in line with the notion that in glia Glu and GABA are converted to Gln, owing to glial glutamine synthetase (Norenberg, Martinez-Hernandez 1979; Norenberg, these Proceedings). While Glu-LI may not be restricted to putative Glu-ergic neurones in perfusion fixed material, it appears to demonstrate Glu-ergic nerve terminals in slices fixed in vitro.

It seems likely that the microscopic demonstration of amino acid-like immunoreactivities in the tissue could be used to investigate compartmentation and changes in the local concentrations of the amino acids induced by drugs, physiological stimuli, and pathological conditions. Possibly even the release process could be visualized. The present approach should be applicable to any small molecule that can be bound to tissue macromolecules by a suitable fixative in such a way that the structure of the fixation product is characteristic of the molecule in question.

We would like to acknowledge the help of AT Bore, P Edminson, T Eliassen, S Fossum, I Fridstrøm, E Gregersen, F-MS Haug, JH Johansen, AK Leknes (deceased), G Lothe, E Risnes, J Line Vaaland, and K Ruud Øztürk. Supported by the Norwegian Research Council for Science and the Humanities.

Balcom GJ, Lenox RH, Meyerhoff JL (1975). Regional y-aminobutyric acid levels in rat brain determined after microwave fixation. J Neurochem 24:609-613.

Balcom GJ, Lenox RH, Meyerhoff JL (1976). Regional glutamate levels in rat brain determined after microwave fixation. J Neurochem 26:423-425.

Barber R, Saito K (1976). Light microscopic visualization of GAD and GABA-T in immunocytochemical preparations of rodent CNS. In: Roberts E, Chase TN, Tower DB (eds), "GABA in Nervous System Function," Raven Press, New York, pp 113-132.

Barber RP, Vaughn JE, Roberts E (1982). The cytoarchitecture of GABAergic neurons in rat spinal cord. Brain Res 238:305-328.

Geddes JW, Newstead JD, Wood JD (1980). Stability of the glutamate content of synaptosomes during their preparation. Neurochem Res 5:1107-1116.

Goldowitz D, Vincent SR, Wu J-Y, Hökfelt T (1982). Immunohistochemical demonstration of plasticity in GABA neurons of the adult rat dentate gyrus. Brain Res 238:413-420.

Houser CR, Vaughn JE, Barber RP, Roberts E (1980). GABA neurons are the major cell type of the nucleus reticularis thalami. Brain Res 200:341-354.

Kvamme E, Lenda K (1981). Evidence for compartmentalization of glutamate in rat brain synaptosomes using the glutamate sensitivity of phosphate-activated glutaminase as a functional test. Neurosci Lett 25:193-198.

Nadler JV, Smith EM (1981). Perforant path lesion depletes glutamate content of fascia dentata synaptosomes. Neurosci Lett 25:275-280.

Naito S, Ueda T (1983). Adenosine triphosphate-dependent uptake of glutamate into protein I-associated synaptic vesicles. J Biol Chem 258:696-699.

Norenberg MD, Martinez-Hernandez A (1979). Fine structural localization of glutamine synthetase in astrocytes of rat brain. Brain Res 161:303-310.

Oertel WH, Schmechel DE, Mugnaini E, Tappaz ML, Kopin IJ
(1981). Immunocytochemical localization of glutamate
decarboxylase in rat cerebellum with a new antiserum.
Neuroscience 6:2715-2735.
Ornstein L (1952). The distributional error in
microspectrophotometry. Lab Invest 1:250-265.
Ottersen OP, Storm-Mathisen J (1984). Neurones con-
taining or accumulating transmitter amino acids. In:
Björklund A, Hökfelt T (eds), "Handbook of Chemical
Neuroanatomy," Elsevier/North-Holland, Amsterdam, Vol 2,
Chapter 10, in press.
Perez de la Mora M, Possani LD, Tapia R, Teran L,
Palacios R, Fuxe K, Hökfelt T, Ljungdahl Å (1981).
Demonstration of central y-aminobutyrate-containing nerve
terminals by means of antibodies against glutamate
decarboxylase. Neuroscience 6:875-895.
Ribak CE, Vaughn JE, Saito K, Barber R, Roberts
E (1977). Glutamate decarboxylase localization in neurons
of the olfactory bulb. Brain Res 126:1-18.
Ribak CE, Vaughn JE, Saito K (1978). Immunocytochemical localization of glutamic acid decarboxylase in
neuronal somata following colchicine inhibition of axonal
transport. Brain Res 140:315-332.
Ribak CE, Vaughn JE, Roberts E (1979). The GABA
neurons and their axon terminals in rat corpus striatum as
demonstrated by GAD immunocytochemistry. J Comp Neurol
187:261-284.
Ribak CE, Vaughn JE, Roberts E (1980). GABAergic
nerve terminals decrease in the substantia nigra following
hemitransections of the striatonigral and pallidonigral
pathways. Brain Res 192:413-420.
Seress L, Ribak CE (1983). GABAergic cells in
the dentate gyrus appear to be local circuit and projection
neurons. Exp Brain Res 50:173-182.
Steinbusch HWM, Verhofstad AAJ, Joosten HWJ
(1978). Localization of serotonin in the central nervous system by immunohistochemistry: description of a
specific and sensitive technique and some applications.
Neuroscience 3:811-819.
Sternberger LA (1979). "Immunocytochemistry, Second
Edition." John Wiley, New York, pp 354.
Storm-Mathisen J (1972). Glutamate decarboxylase in rat hippocampal region after lesions of the afferent fibre systems. Evidence that the enzyme is localized in intrinsic
neurones. Brain Res 40:215-235.

Storm-Mathisen J, Leknes AK, Bore AT, Vaaland, JL,
  Edminson P, Haug F-MŠ, Ottersen OP (1983). First
  visualization of glutamate and GABA in neurones by immunocytochemistry. Nature 301:517-520.
Taxt T, Storm-Mathisen J (1979). Tentative localization
  of glutamergic and aspartergic nerve endings in brain.
  J Physiol (Paris) 75:667-684.
Taxt T, Storm-Mathisen J (1983). Uptake of D-aspartate
  and L-glutamate in excitatory axon terminals in hippocampus: autoradiographic and biochemical comparison with
  y-aminobutyrate and other amino acids in normal and
  lesioned rats. Neuroscience, in press (accepted 7 July
  1983).
Ulmar G, Ljungdahl Å, Hökfelt T (1975). Enzyme changes after
  undercutting of cerebral cortex in the rat. Exp Neurol
  46:199-208.
Vincent SR, Hökfelt T, Skirboll LR, Wu J-Y (1983). Hypothalamic y-aminobutyric acid neurons project to the neocortex.
  Science 220:1309-1311.

METABOLISM OF GLUTAMINE, GLUTAMATE, AND GABA AT THE CELLULAR AND SUBCELLULAR LEVEL

Glutamine, Glutamate, and GABA
in the Central Nervous System, pages 205–217
© 1983 Alan R. Liss, Inc., 150 Fifth Avenue, New York, NY 10011

THE METABOLIC COMPARTMENTATION CONCEPT

S. Berl and *D.D. Clarke

Mt. Sinai School of Medicine, Bronx,
N.Y. 10458; *Department of Chemistry,
Fordham University, New York, N.Y. 10029.

The concept of metabolic compartmentation describes the presence in a tissue of functionally different and chemically distinct pools of a given substrate. These separate pools equilibrate only very slowly, if at all, and exhibit different turnover and flux rates. Such heterogeneous functional pools of amino acids were coming under investigation in microorganisms (Britten et al. 1955; Cowie, Walton 1956; Cowie, McClure 1959), plants (Steward et al. 1956; MacLennan et al. 1963), and animal tissues (Korner, Tarver 1957; Green, Lowther 1959; Kipnis et al. 1961) at about the same time that we began our studies on glutamate-glutamine metabolism in brain. The first reference to the term metabolic compartmentation that we have noted is in the work of Stuart et al. (1956). In their studies on the carrot root explant, they found tht glutamic acid derived from [U-^{14}C]glutamine had a higher specific activity (counts/min/μmol, SA) than the glutamine isolated from the tissue, a situation opposite to that which prevails in brain. They deduced that there were two separate pools of glutamine, only one of which was active in glutamate synthesis. Their studies with the growing carrot root also demonstrated that [^{14}C]glucose labeled more readily protein glutamic acid than did [^{14}C]glutamine. GABA was also shown to be readily converted to glutamic acid and glutamine. Our studies with brain led to the conclusion that compartmentation of metabolic events was the most logical explanation of the phenomena we were observing.

I.V. Administration of [^{14}C]Glutamate

The earliest results which suggested this idea came from short-term experiments in which [^{14}C]glutamate was injected intravenously into rats and mice and the specific activities of the glutamate and glutamine were measured in various organs and plasma (Lajtha et al. 1959). It was noted that the SA of the glutamine isolated from the plasma was usually greater than that of tissue glutamine or glutamic acid (Table 1). It was postulated that the administered labeled glutamate did not mix with total tissue glutamate but was in part converted to glutamine which returned to the blood without prior equilibration with tissue glutamate. In these studies, very little of the administered labeled glutamate entered the brain although some exchange between plasma and brain glutamate appeared to occur.

Table 1. I.V. Administration of [^{14}C]glutamic acid in rat

Organ	Specific Activity (SA)	
	Glutamic Acid	Glutamine
Plasma	3200	670
Brain	43	17
Liver	1800	470
Kidney	860	470
Muscle	400	46

[U-^{14}C-]-L-Glutamic acid (0.5 μCi, 0.1 ml) was injected via the tail vein. Animals were decapitated 5 min after administration of the radioactivity. Specific activity: counts/min/μmole.

Intracisternal Administration of [^{14}C]Glutamate

To bypass the blood-brain barrier [^{14}C]L-glutamate was injected intracerebrally and its conversion to glutamine was examined (Berl et al. 1961). Radioactive glutamate rapidly left the brain and was metabolized in other organs. In plasma and liver, the expected product-precursor relationship was seen (Table 2). However in brain it was evident that the expected product-precursor relationship of glutamine to glutamate did not occur since, within minutes,

Table 2. Intracisternal administration of [¹⁴C]glutamic acid in rat

Time (min)	Substrate	Specific Activity			RSA
		Plasma	Brain	Liver	
0.25	GA		7,700		
	Gm		3,300		0.43
1	GA	180,000	5,500	200	
	Gm	1,200	7,300	66	1.3
2	GA	130,000	3,200	800	
	Gm	2,200	12,000	600	3.8
5	GA	34,000	2,700	700	
	Gm	6,100	14,000	760	5.2
15	GA	8,900	2,200	190	
	Gm	6,500	11,000	280	5.0
30	GA	3,300	2,100	180	
	Gm	870	7,300	240	3.5

[U-¹⁴C]L-Glutamic acid (0.8 μCi in 0.02 ml of normal saline) was injected into the cisterna magna. GA: glutamic acid; Gm: glutamine; RSA: relative specific activity of the glutamine in brain, glutamate = 1.

the radiospecific activity of the isolated glutamine was several times that of the isolated glutamic acid. In a homogenous one compartment system in which an immediate precursor is administered, it is anticipated that, as the SA of the precursor falls, that of the product rises and achieves a SA equal to or slightly greater than that of the precursor (Reiner 1953). In brain the relative specific activity (RSA) of glutamine (glutamate = 1) was 5 or more. In fact, when the RSA of glutamine to that of glutamate was highest (at 5 min), its SA was greater than that present in the highest glutamic acid SA measured at 15 sec. This was equally true in several different parts of the brain (Berl et al. 1961)(Table 3).

Another indication of the heterogeneity of the gluta-

mate pools in brain can be seen in the finding that the RSA
of GABA was much less than 1. Hence the glutamate pool
active in making glutamine is not the same as the one active
in the synthesis of GABA.

Table 3. Intracisternal administration of [^{14}C]glutamic
acid: labeling of glutamine and GABA in brain areas

Brain Area	SA	RSA	
	Glutamate	Glutamine	GABA
Posterior Cerebrum	4,600	3.9	0.12
Cerebellum	7,000	5.3	0.34
Pons-medulla	14,000	5.0	0.23

[U-^{14}C]-L-Glutamic acid (0.02 ml, 0.8 µCi in normal saline)
was injected into the cisterna magna of rats. Animals decapitated 2 min after injection, the brain dissected and frozen
on dry ice. SA: counts/min/µmole; RSA: SA/SA glutamate.

Intracisternal Administration of ^{14}C-Aspartate

The metabolism of [^{14}C]-L-aspartic acid as the tracer
was similarly studied following intracisternal administration (Berl et al. 1961). Again the specific radioactivities
of the glutamine relative to that of glutamic acid were in
the range of 4-5.5 (Table 4). Under these circumstances, in
a homogeneous system, it would have been expected that, as

Table 4. Intracisternal administration of [^{14}C]aspartate:
labeling of glutamine and GABA in brain areas

Brain Area	SA	RSA		
	Glutamate	Glutamine	GABA	Aspartate
Posterior Cerebrum	1700	5.5	0.15	34.1
Cerebellum	3400	4.7	0.20	47.1
Pons-Medulla	4500	4.0	0.07	15.6

U-^{14}C-L-Aspartate (0.02 ml, 1 µCi in normal saline) was
injected into the cisterna magna of rats. The animals were
decapitated after 2 min, the brain dissected and frozen on
dry ice.

the SA of the glutamate rises, that of the glutamine would also rise but at a slower rate and eventually equal or slightly exceed that of the glutamic acid (Reiner 1953) but not exceed it by a factor of 5. The explanation offered for these phenomena was that the administered or newly formed glutamate mixed only with a small part of the total tissue glutamate before being converted to glutamine. When the total tissue content of the amino acids was extracted, the SA of the glutamate was greatly decreased and was measured as less than that of the glutamine.

Intracisternal Administration of ^{14}C-Glutamine

When [^{14}C]glutamine was the labeled precursor administered intracisternally, the RSA of GABA (glutamate = 1) ranged from 0.5-0.9 (Table 5; Berl et al. 1961). This should be compared to values of 0.12-0.34 attained when ^{14}C-glutamate was administered (Table 3). It is clear that the glutamate formed from glutamine labels the GABA pool more

Table 5. Intracisternal administration of ^{14}C-glutamine: labeling of glutamate, aspartate and GABA in brain areas

Brain Area	SA		RSA	
	Glutamate	Glutamine	GABA	Aspartate
Posterior Cerebrum	330	12	0.5	0.7
Cerebellum	860	12	0.9	0.7
Pons-Medulla	930	13	0.6	0.5

U-^{14}C-L-Glutamine (0.02 ml, 1 µCi in normal saline) was injected into the cisterna magna of rats. The animals were decapitated after 2 min, the areas dissected and frozen on dry ice.

readily than does administered glutamate. More recently, it has been shown that glutamine can serve more readily as a source of releasable glutamate than glucose (Hamberger et al. 1979a,b). Formation of glutamine probably functions, not only to neutralize released transmitter glutamate, but also to recycle the carbon skeleton for reuse as transmitter glutamate or GABA at nerve endings (Bradford et al. 1978).

Metabolism of [1-¹⁴C]Acetate

Peripherally administered [1-¹⁴C]acetate is readily converted to amino acids in brain (Busch 1953). Following saphenous vein injections in the cat of tracer amounts of labeled acetate, the glutamate, glutamine, aspartate and GABA were rapidly labeled in the cortex, thalamus and caudate nucleus (Berl, Frigyesi 1969). The decay rates of the amino acids showed two exponential decrements, one with a half-life of approximately 11-16 min and a slower one with a half-life of approximately 3-4 hr. In addition, the specific activity of the isolated glutamine was always greater than the SA of the isolated glutamic acid and the peak SA of the former was greater than the peak SA of the latter. These phenomena require a heterogeneous compartmented system for explanation.

Metabolism of ¹⁵N-Ammonium Acetate

In brain, metabolism of ammonia is closely associated with the synthesis of glutamate and glutamine and, therefore, studies on ammonia detoxification provided other information on the metabolic compartmentation of this system (Berl et al. 1962). [¹⁵N]Ammonium acetate was infused at a constant rate into the carotid artery of the cat for varying periods of time; this constant feed provided data on the accumulation of isotope rather than decay of isotope in the amino acids. The results of a representative experiment of 25 min duration is seen in Table 6. In brain, aside from the free ammonia, the amide moiety of glutamine had the highest concentration of ¹⁵N. The α-amino moiety of the glutamine was approximately 10 times higher in ¹⁵N content than the α-amino moiety of glutamate. The cerebral glutamine must have been derived from a pool of glutamate that did not equilibrate with the total tissue glutamate. It was also apparent that blood glutamate was not the source of glutamine formation in the cortex since the α-amino group of the brain glutamine had a higher concentration of ¹⁵N than that of the blood glutamic acid. Also, the amide and α-amino nitrogen of the brain glutamine was higher in ¹⁵N than that of the amino acid isolated from the blood. Since glutamate dehydrogenase is required for the direct incorporation of ¹⁵NH₃ into α-ketoglutarate for the formation of glutamate, the data point to the association of this enzyme with the synthesis of that small pool of glutamate which functions in

Table 6.   Intravenous infusion of [^{15}N]ammonium acetate into the cat: isotope distribution in amino acids

	Cerebral Cortex		Blood	
	μmol/g	^{15}N	μmol/g	^{15}N
Glutamate	9.3	0.87	0.08	3.1
Glutamine α-amino	7.8	8.6	0.32	1.8
amide	7.8	38.7	0.32	21.4
Aspartate	1.9	0.67	--	--
GABA	1.2	0.22	--	--
Urea	5.9	1.3	7.7	15.0
Ammonia	1.8	66.0	2.8	82.0

^{15}N-Ammonium acetate (99.6 atom % excess; 1 mmol/ml) was infused into the carotid artery of the cat at a uniform rate of 0.67 ml/min for 24 min. ^{15}N-content expressed as atom % excess.

the formation of glutamine, at least in the presence of relatively high levels of ammonia. In more recent studies Cooper et al. (1979) infused radioactive [^{13}N]ammonia at physiological concentrations of ammonia via the internal carotid artery of the rat. Their data corroborated our findings and were consistent with the concept that ammonia entering the brain from the blood is metabolized in a small pool of glutamate that is turning over very rapidly and distinct from a larger tissue pool of glutamate. Therefore, the compartmentation of glutamate metabolism seen with ^{15}NH$_3$ could not be ascribed to the toxic effect of NH$_3$.

Metabolism of NaH^{14}CO$_3$

     In our series of experiments with toxic levels of ammonia, it was evident, as previously reported by others (Flock et al. 1953; Eisman, Clark 1958), that glutamine levels increased in brain without a concomitant decrease in glutamate concentration. For this to occur, 4-carbon units must have been replenished in the Krebs' tricarboxylic acid cycle; a likely pathway for such replacement would be CO_2 fixation in the brain tissue. Intravenous infusion of NaH^{14}CO$_3$ in the cat resulted in incorporation of labeled CO_2 into aspartic acid, glutamic acid and glutamine (Berl et al. 1962; Waelsch et al. 1964). A representative experiment is shown in Table

Table 7. Intravenous infusion of $NaH^{14}CO_3$ into the cat: isotope distribution in amino acids of the cerebral cortex

Duration	SA	RSA		
Min	Glutamate	Glutamine	Aspartate	α-KG
4.5	250	1.9	8.6	4.4
8.5	840	1.1	4.6	2.1
17.0	1380	1.8	3.3	1.56

1.7 ml of bicarbonate solution (0.06 M, 0.29 mCi/ml in saline) was given during the 1st ten seconds to bring the SA of the blood CO_2 to a precalculated level. Infusion was then continued at a rate of 0.2 ml/min. Infusion was into the inferior vena cava via a cannula inserted into the femoral vein.

7. CO_2 fixation occurred at the oxaloacetate level since aspartic acid had the highest SA. The SA of the glutamine was again higher than that of its precursor glutamic acid. Following simultaneous infusion of ammonium acetate and labeled bicarbonate, the SA of the glutamine increased, although there was little change in the SA of the glutamate or aspartate (Table 8). It appeared that the newly formed oxaloacetate was rapidly channelled into glutamine synthesis. The SA of the ketoglutarate was also higher than that of the glutamate. This suggests that the Krebs' cycle intermediates are also compartmented.

Table 8. Intravenous infusion of $NaH^{14}CO_3$ and ammonium acetate into the cat: isotope distribution in amino acids of the cerebral cortex

Duration	SA	RSA		
Min	Glutamate	Glutamine	Aspartate	α-KG
15.5	1520	5.2	3.9	2.1
16.0	1320	4.1	1.8	1.9

1.7 ml of bicarbonate solution (0.06 M, 0.29 mCi/ml) was rapidly injected and immediately followed by a constant infusion at 0.2 ml/min of ammonium acetate (2.5M) containing $NaH^{14}CO_3$ (0.6M, 0.29 mCi/ml). See Table 7 for other details.

Specific Activity Less Than 1

There are several substrates which do not demonstrate compartmentation as shown by the glutamate-glutamine system. These are glucose (Cremer 1964; Gaitonde 1965; O'Neal, Koeppe 1966; O'Neal et al. 1966), lactate and glycerol (O'Neal, Koeppe 1966; O'Neal et al. 1966): substances which probably enter all compartments and thereby give an RSA of glutamine to glutamate of <1. Acetoacetate and β-hydroxy-butyrate (Cremer 1971) have been added to this list. The latter two substances probably preferentially label the large pool of glutamate and therefore the RSA of glutamine is 1.

In Vitro Studies

If metabolic compartmentation of the glutamate-glutamine system demonstrable in vivo is a cellular event occurring in the brain tissue, it should also be demonstrable in brain slice preparations. Results similar to those obtained in vivo were obtained in vitro with [^{14}C]-labeled glutamate, aspartate, acetate, bicarbonate and GABA (Berl et al. 1968; 1970). With all of these substrates, the SA of the isolated glutamine was higher than the SA of the isolated glutamate.

Development of Compartmentation

The glutamate-glutamine compartmentation system is not evident at birth but develops in the brain with maturation (Berl 1965). This was studied in kittens by the application of [U-^{14}C]-L-glutamate to the surface of the cortex. During the first three weeks of life, the SA of the glutamine was below that of the glutamate. During the fourth week, the RSA of the glutamine rose to values approaching 3 and to values of 4 in animals six weeks of age. In rats, similar developmental aspects were seen with the RSA of glutamine becoming greater than 1 during the critical period of development of two-three weeks (Patel, Balazs 1970). In these experiments, labeled leucine was injected subcutaneously and the radioactivity in the isolated amino acids measured.

Location of Compartments

The obvious question which arises is where is the

anatomical localization of these compartments since cellular
or subcellular organizations are the most likely basis for
such compartmentation.

Most of the data can be explained by the oversimplified
assumption of 2 or 3 compartments. It would place the small
pool of glutamate active in glutamine formation in the glia,
the large pool of glutamate in neurons and their extensions,
with a subpool of the larger glutamate pool in nerve endings.
Such a localization could be supported by the maturational
studies since the manifestation of compartmentation occurs
during the development of neuronal cell bodies and the neuropil, which comprises the axons and dendrites. However, the
glia are also developing at this time. The small pool would
be expected to be associated with glutamine synthetase, glutamate dehydrogenase and with acetyl CoA synthase, the enzyme
which converts acetate to acetyl CoA. In animals in which
ammonia was infused or a hepato-portal shunt was performed
(Cavanagh 1974), the astrocytes, rather than the neurons,
were most severely affected and histochemical studies showed
increased glutamate dehydrogenase activity localized to the
astrocytes (Norenberg 1976). In humans with hepatic encephalopathy, the astrocytes again are the cells showing the
greatest changes (Cavanagh 1976). In addition, glutamate
dehydrogenase has been reported to be low in synaptosomes
(Neidle et al. 1969; Wilson, Barch 1971) and in nerve cell
bodies (Kuhlman, Lowry 1956). A major support for the place-
ment of the small compartment in the glia came from an
immunohistochemical study which indicated that glutamine
synthetase was concentrated in the glia and not evident by
this technique in neuronal cell bodies, endothelial cells or
choroid epithelium (Martinez-Hernandez et al. 1977). In retina, the metabolism of glutamate and GABA is compartmentalized as in brain (Starr 1974; Kennedy et al. 1974). Immunohistochemical techniques have also shown that, in rat retinal
tissue, glutamine synthetase is localized in the Muller cells
which are considered to be the retinal glia (Riepe, Norenberg
1977). Gombos (personal communication), by similar methods,
has also found glutamine synthetase to be concentrated in the
glial Bergmann cells of the cerebellum. In other supportive
studies, glutamate dehydrogenase and acetyl CoA synthase were
demonstrated to be enriched in a fraction of brain mitochondria that sedimented more rapidly in a sucrose density gradient than the average of all brain mitochondria (Reijnierse
et al. 1975). This fraction of mitochondria may be characteristic of glial cells but there is no direct evidence for
this.

Thus, the many studies on metabolic compartmentation of amino acids in brain support the supposition that glia function in the rapid uptake and metabolism of exogenous or extracellular transmitter amino acids and ammonia. As a corollary to this function, carbon skeleton and amino nitrogen are conserved and recycled.

REFERENCES

Berl S (1965). Compartmentation of glutamic acid metabolism in developing cerebral cortex. J Biol Chem 240:2047.

Berl S, Frigyesi TL (1969). The turnover of glutamate, glutamine, aspartate and GABA labeled with 1-^{14}C-acetate in caudate nucleus, thalamus and motor cortex (cat). Brain Res 12:444.

Berl S, Lajtha A, Waelsch H (1961). Amino acid and protein metabolism - VI. Cerebral compartments of glutamic acid metabolism. J Neurochem 7:186.

Berl S, Nicklas WJ, Clarke DD (1968). Compartmentation of glutamic acid metabolism in brain slices. J Neurochem 15:131.

Berl S, Nicklas WJ, Clarke DD (1970). Compartmentation of citric acid cycle metabolism in brain: Labeling of glutamate, glutamine, aspartate and GABA by several radioactive tracer metabolites. J Neurochem 17:1009.

Berl S, Takagaki G, Clarke DD, Waelsch H (1962a). Metabolic compartments in vivo. Ammonia and glutamic acid metabolism in brain and liver. J Biol Chem 237:2562.

Berl S, Takagaki G, Clarke DD, Waelsch H (1962b). Carbon dioxide fixation in the brain. J Biol Chem 237:2570.

Bradford HF, deBelleroche JS, Ward HK (1978). On the metabolic and intrasynaptic origin of amino acid transmitters. In Fonnum F (ed): " Amino Acids as Chemical Transmitters," New York: Plenum Press, p 367.

Britten RJ, Roberts RB, French EF (1955). Amino acid absorption and protein synthesis in Escherichia coli. Proc Natl Acad Sci USA 41:863.

Busch H (1953). Studies on the metabolism of acetate-1-^{14}C in tissues of tumor-bearing rats. Cancer Res 15:365.

Cavanagh JB (1975). Liver bypass and the glia. In Plum F (ed): "Brain Dysfunction in Metabolic Disorders," New York: Raven Press, p 13.

Cooper AJL, McDonald JM, Gelbard AS, Gledhill RF, Duffy TE (1979). The metabolic fate of ^{13}N-labeled ammonia in rat brain. J Biol Chem 254:4982.

Cowie DB, McClure FT (1959). Metabolic pools and the

synthesis of macromolecules. Biochim Biophys Acta 31:236.

Cowie DB, Walton BP (1956). Kinetics of formation and utilization of metabolic pools in the biosynthesis of protein and nucleic acid. Biochim Biophys Acta 21:211.

Cremer JE (1964). Amino acid metabolism in rat brain studied with ^{14}C-labeled glucose. J Neurochem 11:165.

Cremer JE (1971). Incorporation of label from D-β-hydroxy-[^{14}C]butyrate and [3-^{14}C]acetoacetate into amino acids in rat brains in vivo. Biochem J 122:135.

Eisman B, Clark GM (1958). Studies in ammonia metabolism. III. The experimental production of coma by carotid arterial infusion of ammonium salts. Surgery 43:476.

Flock EV, Block MA, Grindlay JH, Mann FC, Bollman JL (1953). Changes in free amino acids of brain and muscle after total hepatectomy. J Biol Chem 200:529.

Gaitonde MK (1965). Rate of utilization of glucose and compartmentation of α-oxoglutarate and glutamate in rat brain. Biochem J 95:803.

Green NM, Lowther DA (1959). Formation of collagen hydroxyproline in vitro. Biochem J 71:55.

Hamberger A, Chiang GH, Nylen ES, Scheff SW, Cotman CW (1979a). Glutamate as a CNS transmitter. I: Evaluation of glucose and glutamine as precursors for the synthesis of preferentially released glutamate. Brain Res 168:513.

Hamberger A, Chiang GH, Sandoval E, Cotman CW (1979b). Glutamate as a CNS transmitter. II. Regulation of synthesis in the releasable pool. Brain Res 168:531.

Kennedy AJ, Voaden MJ, Marshall J (1974). Glutamate metabolism in the frog retina. Nature 252:50.

Kipnis DM, Reis E, Helmreich E (1961). Functional heterogeneity of the intracellular amino acid pool in mammalian cells. Biochim Biophys Acta 51:519.

Korner A, Tarver H (1957). Studies in protein synthesis in vitro. VI. Incorporation and release of amino acids in particulate preparations from livers of rats. J Gen Physiol 41:219.

Kuhlman RE, Lowry OH (1956). Quantitative histochemical changes during the development of the rat cerebral cortex. J Neurochem 1:173.

Lajtha A, Berl S, Waelsch H (1959). Amino acid and protein metabolism of the brain - IV. The metabolism of glutamic acid. J Neurochem 3:322.

MacLennan DH, Beevers H, Harley JL (1963). "Compartmentation" of acids in plant tissues. Biochem J 89:316.

Martinez-Hernandez A, Bell KP, Norenberg MD (1977). Glutamine synthetase: Glial localization in brain. Science 195:1356.

Neidle A, Van den Berg CJ, Grynbaum A (1969). Heterogeneity of rat brain mitochondria isolated in continuous sucrose gradients. J Neurochem 16:225.

Norenberg MD (1976). Histochemical studies in experimental porto-systemic encephalopathy. Arch Neurol 33:265.

O'Neal RM, Koeppe RE (1966). Precursors in vivo of glutamate, aspartate and their derivatives of rat brain. J Neurochem 13:835.

O'Neal RM, Koeppe RE, Williams EI (1966). Utilization in vivo of glucose and volatile fatty acids by sheep brain for the synthesis of acidic amino acids. Biochem J 101:591.

Patel AJ, Balazs R (1970). Manifestation of metabolic compartmention during the maturation of the rat brain. J Neurochem 17:955.

Reijnierse GLA, Veldstra H, Van den Berg CJ (1975). Short-chain fatty acid synthesis in brain. Biochem J 152:477.

Reiner JM (1953). The study of turnover rates by means of isotopic tracers. Arch Biochem Biophys 46:53.

Riepe RE, Norenberg MD (1977). Muller cell localization of glutamine synthetase in rat retina. Nature 268:654.

Starr MS (1974). Evidence for compartmentation of glutamate metabolism in isolated rat retina. J Neurochem 23:337.

Steward FC, Bidwell GS, Yemm EW (1956). Protein metabolism, respiration and growth. Nature 178:734.

Waelsch H, Berl S, Rossi CA, Clarke DD, Purpura DD (1964). Quantitative aspects of CO_2 fixation in mammalian brain in vivo. J Neurochem 11:717.

Wilson JE, Barch D (1971). Heterogeneity of rat brain mitochondria. Fed Proc 30:1139 (abst.).

**Glutamine, Glutamate, and GABA
in the Central Nervous System, pages 219–231**
© **1983 Alan R. Liss, Inc., 150 Fifth Avenue, New York, NY 10011**

RELATIVE CONTRIBUTIONS OF NEURONS AND GLIA TO METABOLISM OF
GLUTAMATE AND GABA

William J. Nicklas, Ph.D.

Department of Neurology
UMDNJ-Rutgers Medical School
Piscataway, N.J.   08854

The current working hypothesis, for which a great deal
of evidence has been obtained, is that glia, in addition to
neurons, contribute significantly to the metabolism and,
therefore, the regulation of the neurotransmitter amino
acids, glutamate/aspartate and GABA (for reviews of glial
contributions to neurotransmitter function, see
Schoffeniels et al., 1978; Varon and Somjen, 1979; Hertz,
1979; Bradford, 1982). For the most part, these conclusions are consistent with the earlier studies on the
biochemical compartmentation of glutamate metabolism in
brain (see Berl et al., this volume, for review of these
pioneering studies). Such studies have indicated that
exogenously supplied glutamate, aspartate and GABA appear
to be metabolized largely in a "small" compartment which,
in recent years, has been suggested to be the astroglial
cell. Since glial cells do have high affinity uptake sites
for these amino acids (see Hertz, 1979), it may be that one
of the functions of the glial cell is to aid in the rapid
removal of neuroactive amino acids released into the
synaptic cleft. A central datum in the "compartmentation" theory was the experimentally-observed rapid
conversion, in vivo and in vitro, of exogenous glutamate
and ammonia to glutamine which suggested a disparate
distribution of the synthesizing enzyme, glutamine
synthetase in brain tissue. This hypothesis was experimentally confirmed by Norenberg and Martinez-Hernandez
(1979) who localized glutamine synthetase to astrocytes in
rat brain by immunohistochemistry. In adult avian and
mammalian retinas, glutamine synthetase has been shown to
be confined to Müller cells (see Linser, Moscona, 1981).

This singular distribution in astroglial cells has also been found in human CNS (Pilkington, Lantos, 1982).

It has become obvious in the past few years than an understanding of the metabolism of glutamine is probably pivotol to elaborating the regulation of the metabolism of the neuroactive amino acids. Glutamine has been postulated to be a major precursor of neuronal, i.e., transmitter, pools of these amino acids (Van den Berg, Garfinkel, 1971; Benjamin, Quastel, 1974; Bradford, Ward, 1976; Weiler et al., 1979), as well as being a deactivated form of the neuroexcitatory, and potentially neurotoxic, glutamate (Nicklas et al., 1980; Krespan et al., 1982). In this hypothesis, glutamate and GABA levels within their respective nerve terminals are maintained by glutamine derived from the extracellular space which in turn can be replenished by synthesis in the glia via glutamine synthetase. Phosphate-stimulated glutaminase does not appear to have a singular localization, although there may be more or less activity in synaptic mitochondria than in mitochondria from elsewhere (glia, neuronal perikarya) (Dennis et al., 1977; Weiler et al., 1979). However, whether glutaminase is or is not preferably localized in neurons, or whether glutamine is or is not preferentially accumulated by nerve endings (Hertz, 1979) may not be overriding considerations. What is important is the functional activity of glutaminase in situ. The primary brain enzyme has been shown to be of the kidney type, both immunologically and kinetically (see review by Kovacevic and McGivan, 1983 for references and discussion) and is subject to multiple effectors, including product inhibition by glutamate. Thus a decrease of glutamate during neuro-transmission could itself increase the in situ activity of glutaminase (Bradford, Ward, 1976; Benjamin, 1981). In summary, the control of these systems need not depend on a differential distribution of glutaminase between neurons and glia but rather upon a delicate poising of glutamate: glutamine ratios within these cells.

A variety of approaches have been taken to investigate the contribution of neurons and glia to the metabolism of glutamate and GABA. An understanding of the in vivo, functioning nervous tissue is the ultimate goal of these studies and the relevance of all results must be considered in relation to the in vivo state. However, the complexity of the in vivo condition makes a quantitative determination of the relative contribution of each compartment and elaboration of its specific function most difficult. The use of model systems such as the intact tissue slice and isolated cell types allow greater manipulation of the environment. Even with these preparations the lack of agents to interact in specific ways with the metabolism of amino acids has hindered a proper biochemical dissection of the system. This report will illustrate the extent of neuronal-glial interactions with an example of on-going work in this laboratory on the use of specific enzyme inhibitors to test the hypothesis of glial-synthesized glutamine as a precursor of nerve-ending glutamate and GABA.

STUDIES ON FLOW OF GLUTAMINE FROM GLIA TO NERVE ENDINGS.

A principal problem in understanding glutamine metabolism in the CNS has been how to approach the hypothesis of a functional flow of glutamine into transmitter pools of amino acids. One tool that is available is the use of radioactive acetate. ^{3}H- or ^{14}C- acetate has been shown to label preferentially the "small" glutamate compartment in which glutamine is synthesized, both in vivo and in vitro (see Van den Berg et al., 1975). On the other hand, radioactive glucose is ubiquitously metabolized. Therefore, when various CNS preparations are labeled with a combination of ^{14}C-glucose/^{3}H-acetate and then depolarized, there is a preferential efflux of ^{14}C-labeled amino acids (DeBelleroche and Bradford, 1972; Minchin, 1977; Bradford et al., 1978; Hamberger et al., 1979). Studies in this laboratory have observed similar effects with cerebellar slices depolarized with veratridine (Krespan et al., 1982). In specific terms, the "glutamine-flow" hypothesis would suggest that acetate labels glutamine in glial cells and this can form veratridine-releasable glutamate or GABA only after transport into nerve endings and catabolism. Therefore, inhibition of glutamine synthesis, transport of glutamine or glutamine breakdown in the nerve ending should cause a large decrease in acetate-labeled, veratridine-releasable glutamate and/or GABA. The radioactive labeling and release of glucose-derived amino acids should not be so affected. Furthermore, an examination of the kinetics of the changes may furnish quantitative information about the precursor role of glutamine.

Table 1.   Effect of 6-Diazo-5-oxo-L-norleucine (DON) on P_i-Stimulated Glutaminase in Brain Slices.

	Activity (% Control)*
Control	100 ± 10
2 mM DON	61 ± 1
4 mM DON	44 ± 6
6 mM DON	32 ± 2

*Control activity was 5.5 µmoles ^{14}C-glutamate formed per hour mg protein at 37° from 10 mM L-^{14}C-glutamine in a 100 mM phosphate-Tris buffer, pH 8.0. Cerebellar slices were preincubated 30 min with DON in Krebs-Ringer bicarbonate medium with glucose prior to homogenization.

The diazoketone, 6-diazo-5-oxo-L-norleucine (DON), irreversibly inhibits phosphate-activated glutaminases in various tissues, in vivo and in vitro, by interacting with the glutamine binding site on the enzyme (Pinkus, Windmueller, 1977; Shapiro et al., 1979). It also inhibits glutamine-dependent activities of some amido transferases (see Shapiro et al., 1979 for references). In earlier studies it was found that preincubation of rat brain homogenates with 2 mM DON gave a 95% inhibition of phosphate-activated glutaminase activity (Nicklas, Krespan, 1982). In studies to test whether DON could penetrate into rat cerebellar tissue slices and inhibit glutaminase in situ, the slices were preincubated with various concentrations of DON, the DON removed by washing, and glutaminase activity measured in homogenates of the slices. The DON was able to penetrate the tissue and react with glutaminase as illustrated by a time-dependent, dose-dependent decrease in residual glutaminase activity (Table 1).

When cerebellar slices were labeled with a mixture of $[2-^{14}C]$ glucose and ^3H-acetate after a 30 min incubation with 5 mM DON, there was an increase in the specific activity of glutamate labeled by acetate (Table 2). This may reflect a decreased dilution of the acetate-labeled glutamate pool by glutamate derived from glutaminase. The most striking result was the very great decrease in the relative specific activity of GABA labeled by acetate. This was due not only to the increases in glutamate specific activity but also to a diminished specific activity in

Table 2. Effect of DON on Amino Acid Labeling from ^{14}C-Glucose/-^{3}H-Acetate

	Glutamate	
	^{14}C	^{3}H
	dpm ·nmole^{-1} ± S.D.	
Control	21.7 ± 3.7	434 ± 32
DON	21.0 ± 2.5	885 ± 147*

	Relative Spec. Act.			
	GLN		GABA	
	^{14}C	^{3}H (glut=1)	^{14}C	^{3}H
Control	0.82	5.97	0.94	0.41
DON	0.60*	3.57*	0.98	0.15*

*$p < .005$ from control.
Cerebellar slices were preincubated 30 min with 5 mM DON. After washing to remove the extracellular DON, the slices were incubated with $[2\text{-}^{14}C]$ glucose/^{3}H-acetate for 15 min.

Table 3. Effect of DON on Veratridine-Released GABA Labeled from ^{14}C-Glucose/^{3}H-Acetate

	Control	+ DON
	labeled from ^{14}C-glucose	
dpm/nmole	9.5 ± 1.0	11.9 ± 1.2
RSA*	1.14 ± 0.18	1.25 ± 0.06
	labeled from ^{3}H-acetate	
dpm/nmole	161 ± 10	117 ± 8[a]
RSA*	0.33 ± 0.06	0.15 ± 0.05[a]

* relative specific activity with glutamate in tissue taken as 1.
[a] Different from control, $p <.005$ for N=4.
Cerebellar slices were treated as in Table 2, then washed to remove the medium radioactivity. After reincubation for 5 min, 10 μM veratridine was added for 3 min and medium and slices separately analyzed.

the GABA labeled by acetate (controls, 198 dpm/nmole; DON-
treated slices, 131 dpm/nmole. This difference was also
reflected in the specific activity and relative specific
activity of GABA released from the slice by 10 μM veratridine (Table 3).

Similarly DON caused a significant decrease (∼ 35%) in
the acetate-derived RSA of veratridine-released glutamate
(Table 4) with no such changes in glucose-derived,
veratridine-releasable glutamate.

Table 4.   Effect of DON on Labeling of Glutamate Released
           by Veratridine.

	Control	DON
	RSA, medium/tissue ± S.D.	
^{14}C-glucose labeled	1.06 ± 0.20	0.93 ± 0.19
^{3}H-acetate	1.85 ± 0.18	1.23 ± 0.20*

*Different from control, p < 005, N=4.

These results with a glutaminase inhibitor, DON, are
consistent with the hypothesis presented earlier that
labeled acetate finds its way into transmitter pools of
amino acids via glutaminase activity, probably in the nerve
ending. Similar results would be predicted for an
inhibition of glutamine synthesis. The convulsive agent,
L-methionine sulfoximine (MSO), is a good inhibitor of
glutamine synthetase and there is evidence to suggest that
its convulsant activity is related to that property, rather
than its ability to inhibit γ-glutamyl cysteine synthetase
(Griffith and Meister, 1979). Gutierrez and Norenberg
(1977) found in rats injected with MSO that the preictal,
primary effect of MSO is on astrocyte morphology and con-
jectured that abnormalities in astrocytes may play a role
in development of MSO-induced seizures.

Unlike the case with DON, when cerebellar slices are
incubated with MSO (1 mM), there are changes in amino acid
levels which must be taken into account in interpreting the
results (Table 5). Glutamine is substantially decreased as
expected; the extent of inhibition is consistent with
measurements of residual glutamine synthetase activity in
the slice and studies with ^{14}C-glutamate metabolism (data

not shown) which indicate an approximately 75% inhibition
of glutamine synthetase in situ. Aspartate, glutamate and
alanine are increased by MSO. This probably reflects the
observed inhibition of glial glutamine synthetase and,

Table 5. Amino Acid Levels in Cerebellar Slices

	Control	MSO
	μmoles $\cdot$100 mg protein^{-1}	
ASP	1.71	2.54*
GLU	7.05	10.87*
GLN	2.59	0.66*
ALA	0.50	0.92*
GABA	0.55	0.54
MSO	-	2.40

*$p < .01$ from control
Cerebellar slices were preincubated in Krebs-Ringer
bicarbonate medium with glucose for 20 min, 1 mM methionine
sulfoximine (MSO) was then added and slices incubated
another 40 min.

Table 6. Effect of MSO on Amino Acid Labeling in Cerebellar
Slices from ^{14}C-Glucose and ^{3}H-Acetate.

	Sp. Ac. Glutamate	
	^{14}C	^{3}H
	dpm $\cdot$nmole^{-1} $\pm$ S.D.	
Control	18.3 $\pm$ 3.9	272 $\pm$ 19
1 mM MSO	9.9 $\pm$ 1.5	278 $\pm$ 52

	Relative Sp. Ac.			
	GLN		GABA	
	^{14}C	^{3}H	^{14}C	^{3}H
		(glut=1)		
Control	0.33	3.13	1.25	0.23
1 mM MSO	0.12*	0.05*	1.84*	0.08*

*$p < 0.01$, different from control, N=4 slices.
Cerebellar slices were pretreated with 1 mM MSO as in
Table 5. After washing to remove excess MSO they were then
incubated with a mixture of [2-^{14}C] glucose and ^{3}H-acetate
for 15 min.

perhaps, transamination of the MSO. Studies with kainate,
which releases glial stores of amino acids, indicate that
this glutamate is apparently accumulated in the glia
(Nicklas and Richie, 1983). It should be noted that the
tissue seems to take up MSO quite well. When slices
treated with MSO were labeled with $[2\text{-}^{14}C]$ glucose/^{3}H-
acetate, the specific activity of glutamate labeled from
glucose was decreased by half with no effect on the
specific activity of acetate-derived glutamate (Table 6).
Glutamine labeling is severely depressed. GABA labeling
from acetate is greatly inhibited. Relative to the specific
activity of glutamate (which was decreased by MSO), the
labeling of GABA from ^{14}C-glucose was increased.

These differences are also seen in the veratridine-
releasable GABA and glutamate (Table 7). Since the acetate-
derived specific activity of tissue glutamate was not
significantly altered by MSO, these changes in relative
specific activity (RSA) of medium amino acids represents a
genuine decrease in labeling from acetate.

Table 7. Veratridine-Released GABA and Glutamate Labeled by
^{14}C-Glucose and ^{3}H-Acetate in Cerebellar Slices.

	^{14}C	^{3}H
	Medium GABA RSA[a]	
Control	1.33	0.38
MSO	2.05*	0.05*
BSO	1.09	0.28
	Medium GLUT RSA[a]	
Control	0.94	1.79
MSO	0.89	0.50*
BSO	1.04	1.85

[a]Specific activity of glutamate in tissue taken as one.
*$p < 0.01$ different from corresponding control or BSO
treatment.
Slices were pretreated with either 1 mM L-methionine
sulfoximine (MSO) or 1 mM D,L-buthioninine-S,R-sulfoximine
(BSO) and incubated with ^{14}C-glucose/^{3}H-acetate as in Table
6. After washing to remove the medium radioactivity, the
slices were treated for 3 min with 10 µM veratridine and
medium and tissue rapidly separated.

As noted previously, both DON and MSO are known to
inhibit other enzymes, e.g., γ-glutamyl-transpeptidase and
γ-glutamyl cysteine synthetase, respectively. The latter
two enzymes are part of the γ-glutamyl cycle which is
present in nervous tissue but whose function is not understood (for review see Pruisner, 1981). Thus the two agents
used in these studies may well have acted by inhibiting
the γ-glutamyl cycle. To test this possibility, cerebellar
slices were also incubated with 1 mM buthionine sulfoximine
(BSO) which, like MSO, is an excellent inhibitor of γ-
glutamyl cysteine synthetase but, unlike MSO, it is not
convulsive and does not inhibit glutamine synthetase
(Griffith and Meister, 1979). The BSO did not alter tissue
amino acid levels as did MSO (data not shown) nor did it
alter the labeling pattern of veratridine-releasable
glutamate and GABA (Table 7). Like MSO, tissue levels of
BSO can be quantitated since it is separated in the HPLC
system used to measure amino acids. After the initial
incubation and washing, 1.0 μmol/100 mg protein were found
in the tissue slices. In other experiments, we have found
that neither DON nor MSO (at concentrations used in these
studies) had any effect on the activity of glutamate decarboxylase or the cytoplasmic or mitochondrial isozymes of
aspartate aminotransferase. Thus, the data are consistent
with the sites of action of DON and MSO being glutaminase
and glutamine synthetase, respectively.

These studies reinforce the notion that when examining
release of "neurotransmitter" amino acids in the presence
of activators or inhibitors, one should always do so by
comparing that which is released with that initially in or
remaining in the tissue. Unfortunately that is not usually
done in release studies. These comparisons often can give
further insight into basic mechanistic problems. For example, we have found that the excitotoxic glutamate analog,
kainic acid, causes a large efflux of glutamate (and, to a
lesser extent, aspartate) from brain tissue slices into the
medium (Nicklas et al., 1980; Krespan et al., 1982). This
has recently been confirmed (Ferkany and Coyle, 1983). Our
data indicated that a large portion of the glutamate came
from non-synaptic sites, perhaps glial cells. The use of
MSO offers the possibility of further testing this hypothesis. As is seen in Table 5, MSO by inhibiting glutamine
synthetase, gives rise to higher levels of glutamate and
aspartate. Presumably a goodly portion of this should be
glial. Therefore, one would expect that kainate, a glial

glutamate releaser, would release this increased glutamate, whereas, veratridine, a nerve ending glutamate releaser (at low concentrations) should not do so. In Table 8, the release of endogenous amino acids are tabulated as a per cent of the total amino acids in the tissue and medium after adding either kainate or veratridine to control or MSO-treated slices.

Table 8.   Veratridine and Kainate-Releasable Amino Acids in Cerebellar Slices Treated with Methionine Sulfoximine

	ASP	Amino Acids in Medium GLUT	GABA
		% Total in Tissue + Medium	
Control	1.3	1.2	2.3
+ MSO	1.4	1.0	3.1
+ KA	14.4[a]	8.6[a]	2.8
+ MSO + KA	14.7[a]	11.3[a]	3.6
+ Ver	3.1[a]	3.7[a]	12.8[a]
+ MSO + Ver	1.5[b]	2.1[b]	9.8[a]

[a] Different from control at p < .02 or better.
[b] Different from corresponding no MSO at p < .02 or better.

Cerebellar slices were pretreated with and without 1 mM methionine sulfoximine (MSO) as in Table 5. The slices were then washed and transferred to fresh Krebs-Ringer bicarbonate medium with glucose. After 5 min incubation at 37°, either control vehicle, 10 μM veratridine or 0.5 mM kainate were added. 5 min later the medium and tissues were separated.

MSO itself causes no change in medium levels of amino acids. 0.5 mM kainate causes a large efflux of aspartate and glutamate but not GABA. In the MSO-treated slices, the same (or higher) relative release of these amino acids is seen. Since tissue levels are higher in MSO-treated slices, this means that in absolute terms more aspartate and gluta-mate are released by kainate. Veratridine enhances the release of glutamate and aspartate and, also, GABA. In MSO-pretreated slices, veratridine releases a lower percentage of the dicarboxylic amino acids, consistent with the site of action of this drug being synaptic. Thus the results are

internally consistent with the hypothesis concerning the
mechanism of action of the compounds used in these studies.

The experiments described above illustrate methods
which can be employed to study the interactions between the
different compartments in nervous tissue which play a role
in the metabolism of neuroactive amino acids. As such they
are experimental evidence for the earlier hypotheses which
suggested that glutamine is a precursor for neuronal stores
of amino acids and that glutamine flows from glia to nerve
endings.

Acknowledgement

The author wishes to thank Mr. Victor Richie for his
dedicated and capable technical assistance in these
studies. This work was supported by NIH grant NS 17360.

Benjamin A (1981). Control of glutaminase activity in rat
  brain cortex in vitro: Influence of glutamate, phosphate,
  ammonium, calcium and hydrogen ions. Brain Res 208:363.
Benjamin A, Quastel JH (1974). Fate of L-glutamate in the
  brain. J Neurochem 128:631.
Bradford HF (1982). "Neurotransmitter Interactions and Com-
  parmentation." New York: Plenum Press.
Bradford HF, Ward HK (1976). On glutaminase activity in
  mammalian synaptosomes. Brain Res 110:115.
Bradford HF, de Belleroche JS, Ward HK (1978). On the metabolic and intrasynaptic origin of amino acid transmitters.
  In Fonnum F, (ed): "Amino Acids as Chemical Neurotransmitters," New York: Plenum Press, p 367.
de Belleroche JS, Bradford HF (1972). Metabolism of beds of
  mammalian cortical synaptosomes: Response to depolarizing
  influences. J Neurochem 19:585.
Dennis SC, Lai JCK, Clark JB (1977). Comparative studies on
  glutamate metabolism in synaptic and non-synaptic rat
  brain mitochondria. Biochem J 164:727.
Ferkany JW, Coyle JT (1983). Kainic acid selectively stimu-
  lates the release of endogenous excitatory amino acids.
  J Pharmacol Exptl Therap 225:399.
Griffith O, Meister A (1979). Potent and specific inhibition of glutathione synthesis by buthionine sulfoximine
  (S-n-butylhomocysteine sulfoximine). J Biol Chem
  254:7558.

Gutierrez JA, Norenberg MD (1977). Ultrastructural study of methionine sulfoximine-induced Alzheimer Type II astrocytosis. Am J Pathol 86:285.

Hamberger AC, Chiang GH, Nylen ES, Scheff SW, Cotman CW (1979). Glutamate as a CNS transmitter: 1. Evaluation of glucose and glutamine as precursors for the synthesis of preferentially released glutamate. Brain Res 168:513.

Hertz L (1979). Functional interaction between neurons and astrocytes. Prog Neurobiol 13:177.

Kovacevic Z, McGivan JD (1983). Mitochondrial metabolism of glutamine and glutamate and its physiological significance. Physiol Rev 63:547.

Krespan B, Berl S, Nicklas WJ (1982). Alteration in neuronal-glial metabolism of glutamate by the neurotoxin kainic acid. J Neurochem 38:509.

Linser P, Moscona AA (1981). Carbonic anhydrase C in the neural retina: Transition from generalized to glia-specific cell localization during embryonic development. Proc Natl Acad Sci 78:7190.

Minchin MCW (1977). The release of amino acids synthesized from various compartmental precursors in rat spinal cord slices. Exp Brain Res 29:515.

Nicklas WJ, Krespan B, Berl S (1980). Effect of kainate on ATP levels and glutamate metabolism in cerebellar slices. Eur J Pharmacol 62:209.

Nicklas WJ, Krespan B (1982). Studies on neuronal-glial metabolism of glutamate in cerebellar slices. In Bradford H (ed): "Neurotransmitter Interaction and Compartmentation," New York: Plenum Press, p 383.

Nicklas WJ, Richie V (1983). Further studies on kainate-induced efflux of glutamate. Trans Am Soc Neurochem 14:130.

Norenberg MD, Martinez-Hernandez A (1979). Fine structural localization of glutamine synthetase in astrocytes in brain. Brain Res 161:303.

Pilkington GJ, Lantos PL (1982). The role of glutamine synthetase in diagnosis of cerebral tumors. Neuropathol Appl Neurobiol 8:866.

Pinkus LM, Windmueller HG (1977). Phosphate-dependent glutaminase of small intestine: Localization and role in intestinal glutamine metabolism. Arch Biochem Biophys 182:506.

Pruisner SB (1981). Disorders of glutamate metabolism and neurological dysfunction. Ann Rev Med 32:521.

Schoffeniels E, Franck G, Hertz L, Tower DB (1978). "Dynamic Properties of Glial Cells." Oxford: Pergamon Press.

Shapiro RA, Clarke VM, Curthoys NP (1979). Inactivation of rat renal phosphate-dependent glutaminase with 6-diazo-5-oxo-L-norleucine. J Biol Chem 254:2835.
Van den Berg CJ, Garfinkel D (1971). A simulation study of brain compartments. Biochem J 123:211.
Van den Berg CJ, Reinjierse A, Blockhuis GCD, Kroon MC, Ronda G, Clarke DD, Garfinkel D (1975). A model of glutamate metabolism in brain: a biochemical analysis of a heterogenous structure. In Berl S, Clarke DD, Schneider D (eds): "Metabolic Compartmentation and Neurotransmission," New York: Plenum Press, p 515.
Varon S, Somjen G (1979). "Neuron-Glia Interactions." Neurosci Res Prog Bull 17. Cambridge, Mass: MIT Press.
Weiler CT, Nystrom B, Hamberger A (1979). Glutaminase and glutamine synthetase activity in synaptosomes, bulk isolated glia and neurons. Brain Res 160:539.

**Glutamine, Glutamate, and GABA
in the Central Nervous System, pages 233–240**
© **1983 Alan R. Liss, Inc., 150 Fifth Avenue, New York, NY 10011**

FLUOROACETATE AS A POSSIBLE MARKER FOR GLIAL METABO-
LISM IN VIVO.

Donald D. Clarke, Ph.D. and Soll Berl, M.D.*

Dept. of Chemistry, Fordham Univ. and Dept.
of Neurology, Mt. Sinai School of Medicine*
Bronx, N.Y. 10458 and New York, N.Y. 10029*

Glucose is the major source of energy in all
brain cells and its metabolism is closely coupled to
functional activity. Advantage has been taken of this
by Sokoloff (1977) and Sokoloff et al. (1977) to study
energy metabolism in different brain areas and their
response to a variety of drugs and stimuli. For this
purpose these workers have developed the procedure for
measuring autoradiographically the accumulation of
$[^{14}C]$-deoxyglucose into its phosphate derivative, a
compound which does not differentiate glial from neuronal metabolism. They could be enhanced if one could
differentiate glial from neuronal metabolic response
to the various experimental conditions. Conceivably,
one could then study the effect of glial metabolism
on neuronal metabolism and vice versa.

Studies on the metabolism of glutamate, glutamine, GABA and aspartate utilizing a variety of precursors (including acetate, glucose and others) indicate that these amino acids exist in brain in distinct
metabolic pools which are accessible to specific precursors (Berl and Clarke, 1969). These metabolic
pools have been suggested to be associated with cellular structures, e.g. neuronal cell bodies, nerve
endings and glia (Berl et al., 1975). Considerable
circumstantial evidence from several laboratories,
utilizing radiolabeled acetate, suggest that acetate
may be selectively matabolized in the tricarboxylic
acid cycle in glial cells (Berl et al. 1975) and thus
be a marker for such cells. Several studies have

suggested that fluoroacetate mimics acetate and is
converted to fluorocitrate (Peters, et al., 1960;
Peters, et al, 1972). Unlike the citrate formed from
acetate, any fluorocitrate formed from fluoroacetate is
unlikely to be metabolized and therefore would accumulate in the mitochondria of the cells. If subtoxic
tracer doses of highly radiolabeled fluoroacetate were
administered to an animal, it should lead to the accumulation of the label in the glia and thus be a marker
for glial metabolism. If the labeling were measured
autoradiographically, it would lead to a system similar
to that developed by Sokoloff and collaborators using
$[^{14}C]$-deoxyglucose but only labeling glial cells.
This would lead to a finer resolution of the events
occurring in discrete brain areas.

Some of the experimental evidence in support of
the idea that fluoroacetate affects the small pool of
glutamate active in glutamine synthesis in brain were
achieved in studies with guinea pig brain slices
(Clarke et al., 1970). As can be seen in Table 1, 1mM
fluoroacetate decreased the specific activity   (SA)
of glutamine relative to that of glutamate (RSA)
approximately fifteen fold. Fluorocitrate was approximately one-hundred times more effective than fluoroacetate in lowering the RSA of glutamine. This is
consistent with the hypothesis of "lethal synthesis"
of fluorocitrate proposed by Peters et al. (1960).
Further confirmation of the effect of fluoroacetate
on the metabolism of the small pool of glutamate is
presented in Table 2. Fluoroacetate lowered the RSA
of glutamine when labeled glutamate, aspartate or GABA
served as the labeled precursor. All of these, when
exogenously applied to brain tissue in vivo and in
vitro, have been shown to be preferentially metabolized
in the small pool believed to be associated with glia.

The half life of $[^{14}C]$ which is 5,700 yrs, pre-
cludes obtaining $[^{14}C]$-fluoroacetate of sufficiently
high specific activity to allow for administration of
a subtoxic tracer dose of fluoroacetate and still permit resolution of cellular structures. Because of the
much shorter half life of tritium, viz. 12 yrs., tritium
labeled fluoroacetate can theoretically be obtained
with approximately 450 times greater specific activity
than that of the $[^{14}C]$ labeled compound (Table 3.).

This should make it possible to achieve adequate radio-activity in brain tissue using tracer doses of fluoro-acetate labeled with this isotope.

TABLE 1.

Effect of Fluoroacetate and Fluorocitrate on the Labeling of Glutamate and Glutamine from $[1\text{-}^{14}C]$-Acetate in Guinea Pig Brain Slices.

Inhibitor		SA	RSA
Fluoro-acetate	Fluoro-citrate	Glutamate	Glutamine
0	0	4.69×10^4	5.87
1 mM	-	1.36×10^4	0.40
0.1 mM	-		6.13
-	1 mM	1.45×10^4	0.04
-	0.1 mM		0.08
-	0.01 mM		0.56

The slices were incubated in Krebs-Ringer phosphate buffer containing 55mM glucose and 2 μCi of $[1\text{-}^{14}\text{-}C]$-acetate (58 μCi./μmole). Incubation time was 10 min. at 37°C.
SA: Specific Activity, c.p.m./μmole.; RSA: SA Gluta-mine/SA Glutamate.

TABLE 2.

Effect of Fluoroacetate on the Labeling of Glutamate and Glutamine from Labeled Glutamate, Aspartate and GABA in Guinea Pig Brain Slices.

Precursor	Fluoroacetate	SA Glutamate	RSA Glutamine
L-$[U\text{-}^{14}C]$-Glutamate	0	2.01	1.32
	1 mM	2.08	0.70
L-$[U\text{-}^{14}C]$-Aspartate	0	2.90	3.45
	1 mM	2.66	0.38
γ-Amino-$[1\text{-}^{14}C]$-Butyrate	0	2.04	4.45
	1 mM	2.14	0.60

Incubation conditions as in Table 1. Slices were in-cubated with 0.5 μCi of L-$[U\text{-}^{14}C]$-glutamate or aspar-tate (> 200 mCi./mmole) or 1 mCi. of GABA (2.7 mCi./mmole).

TABLE 3

Half Life of $^{14}_{3}C$	= 5,730 yrs.
Half Life of ^3H	= 12.3 yrs.
Ratio of Half Lives	= 466

Allowing for different
efficiencies in counting
of ^{14}C and ^3H, the ratio $\cong$ 200.

Tritiated fluoroacetate is not available commercially. Several attempts were made by Amersham-Searle and New England Nuclear Corp. to prepare tritiated fluoroacetate of high specific activity and sufficient purity for us. New England Nuclear Corp. succeeded in preparing for us [^3H]-fluoroacetate at a SA of 16 Ci./mmole (pure [^3H] has a SA of 29 Ci./mgm. atom). This was done by exchanging the hydrogen atoms of fluoromalonic acid with tritiated water followed by heating to decarboxylate the fluoromalonate to form fluoroacetate. Before use, the tritiated fluoroacetate supplied to us was purified by liquid chromatography on AG-1 chloride form, (200-400 mesh). The labeled compound was eluted from the column with 0.1N HCl; the main fraction containing 85% of the radioactivity was neutralized with 1.0N NaOH, lyophilized and taken up in physiological saline.

Rats were prepared with indwelling catheters in the femoral vein. The following day three rats were each injected with 0.3 ml of [^3H]-fluoroacetate solution ($\sim$1 mCi.) followed by 0.5 ml of normal saline. At 10, 20 and 30 mins. the rats were decapitated, blood collected from the severed neck, and heart, liver and kidney dissected and frozen in isopentane cooled in liquid N_2 (10 & 30 mins.). These were packed in dry ice and shipped to Dr. Sokoloff for autoradiographic studies. Although the autoradiographs were qualitatively different from those observed with [^{14}C]-deoxyglucose we do not have any quantitative comparisons at this time. The brain from the 20 min. animal was dissected into brain stem, cerebellum, caudate nucleus and cortex and each frozen in liq. N_2.

The tissues were extracted with 0.4N perchloric acid. These extracts were neutralized with 5N KOH

and the supernatants chromatographed on columns of
AG-1-acetate (Berl et al. 1968). The columns were
eluted with 0.05, 0.1 and 0.3N acetic acid followed by
0.1N HCl. Tritiated water was eluted in the 0.05N
acetic acid and aspartate with 0.3N acetic acid.
Fluoroacetate, citrate and fluorocitrate were eluted
with 0.1N HCl. The elution position of acetate and
fluoroacetate were determined with the tritiated compounds and that of citrate and fluorocitrate by their
color reactions developed with acetic anhydride and
pyridine (Hartford, 1962).

The distribution of the radioactivity in the
various organs is summarized in Table 4. It is obvi-
that within the time period of this study very little
of the fluoroacetate was metabolized in any of the organs. In agreement with others, kidney and heart
metabolized fluoroacetate to the greatest extent (Gal,
1972). In brain, unmetabolized fluoroacetate accounted for approximately 95% of the radioactivity in the
tissue. Only trace amounts, if any, of fluorocitrate
appeared to be formed. Metabolic products do not
appear to be accumulating in the serum which makes
transfer of metabolites between organs unlikely.

These results, obtained in different areas of the
brain, raise the question of whether any significant
quantities of fluorocitrate are synthesized in brain.
Even in heart and liver the significance of the extent
of formation of fluorocitrate is open to question. The
accumulation of fluorocitrate in any organ of a fluoroacetate poisoned animal has never been adequately demonstrated by isolation techniques. Several chromatographic identifications have been made. The theory of
"lethal synthesis" of fluorocitrate was based on the
well demonstrated accumulation of citrate in kidney
and heart (Peters et.al., 1960). This has been repeatedly confirmed and corroborated in the brains of
rats by Goldberg, et al. (1966). Accumulation of
fluorocitrate from fluoroacetate to the extent of
about 2% (on a weight basis) of the radioactivity in
brain is suggested by studies using convulsive doses
of [^{14}C]-labeled fluoroacetate (Gal, 1972). The identification of fluorocitrate in those studies was by
paper chromatography. In the studies reported here

TABLE 4.

Distribution of Radioactivity after I.V. Administration of Tritiated Fluoroacetate

	Total c.p.m./gm of Tissue x 10^6	% of Radioactivity in the Tissue						
		^3H_2O	FAc	Ac	Cit.	FCit.	Glu	Asp.
Cortex	2.3	3.7	94.4	<0.02	<0.1	<0.02	~0.05	~0.05
Caudate Nucleus	2.2	3.6	96.3	<0.02	<0.1	<0.02	~0.05	~0.05
Cerebellum	2.2	3.9	94.8	<0.02	<0.1	<0.02	~0.05	~0.05
Pons-Medulla	2.0	3.6	94.5	<0.02	<0.1	<0.02	~0.05	~0.05
Liver	2.6	3.6	92.7	~0.01	~1.0	~0.1	~0.15	~0.15
Heart	4.0	8.0	86.3	~0.4	~1.0	~0.25	~0.6	~0.3
Kidney	2.2	10.3	82.1	~0.4	~1.0	~0.35	~0.5	~0.4
Serum	5.3	0.1	97.2	<0.001	<0.02	<0.001	<0.001	<0.001

Approximately 1 mCi. of purified tritiated sodium fluoroacetate (16 Ci./mmole) was injected via an indwelling catheter in the femoral vein. After 20 minutes the rat was decapitated, blood collected, the tissues dissected and frozen in liquid N_2. The tissues were extracted with 0.4N perchloric acid. The extracts were neutralized with 5N KOH and the supernatants chromatographed on columns of AG-1-X4, 200-400 mesh in the acetate form.

FAc: Fluoroacetate; Ac: Acetate; Cit: Citrate; FCit: Fluorocitrate; Glu: Glutamate; Asp: Aspartate.

tracer doses of labeled fluoroacetate were used. Accordingly these studies need to be repeated using higher doses of fluoroacetate before more definitive statements about the extent of synthesis of fluorocitrate in brain can be made.

Synthetic fluorocitrate has been repeatedly shown to inhibit aconitase and biosynthesis of fluorocitrate from synthetic fluoroacetyl-coenzyme A by mitochondrial preparations has been adequately demonstrated. It therefore seems that it is not the theory of lethal synthesis which should be questioned but the competitive inhibition of aconitase as an explanation for the accumulation of citrate. It would seem more likely that fluorocitrate may be a suicide substrate for mitochondrial aconitase and this leads to the accumulation of citrate. The low rate of synthesis of fluorocitrate and its utilization as a substrate by aconitase accompanied by the concomittant destruction of aconitase would better seem to explain the time dependence of fluoroacetate toxicity and the failure to isolate fluorocitrate from poisoned animals to date.

It therefore seems that one of our starting assumptions is probably not true, viz. that fluorocitrate is a non-metabolizable compound. This however does not invalidate our thesis because fluoroacetate seems to fit the description of a practically non-metabolizable compound. As shown above, in tracer doses, at least 95% of the radioactivity remains unmetabolized. If fluoroacetate is taken up predominantly by glia and its uptake is affected by changes in glial metabolism, then it can still be a useful marker of glial function.

REFERENCES

Berl S, Clarke DD (1969). Compartmentation of amino acid metabolism. In Lajtha A. Handbook of Neurochemistry, Vol 2, New York: Plenum Press, p 447.
Berl S, Clarke DD, Schneider D (1975). "Metabolic compartmentation and neurotransmission: Relation to brain structure and function." New York: Plenum Press, p 1.

Berl S, Nicklas WJ, Clarke DD (1968). Compartmentation of glutamic acid metabolism in brain slices. J. Neurochem. 15: 131.

Clarke DD, Nicklas WJ, Berl S (1970). Tricarboxylic acid cycle metabolism in brain: Effect of fluoro-acetate and fluorocitrate on the labeling of glu-tamate, aspartate, glutamine and γ-amino-butyrate. Biochem J 120: 345.

Gal EM (1972). Effect of fluoro compounds on metabo-lic control in brain mitochondria. In Peters,R (ed). "Carbon-Fluorine Compounds: Chemistry, Bio-chemistry and Biological Activities", New York: Elsevier, p 78.

Goldberg ND, Passoneau JV, Lowry OH (1966). Effect of changes in brain metabolism on the levels of citric acid cycle intermediates. J Biol Chem 241: 3997.

Hartford CG (1962). Rapid spectrophotometric method for the determination of itaconic, citric, aconitic and fumaric acids. Anal Chem 34: 426.

Peters R (1972). Some metabolic aspects of fluoroace-tate especially related to fluorocitrate. In Peters R (ed). Carbon-fluorine compounds: Chemistry, Bio-chemistry and Biological Activities" New York: Elsevier p 55.

Peters R, Hall RJ, Ward PFV, Sheppard N (1960). The chemical nature of the toxic compounds containing fluorine in the seeds of dichapetalum toxicarum. Biochem J 77: 17.

Sokoloff L (1977). Relation between physiological function and energy metabolism in the central ner-vous system. J Neurochem 29: 13.

Sokoloff L, Reivich M, Kennedy C, Des Rosiers MH, Patlak CS, Pettigrew KD, Sakurada O, Shinohara M. (1977). The [^{14}C]-deoxyglucose method for the measurement of local cerebral glucose utilization: theory, procedure and normal values in conscious and anesthesized albino rats. J Neurochem 28: 897.

Glutamine, Glutamate, and GABA
in the Central Nervous System, pages 241–247
© 1983 Alan R. Liss, Inc., 150 Fifth Avenue, New York, NY 10011

TRANSMITTER AND METABOLIC GLUTAMATE IN THE BRAIN

Frode Fonnum, and Bernt Engelsen

Norwegian Defence Research Establishment
Division of Environmental Toxicology
PO Box 25, N-2007 Kjeller, Norway

Metabolic studies have identified different pools of
glutamate, probably neuronal and glial, in the brain
(Balazs, Cremer, 1972; Van den Berg et al, 1975), but have
been unable to differentiate between the metabolic and
transmitter pool of glutamate (Fonnum, 1980). The contribution of glucose and glutamine as transmitter precursor in
vivo is not fully understood although glutamine dominates in
vitro (Hamberger et al, 1979a, 1979b; Bradford, Ward, Tomas,
1978). Although phosphate activated glutaminase is present
in high concentrations in nerve terminals it is not highly
concentrated in glutamergic terminals only (Walker, Fonnum &
Sterri, to be published).

In the present communication we have made an attempt
to differentiate between the turnover of the transmitter and
metabolic pools of glutamate. We have taken advantage of
the fact that unilateral cortical ablation will provide a
neostriatum almost devoid of the transmitter pool of glutamate on the ipsilateral side whereas the contralateral
neostriatum is almost unaffected and may be used as a
control (Fonnum, Storm-Mathisen, Divac,1981; Hassler et al,
1982). The aim of the present investigation was to study
the effect of different pharmacological tools on the glutamate contents of intact (transmitter and metabolic pool) and
of decorticated (metabolic pool only) neostriatum. The
pharmacological tools were insulin (to decrease glucose),
methionine sulphoxime (inhibitor of glutamine synthetase)
(Tews, Stone, 1964; Van den Berg, Van den Velden, 1970)
and ammonia (activator of glutamine formation) (Benjamin,
1981, 1982).

Adult albino Wistar rats, weighing 220–250 g, were obtained from Dr Møllergaard–Hansens Avlslaboratorium, Vejby, Denmark. The animals were anaesthesized with diazepam 0.2 ml (5 mg/ml) i.p. and fentanyl 0.2 mg/ml (Hypnorm 0.2 ml) s.c. The skull was opened and a frontal cortical ablation was made by suction of cortex down to the white matter from the frontal pool to the frontal–parietal suture. Subsequently the lesions were inspected microscopically and in none of the animals the lesion penetrated into the striatum.

One day after the operation i e when neurotransmission of glutamergic terminals had stopped or seven days after i e when the glutamergic terminals had degenerated, the animals received the pharmacological tools, intraperitoneally. The animals were killed by decapitation and their heads dropped into liquid nitrogen for 10 sec to cool the brain to near freezing point. The corresponding neostriatal tissue samples were rapidly dissected from transverse brain slices about 600 µm thick. The tissue samples were homogenized in 1 ml 2.5% trichloroacetic acid and the samples analyzed on an automatic amino acid analyzer (Kontron) as described (Fonnum et al, 1981). In all cases the samples from operated and non–operated sides were from the same batch analyzed. Blood samples for serum glucose concentrations were taken immediately following decapitation and determined by hexokinase method.

The animals injected with insulin 7 days after operation were separated into normoglycemic (saline injected), hypoglycemic animals (killed 65 min after insulin injection) and severely hypoglycemic rats (120–150 min after insulin injection). The mean blood glucose concentration was 5.6 mmol/l, 1.7 mmol/l and 0.9 mmol/l respectively.

The results show that in normoglycemic rats there was a larger fall in glutamate (glu) than in aspartate (asp) and an increase in glutamine (gln) on the operated compared to the unoperated side. The glu/asp and glu/gln ratios are consequently decreased on the operated side, (Table I). In hypoglycemic animals there were an increase in asp on both sides, but predominantly on the unoperated side. Under these conditions there were only small changes in glu and gln levels compared to those of the normoglycemic animals. The glu/asp ratios are significantly decreased on both sides, but most clearly on the unoperated side. During severe hypoglycemia the changes in amino acid levels were even more pronounced. On the unoperated side there were considerable decreases in glu and gln levels and a very large increase in asp level. On the operated side there was decrease in glu level and an increase in the asp level. The changes were significantly less than on the unoperated side. The glu/asp ratio and the glu/gln ratio on both side were significantly changed compared to normoglycemia ratio.

TABLE 1   AMINO ACID RATIOS IN RAT NEOSTRIATUM

AMINO ACID RATIO	GLU/ASP		GLU/GLN	
	N	O	N	O
NORMOGLYCEMIC	6.7 ± 1.2	5.3 ± 0.9	2.7 ± 0.5	1.4 ± 0.2
HYPOGLYCEMIC	3.2 ± 0.6	3.7 ± 0.4	3.4 ± 1.4	1.4 ± 0.5
SEVERE HYPOGLYCEMIC	0.7 ± 0.2	2.2 ± 0.7	9.3 ± 3.0	2.0 ± 0.8
METHIONINE SULPHOXIMINE				
CONTROL	5.6 ± 1.1	5.1 ± 1.2	1.9 ± 0.5	1.1 ± 0.2
MET SULPHOXIME 2 h	–	–	1.7 ± 0.3	2.3 ± 1.3
MET SULPHOXIME 4 h	7.2 ± 2.3	6.2 ± 1.6	4.0	10.5
MET SULPHOXIME 8 h			∞	∞
AMMONIA				
CONTROL	5.6 ± 1.1	5.1 ± 0.4	1.9 ± 0.5	1.1 ± 0.2
AMMONIUM CHLORIDE 7–14 min	6.8	7.0	1.0	0.6

N = NOT OPERATED SIDE

O = OPERATED SIDE

In animals treated with insulin 1 day after the operation the changes between control and hypoglycemic animals were similar although not as striking (Table 2).

The increase in asp and decrease in glu and gln during hypoglycemia are in general agreement with previous investigations in unoperated animals (Butterworth, Merkel, Landrevelle, 1982; Lewis et al, 1979). The important new finding is the different effect of hypoglycemia on amino acid levels in unoperated and operated brains. The results indicate a higher turnover of glu in the intact neostriatum i e where the transmitter pool of glu is present.

We then wanted to test this hypothesis with another drug which have an effect on the glu-gln system. For this purpose we selected methionine sulphoxime, a well-known inhibitor of glutamine synthetase, the enzyme synthesizing glutamine. The animals were then examined about 2 hrs after being given methionine sulphoxime. At this time the most striking difference was a reduction of glutamine on the operated side only. Later, at 4 hrs after giving methionine sulphoxime, there were small reduction in glu on the unoperated side and reductions in asp on both sides. In this case the gln level on the operated and unoperated sides were reduced to 10 and 40 per cent of that in uninjected animals respectively. These results could also be interpreted as if the glutamate turn-over is severely reduced on the operated side so that there is less glutamate being released and taken into glial cell, and consequently less glu available for gln formation on that side.

An alternative drug was ammonia which leads to an increase in gln. This may be caused both by increased synthesis and by inhibition of glutaminase. The animals examined between 7 and 15 min after being injected with an ammonium salt showed a decrease in glu and asp, and an increase in gln on both sides. This is in agreement with investigations on unoperated rats (Benjamin, 1982). There were no striking differences between the operated and nonoperated sides.

The results clearly indicate that the turnover of glutamate in the intact and deafferented neostriatum are quantitatively different. The results, particularly those based on hypoglycemia, indicate a higher turnover in the intact neostriatum which contains the transmitter pool of glu. We

TABLE 2 AMINO ACID CONCENTRATIONS IN RAT NEOSTRIATUM

	CONTROL			HYPOGLYCEMIC RATS			
	Unoperated	Operated		Unoperated	Percent of control	Operated	Percent of control
	(n=8)	(n=8)		(n=13)		(n=13)	
	μmole/gm protein			μmole/gm protein		μmole/gm protein	
GLUTAMATE	106.0 ± 23.4	80.6 ± 11.0		58.2 ± 10.4	− 40.1%	69.9 ± 10.5	− 28.1%
ASPARTATE	10.9 ± 2.5	8.6 ± 3.1		34.6 ± 7.8	+217.4%	21.2 ± 5.1	+ 94.5%
GLUTAMINE	77.3 ± 22.6	64.8 ± 11.6		29.3 ± 10.6	− 62.1%	65.8 ± 25.4	− 14.9%
GABA	11.3 ± 4.0	10.6 ± 6.9		9.6 ± 2.4	− 15.0%	10.6 ± 3.2	− 6.2%
TAURINE	61.1 ± 8.2	56.8 ± 6.4		57.3 ± 4.9	− 6.2%	62.5 ± 12.1	+ 2.3%

therefore tentatively conclude that the turnover of transmitter glu is much faster than the metabolic glu. We are,
however, fully aware of the fact that other explanations are
possible. Thus the cortical input could be of major importance for maintaining the activity and thereby the metabolism for the whole neostriatum.

Balazs R, Cremer IE (1972). Metabolic compartmentation in
the brain. London McMillan.

Benjamin AM (1981). Control of glutaminase activity in rat
brain cortex in vitro: influence of glutamate, phosphate,
ammonium, calcium and hydrogen ions. Brain Research 208:
363.

Benjamin AM (1982). Ammonia. In A Lajtha (eds) "Handbook
of Neurochemistry" 2nd Ed, Vol 1. Plenum Press, New York
p 117.

Bradford HF, Ward HK & Tomas AJ (1978). Glutamine - a major
substrate for nerve endings. J Neurochem 30:1453.

Butterworth RF, Merkel AD & Landreville F (1982). Regional
Amino Acid Distribution in Relation to Function in Insulin Hypoglycaemia. J Neurochem 38:1483.

Fonnum F (1980). Tunover of transmitter amino acids, whith
special reference to GABA. In Pycock CJ, Tabernes PV:
Central neurotransmitter turnover. Bristol Univ Park
Press p 105.

Fonnum F, Storm-Mathisen J & Divac J (1981). Biochemical
evidence for glutamate as neurotransmitter in corticostriatal and corticothalamic fibres in rat brain.
Neuroscience 6:863.

Hamberger AC, Chiang GH, Nylen ES, Scheff SW & Cotman CW
(1979a). Glutamate as a CNS transmitter. I. evaluation
of glucose and glutamine as precursors for the synthesis
of preferentially released glutamate. Brain Research
168:513.

Hamberger AC, Chiang GH, Sandoval E & Cotman CW (1979b).
Glutamate as a CNS transmitter. II. regulation of synthesis in the releaseable pool. Brain Research 168:531.

Hassler R, Haug P, Nitch C, Kim JS & Paik K (1982). Effect
of motor and premotor cortex ablation on concentrations of
amino acids, monoamines, acetylcholine and on the ultrastructure in rat striatum. A confirmation of glutamate as
the specific cortico-striatal transmitter. J Neurochem
38:1087.

Lewis LD, Ljunggren B, Norberg K & Siesjø BK (1974).
Changes in Carbohydrate Substrates, Amino Acids and Ammo-
nia in the Brain during Insulin-Induced Hypoglycemia.
J Neurochem 23:659.
Tews JK & Stone WE (1964). Effects of methionine sulfoxi-
mine on levels of free amino acids and related substances
in brain. Biochem Pharmacol 13:543.
Van den Berg CJ, Matheson DF, Ronda G, Reijnierse GLA,
Blokhuis GGD, Kroon MC, Clarke DD & Garfinkel D (1975).
A Model of Glutamate Metabolism in Brain. A Biochemical
Analysis of a Heterogenous Structure. In Berl S,
Clark DD, Schneider AD (eds): "Metabolic Compartmentation
and Neurotransmission". Plenum Press p 515.
Van den Berg CJ & Van den Velden J (1970). The effect of
methionine sulphoximine on the incorporation of labelled
glucose, acetate, phenylalanine and proline into glutamate
and related amino acids in the brains of mice.
J Neurochem 17:985.

Glutamine, Glutamate, and GABA
in the Central Nervous System, pages 249–260
© 1983 Alan R. Liss, Inc., 150 Fifth Avenue, New York, NY 10011

GLUTAMINE AS A NEUROTRANSMITTER PRECURSOR: COMPLEMENTARY
STUDIES IN VIVO AND IN VITRO ON THE SYNTHESIS AND RELEASE OF
TRANSMITTER GLUTAMATE AND GABA.

H.F. Bradford, H.K. Ward and C.M. Thanki

Department of Biochemistry, Imperial College,
London SW7 2AZ, United Kingdom.

Studies with brain slices and synaptosomes at the biochemical level bring considerable advantages through control
of the environment of the preparation. However, gains in
simplicity are necessarily losses in complexity and with
this may come distortions in the isolated system under
scrutiny.

Thus, in vivo evidence which will complement and vali-
date in vitro results has always been an important require-
ment. We have made studies of amino acid neurotransmitter
synthesis, storage and release at both levels over the years
(Bradford 1981a,b) and this paper presents recent data which
bear on the possible transmitter function of glutamic acid
in mammalian brain. A cortical 'washing' or superfusion
system was employed for rat brain which allows the collection of amino acids and other neurotransmitters released by
direct surface depolarizations, or by specific sensory
stimulation from localized (4 mm diam) cortical regions
(Abdul-Ghani et al. 1978,1980; Coutinho-Netto et al. 1980).
Thus, application of the depolarizing peptide tityustoxin
isolated from scorpion venom, or application of the plant
alkaloid mixture veratrine to the cortical surface causes
release of putative amino acid neurotransmitters including
acetylcholine (Abdul-Ghani et al. 1980).

These responses may be entirely prevented by the Na^+-
channel blocker tetrodotoxin (Fig. 1 & 2) indicating their
neuronal origin. In addition transmitter release evoked by
topically applied agents or by sensory stimulation can be
prevented by morphine given by intraperitoneal injection,

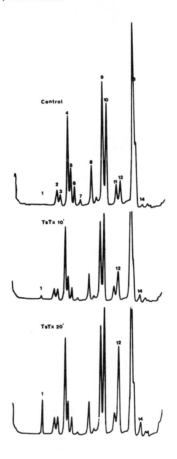

Fig. 1. Patterns of amino acids released from superfused rat sensorimotor cortex. Representative chromatograms of control and stimulated samples collected 10 and 20 min after beginning superfusion with saline containing tityustoxin (TsTx) (1 μM) are shown. Amino acids: 14, aspartate; 13, threonine, glutamine and serine; 12, glutamate; 11, citrulline; 10, glycine: 9, alanine; 8, valine; 7, methionine: 6, isoleucine; 5, leucine; 4, norleucine (50 pmol/100 μl of sample): 3, tyrosine; 2, phenylalanine; 1, GABA (from Coutinho-Netto et al. 1980).

and this effect is in turn prevented by naloxone (Coutinho-Netto et al. 1980, 1982). This sensitivity increases the likelihood that the evoked release of transmitter is the direct result of neuronal activity.

Collection and analysis of the released neurotransmitter allows study of its modulation by various added
drugs, but also allows investigation of its likely
biosynthetic precursors.

In particular, we have attempted to establish the
nature of the precursors for the pool of glutamate which
serves a neurotransmitter function.

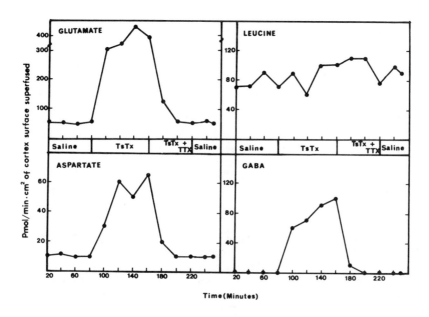

Fig. 2. Effect of tetrodotoxin on the amino acid-releasing
action of tityustoxin. In each animal eight 1-ml control
samples were collected (10 min each) from sensorimotor
cortex before tityustoxin (1 μM final concentration) was
added to the superfusion fluid for 80 min. Then, both
tetrodotoxin (0.1 μM) and tityustoxin (1 μM) were introduced for 60 min. This superfusate mixture was then
replaced by saline. The values given represent the mean of
three values from three animals superfused. Only alternate
samples were analysed for amino acid content (from
Coutinho-Netto et al. 1980).

A body of evidence now exists which indicates that while both glutamine and glucose can readily label the pools of tissue glutamate in the brain when presented to in vitro preparations, glutamine appears to label preferentially glutamate released by depolarizing stimuli.

These findings indicate that glutamate released to serve a neurotransmitter function is largely derived directly from glutamine through the activity of the enzyme glutaminase. The glutamate pool generated from glucose by transamination of 2-oxoglutarate appears therefore to be partially separated from the glutamine-derived pool. The connection between these two pools would be by way of con-version of the glucose-derived glutamate to glutamine (Fig. 3).

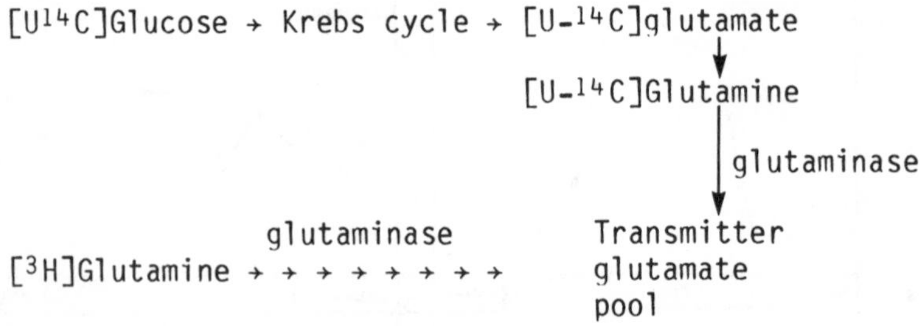

$[U^{14}C]$Glucose → Krebs cycle → $[U-^{14}C]$glutamate

$[U-^{14}C]$Glutamine

glutaminase

$[^3H]$Glutamine → → → → → → → →   glutaminase   Transmitter glutamate pool

Fig. 3. Scheme showing two routes of labelling of transmitter glutamate pool.

However, much of this evidence was derived from studies of in vitro labelling and release of glutamate in various isolated preparations such as slices of hippocampus (Hamberger et al. 1979a,b), cerebrocortical synaptosomes (Bradford et al. 1978) and slices of pigeon optic tectum (Reubi et al. 1978). In order to examine the extent to which such preferential labelling of glutamate transmitter stores by glutamine occurs in vivo, the endogenous pools of glutamate and other transmitter amino acids of cerebral cortex and hippocampus were radiolabelled in vivo by intra-cerebral injection of isotopic glutamine or glucose in both single- and double-labelling experiments. The patterns of radiolabelling of glutamate, glutamine, γ-aminobutyric acid (GABA) and aspartate released in vitro from brain slices subsequently prepared were then monitored (Ward et al. 1982). This is the so-called ex-vivo approach.

Incubations

Slices (30-60 mg) were incubated at 37°C for 10 min in Krebs-Tris medium under a gas phase of 100% O_2. The Krebs-Tris medium had the following composition (mM): NaCl 124; KCl 5.0; KH_2PO_4 1.25; $MgSO_4$ 1.2; $CaCl_2$ 0.75; Tris-HCl 35; glucose 10; pH 7.2. After brief rinsing in medium, the slices were incubated for a further 8 min in 1 ml fresh medium. Veratrine (75 µM) was present in all vessels, and tetrodotoxin (1 µM) in all control media.

Ex Vivo Studies: Single labelling experiments

Slices of hippocampus or cerebral cortex labelled in vivo by intracerebral injection of [U-^{14}C] glucose (0.8 mM) or [U-^{14}C] glutamine (1.25 mM), were subsequently incubated (Ward et al. 1982) and stimulated by addition of veratrine (75 µM). The amounts and the extent of labelling of the amino acids released by this treatment were measured, and the specific radioactivities of amino acids generated from [U-^{14}C] glucose and [U-^{14}C] glutamine were compared (Table 1). Corrections (about 5%) were made for the small amounts of counts and nanomoles of amino acids released by unstimulated slices. It can be seen that for hippocampal slices with [U-^{14}C] glutamine as in vivo precursor, the specific radioactivity of glutamate released by the depolarizing stimulus of veratrine was about equal to that shown by these amino acids in the tissue; for GABA it was double. With [U-^{14}C] glucose as the in vivo precursor, the specific radioactivity of these two amino acids in the medium was about half that found in the tissue. Thus, in comparative terms, glutamine appeared to be more effective than glucose in labelling releasable glutamate formed in vivo by hippocampus.

Employing this single label approach, glutamine also appeared to label releasable glutamate and GABA of cortical slices preferentially, the labelling of GABA being the greater (Table 1).

Ex Vivo Studies: Double labelling experiments

Slices of hippocampus previously labelled in vivo simultaneously with [U-^{14}C] glucose (3.7 mM) and [^{3}H]

Table 1. In vivo labelling and in vitro release from slice

Precursor	Ratio of specific radioactivities (medium:tissue)	
	Glutamate	GABA
A.		
Hippocampus		
[U-14C] glucose	0.61±0.07 (4)	0.61±0.08 (4)
[U-14C] glutamine	1.04±0.11 (4)	2.56±0.21 (4)
Cortex		
[U-14C] glucose	0.76±0.09 (7)[a]	1.19±0.45 (7)[b]
[U-14C] glutamine	1.69±0.23 (11)	1.96±0.49 (11)
B.		
Hippocampus		
[U-14C] glucose	0.772±0.05 (7)[c]	1.24±0.13 (7)[c]
[3H] glutamine	1.009±0.19 (7)	1.23±0.14 (7)
C.		
[3H] glutamine	13.82±1.4 (8)	21.8±1.79 (7)
[U-14C] glucose	11.80±0.63 (7)	18.8±0.93 (7)

A: Single label. B: Double label (hippocampal slices)
C: Percentage release (hippocampal slice). After labelling
in vivo for 1.5h with the substrates indicated, slices were
stimulated in vitro with veratrine as described in
Experimental Procedures. Values are mean ± SEM for the
number of values given in parentheses.
a,b Values for glucose different from values for
glutamine; a: $p < 0.025$; b: $p < 0.05$; c: Not significant

glutamine (0.54 mM), were stimulated by veratrine as des-
ribed above. On the whole, the findings were in accord
with those from hippocampal slices employing the single
labelling approach (Table 1 & 2). Thus, the ratio of
specific radioactivities of glutamate recovered in medium
compared with that in tissue was close to unity when [3H]
glutamine was the substrate. In contrast to the single-
label experiments described above, [U-14C] glucose was
equally effective in labelling glutamate recovered in
medium and tissue, since the apparently lower extent of
labelling by glucose (0.77) was not significant and
represented only a trend (Table 1). In addition,
equivalent proportions of the total [3H]-labelled and

[^{14}C]-labelled aspartate, glutamate and GABA were released by veratrine, which also suggested that the transmitter pools received similar contributions from [^{3}H] glutamine and the [^{14}C] of [U-^{14}C] glucose under these conditions of labelling.

A major limitation in comparing glucose and glutamine as substrates in vivo or in whole tissue slice studies is the background formation of glutamine from radiolabelled glucose. This glutamine is then, in the longer term, able to mix with that applied directly and, at least partially, to mask the contribution due to the glutamate generated (Fig. 3). This is seen to be the case from the data of Table 2, where the specific radioactivity of [^{14}C] glutamine generated from glucose is two- to three-fold higher than that of [^{3}H] glutamine. There is evidence that two species of glutaminase having different regulatory properties may exist in mitochondria, one in the inner matrix yielding glutamate for energy production and a second type in the outer matrix which could supply glutamate for transmitter and other functions in the cytosol (Kvamme & Olsen 1981).

Table 2. Relative specific radioactivities of glutamate, glutamine and GABA after double isotope labelling in vivo

Compound	^{14}C Specific radioactivity / ^{3}H Specific radioactivity
Glutamate	4.28 ± 0.61 (8)
Glutamine	2.55 ± 0.43 (8)
GABA	2.81 ± 0.19 (6)

Values are for whole tissue and represent the mean ± SEM for the number of values in parentheses. Allowance has been made for the sevenfold difference in specific radioactivities between [^{3}H] glutamine and [U-^{14}C] glucose present in the infusate.

However, in spite of this possibly exaggerated contribution from glucose to transmitter glutamate pools, glutamine appears to be at least as effective as glucose as precursor in vivo when judged on the basis of contribution to specific labelling of tissue and 'releasable' glutamate, or by the percentage of total pool released by depolariza-

tion. This is the case in spite of the fact that the concentration of glutamine in the intracerebrally infused
solutions - and in the cerebrospinal fluid - is 7 to 10
times less than that of glucose.

Thus, these results from ex vivo experiments support
the contention that glutamine is a major in vivo precursor
of transmitter glutamate and GABA. The single-label experiments show a clear preference for glutamine as precursor,
while the double-label approach indicates equal contributions from both glutamine and glucose. The results differ
from those from experiments with synaptosomes, which
unequivocally showed a three- to four-fold greater contribution from glutamine than from glucose (Bradford et al.
1978). However, the absence of glutamine synthetase in
synaptosome preparations eliminates the contribution to
releasable glutamate from glucose-derived glutamine. In
vitro experiments with slices of hippocampus also firmly
indicate the preferential role of glutamine rather than
glucose as precursor (Hamberger et al. 1979a,b). Radiolabelling under these conditions allows precise control of
the concentrations and specific radioactivities of
precursors added to the incubation medium.

Other evidence from in vitro preparations indicates
the substantial role of glutamine as precursor of transmitter glutamate. This includes studies on the inhibition
of glutaminase in cerebellar (Nicklas & Krespan 1982;
Hamberger et al. 1979) and hippocampal slices, which
results in decreased release of glutamate. Slices of
pigeon optic tectum also show a high degree of labelling of
releasable glutamate and GABA by glutamine given as
precursor (Reubi et al. 1978).

The Labelling of GABA

In single-label experiments, GABA released to the
medium by veratrine was of approximately twice the specific
radioactivity of that remaining in the tissue. In double-
label experiments, these were very similar. The same
limitations apply concerning the comparative labelling of
GABA by glucose and glutamine as applied to glutamate
formation in vivo. It is clear, however, that glutamine,
as well as glucose, can efficiently label transmitter GABA
in vivo. Others have shown a similar high degree of label-

ling of GABA by glutamine continuously infused into the
substantia nigra and pallidoentopeduncular nuclei in vivo
(Gauchy et al. 1980; and in vitro, Kemel et al. 1979).

In Vivo Studies

The cerebral cortex of awake, unrestrained and
behaviourally normal rats was superfused continuously as
described above. Following infusion (20 min) of [$U^{14}C$]
glutamine at the cerebrospinal fluid level (0.5 mM) onto
localized areas of cortex (sensorimotor area) and a
subsequent washing period, a depolarizing stimulus was
delivered to the cortex (tityustoxin 1 μM for 45 min).
This caused considerable, selective, and tetrodotoxin-
sensitive, release of transmitter amino acids (Figs. 1,2,4
and 5), particularly of glutamate. When these were

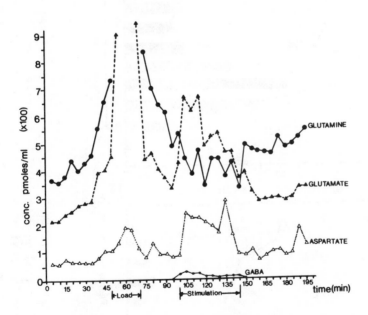

Fig. 4. Release in vivo of glutamate, aspartate and GABA
from superfused sensorimotor cerebral cortex of rats.
Stimulation was with tityustoxin (1 μM) for 45 min.
[$U^{14}C$] Glutamine at 0.5 mM was loaded for 20 min. Flow
rate 1.2 ml/h. Data from one experiment typical of five
(from Thanki et al. 1983).

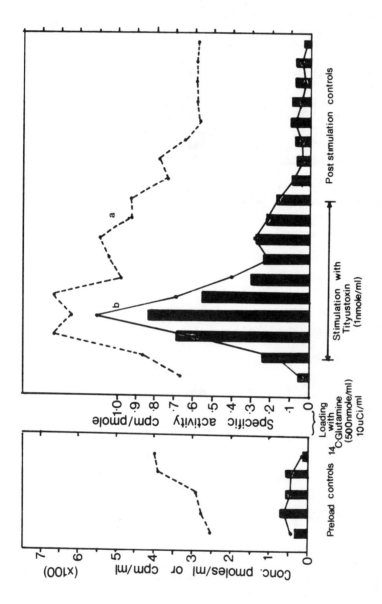

Fig. 5. Release of [¹⁴C] glutamate from superfused sensorimotor cerebral cortex of rat after loading with [U¹⁴C] glutamine (see Fig. 4). Residual activity (0–50 min) is due to previous experiments. Key: a, total nmol; b, total counts; histobars, specific radioactivity of glutamate (from Thanki et al. 1983).

separated and their radioactivity counted it was found that the glutamate released was of the "newly synthesized" category, being of much higher specific radioactivity than that released before or after the induced release signal (Figs. 4 & 5). [U^{14}C] Glutamate infused alone at 20-50 μM was released in much smaller quantities (6-8%) and could not account for the [^{14}C] glutamate released after infusion of [U^{14}C] glutamine (Thanki et al. 1983). Thus, once again, the likely importance of glutamine as the principal and direct precursor of transmitter glutamate is high-lighted; and, in this series of experiments, both labelling and release were responses of normal intact, fully functioning, sensorimotor cortex in vivo.

REFERENCES

Abdul-Ghani AS, Bradford, HF, Cox DWG, Dodd PR (1978). Peripheral sensory stimulation and the release of transmitter amino acids in vivo from specific regions of cerebral cortex. Brain Res 171:55.

Abdul-Ghani AS, Coutinho-Netto J, Bradford HF (1980). In vivo release of acetylcholine evoked by brachial plexus stimulation and tityustoxin. Biochem Pharmacol 29:2179.

Bradford HF (1981). Glutamate as a neurotransmitter: Studies on its synthesis and release. In Rodnight RB (ed): "Chemisms of the Brain," Churchill Livingstone, Edinburgh.

Bradford HF (1981). GABA release in vivo and in vitro: Responses to physiological and chemical stimuli. In Tapia R, Cotman CW (eds): "Regulatory Mechanisms of Synaptic Transmission," Plenum Press, New York.

Bradford HF, Ward HK, Thomas AJ (1978). Glutamine - A major substrate for nerve endings. J Neurochem 30: 1453.

Coutinho-Netto J, Abdul-Ghani AS, Norris PJ, Thomas AJ, Bradford HF (1980). The effects of scorpion venom toxin on the release of amino acid neurotransmitters from cerebral cortex in vivo and in vitro. J Neurochem 35:558.

Coutinho-Netto J, Abdul-Ghani AS, Bradford HF (1982). Morphine suppression of neurotransmitter release evoked by sensory stimulation in vivo. Biochem Pharmacol 31:1019.

Coutinho-Netto J, Abdul-Ghani AS, Bradford HF (1980). Suppression of evoked and spontaneous release of neurotransmitters in vivo by morphine. Biochem Pharmacol 29:2777.

Cotman CW (1981). Plenary lecture published in "Glutamate as a Neurotransmitter." Di Chiara G, Gessa GL (eds) Raven Press, New York.

Gauchy ML, Kemel ML, Glowinski J, Besson MJ (1980). In vivo release of endogenously synthesized [^{3}H] GABA from the cat substantia nigra and the pallidoentopenducular nuclei. Brain Res 193:129.

Hamberger A, Chiang C, Nylen ES, Scheff SW, Cotman CW (1979). Glutamate as a CNS transmitter I. Evaluation of glucose and glutamine as precursors for the synthesis of preferentially released glutamate. Brain Res 168:513.

Hamberger A, Chiang GH, Sandoval E, Cotman CW (1979). Glutamate as a CNS transmitter II. Regulation of synthesis in the releasable pool. Brain Res 168:531.

Kvamme E, Olsen BE (1981). Evidence for compartmentation of synaptosomal phosphate-activated glutaminase. J Neurochem 36:1916.

Kemel ML, Gauchy C, Glowinski J, Besson MJ (1979). Spontaneous and potassium-evoked release of ^{3}H-GABA newly synthesized from ^{3}H-glutamine in slices of the rat substantia nigra. Life Sci 24:2139.

Nicklas WJ, Krespan B (1982). Studies on neuronal-glial metabolism of glutamate in cerebellar slices. In Bradford HF (ed): "Neurotransmitter Interaction and Compartmentation," Plenum Press New York, p. 370.

Reubi JC, Van Den Berg C, Cuenod M (1978). Glutamine as precursor for the GABA and glutamate transmitter pools. Neurosci Lett 10:171.

Thanki CM, Sugden D, Thomas AJ, Bradford HF (1983). In vivo release from cerebral cortex of [^{14}C]-glutamate synthesized from [U^{14}C]-glutamine. J Neurochem 41:611.

Ward HK, Thanki CM, Bradford HF (1982). Glutamine and glucose as precursors of transmitter amino acids: Ex vivo studies. J Neurochem 40:855.

Glutamine, Glutamate, and GABA
in the Central Nervous System, pages 261–272
© 1983 Alan R. Liss, Inc., 150 Fifth Avenue, New York, NY 10011

GLUTAMATE, ASPARTATE AND GABA METABOLISM IN THE RAT RETINA:
COMPARTMENTATION AND EFFECTS OF LIGHT.

Mary J. Voaden

Reader in Biochemistry
Department of Visual Science,
Institute of Ophthalmology,
Judd St, London WC1H 9QS, U.K.

It has been recognized for many years that a typical
'Chain' pattern is observed when ^{14}C-glucose is metabolised
by the rat retina (Catanzaro et al 1962). Thus after
1 hr. incubation, radioactivity is seen, in order of
decreasing amounts in lactate, CO_2, glutamate, GABA,
aspartate, glutamine and alanine. Subsequent studies,
confirming and extending this observation, have provided
evidence for close similarities in metabolic organization
between the inner neuronal layers of the rat retina and
brain (Starr 1974, 1975;Voaden et al 1977;Voaden 1978).
However, it has also become apparent that there may be
fundamental species differences in,principally, GABA
homeostasis within the retina, and the aim of this
communication is to not only consider metabolism and function
in the rat but to also outline species differences where they
are known.

ENDOGENOUS LOCALIZATION AND SITES OF UPTAKE

Aspartate, glutamate and GABA are present in the rat
retina at concentrations of about 1.0 - 2.0, 3.0 - 6.0
and 1.5 - 3.0 μmol / gm wet wt respectively, but whereas
in the rat the former are fairly evenly distributed between
the photoreceptor cells and inner retinal neurones /glia,
GABA is considerably more concentrated in the inner neuronal
layers (Kennedy et al 1977; Morjaria, Voaden 1979;
Voaden 1979). Correlating with the latter, immunohistochemical studies have localized glutamate decarboxylase
to amacrine cells that appear to have a narrow-field,
multi-stratified distribution and that receive approximately

80% of their synaptic input from bipolar cells (Vaughn et al 1981; Famiglietti, Vaughn 1981). In addition, GABA formation from both glucose and glutamine has been shown to occur predominantly in a location consistent with this distribution (Voaden et al 1978; Morjaria, Voaden 1979). However, in both direct localization, and metabolic studies, evidence has also been obtained for the presence of a small but active GABA pool in the photoreceptor cell layer of the tissue. More work is needed to establish the site of this, but it may reflect the presence of the GABA bypath in rat photoreceptor cells (Morjaria, Voaden 1979; Voaden, Morjaria 1980)

It is now generally recognized that most if not all neuroactive amino acids, that are fulfilling a function based on their release from a neurone, can be taken up again into the cells releasing them by active, high-affinity mechanisms. When rat retinas are incubated with μM concentrations of glutamate or aspartate, identifiable uptake occurs into photoreceptors (>95% rods in the rat retina), and into the glial Müller cells (White, Neal 1976; Marshall, Voaden unpublished). As yet we do not know the preferred substrate for the photoreceptor carrier, but cell specificity does exist in other species (vide infra) and it is recognized that in the brain there is specificity between the carriers for cysteine sulphinic and glutamic acids in synaptic membranes (Recasens et al 1983).

Exogenously - applied GABA is taken up predominantly into Müller cells in the rat retina (Neal, Iversen 1972; Marshall, Voaden 1974). However, a GABA carrier is also present in a subpopulation of amacrine interneurones (Bauer, Ehinger 1978).

Species Differences:

As well as entering into glia, glutamate and/or aspartate (including D-aspartate) have been shown to be taken up into rod photoreceptor cells in man (Bruun, Ehinger 1974; Lamb, Hollyfield 1980; Marshall, Voaden unpublished), Cynomolgus monkey (Bruun, Ehinger 1974), baboon (Voaden et al 1981) and goldfish (Marc, Lam 1981), and into cones in guinea pig (Voaden et al 1981; Ehinger 1981),pigeon and rabbit (Ehinger 1981) and again goldfish (Marc, Lam 1981). In the latter study a unit area of rod membrane transported glutamate 30 times better than aspartate but little selectivity was seen in the subpopulation of active cones. Turtle cones may be cholinergic (Sarthy, Lam 1979).

All species thus far examined appear to have subpopulations of GABAergic amacrine cells which, in cyprinid fish and mudpuppy retinas may contact 'on' rather than 'off' centre bipolar cells (see Famiglietti, Vaughn 1981). In the cat retina, exogenously-applied GABA is also accumulated by some interplexiform neurones (Nakamura et al 1980; Pourcho 1981) and in lower order species such as amphibia, fish and birds, some horizontal cells are GABAergic (see Lam 1975; Voaden 1979). In addition, 'uptake' suggests a population of GABAergic bipolar cells in frog (Voaden 1976). There is no evidence for glial uptake of GABA in retinas from goldfish, turtle, frog, pigeon and chicken. In contrast it has been seen in skate, axolotl and salamander retinas and in all the mammalian retinas that have been studied.

METABOLISM AND EFFECTS OF LIGHT STIMULATION

In line with the observations of a predominant neuronal localization of endogenous GABA in the rat retina, and the uptake of exogenous GABA, principally by Müller cells (a major site of GABA-α-oxoglutarate transaminase activity: Hyde, Robinson 1974), the metabolism of radiolabelled GABA shows typical 'small compartment' characteristics – glutamine of higher specific activity than the total tissue glutamate being produced (Starr 1975a; Voaden et al 1977). The reverse is seen in frog and pigeon retinas (Voaden et al 1977; but cf Starr 1975a and discussion by Voaden 1978), where GABA enters predominantly if not solely into neurones (vide supra). Consistent with the presence of a glutamine 'cycle' in the rat retina, glutamine is metabolized alongside glucose to form glutamate, aspartate and GABA (Morjaria, Voaden 1979), the latter predominating in label and chase studies and autoradiography suggesting that the formation occurs in a subpopulation of amacrine cells (Voaden et al 1978).

A major advantage of the retina is that it can be functionally stimulated, both in vivo and in vitro, with light. It was, therefore, a natural progression from the above studies to investigate effects of illumination on the metabolism of glucose and glutamine.

Table 1 summarizes our findings as they relate to the turnover of aspartate, glutamate and GABA. In these studies 'dim light' refers to ambient daylight attenuated to approximately 5×10^{-3} lux : our aim in using this was to be within the working range of the rod photoreceptors. In vivo the amount of light reaching the retina will be further attenuated by about 50%. 'Day light' refers to a combination of actual daylight and ceiling fluorescent lights. These gave an average illumination, on the bench, of about 40 lux. For both in vitro and in vivo (Fig 1) studies with dim light, the rats were dark-adapted for 24 hrs and the retinas exposed at the start of the experimental period: photolabile pigment was still present at the end of incubations. In contrast, the visual pigment in light-adapted retinas, incubated in day light, rapidly bleached.

In general, distribution through the rat retina of the sites of synthesis of aspartate, glutamate and GABA from both glucose and glutamine appeared similar, the major difference being a relatively greater production of aspartate and glutamate from glutamine in the inner-most retinal layers (Morjaria, Voaden 1979). However, stimulation with dim light significantly reduced specific activities in the 'pools' derived from glutamine but not glucose (Table 1), suggesting that they were distinct.

The preferential turnover and release of neuroactive, amino acids derived from glutamine as compared with those from glucose has been noted in studies of several regions of the CNS (eg Bradford et al 1978; Hamberger et al 1979). Therefore, although decreased specific activities might reflect decreased turnover, they might also arise because increased turnover has led to the preferential release of newly-formed, more highly-labelled pools that have not equilibrated with the general tissue stores.

As regards glutamate and aspartate, the decreased activities were seen in both the photoreceptor cell and inner retinal layers (Voaden, Morjaria 1980). Apart from localization within, and high-affinity uptake into photoreceptors (vide supra), several neurophysiological studies involving postsynaptic receptor sensitivity have provided additional evidence that glutamate and/or aspartate are photoreceptor neurotransmitters (eg Wu, Dowling 1978; Kondo, Toyoda 1980). Photoreceptors release their neuro-transmitters in the dark and the release is curtailed

Table 1   The relative effects of light stimulation on the production of glutamate, aspartate and GABA from radiolabelled glucose and glutamine in the rat retina.

| | Relative Specific Activity[#] | | | | |
| | ^{14}C-glucose & glutamine | | ^{14}C-glutamine & glucose | | |
	DARK	DIM LIGHT	DARK	DIM LIGHT	DAY LIGHT
Aspartate	10.6	8.0	9.4	4.4***	5.0*
Glutamate	24.0	19.4	22.5	12.8**	19.3
Glutamine	8.8	8.2	81.0	76.2	73.4
GABA	6.7	5.7	12.1	7.0***	14.1

[#] specific activity of the amino acid relative to that of the precursor at the beginning of the incubation.
Asterisks denote the probabilities found when the original values for dpm/amino acid/3mm dia. disc retina (Voaden, Morjaria 1980; Voaden et al 1981, 1983) were t-tested against dark-adapted values.
* p < .05   ** p < .02   *** p < .01
Data for dark and dim light were obtained from 200 gm ♀, and for daylight from 300gm ♂, albino rats.
All retinas were incubated at 37°C, for 30 min, in Krebs' bicarbonate medium containing 5.5 mM glucose and 600 μM glutamine, plus either 30 μCi/ml ^{14}C-glucose or 15 μCi/ml ^{14}C-glutamine: they were then processed for the isolation of amino acids as described by Voaden et al (1978). Each value represents the mean of 4 estimations, three 3.0 mm discs of retina being combined for each one.
For the present evaluation endogenous amino acids were remeasured by HPLC (see Voaden et al 1983 for programme). Values were 20-30% lower than those obtained previously by double-label dansylation - glutamine being reduced by about 50%.
GABA levels were approx 50% higher than starting levels and, after incubation, did not show significant differences between light- and dark-adapted retinas (cf. Fig 1).

by light (eg Dowling Ripps 1973; Schacher et al 1976). In
line with this, evidence has been obtained for a decreased
output of aspartate from mud-puppy photoreceptors on light
stimulation (Miller et al 1982). Therefore, if we attempt
to relate the decreased specific activities in glutamate
and aspartate, which we saw in the light-stimulated retina,
to transmitter output, the result in the photoreceptor cell
layer is much more likely to be reflecting decreased output
and, consequently, decreased turnover. As for the inner
retina, however, we do not know the location of the changes.
Autoradiography has not, as yet, shown decipherable, specific
uptake of glutamate or aspartate into any inner retinal
neurones in the rat, and there are no clues from neurophysiology. For want of other candidates, it is often
proposed that some bipolar cells use glutamate or aspartate
as neurotransmitter, and, indeed, there is good evidence
for aspartatergic bipolars in cats (Ikeda, Sheardown 1982).
It is, in addition, possible that the changes seen in,
glutamate and aspartate followed from a decrease in GABA
turnover, since the specific activity of GABA was also
reduced when dark-adapted retinas were incubated in dim light
(Table 1).

An alternative index of GABA synthesis is its initial
rate of accumulation following inhibition of GABA-α-
oxoglutarate transaminase (GABA-T: see Bernasconi et al
1982, for references). As this approach potentially
provides a means of studying GABA turnover in vivo and is,
therefore, a useful if not vital adjunct to our in vitro
studies, we decided to include it in our investigations
(Voaden et al 1983). Initially, we have chosen as our
transaminase inhibitor the GABA analogue, ʃ-vinyl GABA,
thought to be highly specific and known to be essentially
without action on brain glutamate decarboxylase (Löscher
1980). The drug was administered intraperitoneally at a
dose of 1,500 mg/kg body wt to 180-230 gm female rats that
were either dark-adapted 24 hrs, dark-adapted 20 hrs
followed by exposure to 'dim light' for 4 hrs (vide supra),
or normally light-adapted, injections being given at
midday. The preliminary results are summarized in Fig 1.
Inhibition of GABA-T led to a non-linear increase in GABA
levels in the retina (cf Rando et al 1982) which, over
approximately 4 hrs, was significantly greater in dark-
adapted retinas than in tissue exposed to dim light.
Considering the similar starting levels, and our previous
observations (Table 1), this result supports the conclusion

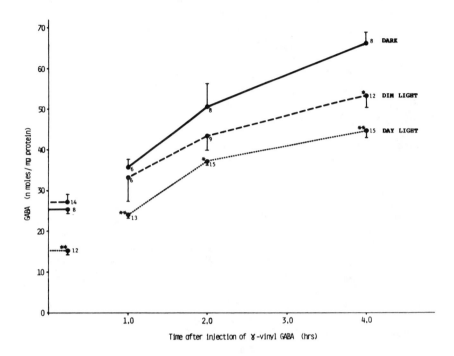

Fig 1. Accumulation of GABA in the rat retina following
intraperitoneal injection of ɣ-vinyl GABA.
* p<.01 ** p<.001 relative to dark-adapted values.
At the times indicated retinas were adsorbed directly from
the back of the eye onto filter paper and the amino acids
analysed by HPLC as described by Voaden et al (1983). GABA
was separated from all the common amino acids. The concentration of ɣ-vinyl GABA in the retina 1-4 hrs after
administration was approximately 30 nmoles/mg retinal protein.

that GABA turnover decreases on light-stimulation. Individual
values, plotted against time, 'best-fitted' rectangular
hyperbolae, (dark, r=0.85, p<.001; dim light, r=0.65,
p<.001; light, r=0.92, p<.001). From these we were able to
estimate initial turnover rates as 0.51 nmol/min/mg protein
in the dark and 0.38 nmol/min/mg protein in dim light
(Voaden et al 1983). The former agrees closely with the value
obtained by Proll and Morgan (1982), who applied a similar

approach but injected the GABA-T inhibitor, gabaculine, intravitreally: recalculating their result on the basis of a 10 mg wet wt rat retina, containing 10% protein, gives 0.52 nmol/min/mg protein.

Several observations provide evidence for the synaptic release of GABA in the dark-adapted rat retina (see Marshburn, Iuvone 1981; Biggio et al 1981; Proll, Morgan 1982). In particular, there is direct evidence suggesting that GABAergic neurones synapse directly onto dopaminergic ones and sustain a tonic inhibition in the dark (Marshburn, Iuvone 1981). Dopamine is the principal catecholamine in the retina where, in several species including the rat, it is located in a subpopulation of amacrine interneurones. Light exposure increases the rate of dopamine biosynthesis and release (eg Kramer 1971; Marshburn, Iuvone 1981), and it can, therefore, be predicted that GABA turnover will be decreasing in the neurones directly controlling the dopaminergic cells. However, apart from a tonic inhibition in the dark, Marshburn and Iuvone (1981) have also obtained data which suggests that, in the rat retina, another subpopulation of GABAergic neurones are involved in a pathway augmenting tyrosine hydroxylase activity in the light-adapted tissue. This observation may explain why, in the rat, intravitreal GABA appears to mimic a background of light and raises the retinal threshold for response to a light flash - picrotoxin and bicuculline having the reverse effect (Graham 1974).

Proll and Morgan (1982) found similar rates of GABA accumulation in fully light- and dark-adapted rat retinas when GABA-T was inhibited with gabaculine, and Starr (1975b) saw no difference in the specific activity of GABA in light and dark, following whole body labelling of rats with ^{14}C-glucose (although, in coincident experiments, GABA labelling was increased in light-exposed retinas of frogs). In addition, the results summarized in Table 1, also show that GABA turnover may be increasing again in the light-adapted (bleached) retina in vitro. However, we are unable to draw a definite conclusion from our preliminary findings with ɣ-vinyl GABA (Fig 1) as, at all the times studied, both before, and after ɣ-vinyl GABA administration, we have found significantly lower levels of GABA in light- as compared with dark-adapted retinas. This contrasts with our previous estimates, using double label dansylation, of about 25 nmoles GABA/mg retinal protein in the dark (a value close to the present one) and 29 nmoles GABA/mg retinal protein in the light (Voaden et al 1980). Others have found no difference between the GABA levels in light- and dark-adapted rat retinas (Starr 1973; Biggio et al 1981; Proll, Morgan 1982). Thus the present results, although highly significant, appear anomalous, and more investigations are needed to resolve the discrepancy.

The initial rate of GABA turnover in the light, obtained by extrapolation of the data shown in Fig 1, was estimated to be 0.38 nmol /min/ mg protein: identical to that found in dim light, but lower than the value reported by Proll and Morgan (1982). However, if the lower endogenous level in the light-adapted tissue proves correct, and if this accurately reflects content of the active GABA pool(s) then these may well be turning over faster than the pool(s) active in darkness.

ACKNOWLEDGEMENTS

I am grateful to Miss Yvette de Souza for typing this manuscript, and to Mr Ali Hussain for remeasuring endogenous amino acid levels in incubated retinas (Table 1). The ɣ-vinyl GABA was a gift from the Centre de Recherche Merrell International, Strasbourg (France).

REFERENCES

Bauer B, Ehinger B (1978). Retinal uptake and release of [^{3}H] DABA. Exp Eye Res 26:275.
Bernasconi R, Maitre L, Martin P, Raschdorf F (1982). The use of inhibitors of GABA-transaminase for the determination of GABA turnover in mouse brain regions: an evaluation of aminooxyacetic acid and gabaculine. J Neurochem 38:57.
Biggio, Guarneri P, Corda MG (1981). Benzodiazepine and GABA receptors in the rat retina: effect of light and dark adaptation. Brain Research 216:210.
Bradford HF, Ward HK, Thomas AJ (1978). Glutamine - a major substrate for nerve endings. J Neurochem 30:1453.
Bruun A, Ehinger B (1974). Uptake of certain possible neurotransmitters into retinal neurons of some mammals. Exp Eye Res 19:435.
Catanzaro R, Chain EB, Pocchiari F, Reading HW (1962). The metabolism of glucose and pyruvate in rat retina. Proc Roy Soc B 156:139.
Dowling JE, Ripps H (1973). Effect of magnesium on horizontal

cell activity in the skate retina. Nature 242:101.

Ehinger B (1981). [³H] —D-Aspartate accumulation in the retina of pigeon, guinea-pig and rabbit. Exp Eye Res 33:381.

Famiglietti EV, Vaughn JE (1981). Golgi-impregnated amacrine cells and GABAergic retinal neurons: a comparison of dendritic, immunocytochemical, and histochemical stratification in the inner plexiform layer of rat retina. J Comp Neurol 197:129.

Graham LT (1974). Comparative aspects of neurotransmitters in the retina. In Davson H, Graham LT (eds): "The Eye: Comparative Physiology,"Vol 6, NY and London: Academic Press, P 283.

Hamberger AC, Chiang GH, Nylén ES, Scheff SW, Cotman CW (1979). Glutamate as a CNS transmitter 1. Evaluation of glucose and glutamine as precursors for the synthesis of preferentially released glutamate. Brain Research 168:513.

Hyde JC, Robinson N (1974). Localization of sites of GABA catabolism in the rat retina. Nature 248:432.

Ikeda H, Sheardown MJ (1982). Aspartate may be an excitatory transmitter mediating visual excitation of 'sustained' but not 'transient' cells in the cat retina: iontophoretic studies in vivo. Neuroscience 7:25.

Kennedy AJ, Neal MJ, Lolley RN (1977). The distribution of amino acids within the rat retina. J Neurochem 29:157.

Kondo H, Toyoda J-I (1980). Dual effect of glutamate and aspartate on the on-center bipolar cell in the carp retina. Brain Research 199:240.

Kramer SG (1971). Dopamine: a retinal neurotransmitter 1. Retinal uptake, storage and light-stimulated release of ³H-dopamine in vivo. Invest Ophthalmol 10:438.

Lam DMK (1975). Synaptic chemistry of identified cells in the vertebrate retina. Cold Spr Harb Symp Quant Biol 40:571.

Lam DMK, Hollyfield JG (1980). Localization of putative amino acid neurotransmitters in the human retina. Exp Eye Res 31:729.

Löscher W (1980). Effect of inhibitors of GABA aminotrans- ferase on the metabolism of GABA in brain tissue and synaptosomal fractions. J Neurochem 34:1603.

Marc RE, Lam DMK (1981). Uptake of aspartic and glutamic acid by photoreceptors in goldfish retina. Proc Natl Acad Sci USA 78:7185.

Marshall J, Voaden MJ (1974). An investigation of the cells incorporating ³H glycine in the isolated retina of the rat. Exp Eye Res 18: 367.

Marshburn PB, Iuvone PM (1981). The role of GABA in the

regulation of the dopamine/tyrosine hydroxylase – containing neurons of the rat retina. Brain Research 214: 335.

Miller RF, Slaughter NN, Massey SC (1982). Light and dark dependent release of glutamate and aspartate in the isolated retina of the mudpuppy. Abstracts Soc.Neurosci: 12th annual meeting, Minneapolis USA, P 131.

Morjaria B, Voaden MJ (1979). The formation of glutamate, aspartate and GABA in the rat retina; glucose and glutamine as precursors. J Neurochem 33:541.

Nakamura Y, McGuire BA, Sterling P (1980). Interplexiform cell in cat retina: identification by uptake of γ-[^{3}H] aminobutyric acid and serial reconstruction. Proc Natl Acad Sci USA 77:658.

Neal MJ, Iversen LL (1972). Autoradiographic localization of ^{3}H-GABA in rat retina. Nature New Biol 235:217.

Pourcho RG (1981). Autoradiographic localization of [^{3}H] muscimol in the cat retina. Brain Research 215:187.

Proll MA, Morgan WW (1982). The use of gabaculine-induced accumulation of GABA for an index of synthesis of GABA in the retina. Neuropharmacology 21:1251.

Rando RR, Coburn J, Parkinson D (1982). The differential effects of GABA-transaminase inactivation in the chick retina and brain. J Neurochem 39:1147.

Recasens M, Saadoun F, Varga V, De Feudis FV, Mandel P, Lynch G, Vincendon G (1983). Separate binding sites in rat brain synaptic membranes for L-cysteine sulfinate and for L-glutamate. Neurochem Int 5:89.

Sarthy PV, Lam DMK (1979). Endogenous levels of neuro-transmitter candidates in photoreceptor cells of the turtle retina. J Neurochem 32:455.

Schacher S, Holtzman E, Hood DC (1976). Synaptic activity of frog retinal photoreceptors. A peroxidase uptake study. J Cell Biol 70:178.

Starr MS (1973). Effect of dark adaptation on the GABA system in retina. Brain Research 59:331.

Starr MS (1974). Evidence for the compartmentation of glutamate metabolism in isolated rat retina. J Neurochem 23:337.

Starr MS (1975a). A comparitive study of the utilization of glucose, acetate, glutamine and GABA as precursors of amino acids by retinae of the rat, frog, rabbit and pigeon. Biochem Pharmacol 24:1193.

Starr MS (1975b). Effect of light stimulation on the synthesis and release of GABA in rat and frog retinae. Brain Research 100:343.

Vaughn JE, Famiglietti EV, Barber RP, Saito K, Roberts E, Ribak CE (1981). GABAergic amacrine cells in rat retina: immunocytochemical identification and synaptic connectivity. J Comp Neurol 197:113.

Voaden MJ (1976). γ-Aminobutyric acid and glycine as retinal neurotransmitters. In Bonting SL (ed): "Transmitters in the Visual Process", Oxford: Pergamon Press, p 107.

Voaden MJ (1978). The localization and metabolism of neuro-active amino acids in the retina. In Fonnum F(ed): "Amino Acids as Chemical Transmitters", NY-London: Plenum Press, p 257.

Voaden MJ (1979). The chemical specificity of neurones in the retina. Progr in Brain Res 51:389.

Voaden MJ, Hussain AA, Taj M, Oraedu ACI (1983). Light and retinal metabolism. Biochem Soc Trans 11, No 6: In press.

Voaden MJ, Lake N, Marshall J, Morjaria B (1978). The utilization of glutamine by the retina: an autoradiographic and metabolic study. J Neurochem 31: 1069.

Voaden MJ, Lake N, Nathwani B (1977). A comparison of γ-aminobutyric acid metabolism in neurones versus glial cells using intact isolated retinae. J Neurochem 28:457.

Voaden MJ, Marshall J, Oraedu ACI (1981). The biochemistry of photoreceptor cells: metabolic effects of light stimulation and light damage. Docum Ophthal Proc Series 25:107.

Voaden MJ, Morjaria B (1980). The synthesis of neuroactive amino acids from radioactive glucose and glutamine in the rat retina: effects of light stimulation. J Neurochem 35:95.

Voaden MJ, Morjaria B, Oraedu ACI (1980). The localization and metabolism of glutamate, aspartate and GABA in the rat retina. Neurochem Int 1:151.

White RD, Neal MJ (1976). The uptake of L-glutamate by the retina. Brain Research 111:79.

Wu SM, Dowling JE (1978). L-Aspartate: evidence for a role in cone photoreceptor synaptic transmission in carp retina. Proc Natl Acad Sci, USA 75:5205.

**Glutamine, Glutamate, and GABA
in the Central Nervous System, pages 273–286**
© **1983 Alan R. Liss, Inc., 150 Fifth Avenue, New York, NY 10011**

The GABA Uptake System in Rabbit Retina

D.A. Redburn, S.C. Massey* and P. Madtes**

Department of Neurobiology and Anatomy
University of Texas Medical School
Houston, Texas 77030

There are many lines of evidence which suggest that chemical transmission in the retina occurs by the same basic mechanisms which operate in other parts of the central nervous system. Most of the classical neurotransmitter agents previously found in other nervous structures, have been found in retina where they are thought to be synthesized and stored in specific sets of pre-synaptic neurons, and released upon stimulation. The released neurotransmitters interact with receptors to excite or inhibit post-synaptic neurons [For recent reviews see Daw et al (1983) and Ehinger (1983)]. Many classical neurotransmitters, particularly biogenic amines and amino acids are inactivated by removal from the synaptic cleft via specific uptake mechanisms.

These widely-held notions concerning the interactions of neurotransmitter synthesis, release, receptor binding and uptake mechanisms are supported by substantial experimental evidence and they have contributed much to our overall understanding of neuronal circuitry and interaction. However, many questions remain as to the precise role each component mechanism may play in determining the overall efficacy of individual trans-

*Present address: Department of Ophthalmology
                   Washington University School of Medicine
                   St. Louis, MO 63110
**Present address: Laboratory of Vision Research National
                   Eye Institute
                   Bethesda, MD 20205

mission events. The anatomy and cellular architecture of the retina offer certain advantages which may allow an analysis of the relative importance of specific components of transmission associated with identified neuronal populations. In addition, the physiological stimulus, light, can be applied in a precisely controlled and non-invasive manner so that relatively direct correlations can be made between specific chemical events and the physiological response.

Electrophysiological and morphological studies in the vertebrate retina suggest that the visual pathway in the vertebrate retina is composed of five major cell types. Photoreceptors, bipolar and ganglion cells represent primary, secondary and tertiary sensory neurons respectively. The two remaining major cell types function as "interneurons". Horizontal cells provide feedback loops associated with photoreceptor to bipolar synapses, all of which are confined to the outer plexiform layer. Likewise, amacrine cells provide feedback loops associated with bipolar to ganglion cell synapses in the inner plexiform layer.

A further analysis of the functional aspects of retinal circuitry suggests that one specific component of synaptic transmission, namely the uptake system, may play a particularly important role in information processing. One well-established principle of retinal circuitry is that most synaptic transmission which occurs in the retina is stimulated by graded, synaptic potentials rather than all-or-nothing action potentials [For review see Rodieck 1973]. As a result, the flow of visual information through chemical synaptic pathways in the retina is a direct reflection of changes in the concentration of neurotransmitter in each synaptic cleft. Many retinal neurons are tonically active and maintain a partial depolarization which increases or decreases in magnitude in direct response to an increase or decrease in excitatory or inhibitory input. For example, photoreceptors are partially depolarized in the absence of light stimulation and thus continually release transmitter in the dark. At the onset of light, the photoreceptor becomes re-polarized and the rate of transmitter is decreased. Under these circumstances an efficient, high affinity uptake system for the neurotransmitter would play a key role in determining the efficacy of chemical transmission by directly influencing the level of transmitter tonically present in the cleft. In addition the uptake mechanism could be one of the major factors in determining response time of second order neurons. Since the light stimulus causes a decrease in the amount of transmitter released by the photoreceptor cell, the uptake system must remove previously released transmitter before the second order neuron can receive the "signal" from the photoreceptors.

The flow of synaptic transmission through the neurons which comprise the remaining retinal circuitry operates under much the same principle as that described for photoreceptor synapses. In bipolar and amacrine cell synapses both the presence as well as the absence of neurotransmitters in the cleft are important signals in the transfer and processing of visual information. Thus, it is reasonable to assume that mechanisms responsible for removal of transmitter are particularly important in the overall functioning of the retina.

Our studies of the uptake systems for a number of retinal neurotransmitters are consistent with this suggestion. In this chapter, we review our work on the uptake system for GABA in the rabbit retina. Using autoradiographic studies we have demonstrated the cellular sites of GABA transport and the relative metabolic rates of various intracellular pools of GABA. Using release studies, we have demonstrated at least one important function of GABA transmission and the impact of the GABA uptake system on that function. Finally, we have demonstrated that the time of postnatal development of the GABA uptake system precedes other synaptic components of the GABA system and furthermore, that the rate of internalization of extracellular GABA early in development, may influence the overall maturation rate of GABAergic synapses.

BIOCHEMICAL ANALYSIS OF ^{3}H-GABA UPTAKE

An avid uptake system for ^{3}H-GABA has been well-established in the rabbit retina. Biochemical studies using subcellular fractions from rabbit retina show the uptake system to be sodium and temperature dependent, and to have a high affinity for GABA (Redburn,

1977). Retinal fractions which contain the highest concentration of conventional synaptic endings primarily from amacrine cells, exhibit the highest level of GABA uptake activity. A three-fold enhancement of specific uptake activity is seen in these fractions as compared to whole retina homogenates. The sequestered GABA has a low leakage rate (2% per min) from retinal synaptosomes when perfused with a modified Ringer's solution. In contrast, greater than 90 percent of the GABA is released when fractions are lysed with icecold distilled water.

Efflux rates of the previously accumulated $[^{14}C]$ GABA were determined by perfusing retinal samples which were immobilized on a filter. In Ca^{++}-free buffer, the amount of $[^{14}C]$ GABA released per min declined with each succeeding wash until a relatively stable efflux rate was reached after three or four, 1 min washes. Addition of depolarizing levels of K^{+} caused a significant increase in the amount of GABA released per minute. Subsequent addition of 6 mM-Ca^{++} caused an additional increase in the release rate of $[^{14}C]$ GABA from the fraction to about 4-5% of the available $[^{14}C]$ GABA pool. Addition of 10 mM-$MnCl_2$ to all perfusates blocked the Ca^{++} stimulated release of ^{3}H-GABA.

These experiments demonstrate that retinal fractions take up ^{3}H-GABA and store it in a relatively stable pool which is released in a calcium-dependent manner during a depolarizing stimulus. Thus, it seems likely that the GABA uptake system could function in retina to terminate or decrease GABAergic transmission by internalizing GABA which had been previously released. Furthermore, the uptake system might serve to replenish releaseable stores of GABA.

AUTORADIOGRAPHIC LOCALIZATION OF ^{3}H-GABA ACCUMULATION

Autoradiographic analysis has demonstrated two sites of ^{3}H-GABA accumulation (Hampton and Redburn, 1983). One is associated with Muller cells, the major glial element of the retina; the other is associated with a specific set of amacrine and displaced amacrine cell neurons. Glial uptake appears to dominate since the number and size of Muller cells far exceed those of amacrine cells. Autoradiographs of rabbit retinas incubated in vitro for 15 min in ^{3}H-GABA are densely labeled with grains over Muller cell bodies and their processes which form the inner and outer limiting membranes. Labeling of amacrine cells is obscured under these conditions. However, further incubation of the tissue for 30 min in buffer alone results in a preferential loss of label associated with Muller cells and retention of label (chromatographically verified as authentic ^{3}H-GABA), associated with a specific set of amacrine cells. The loss of label by Muller cells during post incubation is presumably via metabolism of ^{3}H-GABA by GABA-transaminase to succinate and other Krebs' cycle intermediates which are not preserved during the autoradiographic process. Consistent with this interpretation, Ehinger (1977) has shown that loss of glial labeling is prevented by amino-oxyacetic acid, a GABA-transaminase inhibitor.

Thus, Muller cells provide a very effective sink for the removal and disposal of extracellular GABA. GABAergic neurons on the other hand also provide an active mechanism of clearance but in contrast to Muller cells, the GABA is not metabolized and is thus presumably available for subsequent recycling through the release system.

One intriguing finding is that brief in vitro exposure of the rabbit retina to kainic acid, a potent excitotoxic agent, causes a dramatic enhancement of ^{3}H-GABA accumulation by amacrine cells. Although the exact mechanism of action of this effect is unknown, it nevertheless has provided a clearer view of GABA-accumulating terminals than has previously been attainable in mammalian retinas (Marshall and Voaden, 1975). Four labeled sublamina are discernible within the inner plexiform layer. The outermost band appears as a continuous lateral arborization whereas the other bands are more punctate. Labeling in the middle of the inner plexiform layer appears as two bands with distinct patches of label. The innermost band is the thickest of the bands and comprises approximately 20% of the inner plexiform layer. It forms an interlacing network of punctate accumulations surrounding rather large, distinct, label-free areas. The broad distribution of GABA terminals within the inner plexiform layer and the relatively large number of GABA accumulating neurons suggests that GABA may be a very prominent neurotransmitter system in the rabbit retina.

INTERACTION OF GABA WITH THE CHOLINERGIC SYSTEM

We have also examined the influence of GABA on the cholinergic neurons of the rabbit retina which have been identified as conventional and displaced amacrine cells bordering the inner plexiform layer in a mirror-symmetrical fashion (Masland and Mills, 1979; Famiglietti, 1983a,b). The exact function of the cholinergic amacrine cells is presently unknown but they provide excitatory input to ganglion cells and appear to be an essential part of the circuitry responsible for directional sensitivity (Ariel and Daw, 1982). ACh is released from these neurons in response to light stimulation and may be detected in the retinal perfusate. This represents a method to monitor the activity of the cholinergic system in the retina and thereby to identify the synaptic inputs. Following this strategy, we have demonstrated that the cholinergic amacrine cells of the rabbit retina are tonically inhibited by GABA amacrines (Massey and Redburn, 1982).

The release of ACh was studied using the superfused in vivo rabbit eye-cup which has been previously described in detail (Massey and Redburn, 1982). The direct measurement of GABA efflux has not been possible using this preparation possibly due to the efficiency of the uptake system(s) responsible for the clearance of released GABA. In contrast, ACh is rapidly removed from the extracellular space not by uptake but through enzymatic hydrolysis by acetylcholinesterase. In our experiments this process is blocked with eserine and therefore ACh diffuses out of the retina to be carried away in the perfusate.

Early results showed that light stimulation of 3 Hz caused a Ca^{++}-dependent tenfold increase in ACh release (See Fig. 1). Some labelled choline was also released but this was not affected by light. Exposure of the retina to 1 mM GABA caused a marked depression in the light-evoked release of ACh with a small but consistent drop in basal efflux. At low concentrations the GABA antagonists bicuculline (5 uM) and picrotoxin (20 uM) caused a striking increase in basal efflux and greatly potentiated the light evoked release of ACh. In contrast the glycine

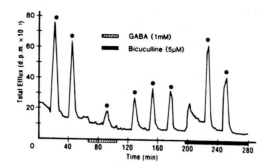

Figure 1. The effect of GABA (1 mM) and bicuculline (5 uM) on the light-evoked release of ACh. The asterisks indicate light stimulation for 4 min at 3 Hz. The light-evoked release of ACh was inhibited by GABA but enhanced by bicuculline. A similar result was seen when bicuculline was replaced with picrotoxin (20 uM). The peak immediately after the addition of bicuculline represents a change in the spontaneous release which we ascribe to GABA disinhibition. Data is from Massey and Redburn (1982a).

antagonist strychnine (5 uM) had no effect on ACh release.

We also examined the effects of the GABA agonist muscimol which in this system was approximately 2000 times more potent than GABA. At a concentration of 1 uM muscimol caused a 90% reduction in the light evoked release of ACh and abolished the basal efflux. We were surprised by the efficacy of muscimol (2000 times more potent than GABA), especially since muscimol is only 5 times more potent than GABA in displacement of receptor binding in retinal membrane preparations (Redburn and Mitchell, 1981). Preferential and rapid GABA transport by the avid glial and neuronal uptake systems, for which muscimol is a poor substrate, may be responsible for this apparent discrepancy, especially if there are many transport sites close to the region of the synapse to terminate the action of released GABA.

In support of this hypothesis 1 mM nipecotic acid, a substance known to block GABA transport without activating the GABA receptor, inhibited the light-evoked release of ACh and decreased the basal efflux in a way similar to the

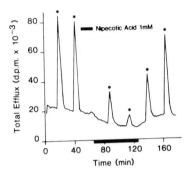

Figure 2. The effect of nipecotic acid on the light-evoked release of ACh. The asterisks indicate light stimulation for 4 min at 3 Hz. Nipecotic acid (1 mM) caused a slow depression in basal efflux and inhibited the light-evoked release of ACh. In contrast to GABA or muscimol, the recovery on washout was prompt. (Data are from Massey and Redburn 1982).

depression seen with GABA or muscimol (See Fig. 2). However, in comparison to these direct receptor agonists, nipecotic acid inhibition was relatively slow in onset but rapid in recovery. We suggest that these effects may be attributed to the slow accumulation of extracellular GABA caused by a block of GABA transport. When nipecotic acid is removed a rapid clearance of GABA should cause a prompt recovery as seen in these experiments. These results indicate the possible importance of the GABA uptake system and appear to be consistent with a tonic GABA release.

DEVELOPMENTAL STUDIES OF THE GABA TRANSPORT SYSTEM

The uptake system for GABA is active prenatally since ^3H-GABA is accumulated by presumptive amacrine cells as early as embryonic day 22 (Fong et al., 1982). Biochemical studies demonstrate that the uptake rate of ^3H-GABA at birth is approximately 60-70% of adult levels. The early appearance of uptake activity during development is in contrast to other components of the GABA system including stimulated release, synthesis and receptor binding, which emerge from postnatal day 6 to day 12, a time coincident with the period of rapid synaptogenesis (Lam et al (1980); Madtes and Redburn,

1982; Redburn and Mitchell, 1981).

Autoradiographic analysis demonstrates that accumulation of ^{3}H-GABA by Muller cells is very limited at birth and that the majority of ^{3}H-GABA accumulated by immature retina is associated with presumptive amacrine cells (Madtes and Redburn, 1983c). When retinas from one or two day old rabbits are incubated for 15 min in ^{3}H-GABA, there is no discrete labeling of cells which possess a mature Muller cell profile although Muller cells are present in substantial number at this developmental stage. In contrast, heavy labeling of amacrine cell bodies is readily apparent at birth along with a band of label in the inner plexiform layer associated with undifferentiated neurites. Glial uptake of ^{3}H-GABA is not observed until postnatal day 4 or 5.

The rate of GABA synthesis in retina is quite low at birth resulting in an endogenous concentration of only 0.2 uM (Lam et al., 1980). However, this level is within the range of the affinity of the GABA transport site, which is approximately 1 uM. Therefore, it is reasonable to assume that the neuronal GABA transport system is active at birth in the rabbit retina and thus may be a major factor in establishing the concentration of extracellular GABA during the developmental period which preceeds synaptogenesis.

However, we questioned the physiological role of the transport system in a tissue virtually devoid of GABAergic transmission. As a test of its possible functional importance, we examined the effects of blocking uptake with nipecotic acid in retinas during early postnatal development (See Fig. 3). Our results showed that a single in vivo injection of nipecotic acid was effective in inhibiting ^{3}H-GABA uptake measured in vitro 24 hours post-injection (Madtes and Redburn, 1983a). Following a transient and as yet unexplained increase in uptake approximately 48 hrs post injection, there was a prolonged inhibition of uptake activity at least up to postnatal day 14.

Another effect on the GABA system was also noted when GABA uptake was blocked in vivo by nipecotic acid (See Fig. 3). Using ^{3}H-muscimol binding as a measure of GABA receptor activity, we demonstrated a significant

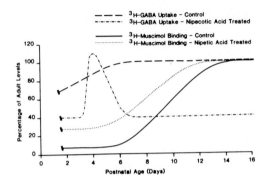

Figure 3. The effect of nipecotic acid on specific ^{3}H-GABA uptake and ^{3}H-muscimol binding during development. Pups were given a unilateral intraocular injection (40 ul) of nipecotic acid (final concentration = 10 mM) one day after birth. The non-injected contralateral eye served as the control. The tissue was assayed for ^{3}H-GABA uptake by in vitro incubation for 10 min in 10 uM ^{3}H-GABA. Data is expressed as specific uptake (uptake at 37°C in the presence of Na$^+$ minus uptake at 0°C, na$^+$-free) corrected for protein content. The tissue was also measured for ^{3}H-muscimol binding. Data is expressed as specific binding [total binding (the amount bound in the absence of unlabeled muscimol) minus non-specific binding (the amount bound in the presence of unlabeled muscimol)]. Data were taken from Madtes and Redburn (1983a).

alteration in the postnatal development of GABA receptors (Madtes and Redburn, 1983a). Normally, the level of GABA receptor binding is low shortly after birth. A rapid rise follows from day 6 to day 12 after birth at which time adult levels are reached. This change coincides with the period of rapid synapse formation. Twenty-four hours after a single injection of nipecotic acid, there was a four fold increase in ^{3}H-muscimol binding to the receptor compared to control values. However, the increase in receptor binding was not maintained beyond day 12 when adult levels are normally reached. The overall effect of the nipecotic acid treatment therefore was to shift the developmental curve to the left without significantly altering the general shape of the curve.

In a subsequent series of experiments we analyzed the

effects of nipecotic acid treatment in vitro, on GABA receptor binding and found them to be identical to those found after in vivo treatment (Madtes and Redburn, 1983b). Exposure of isolated retinas from 1 day old rabbits, to nipecotic acid for 45 min in vitro caused a 4 fold increase in GABA receptor binding compared to controls incubated in buffer only. The increase observed in vitro was determined to be an increase in the number of high-affinity receptors, with no change in the apparent affinity (Madtes and Redburn, unpublished data). The number of receptors present after nipecotic acid treatment is identical to the number observed after Triton X-100 treatment, a method which unmasks all GABA-sensitive binding sites. These results suggests that the induction phenomenon may involve the unmasking of previously synthesized receptors present in the postsynaptic membrane rather than de novo synthesis. In contrast, isolated retinas from adult rabbits showed a decrease in binding after the same in vitro incubation with nipecotic acid. This finding indicates that the observed induction of receptors with neonatal tissue reflects a developmental sensitivity which disappears with maturation.

Several laboratories have shown that nipecotic acid has virtually no affinity for the GABA receptor (Lester and Peck, 1978; Olsen et al., 1978). Therefore, the increase in GABA receptors we observed is probably not due to a direct interaction of nipecotic acid with the receptor. Hence, an indirect effect, such as an increase in GABA concentration, may be a more likely possibility. Nipecotic acid-induced inhibition of endogenous GABA accumulation by retinal cells might reasonably be expected to cause an increase in extracellular GABA concentration since Wood et al (1980) demonstrated that inhibition of GABA uptake by nipecotic acid in vivo caused an increase in the synaptic level of GABA in the adult rat cerebellum. Thus, an increased GABA concentration may be the direct cause of the increase in receptors which we observed.

In order to test this hypothesis, we analyzed the in vitro effects of GABA agonists and found that pre-treatment with GABA, 4,5,6,7-tetrahydroisoxazol [5,4,-c] pyridine-3-ol (THIP) or muscimol mimicked the effect of nipecotic acid on GABA receptor binding. We interpret these results to suggest that receptor agonists may influence the expression of receptor number in immature retina. In addition, the effects of nipecotic acid may be indirectly mediated via its regulation of extracellular levels of GABA which in turn influence receptor binding activity. The induction of GABA receptors by exposure to GABA itself, GABA agonists or treatments which cause an increase in extracellular GABA may suggest that GABA acts as a trophic substance during development by stimulating the functional maturation of post-synaptic GABA receptors.

In support of this hypothesis are the findings in brain which suggest that GABA itself may modulate the development of its own functional capacities (Spoerri and Wolff, 1981; Wolff, 1981). Moreover, the findings of Meier and Schousboe (1982) demonstrate that the addition of GABA to the culture medium of immature cerebellar granule cells resulted in the increase of physiologically active, low-affinity GABA receptors.

While these interpretations are consistent with our findings and those of other laboratories, further experimentation will be necessary in order to fully evaluate the trophic actions of GABA during development. It is important to note, however, that regardless of the actual mechanism of action, our data clearly shows two profound effects of blocking the GABA uptake system in the immature retina. First, there is a permanent inhibition of GABA uptake after only a single exposure to the uptake blocker. Second, there is a transient but substantial increase in GABA receptor binding. Thus, it would appear that the GABA transport system plays a vital role in the maturation of the GABA system as a whole. Since these effects are observed at a time when GABAergic synaptic transmission is virtually absent, we assume that they reflect a functional role for the transport system in developing retina which is distinct from the adult model in which it serves to terminate GABAergic transmission and replenish releasable pools of GABA.

In summary, we have demontrated the presence of GABA transport sites associated with Muller cells and amacrine cells of the rabbit retina. We have also shown that GABAergic neurons are tonically active. Furthermore, the activity of the uptake system has significant influence on GABAergic transmission presumably by regulating the extracellular concentration of GABA. Specifically, we find that blockage of the uptake system by nipecotic acid causes a significant increase in the efficacy of GABAergic inhibition of the cholinergic pathway.

Neonatally, the uptake system for GABA is the first parameter of the GABA system to mature. It appears to be a functionally active system in immature retina and it may influence the overall maturation of GABAergic synapses. Blockage of uptake by a single intraocular injection of nipecotic acid caused a significant decrease in uptake activity and a concomitant increase in GABA receptor binding. Thus, it appears that the transport system is active in immature retina and that its actions in the subsequent maturation of GABAergic synapses represents a function distinct from its role in adult chemical transmission.

Ariel M, Daw NW (1982). Pharmacological analysis of directionally sensitive rabbit retinal ganglion cells. J Physiol 324:161.

Daw NW, Ariel M, Caldwell JH (1983). Function of neurotransmitters in the retina. Retina 2:322.

Ehinger B (1977). Glial and neuronal uptake of GABA, glutamic acid, glutamine and glutathione in the rabbit retina. Exp Eye Res 25:221.

Ehinger B (1983). Neurotransmitter systems in the retina. Retina 2:203.

Famiglietti EV Jr (1983a). Synaptic connections of stardust amacrine cells in rabbit retina. Invest Ophthalmol & Vis Sci 24: Suppl p 260.

Famiglietti EV Jr (1983b). 'Stardust' amacrine cells and cholinergic neurons: mirror-symmetric ON and OFF amacrine cells of rabbit retina. Brain Res 261:138.

Fong SC, Kong YC, Lam DM (1982). Prenatal development of GABAergic, glycinergic and dopaminergic neurons in the rabbit retina. J Neurosci 2:1623.

Hampton CK, Redburn DA (1983). Autoradiographic analysis of ^{3}H-glutamate, ^{3}H-dopamine and ^{3}H-GABA accumulation in rabbit retina after kainic acid treatment. J Neurosci Res 9:239.

Lam DM, Fong SC, Kong YC (1980). Post-natal development of GABA-ergic neurons in the rabbit retina. J Comp Neurol 193:89.

Lester BR, Peck EH (1978). Kinetic and pharmacological characterization of gamma-aminobutyric acid receptor sites from mammalian brain. Brain Res 161:79.

Madtes P, Redburn DA (1982). (^{3}H)-GABA binding in developing rabbit retina. Neurochem Res 7:495.

Madtes P, Redburn DA (1983a). Synaptic interactions in the GABA system during development in retina. Brain Res Bull in press.

Madtes P, Redburn DA (1983b). GABA as a trophic factor during development. Life Sci in press.

Madtes P, Redburn DA (1983c). Postnatal maturation of GABA uptake systems in neurons and glia of the rabbit retina. (Submitted for publication).

Marshall J, Voaden M (1975). Autoradiographic identification of the cells accumulating ^{3}H-gamma aminobutyric acid in mammalian retinae: a species comparison. Vision Res 15:459.

Massey SC, Redburn DA (1982). A tonic gamma-aminobutyric acid-mediated inhibition of cholinergic amacrine cells in rabbit retina. J Neurosci 2:1633.

Meier E, Schousboe A (1982). GABA induces formation of low affinity responses. Amer Soc Neurochem Abstr 13:26.

Masland RH, Mills JW (1979). Autoradiographic identification of acetylcholine in the rabbit retina. J Cell Biol 83:159.

Olsen RW, Greelee D, Van Ness P, Ticku MK (1978). Studies on the gamma-butyric acid receptor/ionophore protein in mammalian brain. In Fonnum F (ed.): Amino Acids as Neurotransmitters: New York: Plenum Press p 467.

Redburn DA (1977). Uptake and release of ^{14}C-GABA from rabbit retina synaptosomes. Exp Eye Res 25:265.

Redburn DA, Mitchell CK (1981). ^{3}H-muscimol binding in synaptosomal fractions from bovine and developing rabbit retina. J Neurosci Res 6:487.

Rodieck RW (1973). "The Vertebrate Retina". San Francisco: Freeman and Company.

Spoerri PE, Wolff JR (1981). Effect of GABA-administration on murine neuroblastoma cells in culture. Cell Tiss Res 218:567.

Wolff JR (1981). Evidence for a dual role of GABA as a synaptic transmitter and a promoter of synaptogenesis. In DeFeudis FV, Mandel P (eds.): Amino Acid Neurotransmitters: New York: Raven Press p 459.

Wood JD, Schousboe A, Krogsgaard-Larsen P (1980). In vitro changes in the GABA content of nerve endings (synaptosomes) induced by inhibitors of GABA uptake. Neuropharmcol 19:1149.

**Glutamine, Glutamate, and GABA
in the Central Nervous System, pages 287–295
© 1983 Alan R. Liss, Inc., 150 Fifth Avenue, New York, NY 10011**

PHYSIOLOGICALLY ACTIVE KAINIC ACID-PREFERRING RECEPTORS IN
VERTEBRATE RETINA

Ian G. Morgan and D.R. Dvorak

Department of Behavioural Biology
Research School of Biological Sciences
Australian National University, Canberra, ACT
Australia

Excitatory amino acids are believed to play a central
role in the processing of visual information in the vertebrate retina. The photoreceptor transmitter is generally
believed to be L-glutamic or L-aspartic acid, and the bipolar cell transmitter, largely by default rather than
positive evidence (but see Ikeda and Sheardown 1982;
Slaughter and Miller 1983a for recent evidence), is also
believed to be an excitatory amino acid. The fact that the
photoreceptor transmitter may be an "excitatory" amino acid
raises some problems of nomenclature, since in addition to
depolarizing effects on horizontal cells and OFF-bipolar
cells, the photoreceptor transmitter is believed to *hyperpolarize* ON-bipolar cells. Throughout this paper the term
"excitatory amino acid" will be used to cover L-glutamic and
L-aspartic acid, and related endogenous compounds, if they
exist, even though they appear to exert inhibitory effects
at certain synapses.

Clarification of the nature of the transmitters and
receptors involved at the photoreceptor and bipolar cell
synapses has been hindered by the absence of agonists and
antagonists with clearly defined specificities. Recent work
(for review see Watkins and Evans 1981) has however defined
three agonists selective for three types of receptors, and
some relatively selective antagonists. One receptor is
selectively activated by N-methyl-D-aspartic acid (NMDA) and
selectively blocked by 2-amino-5-phosphonovaleric acid (2APV).
The second is selectively activated by quisqualic acid and
in some situations is blocked by glutamic acid diethyl ester

(GDEE) and γ-D-glutamylglycine (DGG). The third is selectively activated by kainic acid, and blocked by cis-2,3,-
piperidine dicarboxylic acid (PDA) and to a lesser extent by
DGG.

NEUROTOXICITY STUDIES USING AGONISTS AND ANTAGONISTS

The selective excitatory amino acid agonists cause
distinct patterns of toxicity in the chicken retina when
injected intravitreally. Injections of 10μl of 2-6mM kainic
acid cause distinct lesions which involve both the inner and
outer plexiform layers (Morgan and Ingham 1981). There is a
clearly defined hierarchy of cellular sensitivity to kainic
acid (Ingham and Morgan 1983; Morgan 1983; Morgan in press),
with most of the amacrine cells and approximately two thirds
of the bipolar cells being by far the most sensitive to
kainic acid. At concentrations 200-fold those of kainic
acid, none of the other agonists appeared to affect cells in
the outer part of the inner nuclear layer. Instead their
effects seemed to be restricted to the amacrine cells of the
inner part of the inner nuclear layer (unpublished results).

Based on the greater potency of kainic acid in causing
destruction of bipolar cells, there appeared to be some form
of kainic acid-preferring receptor at the level of the second-
order neurons in the outer plexiform layer. This was confirmed by using the antagonists (Fig. 1), where kainic acid-
induced toxicity was clearly blocked very effectively by PDA
and to a lesser extent DGG, while 2APV and GDEE were almost
without effect. It is difficult to estimate the effective
concentrations of kainic acid in the experiments performed
in vivo, but preliminary experiments using perfusion of isolated retinas suggest that toxic effects can be clearly
observed with concentrations of kainic acid of 100nM. This
figure is slightly higher than the K_D's (2nM and 44nM)
determined for kainic acid-binding sites in chicken retina
(Biziere and Coyle 1979). 100-fold molar concentrations of
PDA were needed to clearly block morphological toxicity.

To explain the partial destruction of bipolar cells,
we suggested that kainic acid might mimic the effect of the
photoreceptor transmitter, depolarizing and destroying the
OFF-bipolar cells and horizontal cells (which are indeed
destroyed by larger doses of kainic acid), while hyperpolarizing and sparing the ON-bipolar cells (Ingham and Morgan
1983). This hypothesis was confirmed by the demonstration

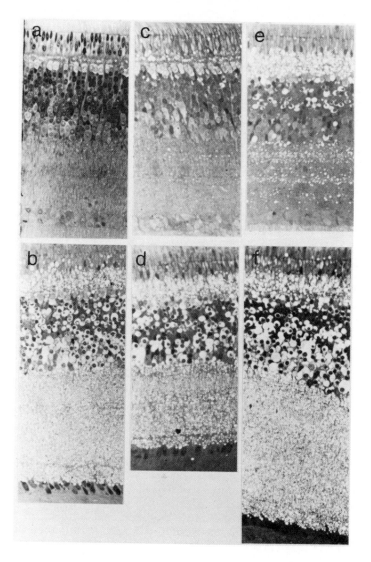

Figure 1. Antagonism of kainic acid-induced neurotoxicity in chicken retina. Transverse sections of chicken retina fixed 1h after 10μl intravitreal injections of a: water, b: 2mM kainic acid, c: 2mM kainic acid + 200mM PDA, d: 2mM kainic acid + 200mM 2APV, e: 2mM kainic acid + 200mM DGG, f: 2mM kainic acid + 1M GDEE.

that the OFF-responses of the ganglion cells were permanently abolished (Dvorak and Morgan 1983), for the simplest interpretation of the morphological and physiological results is that the OFF-bipolar cells, believed to be essential for generating OFF-responses, had been eliminated from the retinal circuits. Thus, from the neurotoxicity studies, it is possible to conclude that there is a kainic acid-preferring receptor, with PDA as a preferential antagonist, on the OFF-bipolar cells and on the horizontal cells. On these cells kainic acid mimics the effect of the photoreceptor transmitter.

At the level of the amacrine cells the situation is more complex, since the three agonists appeared to affect amacrine cells. However the effects of kainic acid on the amacrine cells appear to be indirect, mediated by its effects on the bipolar cells (Morgan 1983; Morgan in press). The effects on NMDA were effectively antagonised by 2APV, while none of the antagonists (including GDEE and DGG) significantly reduced the effects of quisqualic acid. These results suggested that in the chicken retina there are separate populations of NMDA-preferring and quisqualic acid-preferring receptors on the amacrine cells, while kainic acid-preferring receptors are probably restricted to the outer plexiform layer.

ELECTROPHYSIOLOGICAL STUDIES USING AGONISTS AND ANTAGONISTS

Using intracellular recording techniques in fish and amphibia, kainic acid has been shown to be a powerful agonist of the photoreceptor transmitter, depolarizing horizontal cells and OFF bipolar cells and hyperpolarizing ON-bipolar cells (Shiells et al. 1981); Lasater and Dowling 1982; Rowe and Ruddock 1982a; Slaughter and Miller 1983b). Another excitatory amino acid analogue, 2-amino-4-phosphonobutyric acid (2APB) has the interesting property of acting as a selective agonist at the ON-bipolar cells (Slaughter and Miller 1981; Shiells et al. 1981). It is difficult to record intracellularly from the small cells of the avian and mammalian retinas, so extracellular recordings were made from the ganglion cells of the chicken retina. The results obtained were consistent with the picture obtained on lower vertebrates, since 2APB selectively eliminated ON-responses, whereas kainic acid eliminated both ON- and OFF-responses.

In fish, Rowe and Ruddock (1982b) found that GDEE, DGG and PDA hyperpolarized horizontal cells and blocked light-evoked responses. In mud-puppy, Slaughter and Miller (1983b) reported that PDA was an effective and relatively selective antagonist of cone input to OFF-bipolar and horizontal cells, but other antagonists were not tested. Using extracellular recordings of ganglion cell responses in the chicken retina intravitreal PDA (10µl, 400mM) gradually increased the latency of the OFF-responses and after approximately 30 min suppressed the OFF-responses, leaving the ON-responses intact (Fig. 2).

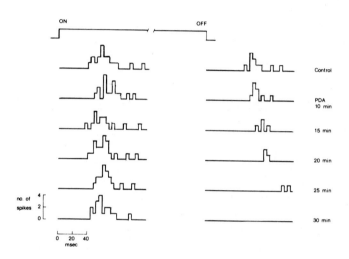

Figure 2. Effect of PDA on ON- and OFF-responses of a ganglion cell in the chicken retina. The results are the summed responses to 4 light flashes. Note the gradual increase in latency and eventual abolition of the OFF-responses.

In conformity with the neurotoxicity data DGG was less effective than PDA, and GDEE was completely ineffective. 2APV appeared to have unusual effects, since it rapidly eliminated the ON-responses, and more slowly eliminated the OFF-responses. Slaughter and Miller (1983a) claimed that while PDA interfered selectively with the OFF-bipolar and horizontal cells rather than the ON-bipolar cells, it also blocked both ON- and OFF-responses in ganglion cells. No evidence to support this idea was obtained in our experiments.

TWO TYPES OF PHYSIOLOGICALLY ACTIVE KAINIC ACID-PREFERRING
RECEPTOR?

Putting together these results, a picture of some general
properties of excitatory amino acid receptors in the outer
plexiform layer of vertebrate retinas can be constructed
(Table 1). Horizontal cells and OFF-bipolar cells are
depolarized preferentially by kainic acid. PDA, and to a
lesser extent DGG are effective antagonists. 2APB is inactive. The photoreceptor transmitter appears to open Na^+
channels on horizontal cells (Kaneko and Shimazaki 1976).
Since PDA blocks OFF-light responses and the effects of
kainic acid on the OFF-bipolar cells, the kainic acid-preferring receptor may be involved in the physiological transmission of information between photoreceptors and OFF-bipolar
and horizontal cells.

TABLE 1: PROPERTIES OF KAINIC ACID-PREFERRING RECEPTORS ON
SECOND-ORDER NEURONS OF VERTEBRATE RETINAS.

	TYPE 1	TYPE 2
Cellular location	OFF bipolar cells, horizontal cells	ON-bipolar cells
Linked response	depolarization, open Na^+ channels	hyperpolarization, closed Na^+ channels
Effect of kainic acid	agonist	agonist
Effect of 2APB	inactive	agonist
Effect of PDA	antagonist	inactive
Effect of DGG	antagonist	inactive

Both 2APB and kainic acid hyperpolarize the ON-bipolar
cells. Whether they act at the same receptor is unclear.
Shiells et al. (1981) have shown that the photoreceptor
transmitter, kainic acid and 2APB close sodium channels on
the ON-bipolar cells. PDA and DGG are not effective antagonists. The lack of effective antagonists makes it difficult
to test the physiological role of the receptor or receptors
on these cells, but they are the most likely candidates for
a physiological role.

WHAT IS THE PHOTORECEPTOR TRANSMITTER?

The greater ability of kainic acid as compared to L-glutamic acid and aspartic acid to activate second order neurons in neurotoxicity and electrophysiological studies suggests that neither of the amino acids is a good candidate as the photoreceptor transmitter. It has been suggested that the low potency of L-glutamic and L-aspartic acid may be due to effective uptake mechanisms (Ishida and Fain 1981; Rowe and Ruddock 1982a) but even in experiments involving perfused eye-cup sectors, kainic acid was found to be much more effective (Shiells et al. 1981). Furthermore, in our toxicity studies, clear evidence of toxicity induced by L-glutamic acid and L-aspartic acid was observed, but only at the level of the inner plexiform layer. Finally, L-glutamic acid does not appear to have a high affinity for the kainic acid-binding sites detected in chicken retina (Biziere and Coyle 1979). It therefore seems to be necessary to consider other possibilities, and specifically the possibility that an as yet unidentified naturally-occurring compound with a high affinity for kainic acid-preferring receptors is the real photoreceptor transmitter. Folic acid derivatives do not act as agonists (Morgan and El-Lakany 1982; Rowe and Ruddock 1982b) although they appear to be effective antagonists (Rowe and Ruddock, 1982b).

One complication which must be borne in mind is the possibility that the transmitters released by rods and cones may be different (Saito et al. 1978). However kainic acid appears to affect horizontal and bipolar cells in both cone-dominated and rod-dominated retinas (Yazulla and Kleinschmidt 1980; Hampton et al. 1981; Ingham and Morgan 1983) and has indeed been claimed to affect cone pathways preferentially (Yazulla and Kleinschmidt 1980; Hampton et al. 1981). Therefore if it does prove to be correct that the rod and cone transmitters are different, they may operate via post-synaptic receptors which share some pharmacological properties, but not others, just as the kainic acid-preferring receptors on ON- and OFF-bipolar cells appear to be pharmacologically distinct.

Biziere K, Coyle JT (1979). Localization of receptors for kainic acid on neurons in the inner layer of retina. Neuropharmacol 18:409-413.
Dvorak DR, Morgan IG (1983). Intravitreal kainic acid permanently eliminates OFF-pathways from chicken retina. Neuroscience Letters 36:249-253.

Hampton CK, Garcia C, Redburn DA (1981). Localization of kainic acid-sensitive cells in mammalian retina. J Neurosci Res 6:99-111.

Ikeda H, Sheardown MJ (1982). Aspartate may be an excitatory transmitter mediating visual excitation of 'sustained' but not 'transient' cells in the cat retina: Iontophoretic studies in vivo. Neuroscience 7:25-36.

Ingham CA, Morgan IG (1983). Dose-dependent effects of intra-vitreal kainic acid on specific cell types in chicken retina. Neuroscience 9:165-181.

Ishida AT, Fain GL (1981). D-aspartate potentiates the effects of L-glutamate on horizontal cells in goldfish. Proc Natn Acad Sci USA 78:5890-5894.

Kaneko A, Shimazaki H (1976). Synaptic transmission from photoreceptors to the second-order neurons in the carp retina. In Zettler F, Weiler R (eds): "Neural Principles in Vision," Berlin: Springer-Verlag, p 143-157.

Lasater EM, Dowling JE (1982). Carp horizontal cells in culture respond selectively to L-glutamate and its agonists. Proc natn Acad Sci USA 79:936-940.

Morgan IG (1983). Organization of amacrine cell types which use different transmitters in chicken retina. Progress in Brain Research 58:191-199.

Morgan IG (1983). Kainic Acid as a Tool in Retinal Research. In Osborne N, Chader G (eds): "Progress in Retinal Research" Vol.2, Oxford: Pergamon Press, in press.

Morgan IG, El-Lakany S (1982). Folic acid derivatives do not reproduce the neurotoxic effects of kainic acid on chicken retina. Neuroscience Letters 34:69-73.

Morgan IG, Ingham CA (1981). Kainic acid affects both plexi-form layers of chicken retina. Neuroscience Letters 21: 275-280.

Rowe JS, Ruddock KH (1982a). Hyperpolarization of retinal horizontal cells by excitatory amino acid neurotransmitter agonists. Neuroscience Letters 30:251-256.

Rowe JS, Ruddock KH (1982b). Depolarization of retinal horizontal cells by excitatory amino acid neurotransmitter agonists. Neuroscience Letters 30:257-262.

Saito T, Kondo H, Toyoda J (1978). Rod and cone signals in the on-center bipolar cell: their different ionic mechanisms. Vision Research 18:591-595.

Shiells RA, Falk G, Naghshineh S (1981). Action of glutamate and aspartate analogues on rod horizontal and bipolar cells. Nature 294:592-594.

Slaughter MM, Miller RF (1981). 2-Amino-4-phosphonobutyric acid. A new pharmacological tool for retina research. Science 211:182-185.

Slaughter MM, Miller RF (1983a). Bipolar cells in the mud-puppy retina use an excitatory amino acid neurotransmitter. Nature 303:537.

Slaughter MM, Miller RF (1983b). An excitatory amino acid antagonist blocks cone input to sign-conserving second-order retinal neurons. Science 219:1230.

Watkins JC, Evans RH (1981). Excitatory amino acid trans-mitters. Annu Rev Pharmacol Toxicol 21:165-204.

Yazulla S, Kleinschmidt J (1980). The effects of intraocular injection of kainic acid on the synaptic organization of the goldfish retina. Brain Res 182:287-301.

**Glutamine, Glutamate, and GABA
in the Central Nervous System, pages 297–315
© 1983 Alan R. Liss, Inc., 150 Fifth Avenue, New York, NY 10011**

Uptake and Release Processes for Glutamine, Glutamate and
GABA in Cultured Neurons and Astrocytes.

A. Schousboe[*], O.M. Larsson[*], J. Drejer[*],
P. Krogsgaard-Larsen[†], and L. Hertz[‡].

[*]) Department of Biochemistry A, Panum Institute,
       University of Copenhagen, Denmark.
[*]) Department of Nuclear Medicine, State Univ-
       ersity Hospital, Copenhagen, Denmark.
[†]) Department of Chemistry BC, Royal Danish
       School of Pharmacy, Copenhagen, Denmark.
[‡]) Department of Pharmacology, University of
       Saskatchewan, Saskatoon, Canada.

INTRODUCTION

Due to the dual role of both glutamate and GABA as neurotransmitters and intermediary metabolites it is of importance to gain knowledge about the dynamic interplay between
neurons and astrocytes concerning fluxes of these amino
acids in and out of the cells. Since glutamine may serve as
an important precursor for both of these amino acids it is
obviously necessary to include studies of uptake and release
processes for this amino acid in the different cell types if
a complete picture of the intercellular communication regarding the amino acid neurotransmitters is to be acquired.

The aim of the present review is to provide a picture of
the dynamic and molecular properties of the transport mechanisms for glutamine, glutamate and GABA in neurons as well as
in astrocytes. For additional information the reader is referred to recent extensive reviews on these topics by Hertz
(1979), Schousboe (1981) and Schousboe & Hertz (1983).

CULTURED CELLS

Glutamatergic Neurons

Biochemical as well as electrophysiological evidence
strongly suggest that cerebellar granule cells utilize glutamate as their transmitter (Young et al., 1974; Stone, 1979).
Since culture methods have been available for this cell type
for some time (Messer, 1977) we have chosen such cultured
cerebellar granule cells as a model system for glutamatergic
neurons (Hertz et al., 1980; Yu & Hertz, 1982; Drejer et al.,
1982, 1983a). From studies of stimulus-coupled release of
exogenously supplied L-glutamate or D-aspartate (Drejer et
al., 1982, 1983a) or endogenously synthesized glutamate
(Gallo et al., 1982) it can be concluded that these cells
behave as functionally active glutamatergic neurons in
culture. For a more detailed characterization of these cells,
see Meier et al. (this volume).

GABAergic Neurons

Recent immunocytochemical studies (Ribak, 1978) have indicated that a large fraction of cerebral cortical interneurons (stellate cells) are GABAergic. Methods for cultiv-
ation of cortical interneurons have also recently become
available (Dichter, 1978) and numerous studies of transmitter biosynthesis, uptake and release as well as electrophysiology in such cultures strongly suggest that the majority
of the neurons in these cultures are indeed GABAergic
(Dichter, 1978, 1980; Hauser et al., 1980; Snodgrass et al.
1980; Larsson et al., 1981, 1983a; Yu et al., 1983). This
culture system which is described in detail by Larsson et al.
(1981) and Yu & Hertz (1982) has therefore been employed as
a model system for GABAergic neurons.

Astrocytes

It is by now widely accepted that astrocytes play an
active role in the maintenance of a normal extracellular
milieu of ions as well as of neurotransmitters in the CNS
(for references, see Hertz (1982)). Protocols for primary
cultures of astrocytes have been available for more than a
decade (for references, see Hertz et al. (1982)) and biochemical and functional characterization of these cultures
have suggested that the cultured astrocytes may be well
suited as a model system for their in vivo counterparts
(Hertz, 1982). Although some evidence points to the exist-

ence of a functional heterogeneity of astrocytes originating from different brain regions (Henn, 1976; Schousboe & Divac, 1979; Drejer et al., 1983b) we have used astrocytes cultured from cerebral cortex (Hertz et al., 1982) for the studies of glutamine, glutamate and GABA transport.

GLUTAMINE TRANSPORT

Uptake

Due to the possibility that glutamine among other functions may serve as an inert 'carrier' of transmitter glutamate between different cellular structures in the CNS some attention has recently been focused on characterization of transport processes for this amino acid in neurons and astrocytes. Table 1 summarizes the kinetic characteristics of these processes. It appears that no major difference exists between GABAergic neurons, glutamatergic neurons and astrocytes in the ability of these cells to accumulate glutamine since at an external glutamine concentration of 0.5 mM which reflects the CSF concentration (Wood, 1982) the velocity for glutamine uptake is essentially the same in the different cell types. This does, however, not mean that the transport system may not be different. In a recent study by Ramaharobandro et al.(1982) it was reported that the neuronal and

Table 1. Kinetic constants for transport of glutamine in cultured neurons and astrocytes.

Cell type	K_m (mM)	V_{max} (nmol $\times$ min^{-1} $\times$ mg^{-1})	$V_{0.5}$
Astrocytes[a]	3.3	50.2	6.4
Astrocytes[b]	0.2	2.0	1.5
Cerebr.cort.neur[c]	3.0	28.2	3.9
Cerebr.cort.neur[b]	0.1	1.0	0.8
Cereb.gran.cells[c]	0.7	10.3	4.4

a) Schousboe et al. (1979a); b) Ramaharobandro et al. (1982).
c) Hertz et al. (1980).
$V_{0.5}$ means the velocity at an external glutamine concentration of 0.5 mM.

glial glutamine carriers exhibit differences both in terms of substrate specificity and in terms of dependency on mono- and divalent cations. Thus, neuronal glutamine uptake is dependent upon Na^+ and Ca^{2+} whereas the glial uptake system does not exhibit such dependency. If this is indeed the case neuronal glutamine uptake would be more susceptible than its glial counterpart to fluctuations in the external ionic concentrations occurring during neuronal excitation as suggested by Ramaharobandro et al. (1982).

Release

Only few studies are available concerning the rate of release of glutamine from neurons and astrocytes. From experiments using brain slices it is known that glutamine is rapidly released from brain tissue (Arnfred & Hertz, 1971). Also cultured neurons (Ramaharobandro et al., 1982) and astrocytes (Schousboe et al., 1979a; Ramahabandro et al., 1982) exhibit release of glutamine which in the astrocytes amounts to approx. 2 nmol $\times$ min^{-1} $\times$ mg^{-1}. From Ramaharobandro et al. (1982) it may be estimated that the neuronal release rate is of the same magnitude but no exact value can be calculated, but Yu et al. (1983) have reported a release rate of 1 nmol $\times$ min^{-1} $\times$ mg^{-1} for cerebral cortex neurons. It appears that the neuronal glutamine release is stimulated by potassium in a Ca^{2+}-independent manner whereas no such stimulation is found for astrocytes (Ramaharobandro et al., 1982). It should be noted that no K^+-stimulated glutamine release from cortical neurons could be demonstrated by Yu et al. (1983).

GLUTAMATE TRANSPORT

Uptake

Since the major mechanism for inactivation of transmitter glutamate appears to be high affinity uptake into astrocytes and nerve endings (Schousboe & Hertz, 1983) and since external glutamate appears to be highly neurotoxic (Olney, 1981) it is of great importance to characterize the transport mechanisms for glutamate. Fig. 1 illustrates the general conclusion from numerous studies of the kinetics of glutamate uptake into neurons and astrocytes (for references, see Hertz, 1979; Schousboe, 1981, 1982) that the uptake capacity (V_{max}) is higher in astrocytes than in neurons. On the other hand,

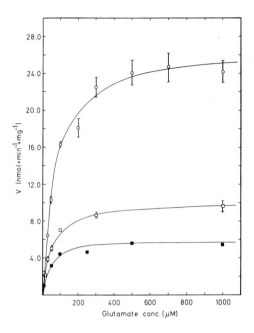

Fig. 1. Glutamate uptake into cultured astrocytes (O) and glutamatergic (□) or GABAergic (■) neurons. Bars represent S.E.M. values. From Drejer et al. (1982).

glutamate uptake into astrocytes does not appear to be electrogenic (Drejer et al., 1982) whereas this seems to be the case for glutamate uptake into neurons (Drejer et al., 1982) as well as into nerve endings (Kanner & Sharon, 1978). This would a priori make the neuronal uptake system more concentrative than the astrocytic uptake system (cf. Schousboe, 1981), but even the latter is able to generate large intra- to extracellular concentration ratios of glutamate (Hertz et al., 1978). This together with an avid glutamate metabolism in this cell type (Hertz et al., this volume) more than adequately enable the astrocytes to function as a sink for neuronally released glutamate (Schousboe & Hertz, 1983). That the apparent difference in Na^+-dependency (Drejer et al., 1982) may not be the only functional difference between the neuronal and glial glutamate carrier is indicated by recent detailed kinetic studies by Drejer et al. (1982, 1983a) of the glutamate carriers on astrocytes and glutamatergic granule cells. It was found that L-glutamate, L-aspartate and

Table 2. Characterization of uptake of D- and L-aspartate and L-glutamate into neurons and astrocytes.

| Transported amino acid | Inhibiting amino acid | | | | | |
| | Neurons | | | Astrocytes | | |
	D-asp	L-asp	L-glu	D-asp	L-asp	L-glu
D-asp	26^a	18	21	83^a	82	75
L-asp	29	32^a	31	70	77^a	73
L-glu	40	40	20^a	106*	68	67^a

The table gives K_m-values (μM, identified by 'a') for uptake of the amino acids and K_i-values (μM) for their mutual inhibition. *Indicates mixed comp./non-comp. inhibition and where not otherwise mentioned the kinetic pattern conforms to linear competitive inhibition.
From Drejer et al. (1983a).

D-aspartate are transported with essentially identical K_m and V_{max} values in both astrocytes and granule cells but unexpectedly, D-aspartate was found to be a complex inhibitor of L-glutamate uptake in astrocytes whereas the remaining mutual inhibitory patterns were strictly competitive with K_i values matching K_m values as shown in Table 2. This indicates that the astrocytic carrier to some extent is able to distinguish between L-glutamate and D-aspartate whereas the neuronal carrier handles these two amino acids in an identical manner. Based on studies of the inhibition of glutamate uptake with different glutamate analogues such as 3-hydroxy-aspartates (erythro-, threo-, D- and L-), D-glutamate, the β- and γ-hydroxamic acid derivatives of D- and L-aspartate and L-glutamate, cysteinate and homocysteinate (Balcar & Johnston, 1972; Roberts & Watkins, 1975; Balcar et al., 1977a,b; Schousboe et al., 1977b; Drejer et al., 1982, 1983a) a model of the glutamate carrier has been proposed (Drejer, 1982). This has 3 binding sites, one for each of the 3 charged groups in L-glutamate and can accomodate the substrates, L-glutamate, D- and L-aspartate, L-aspartate-β-hydroxamate, cysteinate and threo-3-hydroxy-D- or L-aspartate but not e.g. D-glutamate, L-α-aminoadipate, the erythro-3-hydroxy-aspartates, L-glutamate-γ-hydroxamate, D-aspartate-β-hydroxamate or homocysteinate mainly due to steric hindrance at the binding site for the ω-carboxyl group. Small differences between the neuronal and glial carrier particularly at this binding site could explain why D-aspartate behaves slightly different as an inhibitor of L-glutamate uptake in the two cell types. Although such a model obviously has some inherent uncertainties it may serve as a 'working model' for future attempts to design glutamate analogues capable of distinguishing between the neuronal and glial glutamate carrier (cf. below).

Release

Release of glutamate from brain cortex in vivo after activation through neuronal pathways was first demonstrated by Jasper & Koyama (1969). That at least part of this released glutamate originates from glutamatergic nerve endings is suggested by the demonstration that endogenous as well as exogenously supplied glutamate is released in a Ca^{2+}-dependent manner from cultured glutamatergic cerebellar granule cells upon stimulation with potassium (Drejer et al., 1982, 1983a; Gallo et al., 1982). It has, however, also been observed that a substantial release of glutamate occurs from astrocytes (Hertz et al., 1978; Drejer et al., 1982), but this glutamate release is neither stimulated by K^+ (Drejer et al., 1982) nor by glutamate (Hertz et al., 1978). The functional significance of this glial glutamate release is difficult to assess, but it has to be taken into account when fluxes of glutamate between the different cell types are discussed (cf. below).

Pharmacological Aspects

Since it is known that glutamate as well as some of its analogues such as kainic acid and α-aminoadipic acid are highly neuro- and gliotoxic (Olney, 1981; Karlsen et al., 1982) it would be of potential pharmacological interest to be able to manipulate the release and inactivation mechanisms for glutamate. This is further stressed by the observation that some of the neuronal degenerations seen in the basal ganglia of patients dying from Huntington's chorea can be mimicked in experimental animals by local injections of kainic acid (McGeer & McGeer, 1976). It has in fact been suggested that malfunction of the glutamate high affinity transport system may be one of the causal factors in the development of this neurological disorder (Coyle et al., 1977) and the demonstration of an apparently intact glutamate uptake in human brain autopsies may provide an experimental tool for direct examination of this hypothesis (Schwarcz & Whetsell, 1982).

On this basis it appears particularly attractive to place the main emphasis on the development of drugs which can block selectively neuronal reuptake of glutamate. This might lead to a partial depletion of glutamate from nerve endings by channelling a larger fraction of released glutamate into surrounding astroglia provided the astroglial uptake system functions normally. This would subsequently lead to a diminished pool of neurotransmitter glutamate. Another approach may be to develop drugs which interfere with glutamate release. In this context it should be kept in mind that efflux as well as influx of glutamate in nerve endings is dependent on Na^+ and K^+ (Kanner & Sharon, 1978; Kanner & Marva, 1982; Drejer et al., 1982, 1983a) and accordingly different ionophores (Kanner & Marva, 1982) might be of interest as potential agents by which the efflux could be manipulated.

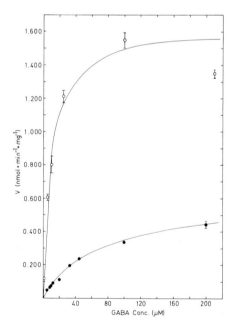

Fig. 2. GABA uptake into cultured astrocytes (●) or GABAergic neurons (O). Bars represent S.E.M. values. From Schousboe et al. (1977a) and Larsson et al. (1981).

GABA TRANSPORT

Uptake

As early as in 1958 it was suggested that cellular transport processes would be likely to be responsible for the inactivation of GABA (Kuffler & Edwards, 1958). Although this
mechanism of inactivation has never been directly proven
experimentally, the notion is supported by a wealth of circumstantial evidence (cf. Curtis & Johnston, 1974; Hertz,
1979; Schousboe, 1981; Schousboe & Hertz, 1983). Fig. 2
shows that high affinity GABA uptake is expressed in both
neurons and glial cells and in contrast to what was found
for glutamate (Fig. 1) the uptake capacity is higher in neurons than in astrocytes. This conclusion is substantiated by

Table 3. Kinetic characterization of neuronal and glial GABA
uptake inhibitors.

GABA Analogue	K_i or IC_{50} (μM)		Inhibition type		Select-ivity
	Neur.	Glia	Neur.	Glia	
3-OH-5-amino-valeric acid	430*	1400*	–	–	N
β-Proline	1200*	400	–	Comp	G
Homo-β-proline	6	16	Comp	Comp	ns
ACHC	69	700*	Comp	Mixed	N
R-Nipecotic acid	20	20	Comp	Comp	ns
Guvacine	25	25*	Comp	–	ns
Cis-4-OH-nipe-cotic acid	40	30	Comp	non-Comp	(G)
N-Methylnipe-cotic acid	100	100	Comp	Comp	ns
Homonipecotic acid	3,000*	700	–	Comp	G
THPO	5,000*	550	–	Comp	G
THAO	> 5,000*	600	–	Comp	G

* Indicates IC_{50} values.
N means neuronal transport and G means glial transport; ns
indicates that the inhibition is non-selective.
ACHC: cis-3-aminocyclohexane carboxylic acid.
THPO: 4,5,6,7-tetrahydroisoxazolo[4,5c]pyridin-3-ol.
THAO: 5,6,7,8-tetrahydro-4H-isoxazolo[4,5c]azepin-3-ol.
From Schousboe et al. (1979b, 1981, 1982) and Larsson et al.
(1981, 1983b).

a large body of literature concerning GABA uptake into brain
slices, synaptosomes and bulk prepared glial cells and cultured cells (cf. Schousboe et al., 1977a; Hertz, 1979; Schousboe 1981, 1982; Schousboe & Hertz, 1983). The driving force
for GABA transport in nerve endings as well as in astrocytes
appears to be the sodium gradient and the transport is electrogenic in both cell types (Martin, 1973; Kanner, 1978;
Larsson et al., 1980, 1983a). This means that both transport
systems are capable of generating and maintaining large intra-
to extracellular ratios of GABA (cf. Schousboe, 1981).

The molecular properties of the neuronal and glial GABA
carrier have been extensively investigated over the past decade and some of the more important findings are summarized
in Table 3. It is clear that the two transport sites exhibit
distinctly different substrate specificities which in all
likelihood means that the carriers accept the GABA molecule
in different conformations. Extensive structure-activity
studies have demonstrated that design of specific GABA uptake inhibitors involves consideration of a variety of structural parameters. This has been tentatively illustrated in
Fig. 3 which may serve as a 'working' model for future
attempts to design cell-specific inhibitors of GABA transport, compounds which may have potential pharmacological
interest (cf. below). While compounds such as homo-β-proline,
nipecotic acid, and guvacine, in which the vicinity of the
amino groups have been conformationally immobilized, are very
potent inhibitors of GABA uptake, a prerequisite for effective interaction with the GABA transport carriers appears to
be a certain degree of rotational freedom of the acid moieties of the compounds. Thus THPO, a rigid analogue of nipecotic acid and guvacine, and its ring homologue THAO are substantially weaker than the cyclic amino acids concerned. The
observation that dihydro-THPO, which has a rigid but L-shap-
ed structure, is virtually inactive as an inhibitor of GABA
uptake strongly suggests that it is the inflexible character
of the acid moiety of for example THPO rather than its planar
structure that makes it a relatively weak inhibitor of GABA
uptake. The data summarized in Fig. 3 seem to indicate that
the different substrate specificities of the glial and neuronal GABA transport system to a certain extent can be explained by a more strict structural specificity of the latter
system. Moreover, recent studies of transport of some of the
GABA analogues such as nipecotic acid, 3-aminocyclohexane
carboxylic acid and cis-4-OH-nipecotic acid have suggested
that the transport system may exhibit heterogeneity not only

COMPOUND	STRUCTURE-CONFORMATIONAL MOBILITY	INHIBITION OF GABA UPTAKE GLIAL	INHIBITION OF GABA UPTAKE NEURONAL	INHIBITION OF GABA RECEPTOR BINDING	GABA AGONIST ACTIVITY
		IC_{50}, μM			Rel. Potency
GABA	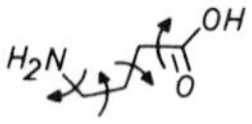	35	15	0.033	— — —
Homo-β-proline	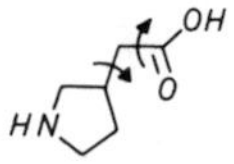	20	75	0.30	— — —
(R)-(—)-Nipecotic acid	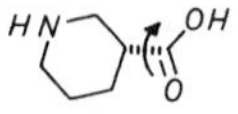	30	70	>100	0
Guvacine	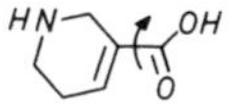	25	100	>100	0
THPO	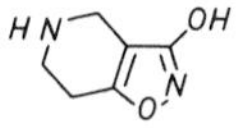	300	5000	72	0
THAO	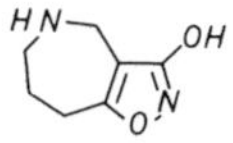	500	>5000	>100	0
Dihydro-THPO	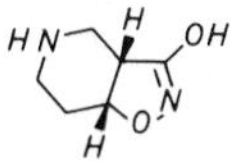	>5000	>5000	>100	0

Fig. 3. Schematic representation of the correlation between the structure-conformational mobility of GABA and some of its analogues and the ability of the compounds to interact with GABA transport sites (neuronal and glial) or GABA receptor sites. The latter was assessed either as the ability of the compounds to inhibit GABA binding or as the approximate potency of the analogues (relative to that of GABA (---)) to produce equal and submaximal depressant effects on cat spinal neurons.
For abbreviations, see legend to Table 3.
From Schousboe et al. (1979b, 1981); Larsson et al. (1981); Krogsgaard-Larsen (this volume), or unpublished data of D.R. Curtis, P. Krogsgaard-Larsen, O.M. Larsson and A. Schousboe.

between different cell types but also within the individual cell types (Larsson et al., 1983a,b). Future studies of this kind will hopefully provide further information about this possibility.

Release.

GABA is released into the fourth ventricle after stimulation of cerebellum (Obata & Takeda, 1969) and there is little doubt that this release is related to the neurotransmitter action of GABA since Ca^{2+}-dependent stimulus coupled GABA release has been demonstrated in numerous brain tissue preparations (cf. Szerb, this volume). Also cultured cerebral cortex neurons exhibit Ca^{2+}-dependent, evoked GABA release (Snodgrass et al., 1980; Hauser et al., 1980; Larsson et al., 1983a; Yu et al., 1983). In contrast to this, cultured astrocytes do not exhibit any evoked GABA release (Pearce et al., 1981; Larsson et al., 1983a) but they have a spontaneous efflux of GABA which amounts to approximately 10% of the neuronally derived spontaneous release of GABA (Larsson et al., 1983a). This is in contrast to glutamate for which the two cell types have non-evoked effluxes of essentially identical magnitude (Drejer et al., 1982).

Pharmacological aspects.

Since malfunction of GABA neurotransmission is thought to be involved in a variety of neurological disorders including epilepsy (cf. Roberts et al., 1976) it is of great interest to be able to manipulate this neurotransmission process at different levels such as the receptor level (cf. Krogsgaard-Larsen, this volume) and the inactivation level (Schousboe et al., 1983). It has been suggested that manipulation of particularly the glial GABA transport system might be beneficial for the function of GABA synapses working at suboptimal levels (Schousboe et al., 1981; Krogsgaard-Larsen et al., 1981) and great effort has been made in producing glial selective GABA transport inhibitors (Schousboe et al., 1979b, 1981). One of these compounds, THPO has been studied in some detail with regard to its ability to increase GABA levels in the transmitter pool of GABA (Wood et al., 1980) which seems to be a prerequisite for an antiepileptic drug acting at the inactivation level (Gale et al., 1982; Wood, this volume). It was found that THPO can indeed increase GABA levels in nerve endings and it has subsequently been shown that this GABA analogue acts as an anticonvulsant after injection intracerebroventricularly (Krogsgaard-Larsen et al., 1981; Meldrum et al., 1982) or intramuscularly under circumstances where it penetrates the blood brain barrier (Wood et al., 1983). Emphasis should accordingly be placed on the design of compounds structurally related to THPO or prodrugs of THPO which more easily than the parent compound penetrates the blood brain barrier.

FUNCTIONAL CONSIDERATIONS

To provide a picture of the dynamic state of release and uptake for the glutamate family of amino acids in astrocytes and glutamatergic and GABAergic neurons the pertinent fluxes of these amino acids in the different cell types have been summarized in Fig. 4. To give also an impression of how these fluxes correlate with actual rates of metabolic interconversions of these amino acids such metabolic fluxes (Hertz et al., this volume) have also been shown. When glutamate release and uptake rates are considered it is apparent that there may be a net uptake into astrocytes of approximately

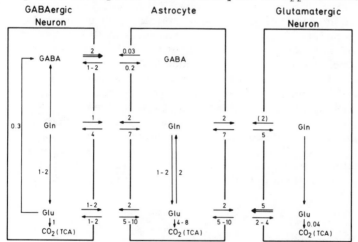

Fig. 4. Schematic representation of the interaction between astrocytes and respectively GABAergic and glutamatergic neurons in Gln, Glu, and GABA homeostasis. Transport as well as metabolic fluxes are given as nmol × min^{-1} × mg^{-1} cell protein. Fluxes across cell membranes have been estimated from kinetic data referred to in the text using an external glutamate and GABA concentration of 50 μM and an external glutamine concentration of 500 μM. Metabolic fluxes (from Hertz et al., this volume) are based on conversion rates measured using ^{14}C-labelled substrates at the same external concentrations (glutamate, 50 μM; glutamine, 500 μM). Double arrows (⇒) indicate release rates measured at elevated potassium concentrations (evoked release). TCA: Tricarboxylic acid cycle.

3-8 nmol $\times$ min^{-1} $\times$ mg^{-1} protein which is higher than the net synthesis of glutamine in the astrocytes amounting to 1 nmol $\times$ min^{-1} $\times$ mg^{-1}, but similar to the rate of oxidative deamination which is 4-5 nmol $\times$ min^{-1} $\times$ mg^{-1}. This means that the net amount of glutamate lost from neurons to astrocytes is unlikely to be quantitatively converted to glutamine in the astrocytes and even if this did occur the prevailing fluxes of glutamine in neurons and astrocytes would not facilitate a net flow of glutamine of this magnitude from astrocytes to neurons (cf. Fig. 4). In case of GABA it is apparent from Fig. 4 that there is only a small loss from neurons to astrocytes (approximately 0.1 nmol $\times$ min^{-1} $\times$ mg^{-1} protein). This could be accounted for by a corresponding flow of glutamine from astrocytes to neurons (Balazs et al., 1972) particularly since GABA is likely to enter the astrocytic glutamate pool from which glutamine is synthesized (Hertz et al., this volume). From the discussion above it is evident that there is an avid communication between neurons and glial cells concerning transfer of glutamine, glutamate and GABA. The central role of astrocytes for the maintenance of low extraneuronal concentrations of glutamate and GABA is underlined by the recent finding, that neurons excrete substances which in a selective manner regulate the capacity for astrocytic high affinity uptake of glutamate and GABA (Drejer et al., 1983b). In this context it should also be emphasized that astrocytes originating in different brain regions being exposed to different neuronal stimuli may have distinctly different properties concerning the transport systems for neurotransmitter amino acids (Henn, 1976; Schousboe & Divac, 1979; Drejer et al., 1983b).

ACKNOWLEDGEMENTS

The technical assistance of Miss Hanne Fosmark and Mrs. Grete Rossing is gratefully acknowledged. The work has been supported financially by the following granting agencies: Danish State Natural Science Research Council (511-20817; 81-3572), Danish State Medical Research Council (12-2322; 12-3967; 12-3419), NOVO Foundation, Hans Lønborg Madsen's Memorial Foundation, King Chr. X's Foundation and MCR of Canada (MT 5957).

REFERENCES

Arnfred T, Hertz, L (1971). Effects of potassium and glutamate on brain cortex slices: uptake and release of glutamic and other amino acids. J Neurochem 18:259.

Balazs R, Patel AJ, Richter D (1972). Metabolic compartments in the brain: their properties and relation to morphological structures. In Balazs R, Cremer JE (eds): "Metabolic Compartmentation in the Brain", London: Macmillan, p 167.

Balcar VJ, Borg J, Mandel P (1977a). High affinity uptake of L-glutamate and L-aspartate by glial cells. J Neurochem 28:87.

Balcar VJ, Johnston GAR (1972). The structural specificity of the high affinity uptake of L-glutamate and L-aspartate by rat brain slices. J Neurochem 19:2657.

Balcar VJ, Johnston GAR, Twitchin B (1977b). Stereospecific inhibition of L-glutamate and L-aspartate high affinity uptake in rat brain slices by threo-3-hydroxyaspartate. J Neurochem 28:1145.

Coyle JT, Schwarcz R, Bennett JP, Campochiaro P (1977). Clinical, neuropathological and pharmacological aspects of Huntington's disease: correlates with a new animal model. Prog Neuropsychopharmac 1:13.

Curtis DR, Johnston GAR (1974). Amino acid transmitters in the mammalian central nervous system. Ergb Physiol 69:97.

Dichter MA (1978). Rat cortical-neurons in cell culture - culture methods, cell morphology, electrophysiology and synapse formation. Brain Res 149:279.

Dichter MA (1980). Physiological identification of GABA as the transmitter for mammalian cortical neurons in cell culture. Brain Res 190:111.

Drejer J (1982). Glutamate-mediated neurotransmission. A review. Studies in neurons and astrocytes in primary cultures. Copenhagen: Ph.D. Thesis, Royal Danish School of Pharmacy, p 1-81.

Drejer J, Larsson OM, Schousboe A (1983a). Characterization of uptake and release processes for D- and L-aspartate in primary cultures of astrocytes and cerebellar granule cells. Neurochem Res 8:231.

Drejer J, Meier E, Schousboe A (1983b). Novel neuron-related regulatory mechanisms for astrocytic glutamate and GABA high affinity uptake. Neurosci Lett in press.

Gale K, Iadarola MJ, Casu M, Keating RF (1982). Relationship between GABA levels in vivo and anticonvulsant activity: Importance of cellular compartments and regional localization in brain. In Okada Y, Roberts E (eds): "Problems in GABA Research from Brain to Bacteria", Amsterdam: Excerpta Medica, p 159.

Gallo V, Ciotti MT, Coletti A, Aloisi F, Levi G (1982). Selective release of glutamate from cerebellar granule cells differentiating in culture. Proc Natl Acad Sci USA 79:7919.

Hauser K, Balcar VJ, Bernasconi R (1980). Development of GABA neurons in dissociated cell culture of rat cerebral cortex. In Lal H, Fielding S, Malick J, Roberts E, Shah N, Usdin E (eds): "GABA-neurotransmission. Current Developments in Physiology and Neurochemistry", Brain Res Bull 5 (Suppl 2) Fayetteville: Ankho International Inc, p 37.

Henn FA (1976). Neurotransmission and glial cells: A functional relationship. J Neurosci Res 2: 271.

Hertz L (1979). Functional interactions between neurons and astrocytes. I. Turnover and metabolism of putative amino acid transmitters. Prog Neurobiol 13:277.

Hertz L (1982). Astrocytes. In Lajtha A (ed): "Handbook of Neurochemistry" 2. ed, Vol 1, New York: Plenum Press, p 319.

Hertz L, Juurlink BHJ, Fosmark H, Schousboe A (1982). Astrocytes in primary culture. In Pfeiffer SE (ed): "Neuroscience Approached Through Cell Culture", Vol 1, Boca Raton FL: CRC Press, p 175.

Hertz L, Schousboe A, Boechler N, Mukerji S, Fedoroff S (1978). Kinetic characteristics of the glutamate uptake into normal astrocytes in culture. Neurochem Res 3:1.

Hertz L, Yu A, Svenneby G, Kvamme E, Fosmark H, Schousboe A (1980). Absence of preferential glutamine uptake into neurons. An indication of a net transfer of TCA constituents from nerve endings to astrocytes? Neurosci Lett 16: 103.

Jasper HH, Koyama I (1969). Rate of release of amino acids from the cerebral cortex in the cat as affected by brainstem and thalamic stimulation. Can J Physiol Pharmacol 47: 889.

Kanner BI (1978). Active transport of γ-aminobutyric acid by membrane vesicles isolated from rat brain. Biochemistry 17:1207.

Kanner BI, Marva E (1982). Efflux of L-glutamate by synaptic plasma membrane vesicles isolated from rat brain. Biochemistry 21:3143.

Kanner BI, Sharon I (1978). Active transport of L-glutamate by membrane vesicles isolated from rat brain. Biochemistry 17:3949.

Karlsen RL, Pedersen OØ, Schousboe A, Langeland A (1982). Toxic effects of DL-α-aminoadipic acid on Müller cells from rats in vivo and cultured cerebral astrocytes. Exp Eye Res 35:305.

Krogsgaard-Larsen P, Labouta I, Meldrum B, Croucher M, Schousboe A (1981). GABA uptake inhibitors as experimental tools and potential drugs in epilepsy research. In Morselli PL, Reynolds EM, Lloyd KG, Löscher W, Meldrum BS (eds): "Neurotransmitters, Seizures and Epilepsy", New York: Raven Press, p 23.

Kuffler SV, Edwards C (1958). Mechanism of γ-aminobutyric acid (GABA) action and its relation to synaptic inhibition. J Neurophysiol 21:589.

Larsson OM, Drejer J, Hertz L, Schousboe A (1983a). Ion dependency of uptake and release of GABA and (RS)-nipecotic acid studied in cultured mouse brain cortex neurons. J Neurosci Res 9:291.

Larsson OM, Hertz L, Schousboe A (1980). GABA uptake in astrocytes in primary cultures: Coupling with two sodium ions. J Neurosci Res 5:469.

Larsson OM, Johnston GAR, Schousboe A (1983b). Differences in uptake kinetics of cis-3-aminocyclohexane carboxylic acid into neurons and astrocytes in primary cultures. Brain Res 260:279.

Larsson OM, Thorbek P, Krogsgaard-Larsen P, Schousboe A (1981). Effect of homo-β-proline and other heterocyclic GABA analogues on GABA uptake in neurons and astroglial cells and GABA receptor binding. J Neurochem 37:1509.

Martin DL (1973). Kinetics of the sodium-dependent transport of gammaaminobutyric acid by synaptosomes. J Neurochem 21:345.

McGeer EG, McGeer PL (1976). Duplication of biochemical changes of Huntington's chorea by intrastriatal injections of glutamic and kainic acids. Nature (Lond) 263:517.

Meldrum BS, Croucher MJ, Krogsgaard-Larsen P (1982). GABA-uptake inhibitors as anticonvulsant agents. In Okada Y, Roberts E (eds): "Problems in GABA Research from Brain to Bacteria", Amsterdam: Excerpta Medica, p 182.

Messer A (1977). The maintenance and identification of mouse cerebellar granule cells in monolayer cultures. Brain Res 130:1.

Obata K, Takeda K (1969). Release of GABA into the fourth
ventricle induced by stimulation of the cat cerebellum.
J Neurochem 16:1043.

Olney JW (1981). Kainic acid and other excitotoxins: A comparative analysis. In Di Chiara G, Gessa GL (eds): "Glutamate as a Neurotransmitter", Adv Biochem Pharmacol 27,
New York: Raven Press, p 375.

Pearce BR, Currie DN, Beale R, Dutton GR (1981). Potassium-
stimulated, calcium-dependent release of [^{3}H]GABA from
neuron- and glia-enriched cultures of cells dissociated
from rat cerebellum. Brain Res 206:485.

Ramaharobandro N, Borg J, Mandel P, Mark J (1982). Glutamine and glutamate transport in cultured neuronal and glial
cells. Brain Res 244:113.

Ribak CE (1978). Aspinous and sparsely-spinous stellate
neurons in the visual cortex of rats contain glutamic
acid decarboxylase. J Neurocytol 7:461.

Roberts E, Chase TN, Tower DB (eds) (1976). "GABA in Nervous
System Function", New York: Raven Press, p 1-554.

Roberts PJ, Watkins JC (1975). Structural requirements for
the inhibition for L-glutamate uptake by glia and nerve
endings. Brain Res 85:120.

Schousboe A (1981). Transport and metabolism of glutamate
and GABA in neurons and glial cells. Int Rev Neurobiol
22:1.

Schousboe A (1982). Metabolism and function of neurotransmitters. In Pfeiffer SE (ed): "Neuroscience Approached
Through Cell Culture", Vol 1, Boca Raton, Fl: CRC Press,
p 107.

Schousboe A, Divac I (1979). Differences in glutamate uptake in astrocytes cultured from different brain regions.
Brain Res 177:407.

Schousboe A, Hertz L (1983). Regulation of glutamatergic
and GABAergic neuronal activity by astroglial cells. In
Osborne NN (ed): "Dale's Principle and Communication
Between Neurones", Oxford: Pergamon Press, p 113.

Schousboe A, Hertz L, Svenneby G (1977a). Uptake and metabolism of GABA in astrocytes cultured from dissociated
mouse brain hemispheres. Neurochem Res 2:217.

Schousboe A, Hertz L, Svenneby G, Kvamme E (1979a). Phosphate
activated glutaminase activity and glutamine uptake in
primary cultures of astrocytes. J Neurochem 32:943.

Schousboe A, Larsson OM, Hertz L, Krogsgaard-Larsen P (1981).
Heterocyclic GABA analogues as new selective inhibitors of
astroglial GABA transport. Drug Dev Res 1:115.

Schousboe A, Larsson OM, Meier E, Hertz L, Krogsgaard-Larsen P (1982). Tissue culture studies of GABA-neurotransmission. In Okada Y, Roberts E (eds): "Problems in GABA-Research from Brain to Bacteria", Amsterdam: Excerpta Medica, p 249.

Schousboe A, Larsson OM, Wood JD, Krogsgaard-Larsen P (1983). Transport and metabolism of GABA in neurons and glia: Implications for epilepsy. Epilepsia in press.

Schousboe A, Svenneby G, Hertz L (1977b). Uptake and metabolism of glutamate in astrocytes cultured from dissociated mouse brain hemispheres. J Neurochem 29:999.

Schousboe A, Thorbek P, Hertz L, Krogsgaard-Larsen P (1979b). Effects of GABA analogues of restricted conformation on GABA transport in astrocytes and brain cortex slices and on GABA receptor binding. J Neurochem 33:181.

Schwarcz R, Whetsell WO jr (1982). Post-mortem high affinity glutamate uptake in human brain. Neurosci 7:1771.

Snodgrass SR, White WF, Biales B, Dichter M (1980). Biochemical correlates of GABA function in rat cortical neurons in culture. Brain Res 190:123.

Stone TW (1979). Glutamate as the neurotransmitter of cerebellar granule cells in the rat: electrophysiological evidence. Br J Pharmacol 66:291.

Wood JD, Johnson DD, Krogsgaard-Larsen P, Schousboe A (1983). Anticonvulsant activity of the glial-selective GABA uptake inhibitor, THPO. Neuropharmacol 22, 139.

Wood JD, Schousboe A, Krogsgaard-Larsen P (1980). In vivo changes in the GABA content of nerve endings (synaptosomes) induced by inhibitors of GABA uptake. Neuropharmacol 19:1149.

Wood JH (1982). Physiological neurochemistry of cerebrospinal fluid. In Lajtha A (ed): "Handbook of Neurochemistry", 2. ed Vol 1, New York: Plenum Press, p 415.

Young AB, Oster-Granite ML, Herndon RM, Snyder SH (1974). Glutamic acid: Selective depletion by viral induced granule cell loss in hamster cerebellum. Brain Res 73:1.

Yu ACH, Hertz E, Hertz L (1983). Biochemical and functional maturation of highly purified cultures of cerebral cortical neurons, a GABAergic preparation. J Neurochem submitted.

Yu ACH, Hertz L (1982). Uptake of glutamate, GABA, and glutamine into a predominantly GABA-ergic and a predominantly glutamatergic nerve cell population in culture. J Neurosci Res 7:23.

Glutamine, Glutamate, and GABA
in the Central Nervous System, pages 317–325
© 1983 Alan R. Liss, Inc., 150 Fifth Avenue, New York, NY 10011

COMPARTMENTATION OF GLUTAMATE AND GLUTAMINE METABOLISM IN CULTURED NERVE CELLS

J. Borg, G. Hamel, B. Spitz and J. Mark

Centre de Neurochimie du C.N.R.S.
5, rue Blaise Pascal, 67084 Strasbourg
Cedex, France.

Several previous studies have described a metabolic compartmentation in the brain which includes glutamate and GABA (Machiyama et al. 1970; Van den Berg et al. 1971). These and other related findings on the localization of enzymes linked to glutamate and GABA metabolism suggested morphological assignments for this compartmentation (Nicklas et al. 1979; Shank, Aprison 1979).

In order to obtain direct information on glutamate metabolism in neuronal and glial cells, we incubated primary cultures with [^{14}C]glutamine or [^{14}C]glutamate and measured the incorporation of radioactivity into related amino acids. Previous studies have shown that these cultures transport glutamate and GABA by high affinity systems (Borg et al. 1980; Ramaharobandro et al. 1982) and glutamine by a low affinity mechanism (Ramaharobandro et al. 1982). These cultures also possess enzymes related to glutamate and GABA metabolism (Borg et al. 1983) and demonstrate, respectively, some characteristics of mature neuronal or glial cells (Borg et al. 1980).

MATERIALS AND METHODS

Primary cultures of neuronal and glial cells were obtained as previously described (Borg et al. 1980), except that neuronal cultures were incubated in a chemically defined medium according to Bottenstein and Sato (1979). Experiments were performed on neurons after 6 days of culture and on glial cells after 21 days.

After removing the growth medium, each culture was incubated at 37°C in a Krebs-Ringer medium as reported previously (Borg et al. 1980). This medium contained 100 μM L-
[U-^{14}C]glutamine (0.3 μCi/dish) or 10 μM U[^{14}C]glutamic acid
(0.3 μCi/dish) and the incubation was continued for the time
period indicated in the text. After incubation, the cultures
were rinsed twice with 3 ml of cold Krebs-Ringer solution and
then scraped off in a small volume of 75% ethanol.

Electrophoretic separation of the amino acids and quantitative determination were performed according to the
method of Sarhan et al. (1979). The extracts were subjected
to another separation which was performed in parallel; this
method consisted of an electrophoretic separation in a pyri-
dine/acetic acid/water (10/4.5/485, v/v/v) buffer, pH 5.2,
for 60 min, followed by ascending chromatography in the same
dimension in 80% ethanol over 3 h. This was necessary to
obtain a glutamine spot which was not contaminated by taurine
or neutral amino acids; the quantitative determination of
glutamate, aspartate and GABA gave similar values with both
the modified and unmodified methods.

After separation, 4 radioactive spots were identified
with a Berthold LB 282 linear analyzer; they corresponded to
aspartate, glutamate, glutamine and GABA. No radioactivity
was detected in any other amino acid spot. The individual
spots were scraped off and counted in a Beckman LS 9000
scintillation spectrometer.

RESULTS

Metabolic Fate of [^{14}C]Glutamine in Neuronal Cells

Figure 1 shows the specific activities of several amino
acids obtained on incubation of neuronal cultures with 100
μM [^{14}C]glutamine for varying periods of time. The specific
activities of aspartate, glutamate and glutamine increased
linearly during the first 80-100 mins and then reached a
plateau. The specific activities of glutamate and aspartate
were already twice that of the precursor after only 10 min
and remained higher during the whole incubation period. This
suggests that [^{14}C]glutamine is rapidly metabolized into glutamate and aspartate and that this metabolism takes place in
a glutamine pool with a high specific activity. On the other

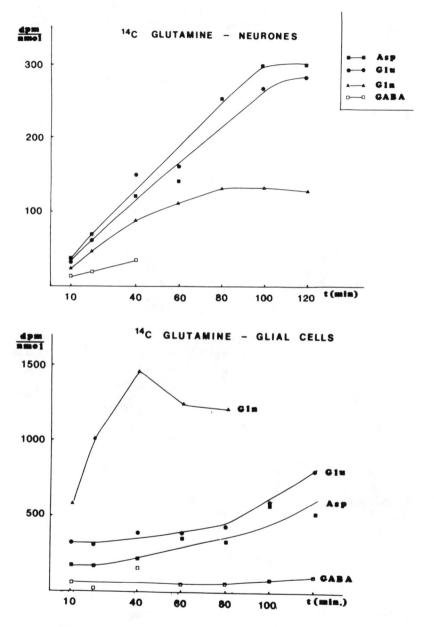

Fig. 1. Specific radioactivities (dpm/nmol) of aspartate, glutamate, glutamine and GABA in neuronal cultures (top) and glial cultures (bottom) as a function of incubation time with 100 μM [U-14C]glutamine. Results are the means of two separate experiments.

hand, the incorporation of radioactivity into GABA was much lower and the specific activity was about half that of the glutamine.

The distribution of radioactivity did not vary much during the incubation: 66% of the total radioactivity was found in glutamine, 25% in glutamate, 8% in aspartate and 1% in GABA. It should be noted that the specific activity of intracellular glutamine (50-100 dpm/nmol) was always much lower than in the medium (2300 dpm/nmol).

Metabolic Fate of [^{14}C]Glutamine in Glial Cells

The pattern of incorporation of radioactivity in glial cultures on incubation with 100 μM [^{14}C]glutamine was strikingly different from that in neuronal cultures. The specific activity of glutamine increased rapidly for 40 min and then leveled off (Fig. 1). The specific activities of glutamate and aspartate increased slowly between 10 and 80 min but then more rapidly and almost linearly when the glutamine specific activity was constant (80-120 min).

It seems that the metabolism of [^{14}C]glutamine in glia is slower than in neurons, as 81% of the radioactivity was still present in glutamine at the end of the experiment, with 15% being found in glutamate, 3% in aspartate and less than 0.5% in GABA. When the specific activity of glutamine was maximal (40 min) the ratio of specific activities was 0.27 for glutamate/glutamine, 0.15 for aspartate/glutamine and 0.11 for GABA/glutamine.

The rate of glutamate synthesis could be estimated during the period 80-100 min when it increased almost linearly, assuming a constant glutamine specific activity. The pool size of glutamate was measured as 14.4 nmoles/mg protein and the amount of glutamate formed per minute could be calculated to be 0.10 nmole/mg protein. This value is about 9% of the glutaminase activity measured in glial cultures (Borg et al. 1983).

Metabolic Fate of [^{14}C]Glutamate in Neurons

The specific activities of glutamate, aspartate and glutamine in neuronal cultures after incubation with 10 μM

[^{14}C]glutamate are shown in Figure 2. It can be seen that the specific activity of glutamate was already maximal after 10 min and then decreased rapidly, reaching a constant level after 40 min. The aspartate values showed a concomitant increase which reached a plateau at the same time. These results suggest a normal precursor/product relationship between glutamate and aspartate. However, the incorporation of radioactivity into glutamine and GABA was low, with maximal values after 20 min of 192 dpm/nmol and 120 dpm/nmol respectively.

Only 3-4% of the total radioactivity was found in glutamine and less than 1% in GABA. After 10 min of incubation, 92% of the radioactivity was present in glutamate and 5% in aspartate; after 60 min these values were 82% and 15% respectively. The relative specific activity of aspartate increased over the same time period from 0.24 to 0.92.

Metabolic Fate of [^{14}C]Glutamate in Glial Cells

Figure 2 shows the incorporation of radioactivity into four amino acids after incubation with 10 μM [^{14}C]glutamate. The specific activities were already maximal after 20 min for al amino acids except glutamine which reached a plateau after 40 min. It can be seen that the specific activities of glutamate, aspartate and GABA decreased after 20 min towards a constant level. [^{14}C]Glutamate seemed to be mainly metabolized into [^{14}C]aspartate since the specific activity of aspartate relative to that of glutamate increased from 0.28 to 0.78 between 10 and 40 min and then remained constant. The relative specific activity of glutamine was lower, reaching 0.23 after 40 min. It should be noted that, at that time, 40% of the total radioactivity was found equally divided between glutamine and aspartate, 60% was still present as glutamate, and GABA accounted for less than 0.5%.

DISCUSSION

The aim of the present study was to investigate the metabolism of glutamate and glutamine in neuronal and glial cells in order to examine the possibility of metabolic compartmentation between these two cell types. When [^{14}C]glutamine is the radioactive precursor, the specific activities

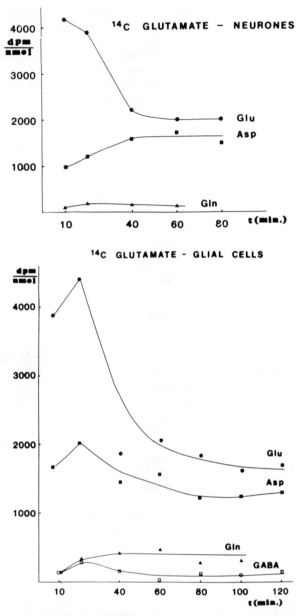

Fig. 2. Specific radioactivities (dpm/nmol) of glutamate, aspartate, glutamine and GABA in neuronal cultures (top) and glial cultures (bottom) as a function of incubation time with 10 µM [U-14C]glutamate.

of glutamine are 10 times higher in glial cells than in neurons; this could be explained by a higher rate of uptake into glial than neuronal cells (Ramaharobandro et al. 1982), coupled with a glutamine pool which is 8 times smaller in glia than in neurons. Moreover, the glutamate specific activity in neurons is twice that of glutamine. This could be due to a compartmentation of the glutamine pool in neurons; i.e., for example, if the exogenous glutamine which is taken up, is accumulated into a small pool with a high specific activity at least equal to that of glutamate. The glutamine from this pool of high specific activity might then be hydrolyzed by glutaminase to produce glutamate which could be converted to aspartate. If we assume that the glutamine compartment, which is labelled by exogenous glutamine, is in equilibrium with glutamine in the incubation medium, the specific activity on both sides of the membrane should be the same (2333 dpm/nmol in our experiments). With a glutamine pool of 190 nmol/mg protein, we can calculate that the pool with high specific activity would be equal to 5% of the total glutamine.

This result suggests that glutamine which is taken up by neurons does not mix with the whole intracellular glutamine pool but is preferentially transformed into glutamate. This mechanism seems to be a direct way for synthesizing glutamate and GABA in neurons. Moreover, the relative specific activities of glutamate, aspartate and GABA are 3 to 4 times higher in neurons than in glial cells. This result suggests that glutamine taken up into neurons is a better precursor for these three amino acids than that taken up into glial cells.

When cultures are incubated with [^{14}C]glutamate, it seems to be taken up rapidly into both glia and neurons. The maximal specific activities of glutamate are very similar in both cell types, while the V_{max} of uptake is about four times higher in glia than in neurons (Ramaharobandro et al. 1982). These results suggest that the glutamate pool labelled by exogenous substrate might be larger in neurons than in glia. Indeed, according to our measurements, the total pool of glutamate is 6 times larger in neurons than in glia (90.2 nmol/mg protein versus 14.4 nmol/mg protein).

It should be pointed out that the initial increase in glutamate specific activity in both types of cultures was followed by a strong decrease between 20 and 40 min of incubation, leading to a plateau. The decrease could be due to an intense metabolism of glutamate after it has reached a certain metabolic pool. It should be noted that the specific activity of aspartate in neurons increases between 20 and 40 min and reaches a plateau at the same time as glutamate, with a relative specific activity equal to 0.92. The decline in glutamate specific activity, as well as strong metabolism through the tricarboxylic acid cycle, have already been reported in other astrocytic cultures (Yu et al. 1982).

The synthesis of glutamine from glutamate seems to be higher in glia than in neurons, as the relative specific activity of glutamine is 3 times higher in glia than in neurons. This result is in accordance with a higher glutamine synthetase activity in astroblasts than in neurons (Borg et al. 1983) and with a preferential localization of that enzyme in glia (Martinez-Hernandez et al. 1977).

In conclusion, our results show that the metabolism of glutamate and glutamine are quite different in neuronal as compared with glial cells. Glutamine seems to be a good precursor for glutamate formation in neurons and further studies will examine the neurotransmitter function of the neosynthesized amino acids.

REFERENCES

Borg J, Ramaharobandro N, Mark J, Mandel P (1980). Changes in the uptake of GABA and taurine during neuronal and glial maturation. J Neurochem 34:1113.

Borg J, Hamel G, Spitz B, Mark J (1983). Glutamine metabolism in mature nerve cells in primary cultures. Proc 9th ISN Meeting, Vancouver (Canada).

Bottenstein JE, Sato GH (1979). Growth of a rat neuroblastoma cell line in serum free supplemented medium. Proc Nat Acad Sciences 76:514.

Machiyama Y, Balázs R, Hammond RJ, Julian T, Richter D (1970). The metabolism of GABA and glucose in potassium ion-stimulated brain tissue in vitro. Biochem J 116:469.

Martinez-Hernandez A, Bell KP, Norenberg MD (1977). Glutamine synthetase: glial localization in brain. Science 195:1356.

Nicklas WJ, Nunez R, Berl S, Duvoisin R (1979). Neuronal-glial contributions to transmitter amino acid metabolism:

studies with kainic acid-induced lesions of rat striatum. J Neurochem 33:839.

Ramaharobandro N, Borg J, Mandel P, Mark J (1982). Glutamine and glutamate transport in cultured neuronal and glial cells. Brain Res 244:113.

Sarhan S, Seiler N, Grove J, Bink G (1979). Rapid method for the assay of GABA, glutamic acid and aspartic acid in brain tissue and subcellular fractions. J Chromatogr 162:561.

Shank RP, Aprison MH (1979). Biochemical aspects of the neurotransmitter function of glutamate. In Filer LJ, Garattini S, Kare MR, Reynolds WA, Wurtman RJ (eds): "Glutamic Acid: Advances in Biochemistry and Physiology," New York: Raven Press, p 139.

Van Den Berg CJ, Garfinkel OA (1971). A simulation study of brain compartments: metabolism of glutamate and related substances in mouse brain. Biochem J 123:211.

Yu AC, Schousboe A, Hertz L (1982). Metabolic fate of ^{14}C-labeled glutamate in astrocytes in primary cultures. J Neurochem 39:954.

Glutamine, Glutamate, and GABA
in the Central Nervous System, pages 327-342
© 1983 Alan R. Liss, Inc., 150 Fifth Avenue, New York, NY 10011

METABOLIC FLUXES FROM GLUTAMATE AND TOWARDS GLUTAMATE IN NEURONS AND ASTROCYTES IN PRIMARY CULTURES

Leif Hertz[1], Albert C.H. Yu[1], Richard L. Potter[1], Thomas E. Fisher[1] and Arne Schousboe[1,2]
Department of Pharmacology, University of Saskatchewan, Saskatoon, S7N 0W0 Canada[1] and Department of Biochemistry, The Panum Institute, University of Copenhagen, DK2200, Denmark[2]

INTRODUCTION

A substantial amount of information is now available about uptake and release rates for glutamate, GABA and glutamine in astrocytes and in glutamatergic and GABAergic neurons (Schousboe et al., this volume). Less information has been compiled about the activities of the enzymes involved in the interconversions between these amino acids in neurons and in astrocytes and about the actual metabolic fluxes leading to their degradation and replenishment. This topic will be dealt with in the present review. It is illustrated in Fig. 1. A key compound in this figure is glutamate which is released from neurons in large amounts and accumulated more intensely into astrocytes than into neurons (Schousboe et al., this volume). Since glutamate is produced from α-ketoglutarate, a tricarboxylic acid (TCA) cycle constituent, this means that TCA cycle constituents become exhausted in neurons unless there is either a neuronal de novo synthesis of TCA cycle constituents or a transfer of one or more glutamate precursor(s) back to the neurons. These precursors could include glutamine, any TCA cycle constituent, or ornithine. In addition to being released, glutamate may be decarboxylated to form GABA which, again, partly is accumulated into astrocytes. This will create similar problems as the glutamate accumulation, but quantitatively to a much less extent since the amounts of released GABA are smaller than those of glutamate (Hertz, 1979; Schousboe, Hertz, 1983) and since GABA is accumulated with considerably higher intensity into neurons than into astrocytes (Schousboe et al., this volume).

GLUTAMATE METABOLISM

   Astrocytes. Whereas no glutamate decarboxylase (GAD)
activity (Table 1) and GABA synthesis (Table 2) are found
in astrocytes, glutamate may be converted to glutamine,
through the action of glutamine synthetase (GS), or to
α-ketoglutarate. The formation of α-ketoglutarate can
conceivably occur either as an oxidative deamination,
catalyzed by glutamate dehydrogenase (GLDH), or as a
transamination, catalyzed by glutamate-oxaloacetic
transaminase (GOT). From Table 1 it can be seen that the
GS activity in astrocytes consistently has been found to be

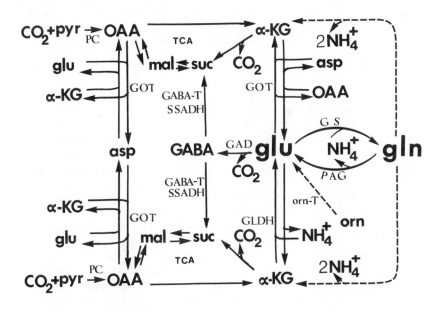

Fig. 1. Scheme of metabolic interconversions between
glutamate (glu); glutamine (gln); γ-aminobutyric acid
(GABA); tricarboxylic acid (TCA) cycle constituents:
succinate (suc), malate (mal), oxaloacetate (OAA), and
α-ketoglutarate (α-KG) ; pyruvate (pyr); aspartate (asp);
ornithine (orn); carbon dioxide (CO_2); and ammonia (NH_4^+).
Some of the enzymes catalyzing these reactions are also
indicated: glutamine synthetase (GS); phosphate activated
glutaminase (PAG); glutamate dehydrogenase (GLDH);
glutamate-oxaloacetic transaminase (GOT); glutamate
decarboxylase (GAD); GABA-transaminase (GABA-T); succinic
semialdehyde dehydrogenase (SSADH); pyruvate carboxylase (PC); and ornithine aminotransferase (orn-T).

about 20 nmol/min per mg protein in the absence of added glucocorticoids and about twice this rate after culturing with glucocorticosteroids, substances known to induce GS activity in vivo (Moscona et al., 1980). Both GOT and GLDH are also found at high activities in astrocytes. With the exception of the larger value determined by Patel et al. (1982) the GLDH activity has generally been found to be about 10 nmol/min per mg protein. The activity of GOT, an almost ubiquitous enzyme, is 10-20 times higher (Table 1).

Enzyme activities do not represent actual metabolic fluxes. In order to obtain information on actual glutamine synthesis rates, cultures of astrocytes were incubated with $[U-^{14}C]$-labeled glutamate, and the time course of alterations in specific activities in glutamate and glutamine was followed (Fig. 2). This, together with measurements of the glutamine pool size, allows calculation of actual fluxes as described by Yu et al. (1982). Such experiments have reproducibly shown a glutamine synthesis of about 2 nmol/min per mg protein (Table 2), calculated on the basis of the specific activity of the total glutamate pool (see below). This metabolic flux is about 10% of the GS activity (Table 1). The availability of ammonia is essential for glutamine synthesis. However, the low amount of ammonia (0.1-0.2 mM) which is present in the cultured cells in the absence of added ammonia (probably originating from glutamine in the medium) is high enough that a minor increase within the physiological range (to about 0.3 mM) or even to pathophysiological levels (1 or 3 mM) has no effect on the transformation rate (Fig. 2). This may well reflect the relatively low K_m for ammonia in glutamine synthesis (Benjamin, 1982). The specific activity of glutamate in the cells becomes, even at equilibrium, only about one-half of that in the medium (Yu et al., 1983c; Fig. 2). This shows that the intracellular pool of glutamate is compartmentalized and that only one-half of the total glutamate pool is readily accessible for exogenous glutamate. This concept of different glutamate pools in astrocytes is compatible with in vivo findings that the two small pool (i.e., probably glial) precursors, acetate and glutamate, label glutamine with different relative specific activities (Krespan et al., 1982). Such a compartmentation of the glutamate pool calls for some caution in the interpretation of the values for glutamine synthesis shown in Table 2. These values were calculated using the average specific activity of the whole intracellular glutamate pool. If glutamine is formed mainly from the readily labeled pool, the specific glutamate activity would be higher and the calculated flux to glutamine accordingly overestimated. Conversely, if glutamine is mainly formed from a pool which is less readily labeled by exogenous glutamate, the specific activity would be lower and the flux towards glutamine underestimated. One way to distinguish between these possibilities is to measure rates of ammonia incorporation into glutamine in astrocytic cultures as has been elegantly done in the brain in vivo (Berl et al., 1962; Cooper et al., 1979). Such studies are underway both in other laboratories (Yudkoff et al., this volume) and in our own (S.-C. Cheng, A.C.H. Yu, D.A. Durden, A. Schousboe, L. Hertz, unpublished) but it is premature to draw any conclusions regarding the quantitative correlation between incorporation of labeled glutamate and of labeled ammonia. However, the fact that the specific activity of

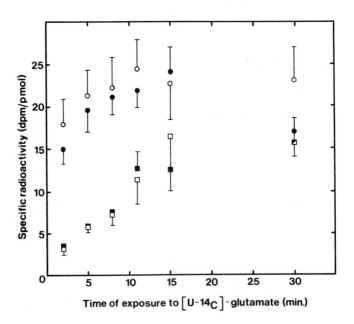

Fig. 2 Specific radioactivities of glutamate (O and ●) and glutamine (□ and ■) in primary cultures of astrocytes incubated for 2-30 min in medium with 50 μM L-[U-14C]-glutamate (47.0 ± 0.8 dpm/pmol) and zero (O and □) or 3 (● and ■) mM ammonia. Results are means of 3-6 experiments and S.E.M. values are shown by vertical bars if they extend beyond the symbols. From Yu et al., 1983c.

Table 1. Enzyme activities (nmol/min per mg protein) in primary cultures of astrocytes or neurons.

	GABA-T	GAD	Orn-T	PAG	GOT	GLDH	GS
Astrocytes	1.6[a]	<0.05[b]	5.3[c]	3.8 (10.7)[d]	206[b]	12.3[b]	25.9[b]
	4.6[e]	N.D.[f]		2.4 (8.9)[g]	154–249[h]	3.0–12.3[h]	22.0–28.1[h]
	6.2[i]	0.2[i]		1.8*[j]	120–140[k]	101.3[j]	41.3**[l]
	5-6[k]	0.009[m]				16.6[n]	43.3**[o]
						10[k]	22.2[j]
							10[k]
Cerebellar Granule Cells	1.2[p]		2.9[c]	21.8*[j]	449[p]	60.8[j]	5.7[j]
				1.1 (4.1)[c]		62.8[p]	
Cerebral Neurons	0.8[p]	13.7[q]	5.0[c]	1.0 (7.9)[c]	367[p]		27.8[p]
	2[r]	1.3[r]					
	0.6[s]	10[s]					

[a] Schousboe et al., 1977a; [b] Schousboe et al., 1977b;
[c] Schousboe et al., 1983; [d] Schousboe et al., 1979;
[e] Hansson, Sellström, 1983; [f] J.-Y. Wu, L. Hertz, A. Schousboe, unpublished; [g] Kvamme et al., 1982; [h] Hertz et al. 1978; [i] Bardakjian et al., 1979; [j] Patel et al., 1982; [k] Tardy et al., 1981; [l] Juurlink et al., 1981; [m] Wilson et al., 1972; [n] Roth-Schechter et al., 1977; [o] Hallermayer et al., 1981; [p] Larsson et al., 1983; [q] Yu et al., 1983b; [r] Hauser, Bernasconi, 1980; [s] Snodgrass et al., 1980.
* The authors' value has been multiplied by 10 since they indicated that only 10% of maximum activity was found at the glutamine concentration used. ** Treated with hydrocortisone or dexamethasone. N.D. not detectable. PAG activities shown in parentheses were measured in the presence of 20 mM phosphate. Abbreviation as in Fig. 1.

glutamine reaches only one-half (Yu et al., 1982) to two-thirds (Fig. 2) of that in glutamate may suggest that glutamine is partly synthesized from a pool which is not readily labeled from exogenous glutamate (see also below). If this is, indeed, the case the flux from glutamate to glutamine would be somewhat higher than that shown in Table 2.

Table 2. Metabolic fluxes (nmol/min per mg protein) in primary cultures of astrocytes or neurons.

	Astrocytes	Cerebellar Granule Cells	Cerebral Neurons
glu → gln	2.4^a 1.7^b		
glu → CO_2	4.1^a 5.9^b 7.4^e	$< 0.1^c$	0.7^d
gln → GABA	$N.D.^d$		0.3^f
gln → glu	2^d		$0.9-2.3^f$
gln → CO_2	2.0^e		1.8^f
mal → glu	0.003^d		0.001^d
mal → CO_2	0.1^e		
GABA → CO_2	0.03^e		

[a]Yu et al., 1982; [b]Yu et al., 1983c; [c]J. Drejer, A. Schousboe, unpublished ; [d]A. Yu, L. Hertz, unpublished; [e]Yu, Hertz, this volume; [f]Yu et al., 1984. N.D. not detectable. Abbreviations as in Fig. 1.

Metabolic fluxes between glutamate and α-ketoglutarate are not easily measured by incorporation of radioactivity into α-ketoglutarate. We have therefore instead measured incorporation of radioactivity from $[1-^{14}C]$-labeled glutamate into carbon dioxide. Since the astrocytes have no GAD activity, this procedure must determine the rate of formation of CO_2 and succinyl CoA via α-ketoglutarate and thus

give a minimum value of fluxes between glutamate and
α-ketoglutarate. It gives <u>per se</u> no information whether
the formation of α-ketoglutarate from glutamate occurs as
an oxidative deamination or as a transamination (Fig. 1).
This distinction is of importance since the high GOT
activity and the equilibrium constant for the transamination
favor rapid exchange between these two compounds. Thus, if
the transformation is catalyzed by GOT the production of
$^{14}CO_2$ from labeled glutamate might simply represent an
isotope exchange of no functional importance. This concern
may be of less importance in the case of the GLDH reaction
(see also Yu, Hertz, this volume).

Carbon dioxide production from glutamate has been
found to occur at a rate of 4-7 nmol/min per mg protein
(Table 2), again on the basis of the specific activity of
the total glutamate pool. It is little, if at all, inhibited by 5 mM AOAA, which completely inhibits transamination (Yu et al., 1982). Thus, it can unequivocally be
concluded that glutamate in astrocytes in primary cultures
can be metabolized to α-ketoglutarate via an oxidative
deamination, and the rate of this process is high compared
to the GLDH activity (Table 1). The concept that the GLDH
reaction operates towards a net synthesis of α-ketoglutarate
may appear to be at variance with the fact that the equilibrium constant for this reaction favors glutamate formation
(Williamson et al., 1967). However, with an intramitochon-
drial NADH/NAD ratio of approximately 1.5 and concentrations
of α-ketoglutarate and ammonia of respectively 0.1 (Chapman
. et al., 1977) and 0.2 mM (see above), this reaction would
be in equilibrium at an intracellular glutamate concentration of 8 mM (approximately 60 nmol/mg protein), i.e., even
less than the glutamate content in astrocytes (Yu et al.,
1983c). That the GLDH reaction does not lead to any major
synthesis of glutamate is also compatible with the <u>in vivo</u>
finding by Cooper et al. (1979) that exogenous ammonia in
the brain at physiologically relevant concentrations is
primarily incorporated as amide nitrogen in glutamine and
only to a very limited extent as amine nitrogen in glutamate and glutamine. It is in further support of this
concept that a small increase in ammonia concentration
(addition of 0.1 mM) has no measurable effect on the rate
of $^{14}CO_2$ production, whereas larger increases (1 mM), which
can be expected to affect the equilibrium and thus the
relative amount of α-ketoglutarate formed from radioactive
glutamate, cause a decrease in production of labeled carbon
dioxide of about 30% (Yu et al., 1983c). A modest increase
in the total amount of glutamate (Yu et al., 1983c) after

exposure to ammonia is also consistent with the expected
effect of this compound on the equilibrium between glutamate
and α-ketoglutarate.

The qualifications mentioned regarding the absolute
magnitude of the glutamine production also apply to the
rate of carbon dioxide formation. Since the subcellular
localizations of glutamine synthetase (a microsomal enzyme,
Sellinger, Verster, 1962) and glutamate dehydrogenase (a
mitochondrial enzyme, McCarthy, Tipton, this volume) are
different, it is unlikely that it is the same glutamate
pool which labels glutamine and carbon dioxide. Thus, if
glutamine is formed to a major extent from the glutamate
pool which is not readily accessible to exogenous glutamate
it seems likely that oxidative deamination occurs mainly
from the accessible pool. This has 2 implications: 1) the
rate of carbon dioxide production given in Table 2 may be
overestimated, although at most by a factor of two (ratio
between the specific glutamate activity in the medium and
in the cells); and 2) exogenous glutamate, including that
released from neurons, is to a large extent used as a
metabolic fuel and thus not available for glutamine
synthesis.

Neurons. Neuronal cultures generally contain a small
amount of astrocytes which can be expected to metabolize
glutamate avidly. However, cultures highly enriched in
the probably glutamatergic cerebellar granule cells
(Schousboe et al., this volume) can be grown in the
absence of serum and are, under these conditions, virtually
free of astrocytes. In such cultures the CO_2 production,
in the presence of AOAA, is only a few percent of that in
astrocytes (Table 2). The high (4-6 times higher than in
astrocytes) GLDH activity in these cells (Table 1) might
therefore conceivably reflect a glutamate synthesis from
α-ketoglutarate in these neurons. The GOT activity is also
higher in cerebellar neurons than in astrocytes, whereas
the glutamine synthetase activity is several fold lower
(Table 1). This is compatible with histochemical in vivo
studies showing that GS is confined to astrocytes
(Norenberg, this volume). It is unknown whether the
non-negligible activity found in cultured neurons indicates
some GS activity in neurons or whether it is due to a minor
contamination with astrocytes.

In cerebral cortical neurons, a predominantly GABA-
ergic preparation (Snodgrass et al., 1980; Yu et al.,

1983b; Schousboe et al., this volume), the GLDH activity is only one-half of that in cerebellar granule cells (but still higher than in astrocytes). GOT activity may also be marginally lower (Table 1) than in the glutamatergic neurons. Again, the CO_2 production is much less than in astrocytes although probably not as low as in cerebellar granule cells (Table 2).

A key process in GABAergic neurons is production of GABA, catalyzed by GAD. This enzyme is present at high activities in cultured cerebral cortical neurons (Table 1), which show higher GAD activities than the brain cortex but only after culturing beyond the age of one week (Yu et al., 1983b). However, exogenous glutamate does not seem to be converted to GABA in cortical neurons (Yu et al., 1983b; Borg et al., this volume). This suggests the presence of more than one glutamate pool also in neurons. In contrast, exogenous glutamine is partly converted to GABA. The actual rate of this GABA production can be measured by labeling with radioactive glutamine and determination of specific activities in glutamate and in GABA as well as the pool size of GABA after different periods of exposure to the radioisotope. Such studies have shown a flux from glutamine via glutamate to GABA of about 0.3 nmol/min per mg protein (Table 2). This value should be compared with a GAD activity of 13.7 nmol/min per mg protein (Table 1).

GLUTAMATE PRECURSORS

Glutamine: From the previous section it follows that glutamate after its transfer to astrocytes is partly, but by no means completely, metabolized to glutamine. This section deals with the subsequent fate of glutamine in the astrocytes themselves and in neurons to which part of the glutamine may be transferred.

The activity of glutaminase (PAG) in astrocytes has consistently been found to be 2-10 nmol/min per mg protein, with the higher values being obtained in the presence of an elevated phosphate concentration. This activity is not negligible compared to that of GS (Table 1). It is unresolved whether it is higher or lower in cultured neurons (Table 1) but it is undoubtedly somewhat higher in synaptosomes, measured under identical conditions (Kvamme et al., 1982). The activities at the cellular level of glutamine transaminase and ω-amidase, the concerted action of which may lead to formation of α-ketoglutarate from glutamine via α-ketoglutaramate (Duffy, Cooper, this volume) are unknown.

The formation of glutamate from glutamine has been investigated in exactly the same manner as the metabolic conversions of glutamate, i.e., by labeling with radioactive glutamine and determination of the time courses for alterations in specific activities of its products. The glutamine pool which is accessible to exogenous glutamine constitutes, in our hands, at least 50% in both astrocytes and neurons; this is far more than the 5% in cultured neurons reported by Borg et al. (this volume), a difference which is possibly due to their use of very young cultures. In astrocytes, the flux from glutamine to glutamate has been found to be about 2 nmol/min per mg protein (i.e., about 20% of the phosphate stimulated PAG activity) and this glutamine can be further metabolized to CO_2 at about the same rate (Table 2). The corresponding fluxes in the cerebral, mainly GABAergic, neurons appear to be rather similar (Table 2). Neither in GABAergic neurons nor in astrocytes does the specific activity ratio between glutamine and glutamate reach unity after 60 min of incubation, again indicating the presence of different amino acid pools. In GABAergic neurons, glutamate which has been formed from glutamine can be further converted to GABA as previously discussed. This is compatible with the concept that glutamine may function as a GABA precursor (e.g., Reubi et al., 1978; Morjaria, Voaden, 1979; McGeer, McGeer, 1979) but it should be kept in mind that the GABA formation (0.3 nmol/min per mg protein) is much slower than the CO_2 production. No corresponding data are available for cerebellar granule cells, but a potassium-induced calcium-dependent release of radioactivity after labeling with glutamine does indicate that glutamine in these cells can be converted to transmitter glutamate (Levi, Ciotti, this volume; J. Drejer, A. Schousboe, unpublished).

Other glutamate precursors. A natural consequence of a less than quantitative return of glutamine from astrocytes to neurons and of the utilization of glutamine in neurons also for other purposes than production of glutamate and/or GABA is that there must exist other precursors which can give rise to a net neuronal synthesis of glutamate. These could comprise TCA cycle constituents (such as α-ketoglutarate or malate (Shank, Campbell, this volume), TCA cycle precursors (such as pyruvate which can be converted to oxaloacetate), or ornithine (which can be converted to

glutamate via glutamate-γ-semialdehyde, McGeer et al.,
this volume). GABA, which is metabolized to succinate, can
similarly be regarded as a TCA cycle precursor.

Malate and α-ketoglutarate are accumulated relatively
slowly (0.05 nmol/min per mg protein) into both astrocytes
and neurons in primary cultures (A.C.H. Yu, A. Schousboe,
L. Hertz, unpublished). The metabolic fate of malate has
been studied in astrocytes and in GABAergic neurons.
Glutamate was labeled, although slowly, in both cell types
(Table 2) and in the neurons there was also incorporation
of radioactivity into GABA. In the neurons, the labeling
of glutamate was not potently reduced by AOAA, showing that
the GLDH catalyzed reaction in these cells may lead to net
synthesis of glutamate, and thus probably of GABA. Such a
net synthesis of glutamate and GABA from a TCA cycle
constituent can only continue provided the relatively small
pools of TCA cycle constituents in neurons are replenished
either by transport from astrocytes or by neuronal de novo
synthesis. The main process leading to de novo synthesis
of TCA cycle constituents in brain is carboxylation of
pyruvate to oxaloacetate (Shank, Campbell, this volume).
This reaction is catalyzed by pyruvate carboxylase (PC), an
enzyme which is present in brain at a non-negligible
activity (Keech, Utter, 1967). However, it is absent in
neurons (Shank et al., 1981; Yu et al., 1983a) annulling
the possibility that neurons could be self-supplying with
TCA cycle constituents. In contrast, astrocytes show a PC
activity (Shank et al., 1981) which amounts to 2 nmol/min
per mg protein (Yu et al., 1983a). Oxaloacetate formed by
this reaction and succinate formed from GABA may both be
glutamate precursors in the astrocytic glutamate pool which
is not readily accessible for exogenous glutamate but
serves for production of glutamine. Such a mechanism would
be compatible with the finding in whole brain that acetate,
a TCA cycle precursor, labels glutamine more readily than
does glutamate (Krespan et al., 1982). It might also
explain suggestions in the literature (Reubi et al., 1978;
Morjaria, Voaden, 1979) that neuronal GABA may be replenished
from glutamine to a larger extent than neuronal glutamate.
It should, however, be kept in mind that GABA and TCA cycle
constituents, such as malate, are also metabolized to CO_2
in astrocytes (Table 2).

A non-TCA-cycle related possible precursor for neuronal
glutamate and GABA is ornithine. Unfortunately, no information is available about fluxes from ornithine in cultured
neurons or astrocytes but it might be in agreement with a

role of this system for GABA formation (Yoneda, Roberts, 1981) that the K_m for the ornithine aminotransferase (Orn-T) is 10-fold lower in cerebral cortical neurons than in astrocytes or cerebellar neurons (J. Drejer, A. Schousboe, unpublished) although the activity is the same in the three cell types (Table 1).

CONCLUDING REMARKS

From the present review, it can be concluded that the observed metabolic fluxes leading towards and away from glutamate in astrocytes and in neurons generally are considerably lower than the activities of the enzymes involved. This can be expected since the enzymatic activities often are studied under optimum conditions and since regulatory mechanisms may be operating in the living cells. However, the AOAA resistant flux from glutamate to α-keto-glutarate in astrocytes may reach values exceeding 50% of the GLDH activity. At the same time, the AOAA sensitive part of this flux is negligible, suggesting that a trans-amination of glutamate does not proceed very actively in spite of the high GOT activity, possibly reflecting a limited availability of oxaloacetate (Yu et al., 1982). The fluxes should also be compared to uptake and release rates, and from Fig. 4 in Schousboe et al. (this volume), it can be concluded that the metabolic fluxes are reason-able when compared to transport rates.

The data also indicate an apparent metabolic compart-mentation in both astrocytes and neurons. This compart-mentation does not resemble classical metabolic compart-mentation in brain, as indicated by specific activity ratios of greater than 1 between products and precursors, but it is characterized by an inaccessibility of part of the pools. In no case was this inaccessibility exceedingly pronounced, indicating that the quantitative errors which may be induced in the calculation of flux rates, remain relatively minor. It appeared that glutamine formation may occur mainly from an endogenously labeled glutamate pool whereas CO_2 formation, which is very pronounced in astrocytes but not in neurons (see also Yu, Hertz, this volume), may especially occur from an exogenously labeled pool. This finding is not in support of the concept (Quastel, 1978) that glutamate accumulated into astrocytes after neuronal release should be quantitatively converted to glutamine and returned to the neurons as such. It does, however, suggest that the release of glutamate from neurons may lead to an enhanced oxidative metabolism in astrocytes and thus gear astrocytic energy metabolism towards the needs evoked by neuronal function, e.g., an active uptake of potassium ions into astrocytes (Walz, Hertz, 1983).

The less than quantitative conversion of glutamate to glutamine in astrocytes and of glutamine to glutamate and GABA in neurons, combined with the fact that there seems to be no net transfer of glutamate or glutamine from other organs to the brain (Lund, 1971; Abdul-Ghani et al., 1978), create the need for a net synthesis of TCA cycle constituents within the brain. Although the neurons are the cells which suffer the immediate loss of glutamate (and GABA), convincing evidence has been obtained that formation of oxaloacetate by aid of PC occurs in astrocytes. The activity of this enzyme is high enough that it may lead to a replenishment of at least part of the neuronal deficit in TCA cycle constituents, provided one or more of these constituents are transferred from astrocytes to neurons. The astrocytic localization of this enzyme seems remarkable since it might provide the possibility for an astrocytic control over the supply of precursors for amino acid transmitter synthesis in neurons. Thus, on one hand, neurons may partly regulate astrocytic metabolism by alterations in the supply of glutamate (see above) and on the other hand, the astrocytes might control the formation of this glutamate. Such a close metabolic interaction between two autonomous cell types might be of fundamental importance for integration of brain function and metabolism.

ACKNOWLEDGEMENTS

The authors' work has been supported by grants from the Canadian Medical Research Council (to L.H.), the NOVO Foundation (to A.S.) and the Saskatchewan Health Research Board (to A.C.H.Y.)

REFERENCES

Abdul-Ghani A-S, Marton M, Dobkin J (1978). Studies on the transport of glutamine in vivo between the brain and blood in the resting state and during afferent electrical stimulation. J Neurochem 31: 541.
Bardakdjian J, Tardy M, Pimoule C, Gonnard P (1979). GABA metabolism in cultured glial cells. Neurochem Res 4: 517.

Benjamin AM (1982). Ammonia. In Lajtha A (ed): "Handbook of Neurochemistry", Vol 1, New York: Plenum Press, p 117.

Berl S, Takagaki G, Clarke DD, Waelsch H (1962). Metabolic compartments in vivo. Ammonia and glutamic acid metabolism in brain and liver. J Biol Chem 237: 2562.

Chapman AG, Meldrum BS, Siesjö BK (1977). Cerebral metabolic changes during prolonged epileptic seizures in rats. J Neurochem 28: 1025.

Cooper AJL, McDonald JM, Belbard AS, Gledhill RF, Duffy TE (1979). The metabolic fate of ^{13}N-labelled ammonia in rat brain. J Biol Chem 254: 4982.

Hallermayer K, Harmening C, Hamprecht B (1981). Cellular localization and regulation of glutamine synthetase in primary cultures of brain cells from new born mice. J Neurochem 37: 43.

Hansson E, Sellström A (1983). MAO, COMT and GABA-T activities in primary astroglial cultures. J Neurochem 40: 220.

Hauser K, Bernasconi R (1980). Rat cortical neurons in dissociated cell culture: changes in GABA and guanyl cyclase activity during development. In Giacobini E, Vernadakis A, Shahar A (eds): "Tissue Culture in Neurobiology", New York: Raven Press, p 205.

Hertz L (1979). Functional interactions between neurons and astrocytes I. Turnover and metabolism of putative amino acid transmitters. Prog Neurobiol 13: 277.

Hertz L, Bock E, Schousboe A (1978). GFA content, glutamate uptake and activity of glutamate metabolizing enzymes in differentiating mouse astrocytes in primary cultures. Dev Neurosci 1: 226.

Juurlink BHJ, Schousboe A, Jørgensen OS, Hertz L (1981). Induction by hydrocortisone of glutamine synthetase in mouse primary astrocyte cultures. J Neurochem 36: 136.

Keech DB, Utter MF (1963). Pyruvate carboxylase. II. Properties. J Biol Chem 238: 2609.

Krespan B, Berl S, Nicklas WJ (1982). Alteration in neuronal-glial metabolism of glutamate by the neurotoxin, kainic acid. J Neurochem 38: 509.

Kvamme E, Svenneby G, Hertz L, Schousboe A (1982). Properties of phosphate activated glutaminase in astrocytes cultured from mouse brain. Neurochem Res 7: 761.

Larsson OM, Hertz L, Schousboe A (1983). Developmental profiles of glutamate and GABA metabolizing enzymes in cultured glutamatergic and GABAergic neurons. J Neurochem 41: S85D.

Lund P (1971). Control of glutamine synthesis in rat liver. Biochem. J. 124: 653.

McGeer EG, McGeer PL (1979). Localization of glutaminase in the rat neostriatum. J Neurochem 32: 1071.

Morjaria B, Voaden MJ (1979). The formation of glutamate, aspartate and GABA in the rat retina: glucose and glutamine as precursors. J Neurochem 33: 541.

Moscona AA, Mayerson P, Linser P, Moscona M (1980). Induction of glutamine synthetase in the neural retina of the chick embryo: localization of the enzyme in Muller fibers and effects of BrdU and cell separation. In Giacobini E, Vernadakis A, Shahar A (eds): "Tissue Culture in Neurobiology", New York: Raven Press, p 111.

Patel AJ, Hunt A, Gordon RD, Balazs R (1982). The activities in different neural cell types of certain enzymes associated with the metabolic compartmentation glutamate. Develop Brain Res 4: 3.

Quastel JH (1978). Cerebral glutamate-glutamine interrelations in vivo and in vitro. In Schoffeniels E, Franck G, Hertz L, Tower DB (eds), "Dynamic Properties of Glia Cells, Oxford: Pergamon Press, p 153.

Reubi JC, Van den Berg C, Cuenod M (1978). Glutamine as precursor for the GABA and glutamate transmitter pools. Neurosci Lett 10: 171.

Roth-Schechter BF, Laluet M, Tholey G, Mandel P (1977). The effect of pentobarbital on the carbohydrate metabolism of glial cells in culture. Biochem Pharmac 26: 1307.

Schousboe A, Drejer J, Hertz L, Svenneby G, Roberg B, Kvamme E (1983). Comparison of ornithine aminotransferase and glutaminase activities in cultured astrocytes and glutamatergic and GABAergic neurons. J Neurochem 41: S86A.

Schousboe A, Hertz L (1983). Regulation of glutamatergic and GABAergic neuronal activity by astroglial cells. In Osborne NN (ed), Dale's Principle and Communication between Neurons", Oxford: Pergamon Press, p 113.

Schousboe A, Hertz L, Svenneby G (1977a). Uptake and metabolism of GABA in astrocytes cultured from dissociated mouse brain hemispheres. Neurochem Res 2: 217.

Schousboe A, Hertz L, Svenneby G, Kvamme E (1979). Phosphate activated glutaminase activity and glutamine uptake in primary cultures of astrocytes. J Neurochem 32: 943.

Schousboe A, Svenneby G, Hertz L (1977b). Uptake and metabolism of glutamate in astrocytes cultured from dissociated mouse brain hemispheres. J Neurochem 29: 999.

Sellinger OZ, Verster F de B (1962). Glutamine synthetase of rat cerebral cortex. Intracellular distribution and structural latency. J Biol Chem. 237: 2836.

Shank RP, Campbell GL, Freyteg SO, Utter MF (1981). Evidence that carboxylase is an astrocyte specific enzyme in CNS tissues. Abst Soc Neurosci 7: 936.

Snodgrass SR, White WF, Biales B, Dichter MA (1980). Biochemical correlates of GABA function in rat cortical
neurons in culture. Brain Res 190: 123.

Tardy M, Fages C, Rolland B, Bardakjian J, Gonnard P (1981).
Effect of prostaglandins and dibutyryl cyclic AMP on
the morphology of cells in primary astroglial cultures
and on metabolic enzymes of GABA and glutamate metabolism. Experientia 37: 19.

Walz W, Hertz L (1983). Functional interactions between
neurons and astrocytes II. Potassium homeostasis at the
cellular level. Progr. Neurobiol. (in press).

Williamson DH, Lund P, Krebs HA (1967). The redox state of
free nicotinamide-adenine dinucleotide in the cytoplasm
and mitochondria of rat liver. Biochem J 103: 514.

Wilson SH, Schrier BK, Farber JL, Thompson EJ, Rosenberg
RN, Blume AJ, Nirenberg MW (1972). Markers for gene ex-
pression in cultured cells from the nervous system.
J Biol Chem 247: 3159.

Yoneda Y, Roberts E (1981). Synaptosomal biosynthesis of
GABA from ornithine and its feedback inhibition by GABA.
In Okada Y, Roberts E (eds), "Problems in GABA Research
from Brain to Bacteria", Amsterdam: Excerpta Medica, p 55.

Yu ACH, Schousboe A, Hertz L (1982). Metabolic fate of
[14]C-labeled glutamate in astrocytes in primary cultures.
J Neurochem 39: 954.

Yu ACH, Drejer J, Hertz L, Schousboe A (1983a). Pyruvate
carboxylase activity in primary cultures of astrocytes
and neurons. J Neurochem (in press).

Yu, ACH, Fisher TE, Hertz E, Tildon T, Schousboe A, Hertz L
(1984). Metabolic fate of [14C]-glutamine in mouse cerebral neurons in primary cultures. Brain Res., submitted.

Yu ACH, Hertz E, Hertz L (1983b). Alterations in uptake
and release rates for GABA, glutamate and glutamine
during biochemical maturation of highly purified cultures
of cerebral cortical neurons, a GABAergic preparation.
J Neurochem, submitted.

Yu ACH, Schousboe A, Hertz L (1983c). Influence of pathological concentrations of ammonia on metabolic fate of
[14]C-labeled glutamate in astrocytes in primary cultures.
J Neurochem, submitted.

Glutamine, Glutamate, and GABA
in the Central Nervous System, pages 343–354
© **1983 Alan R. Liss, Inc., 150 Fifth Avenue, New York, NY 10011**

UPTAKE OF GLUTAMATE AND GABA IN SYNAPTOSOMAL AND ENRICHED
CELL POPULATIONS OF CEREBELLUM

Graham LeM. Campbell and Richard P. Shank*

Department of Neurology, the Graduate Hospital
Philadelphia, PA 19104 *Current Address:
Department of Biological Research, McNeil
Pharmaceutical, Spring House Lane, PA 19477

Glutamate and GABA are two extensively studied amino
acid neurotransmitters (Curtis, Johnston 1974; Krnjevic
1974; Davidson 1976; Shank, Campbell 1983a). Little is
known about the regulation of their uptake, the metabolic
origin of their respective neurotransmitter pools, and the
role of individual cell types in this regulation. It is
difficult to design experiments to answer such questions in
structurally intact tissue. This paper describes one
approach for fractionating tissue into cellular and subcellular components representative of individual cell types.
This approach provides an opportunity to compare the uptake
and metabolism of glutamate and GABA in these cellular and
subcellular compartments of the cerebellum.

The cerebellum is an ideal system for these studies.
Glutamate and GABA are predominant neurotransmitters. The
granule cells (glutamatergic) comprise 70-75% of the total
cell population, whereas the remaining neuronal cell types
Purkinje, Golgi II, stellate and basket cells (~5%) are
inhibitory neurons (GABAergic). Synaptogenesis occurs postnatally beginning around day 10. The tissue is readily
dissociated into single viable cells up to day 14. In the
mouse there are mutants in which there are genetic defects
for neuronal development. Studies have also been performed
in which selective loss of one cell type, the granule cell,
is mediated (Young et al. 1974; McBride et al. 1976).

In this study, we present information primarily focused
on the initial uptake conditions of glutamate and GABA.
Comparisons between cell types, and between cell bodies and

"synaptosomes" are presented. The significance of these results emphasizing cell function in the regulation of amino acid neurotransmitter pools is discussed.

MATERIALS AND METHODS

Preparation and Isolation of Cerebellar Material Enriched in Cell Bodies and Nerve Terminals

Cerebella are removed from 1CR mice (P8-P14) and dispersed as described in Campbell et al. (1977). The resultant suspension of cell bodies and subcellular material is layered onto a preformed 40% Percoll (Pharmacia, Upsala) gradient. Centrifugation at 4,300 g for 15 minutes resulted in two bands of material. The materials in these bands are pelleted by centrifugation at 800 g after dilution with Hank's B.S.S. containing 0.0025% DNAse. The materials from the upper and lower bands are then layered onto 20% and 60% preformed Percoll gradients respectively, and centrifuged as before. Five regional bands are obtained in the two gradients; three in the 20% gradient and two in the 60% gradient. Each band of material is removed, diluted with Hank's B.S.S. and centrifuged to pellet the material. This material is resuspended in incubation medium and maintained at 4°C prior to experimental use.

Percoll continuous gradients are preformed after dilution 9:1 Percoll: 10x Hank's B.S.S. (Gibco #318 4180), dilution with 1x Hank's B.S.S. obtains 20%, 40% and 60% solutions. Gradient formation occurs by centrifugation for 30 minutes at 27,000 g using a fixed angle rotor.

Determination of Initial Rate of Uptake

In general, these experiments are performed using a 50 μl sample containing 5-30 μg protein to which is added 150 μl of incubation medium containing 0.02 to 0.05 μCi of a ^{14}C-labelled compound or 0.1 to 0.2 μCi of a ^{3}H-labelled compound. The incubation period in these experiments was 4, 6 or 10 minutes (uptake of GABA or glutamate is linear for up to 20 minutes). The incubation medium comprises 120 mM NaCl, 3 mM KH_2PO_4, 2 mM $MgCl_2$, 2 mM $CaCl_2$, 5 mM glucose buffered with 24 mM $NaHCO_3$ to pH 7.4. Prior to incubation, the medium is aerated with O_2:CO_2 (95:5). Samples are incubated in polyethylene microfuge tubes (400 μl) at 35°C.

Blank samples are incubated at 4°C. Incubation is terminated by transferring samples to an ice bath. Material is pelleted by centrifugation, the supernatant removed and the pellet is washed 2x with cold incubation medium. The bottom of the microfuge tube containing the pellet is cut off, excess liquid is removed by blotting and the pellet is placed in a scintillation vial for determination of radioactivity.

Protein determinations are made using the Bio-Rad procedure (Technical Bulletin 1051). Bovine serum albumin was used as a standard.

Calculation of Transport Kinetic Constants

The K_m and V_{max} values were calculated using a weighted non-linear regression analysis. This analysis was done by use of the Pennzyme computer program (Kohn et al. 1979). Eadie-Hofstee plots of the data indicated that, in several instances, uptake could have been mediated by two transport systems. In these instances, a regression analysis was performed using rate law equations appropriate for uptake mediated by a single system, and by two carrier systems functioning independently. Uptake was judged to be mediated by one carrier or two carriers based on the criteria specified by Kohn et al. (1979).

RESULTS AND DISCUSSION

Table 1 describes the morphological characteristics of the Percoll gradient fractions obtained from cell suspensions of cerebella from 8 to 14 day old mice. There are five fractions, three from the 20% gradient and two from the 60% gradient. The fraction in which the greatest change is seen in this developmental time period is fraction 2, found in the mid region of the 20% gradient. This fraction contains the subcellular components of the original cell suspension. It increases from a 10% contribution, as measured in mg protein on day 8, to a 50% contribution by day 14. The other four fractions all contain cell bodies predominantly; fraction 1 does contain membraneous and subcellular material. Fraction 5 comprises approximately 70% of the total cellular population and, on the basis of a variety of criteria, is considered to contain 95% granule cells (this fraction compares with the granule enriched population described by Campbell et al. (1977) and by Campbell and Shank (1978)). Fractions 3 and 4

Table 1: Summary of cellular and subcellular content of
Percoll gradient fractions.

Fraction #	No. Cells[a]	Protein[b]	Morphology[c]
1 - 20% Top	0.2	5%	Large cells (neuronal) and membranes
2 - 20% Mid	1.0	50%	Subcellular material (synaptosomes,cytosomes) and cell bodies
3 - 20% Btm	1.0	5%	Cell bodies (glial and other cell types)
4 - 60% Top	2.0	10%	Cell bodies (glial and other cell types)
5 - 60% Btm	8.0	30%	Cell bodies (granule cells)

Taken from Shank, Campbell (1983b).
a) The number of nucleated cell bodies (in millions) is
reported as the approximate number present in each
fraction per cerebellum.
b) Protein values represent the approximate percentage of
the amount accounted for in all five fractions. In mice
less than 10 days old, the percent in fraction 2 was
less than 50%, whereas in mice more than 12 days old,
the percentage was higher than 50%.
c) The term "cytosome" refers collectively to membrane
bounded entities containing identifiable subcellular
organelles such as mitochondria and vesicles. These
entities are presumably derived from dendrites, axons
and glial processes in addition to nerve terminals.

are enriched in glial cell types, i.e. astrocytes (30-40%)
and oligodendrocytes (10%) (Campbell, Shank, unpublished
observations). In some experiments these fractions are
treated separately and in others they are combined,
particularly for the initial uptake studies.

Comparison of uptake for amino acids thought to be neuroactive reveals a wide range of uptake velocities and differential uptake in the five fractions (Fig. 1). Glutamate and

GABA are accumulated most rapidly, while taurine and proline accumulation is much slower. The higher uptake for each amino acid in the synaptosomal fractions (fraction 2) reflects, in part, the increased surface area to volume ratio, and hence an increased density of transport carriers. Comparisons among the cell body fractions indicate similar patterns with some notable exceptions. GABA is taken up fastest by fraction 1, in which large, presumptive neuronal cell bodies are seen, but the uptake by the granule cell fraction is negligible. Proline and taurine are taken up equally well by all cell body fractions.

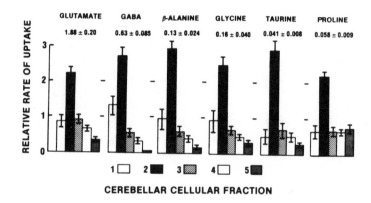

Figure 1: Uptake of six amino acids by the five fractions. The number listed under the name of each compound represents the average uptake values (nmol/min-mg protein). The relative uptake is the ratio between each fraction and the average value (N=6-10 determinations). Each experiment was performed in triplicate. Initial concentration for each compound was 8 µM. Incubation period 4, 6 or 10 minutes.

Figures 2, 3 and Table 2 show the results obtained in experiments designed to measure the K_m and V_{max} for glutamate and GABA in fractions of cerebellar suspensions. In these experiments, fractions 3 and 4 were combined and fraction 1 was not used because of the relatively small amounts of material. These results are based on three fractions: synaptosomal (fraction 2), astrocyte enriched (fraction 3 & 4) and granule (fraction 5). The results in Figures 2 and 3

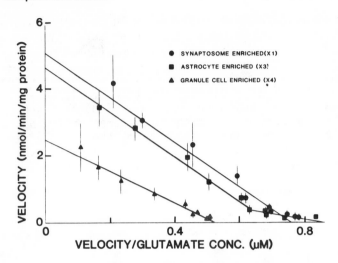

Figure 2: Glutamate uptake by selected fractions of cerebellar material as a function of exogenous glutamate concentration. The uptake velocities for astrocyte enriched
and granule cell fractions have been multiplied by 3 and 4
respectively to facilitate comparison of the data. Each
data point is the mean ± S.E.M. of 3 to 5 experiments.
Lines were drawn based on visual inspection of the data.

are the Eadie-Hofstee plots which, in some cases, are non-
linear; Table 2 summarizes the K_m and V_{max} values calculated using the Pennzyme computer program.

The kinetic constants for glutamate yield several interesting observations. The differences observed in the uptake
capacity of the various fractions seen in Figure 1 are in
large part due to differences in V_{max} values. Specifically,
the uptake by granule cell bodies is around 8x slower than
that by the synaptosomal fraction and 3x slower than that by
the astrocyte enriched fractions. However, the astrocyte
enriched fraction is characterized by two transport affinity
systems; the higher affinity of the two is not seen in the
synaptosomal fraction or in the granule cell body fraction.
Similarly, the GABA uptake system shows marked differences
in the uptake velocities. In this instance, the granule cell
body fraction has a V_{max} 120x slower than the synaptosomal
fraction and 17x slower than the astrocyte enriched fraction.
However, both the astrocyte enriched and granule cell body
fractions contain two high affinity transport systems. We

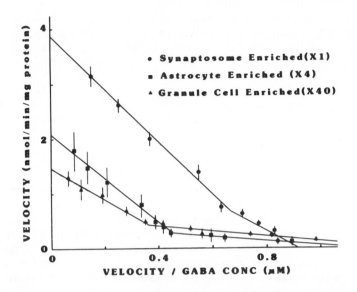

Figure 3: GABA uptake by selected fractions of cerebellar material as a function of exogenous GABA concentration. The uptake velocities for astrocyte enriched and granule cell fractions have been multiplied by 4 and 40 respectively to facilitate comparison of the data. Each data point is the mean ± S.E.M. of 3 to 5 experiments. Lines were drawn based on visual inspection of the data.

Table 2: Kinetic constants for glutamate and GABA uptake

Fraction	Glutamate		GABA	
	K_m	V_{max}	K_m	V_{max}
Astrocyte enriched	0.14±0.04	0.20±0.06	0.21±0.06	0.06 ±0.01
	7.2 ±1.3	1.60±0.1	8.6 ±0.8	0.52 ±0.04
Granule cell	4.7 ±0.3	0.63±0.04	0.30±0.05	0.008±0.001
			8.4 ±2.0	0.03 ±0.01
Synapto-somes	6.7 ±0.3	5.10±0.2	4.3 ±0.2	3.70 ±0.1

K_m is µM; V_{max} is in nmol/min-mg protein. Values were derived using the Pennzyme computer program (Kohn et al. 1979). Essentially from Shank and Campbell (this volume).

know, from previous studies, that the granule cell fraction contains 10-20x fewer astrocytes than the astrocyte fraction. We therefore deduce that the minimal uptake by the granule cell bodies reflect a small contamination by astrocyte cells. Bearing this comparison in mind, we also conclude that, although the granule cell fraction transports glutamate 3x slower than the astrocyte enriched fraction, this difference cannot be accounted for solely on the basis of astrocyte contamination.

The kinetic constants for the uptake of glutamate and GABA have been determined in a variety of preparations of brain tissue (for review see Hertz 1979). These determinations have been made on synaptosomal fractions and cells grown in vitro, normal and tumor cell lines and bulk preparations of enriched cell types. For glutamate, affinity constants range from 2 μM to 50 μM with velocity uptakes in the range 0.02 to 6.0 nmoles/min-mg protein. For GABA, affinity constants range from 0.2 μM to 50 μM with velocity constants 2×10^{-4} to 2.2×10^{-1} nmoles/min-mg protein. These wide ranges reflect differences in cell type and methodologies for measuring these constants. However, in all cases, these measurements relate to a single transport system. In an earlier study using a discontinuous density gradient procedure (Campbell, Shank 1977), we found evidence for two high affinity systems for glutamate in preparations of enriched cerebellar cells, but not in synaptosomes. The results shown here extend those analyses to both glutamate and GABA transport systems. We have used a modified gradient procedure to permit analyses of cellular and synaptosomal fractions from the same preparation.

Current evidence indicates that amino acid transmitters are removed from the interstitial fluid either by uptake into nerve terminals or into astrocytic elements. The basic question is how to account for these differential transport systems, particularly in astrocytes. Data reported by Young et al. (1974) suggest that glutamate is transported by carriers located in granule cell nerve terminals, whereas data reported by East et al. (1980), Gordon et al. (1981) and Wilkin et al. (1982) indicate that uptake is mediated primarily by carriers in astrocyte membranes. These latter data are based on both transport studies and electron microscopic localization. Exogenous GABA is taken up actively in astrocyte enriched populations (Henn, Hamberger 1971; Burry, Lasher 1975; Lasher 1975). Autoradiographic studies indicate that

GABA is accumulated predominantly into GABAergic terminals in most CNS regions (Iversen 1972; Kelly, Dick 1975; Sterling, David 1979). The content of GABA in astrocytes is low, but the activity of GABA transaminase is high (Roberts 1975). Hence, turnover of GABA may be quite high in astrocytes. In studies using ^{3}H-GABA, the tritium label will be rapidly lost and converted to water. Short term in vivo and in vitro studies using the retina (Voaden, this volume; Redburn, this volume) and cerebellar populations (Levi, this volume) clearly show a preferred uptake by astrocytes at concentrations of 1 µM or less. These results are consistent with ours.

Our results provide some additional insight into the metabolic origin of these neurotransmitter pools, based on the concentrations of GABA and glutamate in the extracellular space. The markedly greater sensitivities of the highest affinity astrocyte systems for both GABA and glutamate, some twenty- or forty- fold over the synaptosomal carrier affinity systems, indicate that, at levels below one µM, the majority of the extracellular amino acid will be taken up by astrocytes and subsequently metabolized to potential precursor molecules for reutilization by the nerve terminal carriers. However, at concentrations above 1 µM, the markedly higher velocity constants of the synaptosomal carriers (three-fold for glutamate and seven-fold for GABA) indicate that a corresponding enhancement of uptake into the synaptosomes occurs rather than into astrocytes. It is reasonable to assume, on the basis of a variety of data and their interpretation, that both GABA and glutamate may be at a concentration of around 1 µM or less in the resting state under normal physiological conditions. Increases in these concentrations occur as a result of synaptic activation, in which case the concentration in the synaptic cleft may be as high as 0.1-1.0 mM. In the immediate surrounding area there would be a resultant gradient of concentration. Ideally, therefore, one might expect the greatest uptake to occur in the synaptic terminals to maximize replenishment of the neurotransmitter pool. Obviously, not all the neurotransmitter released can be reutilized and, under these conditions, astrocytic uptake of amino acids is critical, not only to decrease the extracellular concentration, but also to provide the precursors essential for replenishing the depleted transmitter pool. The mechanisms and relative contribution of these precursors in such an anaplerotic process is discussed in detail in the accompanying paper (Shank, Campbell, this volume).

Based on information derived from metabolic studies of glutamate, α-ketoglutarate and glutamine, there are two points worthy of note (Shank, Campbell 1982). Although glutamate is the immediate precursor of GABA, exogenous glutamate is a poor substrate for GABA synthesis. Comparison of GABA:glutamate ratios demonstrate, as shown in Table 3, that glutamine is the preferred precursor source for synthesis of GABA, whereas the conversion of each substrate to aspartate

Table 3. Relative formation of GABA and aspartate in cerebellar synaptosomes

Precursor	RSA x 100	
	(GABA:GLU)	(ASP:GLU)
L-Glutamine	8.9 ± 1.3	18.9 ± 1.1
L-Glutamate	1.2 ± 0.2	9.7 ± 1.5
α-Ketoglutarate	1.4 ± 0.5	16.9 ± 2.7

RSA = Relative Specific Activity of GABA and aspartate in material expressed as a ratio of glutamate formed. Synaptosomes were incubated for four minutes in the presence of the ($U-^{14}C$) labelled precursors. Methodology for labelling and separation on thin layer chromatography as described in Shank, Campbell (1983b)(N=4 experiments).

as mediated through the TCA cycle does not reflect such differences. One possible explanation for this result is that high affinity uptake of glutamate by carriers in the GABAergic membranes is either non-existent or at an extremely low velocity constant. Such an explanation is a striking parallel to the results presented here indicating that GABA is essentially not taken up by carriers in the granule cell membrane. Such selective uptake by individual cell types, coupled with the concentration dependent selective uptake, is consistent with the hypothesis that transport systems in part regulate the metabolic origin of neurotransmitter pools. Such a hypothesis, in conjunction with constraints determined by other regulatory processes known to be cell-specific, such as metabolic compartmentalization (Berl, Clarke 1969; Shank, Campbell 1983a), are key components in the determination of the biochemical processes regulating amino acid neurotransmitter pools.

REFERENCES

Berl S, Clarke DD (1969). Metabolic compartmentation of glutamate in the CNS. In Lajtha A (ed): "Handbook of Neurochemistry," New York: Plenum Press, Vol 1, p 168.

Burry RW, Lasher RS (1975). Uptake of GABA in dispersed cell cultures of postnatal rat cerebellum: an electron microscope autoradiograpic study. Brain Res 88:502.

Campbell GLeM, Schachner M, Sharrow SO (1977). Isolation of glial cell enriched and depleted populations from mouse cerebellum by density gradient centrifugation and electronic cell sorting. Brain Res 127:69.

Campbell GLeM, Shank RP (1978). Glutamate and GABA uptake by granule and glial cell enriched populations. Brain Res 153:618.

Curtis DR, Johnston GAR (1974). Amino acid transmitters in the mammalian central nervous system. Ergebn Physiol 69:97.

Davidson N (1976). "Neurotransmitter Amino Acids." London: Academic Press.

East JM, Dutton GR, Currie DN (1980). Transport of GABA, β-alanine and glutamate into perikarya of postnatal rat cerebellum. J Neurochem 34:523.

Gordon RD, Wilkin GP, Hunt A, Patel AJ, Balazs R (1981). Glutamate high affinity uptake and metabolism in cerebellar cells. Trans Am Soc Neurochem 12:377.

Henn FA, Hamberger A (1971). Glial cell function: Uptake of transmitter substances. Proc Natl Acad Sci (USA) 68:2686.

Hertz L (1979). Functional interactions between neurons and astrocytes. I. Turnover and metabolism of putative amino acid transmitters. Prog Neurobiology 13:277.

Iversen LL (1972). The uptake, storage, release and metabolism of GABA in inhibitory nerves. In Snyder SH (ed): "Perspectives in Neuropharmacology", London: Oxford University Press, p 75.

Kelly JS, Dick F (1975). Differential labeling of glial cells and GABA-inhibitory interneurons and nerve terminals following microinjection of ^{3}H-β-alanine, ^{3}H-DABA and ^{3}H-GABA into single folia of the cerebellum. Cold Spring Harbor Symposium on Quantitative Biology, The Synapse 40:93.

Kohn MC, Menten LE, Garfinkel D (1979). A convenient computer program for fitting enzymatic rate laws to steady data. Computers and Biomed Res 12:461.

Krnjevic K (1974). Chemical nature of synaptic transmission in vertebrates. Physiol Rev 54:418.

Lasher RS (1975). Uptake of GABA by neuronal and nonneuronal cells in dispersed cell cultures of postnatal rat cerebellum. J Neurobiol 6:597.

McBride WJ, Nadi NS, Altman J, Aprison MH (1976). Effects of
selective doses of x-irradiation on the levels of several
amino acids in the cerebellum of the rat. Neurochem Res
1:141.

Roberts E (1975). GABA in nervous system - an overview. In
Tower DB, Brady RO (eds): "The Nervous System: Vol 1 The
Basic Neurosciences," New York: Raven Press p 541.

Shank RP, Campbell GLeM (1982). Glutamine and alpha-ketoglutarate uptake and metabolism by nerve terminal enriched
material from mouse cerebellum. Neurochem Res 7:601.

Shank RP, Campbell GLeM (1983a). Glutamate. In: Lajtha A
(ed) "Handbook of Neurochemistry, 2nd ed, Vol 3, New
York, Plenum Press, p 381.

Shank RP, Campbell GLeM (1983b). Amino acid uptake, content-
and metabolism by neuronal and glial enriched cellular com
ponents from mouse cerebellum. J Neurosci (in press).

Sterling P, David TL (1980). Neurons in cat lateral
geniculate nucleus that concentrate exogenous (^{3}H)amino-
butyric acid (GABA). J Comp Neurol 192:692.

Wilkin GP, Garthwaite J, Balazs R (1982). Putative amino
acid transmitters in the cerebellum. II. Electron microscopic localization of transport sites. Brain Res 244:69.

Young AB, Oster-Granite ML, Herndon RM, Snyder SH (1974).
Glutamic acid: Selective depletion by viral induced
granule cell loss in hamster cerebellum. Brain Res 73:1.

Glutamine, Glutamate, and GABA
in the Central Nervous System, pages 355–369
© 1983 Alan R. Liss, Inc., 150 Fifth Avenue, New York, NY 10011

METABOLIC PRECURSORS OF GLUTAMATE AND GABA

Richard P. Shank* and Graham LeM. Campbell[+]

*Department of Biological Research, McNeil Pharmaceutical, Spring House, PA 19477, and Department of Physiology, Temple University, School of Medicine, Philadelphia, PA 19140. [+]Department of Neurology, The Graduate Hospital, Philadelphia, PA 19104.

For several reasons the identification of the metabolic substrates that are utilized to replenish the neurotransmitter pools of glutamate and GABA is a formidable research problem. These reasons include: (1) the large number of metabolites that are possible precursors, (2) the involvement of glutamate in a variety of biochemical processes, particularly energy metabolism, (3) the dynamic nature of glutamate metabolism, and (4) technical difficulties in separating the neurotransmitter pools of glutamate and GABA from other pools.

COMPOUNDS THAT THEORETICALLY CAN FUNCTION AS METABOLIC PRECURSORS OF THE TRANSMITTER POOLS OF GLUTAMATE AND GABA

A compound may be regarded as a possible metabolic precursor of the transmitter pool of glutamate if it is known to be present in neural tissues, and has the metabolic potential for being utilized as a net source of either the dicarboxylate or amino moieties of glutamate. Assuming that glutamate synthesized within the terminals of GABAergic neurons serves as the immediate precursor of the transmitter pool of GABA, then the list of possible metabolic precursors of the transmitter pool of GABA is the same as that for the transmitter pool of glutamate.

The list of possible precursors can be separated into three groups: (1) those that can supply both the dicarboxylate and amino moieties, (2) those that can supply only the dicarboxylate moiety, and (3) those that can supply only the amino moiety. We have identified six compounds, five amino acids and glutathione as potential sources of both moieties (Table 1). Compounds that can serve as a source of only the dicarboxylate moiety include glucose, glycerol, pyruvate, and the citrate cycle intermediate α-ketoglutarate. Compounds that can supply only the amino moiety include aspartate, alanine and other amino acids that serve as substrates for aminotransferase enzymes that generate glutamate from α-ketoglutarate.

TABLE 1

POTENTIAL METABOLIC PRECURSORS OF THE
NEUROTRANSMITTER POOLS OF GLUTAMATE AND GABA

A. Compounds that can supply the dicarboxylate and
amino moieties

Glutamine*   Proline
Ornithine*   Histidine
Arginine*   Glutathione
Citrulline*

B. Compounds that can supply only the dicarboxylate
moiety

Glucose (glycerol, pyruvate)
Alpha-Ketoglutarate

C. Compounds that can supply only the amino moiety

Aspartate   Ammonia
Alanine
Leucine (and most other α-amino acids)

*These compounds can supply two amino moieties per molecule.

Some compounds not listed in Table 1 that can serve to replenish the neurotransmitter pools of glutamate and GABA indirectly include citrate cycle intermediates and amino acids that can serve an anaplerotic role for the citrate cycle. These compounds can serve to replenish

α-ketoglutarate, and thereby serve as a net source of the dicarboxylate moiety of glutamate. Protein is another possible source of glutamate. Assuming that some of the protein synthesized in the cell soma and transported to the synaptic terminal is hydrolyzed back into the amino acid constituents within the terminal this metabolic turnover of protein could serve as a net source of glutamate for replenishing the transmitter pools of glutamate and GABA.

CRITERIA FOR EVALUATING COMPOUNDS AS PRECURSORS OF THE NEUROTRANSMITTER POOLS OF GLUTAMATE AND GABA

We have formulated a list of five criteria that can be used to establish the identity of compounds that serve as metabolic precursors of the neurotransmitter pools of glutamate and GABA. These criteria include: (1) the availability of the compound to synaptic terminals, (2) the capacity of glutamatergic and GABAergic synaptic terminals to accumulate the compound by a saturable membrane transport process, (3) the ability of synaptic terminals to metabolize the compound to glutamate, and to GABA in GABAergic terminals, (4) the effect that limiting the availability of the compound, or blocking its metabolic conversion, has on the content of glutamate and GABA, and the amount released from synaptic terminals by membrane depolarization, and lastly (5) the degree to which the uptake and metabolism of the compound is subject to biochemical regulation.

The criterion of availability must take into account the permeability of the potential precursor across the blood-brain barrier, and the possibility that astrocytes serve as a source of the precursor, or that the precursor is transported from the cell soma to the synaptic terminal by axoplasmic flow. The capacity of synaptic terminals to take up or accumulate the potential precursor would not be an applicable criterion for compounds likely to be derived from the cell soma via axoplasmic transport. Experimentally this criterion would be applied to a specific compound by determining the kinetic parameters of carrier mediated transport across the cell membrane (uptake of the radiolabelled compound into synaptosomes). Obviously, the enzyme(s) required to convert the potential precursor to glutamate must be present within both glutamatergic and GABAergic terminals; however, the quantitative activity of the enzyme(s) may not serve as a useful index for the relative contribution of the precursor toward replenishing the neurotransmitter pool. The criterion that experimentally induced alterations in the availability and metabolism of the potential precursor should significantly affect on the content of glutamate and GABA, and more importantly, the amount released by a physiological stimulus is probably the most valuable of all the criteria in that it should provide the most definitive information regarding the quantitative relationship between the metabolic precursor and the functional pool of the neurotransmitter.

The criterion stipulating that uptake and metabolic conversion of the precursor should be regulated is predicated on the concept that glutamate and GABA can function effectively as neurotransmitters only if their neurotransmitter pools are controlled within narrow limits. The sites responsible for regulating the neurotransmitter pools are likely to include some aspects of the synthetic process.

GLUTAMINE AS A METABOLIC PRECURSOR OF THE NEUROTRANSMITTER POOLS OF GLUTAMATE AND GABA

During the past ten years several groups of researchers have reported experimental observations relevant to the role of glutamine as a metabolic precursor of the transmitter pools of glutamate and GABA. When evaluated in terms of our five criteria, the data collectively provide compelling evidence that glutamine is a functional precursor of the transmitter pool of both neurotransmitters. However, it is not yet possible to draw a definitive conclusion regarding the quantitative contribution of glutamine to the transmitter pools of either glutamate or GABA.

Based on the knowledge that the concentration of glutamine in blood plasma and cerebrospinal fluid is comparatively high (~ 0.5 mM), and the evidence that glutamine is readily synthesized in, and released from, astrocytes (see Shank, Aprison 1981) it would appear that glutamine is available to synaptic terminals in abundance. Glutamine is rapidly taken up by synaptic terminals by carrier mediated membrane transport (Balcar, Johnston 1975; Baldessarini, Yorke 1974; Shank, Campbell 1982; Kvamme 1983). Current evidence indicates that glutamine is transported primarily by the alanine preferring amino acid carrier, but that the large neutral amino acid (LNAA) carrier, and to a lesser extent the basic amino acid carrier also contribute to the transport of glutamine across synaptic membranes (Shank, Campbell 1982). Kinetic analyses of uptake indicate that most of the glutamine transported under physiological conditions is mediated by one or more carriers possessing a low affinity for glutamine (K_m values between 0.2 and 0.5 mM). However, the results of some studies suggest that glutamine is also transported by a high-affinity, low capacity carrier (Balcar, Johnston 1975; Shank, Campbell 1982).

It is well established that glutamine can be metabolically converted to glutamate in synaptic terminals (Bradford et al. 1978). Current evidence indicates that two phosphate-activated glutaminase isozymes mediate this conversion process (Kvamme, Olsen 1981). Ward et al. (1982) have reported the activity of at least one of these enzymes is selectively decreased subsequent to lesioning of cortico-striatal neuronal fibers. This observation indicates that one or both of these enzymes is concentrated in neurons that project from the cerebral cortex to the striatum, which are thought to utilize glutamate as a neurotransmitter (McGeer et al. 1977).

Experiments conducted on a variety of preparations in vitro have revealed that the addition of glutamine to the incubation medium increases substantially the content of glutamate in CNS tissue slices and synaptosomal preparations, and the amount of glutamate released during membrane depolarization (Bradford et al. 1978; Shank, Aprison 1977; Hamberger et al. 1979). Therefore, at least in CNS preparations in vitro the content of glutamate and amount released correlates directly with the presence of glutamine in the medium. Similarly the amount of GABA released has been found to correlate with the presence of glutamine (Tapia, Gonzalez 1978; Reubi et al. 1978; Gauchy et al. 1979). The effect that a selective inhibition of glutaminase might have on the content of glutamate and the amount released has yet to be determined.

In the series of biochemical events that mediate the formation of glutamate from glutamine one likely site of regulation is the enzyme glutaminase. Glutamate, at physiologically relevant concentrations, inhibits glutaminase activity in CNS tissues (Weil-Malherbe 1950; Kvamme, Olsen 1981). This may function as a feedback inhibitory mechanism regulating the synthesis of glutamate. Other possible regulatory sites include the transport carriers in the synaptic cell membrane and mitochondrial membrane.

METABOLISM OF GLUCOSE AS RELATED TO REPLENISHMENT OF THE NEUROTRANSMITTER POOLS OF GLUTAMATE AND GABA

In the course of normal metabolic activity in CNS tissues, a large portion of the carbon moieties derived from glucose accumulates in glutamate and GABA prior to being oxidized to CO_2 (Berl, Clarke 1969; Van den Berg 1970). This is due in part to a rapid interconversion between α-ketoglutarate and glutamate. The metabolic significance of this metabolic interconversion can be attributed at least partially to the role of α-ketoglutarate and glutamate as intermediates in the malate-aspartate shuttle (Shank, Campbell 1983b). The rapid synthesis of glutamate from α-ketoglutarate is consistent with the possibility that glucose serves as a precursor (albeit metabolically remote) of the dicarboxylate moiety of glutamate molecules used to replenish the neurotransmitter pools of glutamate and GABA. However, the utilization of glucose as a net source of the dicarboxylate moiety requires the existence of an anaplerotic process which must stoichiometrically replenish the α-ketoglutarate (derived from glucose) molecules lost from the citrate cycle due to the net synthesis of glutamate. In CNS tissues nearly all anaplerotic activity can be attributed to pyruvate carboxylase (Patel 1974). Therefore, the net utilization of glucose as a precursor of the transmitter pools of glutamate and GABA at most cannot exceed the rate at which pyruvate is carboxylated to form oxaloacetate (Fig. 1).

The activity of pyruvate carboxylase in CNS tissues is high in comparison to most other non-gluconeogenic tissues (Utter, Scrutton 1970). However, a substantial amount of evidence indicates that this enzyme is selectively expressed in glial cells, particularly astrocytes, and may even be totally absent from neurons. This evidence includes (1) immunocytochemical localization of the enzyme to Bergman glia cells and other glial cells in the cerebellum of rats and mice (Shank et al. 1981 and

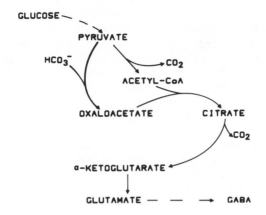

Fig. 1. The anaplerotic metabolic pathway in CNS tissues. Alpha-ketoglutarate generated via this pathway can be utilized as a net source of the dicarboxylate moiety of glutamate, and thereby serve a role in replenishing the neurotransmitter pools of glutamate and GABA. The key reaction in this pathway is the carboxylation of pyruvate, which is catalyzed by pyruvate carboxylase, an ATP dependent enzyme located in the matrix of mitochondria.

unpublished observations), (2) an association of the biochemical activity of the enzyme with glial enriched cellular fractions (Shank et al. 1981), and (3) the results of metabolic compartmentation studies which have demonstrated that CO_2-fixation in CNS tissues is associated with the small (synthetic) metabolic compartment (Berl, Clarke 1969) now known to reside primarily in astrocytes (Shank, Campbell 1983b).

If neurons are indeed devoid of pyruvate carboxylase, it would appear that glucose metabolized to α-ketoglutarate within neurons cannot be utilized as a net source of the dicarboxylate moiety for replenishing the transmitter pools of glutamate and GABA. The apparent absence of pyruvate carboxylase from neurons raises the issue of the mechanism by which a depletion of the pool of citrate cycle intermediates within synaptic terminals is prevented. It is reasonable to expect that some mechanism must exist which serves this function. Based on the compelling evidence that glutamine is synthesized and released by astrocytes, and thereby made available to neurons, it is conceivable that this amino acid via a deamidation and deamination process could act as a net metabolic source of α-ketoglutarate for neurons, and thereby serve an anaplerotic function. However, this process would be cumbersome since it would generate free ammonia within neurons, which would have to be extruded.

Another means by which the pool of citrate cycle intermediates in neurons might be replenished is by the direct transfer of one or more citrate cycle intermediates from astrocytes to neurons. Since oxaloacetate synthesized by the carboxylation of pyruvate can react with acetyl CoA to form citrate, the net synthesis of oxaloacetate by pyruvate carboxylase can result in an effective net synthesis of any citrate cycle intermediate. Consequently any of the citrate cycle intermediates could serve as an anaplerotic carrier from astrocytes to neurons.

ALPHA-KETOGLUTARATE METABOLICALLY DERIVED FROM ASTROCYTES AS A PRECURSOR OF THE TRANSMITTER POOLS OF GLUTAMATE AND GABA

If α-ketoglutarate were to serve such a carrier role, it could also act as a net source of the dicarboxylate moiety of glutamate molecules used to replenish the neurotransmitter pools of glutamate and GABA. An important prerequisite for the effective transfer of α-ketoglutarate, or any other citrate cycle intermediate, from astrocytes to neurons is the existence of biochemical systems that mediate the efflux from astrocytes and influx into neurons. The most likely systems would be transport carriers in the plasma membrane of both types of cells.

To test for the existence of such transport carriers, we have examined cerebral tissue slices and a variety of preparations enriched in synaptic terminals, neuronal cell bodies, and glial cell bodies for their ability to accumulate ^{14}C labelled α-ketoglutarate. In addition, we have determined the ability of some of the preparations to accumulate ^{14}C labelled citrate and malate. Our studies revealed that preparations enriched in synaptic terminals vigorously accumulate ^{14}C-α-ketoglutarate by two or more Na^+-dependent, high-affinity transport systems (Shank, Campbell 1981; 1982; 1983c-e). Furthermore, these systems mediated a rapid net uptake from the incubation fluid. The preparations enriched in astrocyte and neuronal cell bodies also accumulated ^{14}C-α-ketoglutarate by high-affinity carriers; however, the V_{max} was considerably less than for the synaptosomal preparations (Shank, Campbell 1983c). Our studies also revealed that synaptosomal preparations readily accumulate ^{14}C-malate by two or more high-affinity transport systems, whereas ^{14}C-citrate was accumulated quite slowly. The uptake of malate was mediated predominantly by a system that was not dependent on the presence of Na^+ (Shank, Campbell 1983d).

The accumulation of ^{14}C-α-ketoglutarate by slices of guinea pig cerebral cortex was distinguished by a rapid metabolic conversion of a substantial portion of the α-ketoglutarate to glutamine (Shank et al. 1983). This is in sharp contrast to results obtained with synaptosomal preparations in which comparatively little of the α-ketoglutarate was metabolized to glutamine. Since it is now established that the synthesis of glutamine occurs almost exclusively in astrocytes (Norenberg 1979) it is evident that in structurally intact CNS tissues much of the α-ketoglutarate is transported into astrocytes. A similar situation is known to exist for several other compounds, including glutamate, GABA and aspartate. The cellular basis for this is not established with certainty; however, one likely explanation is that the structure of CNS tissue is such that any compound supplied exogenously to the surface of the tissue is selectively exposed to astrocytic cellular processes as compared to synaptic terminals. The results of α-ketoglutarate uptake by tissue slices indicates that the plasma membrane of astrocytes possesses carriers which have the ability to transport α-ketoglutarate into the cell. If there is normally a net efflux of α-ketoglutarate from astrocytes, as stipulated by our hypothesis, the carriers mediating the influx of ^{14}C-α-ketoglutarate into astrocytes might function as the mechanism responsible for the efflux from the astrocytes. Assuming these carriers do serve to facilitate the flux in either direction, then the presumed net efflux would be driven by an electrochemical gradient across the membrane. Unfortunately, we have not yet developed a procedure by which a sufficient quantity of a highly enriched astrocyte cellular preparation can be obtained so that the magnitude and direction of the net flux of α-ketoglutarate can be established.

In addition to the membrane transport studies, we have obtained further information that relates specifically to the five criteria discussed previously for evaluating the metabolic precursor role of a compound. Assuming that the concentration in CSF indicates the availability to synaptic terminals, α-ketoglutarate should be available in ample amounts. The concentration in human CSF has been reported to be 20 μM (Juggi et al. 1979), and we found the average concentration in CSF obtained from the cisterna magna of four anesthetized dogs to be 8 μM (unpublished observations). These concentrations are sufficient to nearly saturate the high-affinity carriers in the membrane of synaptic terminals ($K_m \sim 1$ μM).

Our metabolic studies have revealed that synaptosomal preparations convert α-ketoglutarate into glutamate quite rapidly (Shank, Campbell 1982; 1983d; 1983e). However, the subsequent formation of GABA from the glutamate derived from α-ketoglutarate is slow in comparison to the formation of GABA from glutamate derived from glutamine. The results of our metabolic studies also have shown that the presence of α-ketoglutarate, at a concentration of 1 μM, in the medium in which synaptosomes are incubated results in a statistically significant increase in the content of glutamate within the synaptosomes. Whether the addition of α-ketoglutarate to the incubation medium increases the amount of glutamate or GABA released from synaptic terminals by a membrane depolarization stimulus has yet to be determined.

Taking into account all the steps involved in the utilization of α-ketoglutarate as a metabolic precursor of the transmitter pools of glutamate and GABA, beginning with the carboxylation of pyruvate to the final reaction in which α-ketoglutarate is metabolized to glutamate there are a large number of potential sites of regulation. Pyruvate carboxylase is a highly regulated enzyme. Activating factors include acetyl CoA, K^+, NH_4^+ and Mg^{++}, whereas glutamate inhibits the enzyme (Scrutton, 1971). The results of our studies on the uptake of ^{14}C-α-ketoglutarate indicate that glutamine, glutamate, aspartate and N-acetylaspartate may all function in the regulation of α-ketoglutarate transport across the membrane of synaptic terminals (Shank, Campbell 1981; 1983e). The transport of α-ketoglutarate may be regulated also by a heat-labile substance present in the post-microsomal supernatant of sucrose homogenates prepared from the brain of rats. This substance has an apparent molecular weight greater than 25,000 and is precipitated by ammonium sulfate at 60% saturation. The enzyme glutamate dehydrogenase is another site at which the formation of glutamate from α-ketoglutarate may be regulated (Chee et al. 1979). Aspartate aminotransferase appears to be selectively enriched in neurons that may utilize glutamate (or aspartate) as a neurotransmitter (Altschuler et al. 1981), but this enzyme can mediate a net synthesis of glutamate only if the pool of aspartate is stoichiometrically replenished.

ORNITHINE AND ARGININE AS METABOLIC PRECURSORS OF THE NEUROTRANSMITTER POOLS OF GLUTAMATE AND GABA

Wong et al. (1981) demonstrated that the regional and subcellular activity of ornithine aminotransferase in rat brain is consistent with the possibility that ornithine is a metabolic precursor of the transmitter pool of glutamate. This observation was substantiated and extended by Yoneda et al. (1982), who demonstrated that GABA can be generated from ornithine in crude synaptosomal (P_2 fraction) preparations from rat brain via a pathway in which glutamate is an intermediate. Murrin (1980) reported data indicating that GABA can be rapidly synthesized from ornithine via a pathway in which putrescine is an intermediate, but these data contrast sharply with other observations that indicate this pathway does not contribute significantly to the replenishment of the neurotransmitter pool of GABA (Seiler, Sarhan 1980; Shank, Campbell 1983a).

We have recently investigated the uptake and metabolism of ornithine by several fractions of cellular material enriched either neuronal or glial cell bodies, or synaptic terminals (Shank, Campbell 1983a). Although current information is consistent with a role for ornithine and arginine in replenishing the neurotransmitter pools of glutamate and GABA our observations do not support a major role in this capacity.

Both arginine and ornithine are available to synaptic terminals in that they are present in comparatively high concentrations in blood plasma (Maker et al. 1976), and are readily transported across the blood-brain barrier (Oldendorf 1971). Ornithine is transported across synaptic membranes by a carrier that probably also transports arginine, lysine and glutamine (Shank, Campbell 1983a); however, the affinity for ornithine is comparatively low ($K_m \sim 0.1$ mM). Our metabolic data indicate that ornithine is metabolized to glutamate and GABA rather slowly, and occurs more readily in cell bodies than synaptic terminals. No attempts to determine if the synaptic content of glutamate and GABA, and amount released by membrane depolarization, can be affected by inhibiting the metabolism of ornithine or limiting its availability have been reported. However, Roberts (1979) reported that i.p. administration of massive amounts (1.4 g/kg) of arginine and α-ketoglutarate resulted in a significant increase in the concentration of glutamate and GABA in the brain of rats.

SUMMARY

Although the compounds that serve as the metabolic precursors of the neurotransmitter pools of glutamate and GABA are not yet established with certainty present evidence strongly implicates glutamine (derived from astrocytes) as an important precursor. The results of our recent studies on α-ketoglutarate indicate that this citrate cycle intermediate (also derived from astrocytes) may serve as a source of the dicarboxylate moiety of glutamate molecules incorporated into the transmitter pools of glutamate and GABA. It is tempting to speculate that the metabolic conversion of glutamine and α-ketoglutarate to glutamate is coupled in a way that minimizes the formation of free ammonia within neurons.

The results of recent studies with arginine and ornithine are consistent with a precursor role for these amino acids, but the quantitive contribution may be minor in comparison to that of glutamine and α-ketoglutarate. Other possible precursors, e.g. proline, remain to be investigated.

REFERENCES

Altschuler RA, Neises GR, Harmison GG, Wenthold RJ, Fex J (1981). Immunocytochemical localization of aspartate aminotransferase immunoreactivity in cochlear nucleus of the guinea pig. Proc Natl Acad Sci 78:6553.

Balcar VJ, Johnston GAR (1975). High affinity uptake of L-glutamine in rat brain slices. J Neurochem 24:875.

Baldessarini RJ, Yorke C (1974). Uptake and release of possible false transmitter amino acids by rat brain tissue. J Neurochem 23:839.

Berl S, Clarke DD (1969). Metabolic compartmentation of glutamate in the CNS. In Lajtha A (ed): "Handbook of Neurochemistry" Vol 1, New York: Plenum p 168.

Bradford HF, Ward HK and Thomas AJ (1978). Glutamine - A major substrate for nerve endings. J Neurochem 30:1453.

Chee PK, Dahl JL, Fahien LA (1979). The purification and properties of rat brain glutamate dehydrogenase. J Neurochem 33:53.

Gauchy ML, Kemel ML, Glowinski J, Besson MJ (1980). In Vivo release of endogenously synthesized [^{3}H] GABA from the cat substantia nigra and the pallido entopeduncular nuclei. Brain Res 193:129.

Hamberger AC, Chiang GH, Nylen ES, Scheff SW, Cotman CW (1979). Glutamate as a CNS transmitter. I. Evaluation of glucose and glutamine as precursors for the synthesis of preferentially released glutamate. Brain Res 168:513.

Juggi JS, Iyngkaran N, Prathap K (1979). Hyperammonemia in Reye's Syndrome. In Crocker JFS (ed) "Reye's Syndrome II," New York: Grune and Stratton p 411.

Kvamme E (1983). Glutamine. In Lajtha A (ed): "Handbook of Neurochemistry", 2nd edition, Vol 3, New York: Plenum p 405.

Kvamme E, Olsen BE (1981). Evidence for compartmentation of synaptosomal phosphate activated glutaminase, J Neurochem 36:1916.

Maker HS, Clarke DD, Lajtha A (1976). Intermediary metabolism of carbohydrates and amino acids. In Siegel GJ, Albers RW, Katzman R, Agranoff GW (eds): "Basic Neurochemistry," Boston: Little, Brown and Co p 279.

McGeer PL, McGeer EG, Scherer U, Singh K (1977). A glutamatergic cortico-striatial path? Brain Res 128: 369.

Murrin LC (1980). Ornithine as a precursor for γ-aminobutyric acid in mammalian brain. J Neurochem 34: 1979.

Norenberg MD (1979). The distribution of glutamine synthetase in the rat central nervous system. J Histochem Cytochem 27:756.

Oldendorf WH (1971). Brain uptake of radiolabelled amino acids, amines and hexoses after arterial injection. Am J Physiology 22:1629.

Patel MS (1974). The relative significance of CO_2-fixing enzymes in the metabolism of rat brain. J Neurochem 22:717.

Reubi JC, Van den Berg C, Cuenod M (1979). Glutamine as a precursor for the GABA and glutamate transmitter pools. Neurosci Lett 10:171.

Roberts E (1981). Strategies for identifying sources and sites of formation of GABA-precursor or transmitter glutamate in brain. In DiChiara G and Gessa GL (eds) "Glutamate as a Neurotransmitter," Advances in Biochemical Psychopharmacology, Vol 27, New York: Raven Press p 91.

Scrutton MC (1971). Possible regulatory factors for pyruvate carboxylase with particular reference to enzyme from chicken liver. Metabolism 20:168.

Shank RP, Aprison MH (1977). Glutamine uptake and metabolism by the isolated toad brain: evidence pertaining to its proposed role as a transmitter precursor. J Neurochem 28:1189.

Shank RP, Aprison MH (1981). Present status and significance of the glutamine cycle in neural tissues. Life Sciences 28:837.

Shank RP, Campbell G LeM (1981). Avid Na^+-dependent, high-affinity uptake of alpha-ketoglutarate by nerve terminal enriched material from mouse cerebellum. Life Sciences 28:843.

Shank RP, Campbell G LeM (1982). Glutamine and alpha-ketoglutarate uptake and metabolism by nerve terminal enriched material from mouse cerebellum. Neurochem Res 7:601.

Shank RP, Campbell G LeM (1983a). Ornithine as a precursor of glutamate and GABA: Uptake and metabolism by neuronal and glial enriched cellular material. J Neurosci Res 9:47.

Shank RP, Campbell G LeM (1983b). Glutamate. Lajtha A. (ed): "Handbook of Neurochemistry, 2nd edition, Vol 3," New York: Plenum Press p 381

Shank RP, Campbell G LeM (1983c). Amino acid uptake, content and metabolism by neuronal and glial enriched cellular components from mouse cerebellum. J Neuroscience (submitted)

Shank RP, Campbell G LeM (1983d). Alpha-ketoglutarate and malate uptake and metabolism by synaptosomes: further evidence for an astrocyte to neuron metabolic shuttle. J Neurochem (submitted)

Shank RP, Campbell G LeM (1983e). Glutamine, glutamate and other possible regulators of alpha-ketoglutarate and malate uptake by synaptic terminals. J Neurochem (submitted).

Shank, RP, Campbell G LeM, Freytag SO, Utter MF (1981). Evidence that pyruvate carboxylase is an astrocyte specific enzyme. Soc Neurosci Absts 7:936.

Shank RP, Potashner SJ, Campbell G LeM (1983). On the metabolic origin of transmitter pools of glutamate and GABA. J Neurochem 40S:(in press).

Tapia R, Gonzalez RM (1978). Glutamine and glutamate as precursors of the releasable pool of GABA in brain cortex slices. Neurosci Lett 10:165.

Utter MF, Scrutton MC (1970). Pyruvate carboxylase. In Horecker BL, Stadtman ER (eds): "Current Topics in Cellular Regulation," Vol 1, New York: Academic p 253.

Van den Berg CJ (1970). Glutamate and glutamine In Lajtha A (ed) "Handbook of Neurochemistry," Vol 3, New York: Plenum p 355.

Ward HK, Thanki CM, Bradford HF (1983). Glutamine and glucose as precursors of transmitter amino acids: ex vivo studies. J Neurochem 40:855.

Ward HK, Thanki CM, Peterson DW, Bradford HF (1982). Brain glutaminase activity in relation to transmitter glutamate biosynthesis. Biochem Soc Trans 10:369.

Weil-Malherbe H (1950). Significance of glutamic acid for the metabolism of nervous tissue. Phyiol Rev 30:549.

Wong PTH, McGeer EG, McGeer PL (1981). A sensitive radiometric assay for ornithine aminotransferase:regional and subcellular distributions in rat brain. J Neurochem 36:501.

Yoneda Y, Roberts E, Dietz GW Jr (1982). A new synaptosomal biosynthetic pathway of glutamate and GABA from ornithine and its negative feedback inhibition by GABA. J Neurochem 38:1686.

Glutamine, Glutamate, and GABA
in the Central Nervous System, pages 371–388
© 1983 Alan R. Liss, Inc., 150 Fifth Avenue, New York, NY 10011

CEREBRAL AMMONIA METABOLISM IN VIVO

Thomas E. Duffy, Fred Plum, and
Arthur J.L. Cooper

Departments of Neurology and Biochemistry
Cornell University Medical College
1300 York Avenue, New York, New York   10021

Ammonia[1] is a major product of systemic and cerebral nitrogen metabolism. Like carbon dioxide, one of the main products of carbohydrate metabolism, high concentrations of ammonia in blood and tissue are potentially toxic to the organism, and to the central nervous system in particular. Most of the body's ammonia is generated in the gastrointestinal tract by the action of bacterial ureases and amine oxidases on the colon contents, and by the deamidation of glutamine in the large and small intestines (Walser and Bodenlos, 1959; Summerskill and Wolpert, 1970; Windmueller and Spaeth, 1974; Weber and Veach, 1979). Substantial quantities of ammonia are also generated in the liver by the oxidative deamination of glutamate by glutamate dehydrogenase (Krebs et al., 1978), and in the kidney, by the deamidation of glutamine (Pitts, 1964). Studies by Duda and Handler (1958) with intravenously administered [^{15}N]-ammonia revealed that the principal fate of systemic blood ammonia, in the brain and other organs, was incorporation into the amide group of glutamine. Portal blood ammonia, on the other hand, which is present in 2- to 4-fold higher concentrations than that in peripheral venous blood (White et al., 1955), is largely detoxified by the synthesis of urea in the liver. Portal-systemic shunting of blood past the liver, as occurs in chronic cirrhosis or following the

---

[1]For convenience, ammonia refers to the sum of ammonium ion (NH_4^+) and ammonia base (NH_3). At physiological pH, ~99% of total ammonia exists as ammonium ion.

surgical construction of a portacaval shunt, greatly increases the circulating ammonia concentration (Singh et al., 1954; White et al., 1955) which, in turn, increases the burden on skeletal muscle, brain, and other organs of maintaining ammonia homeostasis (Ganda and Ruderman, 1976; Lockwood et al., 1979). Ammonia is a potent neurotoxin: the administration of ammonium salts to animals will produce lethargy, coma and generalized convulsions (Torda, 1953; Hindfelt and Siesjö, 1971), and the administration of ammonia to patients with liver disease and portal-systemic shunting of blood (Ammonia Tolerance Test) can evoke a response that is indistinguishable from impending hepatic coma (Phillips et al., 1952; McDermott and Adams, 1954). For these reasons, ammonia has long been implicated as a cause of the neurological dysfunction that is a frequent complication of liver failure (see Duffy and Plum, 1982).

CEREBRAL AMMONIA FORMATION IN BRAIN AND UPTAKE FROM BLOOD.

Ammonia is constantly generated in brain by the deamination of aspartate (via the enzymes of the purine nucleotide cycle), glutamate, monoamines, and other nitrogenous substances, and by the deamidation of glutamine (Weil-Malherbe and Gordon, 1971; Weil-Malherbe, 1975; Schultz and Lowenstein, 1978). The concentration of ammonia in brain is higher than that in blood or cerebrospinal fluid (Hindfelt et al., 1977) and appears to be closely linked to the level of neural activity. Brain ammonia increases during afferent stimulation (Tsukada et al., 1958) and generalized seizures (Howse and Duffy, 1975), and declines during anesthesia (Richter and Dawson, 1948). Ammonia is also taken up by the brain from the blood and cerebrospinal fluid (Berl et al., 1962a; Lockwood et al., 1979; Cooper et al., 1979). Transport of ammonia from blood to brain is diffusion-limited, probably owing to the low permeability of the blood-brain barrier to ammonium ion (Carter et al., 1973; Phelps et al., 1977; Raichle and Larson, 1981). At physiological pH, the brain uptake index for [^{13}N]ammonia, i.e., the cerebral uptake of ammonia relative to that of the freely-diffusible indicator, n-[1-^{14}C]butanol, in awake adult rats (Table 1) is constant at approximately 25% and independent of the concentration of ammonia in the injected bolus over a 1000-fold range (Cooper et al., 1979). The brain uptake index for ammonia more than doubled when the pH of the bolus was increased from 7.2 to 8.6 (Cooper et al., 1981; see also Lockwood et al., 1980); this finding agrees with data of Carter et al. (1973) which showed a positive correlation between the pH of arterial blood and the cerebral uptake of systemically administered [^{13}N]-ammonia in dogs. These results indicate that blood-borne ammonia enters brain by diffusion, and not by carrier-mediated transport.

TABLE 1

BRAIN UPTAKE INDEX FOR [^{13}N]AMMONIA RELATIVE TO n-[1-^{14}C]BUTANOL

Ammonia Concentration in the Bolus (mM)	pH of Bolus	(n)	Uptake Index (%)
0.025	7.2	2	22.5, 20.1
2.5	7.2	4	24.5 ± 0.4
26.0	7.2	2	25.1, 20.0
0.10	7.2	6	23.7 ± 4.1
0.10	8.6	5	53.0 ± 4.0

A 0.2 ml bolus containing [^{13}N]ammonia, n-[1-^{14}C]butanol and ^{111}In-DPTA (as a non-permeable vascular marker) in 10 mM potassium phosphate buffer (pH 7.2), or in 10 mM HEPES-HCl buffer (pH 8.6), was injected into the right common carotid artery of awake adult male Wistar rats. After 5 s, the rats were decapitated and the ratio of ^{13}N/^{14}C activity in the right cerebral hemisphere, divided by the ^{13}N/^{14}C activity in the injected bolus, was calculated to obtain the cerebral uptake of ammonia relative to that of n-butanol. Data of Cooper et al. (1979, 1981).

AMMONIA METABOLISM IN BRAIN.

The brain lacks significant activity of carbamyl phosphate synthetase and ornithine transcarbamylase (Jones et al., 1961), the mitochondrial enzymes of the urea cycle, and therefore cannot synthesize urea from precursor ammonia. Brain metabolizes ammonia mainly through two reactions (Figure 1): (1) reductive amination of α-ketoglutarate to form glutamate, and (2) ATP-dependent amidation of glutamate to form glutamine. Glutamine can diffuse out of the brain into venous blood and cerebrospinal fluid (CSF); it can be hydrolyzed by glutaminase to glutamate and ammonia;

it can also transaminate with phenylpyruvate or other appropriate α-keto acids (Cooper and Gross, 1977) to yield α-ketoglutaramate and the corresponding amino acid. Hydrolysis of α-ketoglutaramate to α-ketoglutarate and ammonia completes this cycle. Normally, α-ketoglutaramate formation in brain is probably quite low, but the rate of glutamine transamination may increase in conditions that raise the brain ammonia and glutamine concentrations. For example, in patients with hepatic encephalopathy, the concentrations of ammonia, glutamine and α-ketoglutaramate in lumbar spinal fluid are all substantially increased, and there is a good correlation between the degree of neurological dysfunction and the rise in CSF α-ketoglutaramate in such subjects (Duffy and Plum, 1975, 1981).

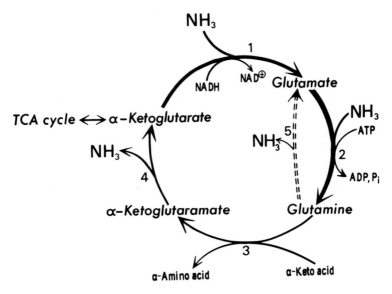

Fig. 1. Pathways of ammonia metabolism in brain. The thickness of the arrows denotes the relative prominence of the reactions catalyzed by: 1, glutamic dehydrogenase; 2, glutamine synthetase; 3, glutamine transaminase; 4, ω-amidase; and 5, glutaminase. The glutaminase reaction is shown as a broken arrow to indicate that it may exist in a different compartment from that of glutamine synthetase, thereby circumventing a futile, energy-wasting cycle of glutamine synthesis and degradation. (Modified from Duffy and Plum, 1982).

TABLE 2

ARTERIAL CONCENTRATIONS, ARTERIAL-VENOUS DIFFERENCES ACROSS THE BRAIN, AND CEREBRAL METABOLIC RATES FOR AMMONIA AND GLUTAMINE IN CONTROL RATS AND IN RATS WITH PORTACAVAL SHUNTS FOR 8 WEEKS.

	Control	Shunted
Ammonia		
Arterial concentration (μM)	80 ± 9	270 ± 32
Cerebral A-V difference (μM)	2 ± 4	48 ± 15*
$CMR_{ammonia}$ (μmol/kg/min)	-3 ± 7	84 ± 35*
Glutamine		
Arterial concentration (μM)	511 ± 20	613 ± 25*
Cerebral A-V difference (μM)	-19 ± 9†	-64 ± 29§
$CMR_{glutamine}$ (μmol/kg/min)	-19 ± 10	-72 ± 33§

Values, expressed as means ± SEM for 6-17 rats per group, are a composite of two studies from the same laboratory (Gjedde et al., 1978; Cruz and Duffy, 1983) in which the preparation of the animals and the methods used to measure cerebral blood flow and to sample cerebral venous blood differed. However, the arterial ammonia concentrations and the arterial-venous differences for ammonia across the brain in the control and shunted groups were virtually identical in the two studies.
*Different from control, $p < 0.01$, §, $p < 0.05$.
†Different from zero, $p < 0.05$.

An increased metabolism of ammonia to glutamine by the brain has been demonstrated directly in hyperammonemic rats (Gjedde et al., 1978; Cruz and Duffy, 1983). The data summarized in Table 2 were obtained with control rats and with moderately hyperammonemic rats that had a portacaval shunt constructed surgically, 8 weeks earlier. At physiological concentrations of ammonia in blood, there was no detectable net uptake of ammonia by the rat brain; however, there was a suggestion (from the negative arterial-venous difference) that rat brain normally releases a small amount of glutamine to the venous blood, a finding that agrees with data obtained in other species (Hills et al., 1972; Abdul-Ghani et al., 1978). In the shunted rats, ammonia was taken up by the brain and glutamine was released to cerebral venous blood in near equimolar amounts. Because glutamine contains two nitrogen atoms, however, some other nitrogen source (in addition to the ammonia taken up from the blood) must have contributed to the glutamine that was released (see below).

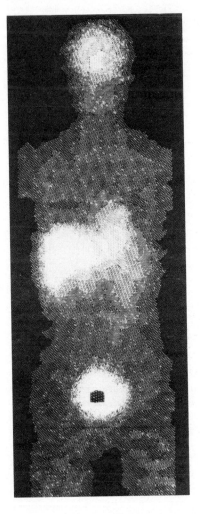

Fig. 2. Distribution of [13N] activity to the head and trunk of a normal individual following the intravenous adminis-tration of [13N]ammonia. The brain, liver and urinary bladder are well-demarcated in this 2-dimensional scan; the "recycled" dark area within the bladder image repre-sents the region of highest radioactivity in this scan. (Reproduced from Lockwood et al., 1979)

AMMONIA METABOLISM IN VIVO, STUDIED WITH [^{13}N]AMMONIA.

The intermediary metabolism of ammonia in vivo can be studied with the aid of isotopically-labeled ammonia tracers. Depicted in Figure 2 is a 2-dimensional ^{13}N-radioactivity scan of a normal individual who received a bolus injection, 20 min previously, of 10 mCi of [^{13}N]ammonia into an arm vein. Most of the ^{13}N activity is distributed to the liver, urinary bladder, and skeletal musculature, but about 8% of the label is consistently taken up by the brain (Lockwood et al., 1979). The radioactivity is thought to enter the brain as [^{13}N]ammonia, and not as a

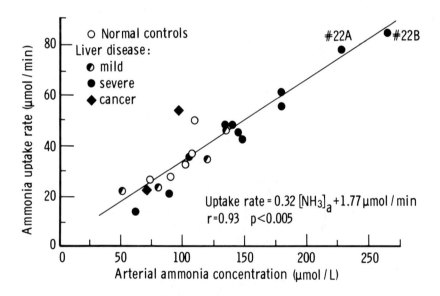

Fig. 3. Cerebral uptake of ammonia from arterial blood in healthy volunteers and in patients with liver disease. Rates of ammonia uptake are expressed per whole brain for each subject. For purposes of calculation, all of the ammonia that entered the brain was assumed to be irreversibly trapped during the time required to complete the measurements. Undoubtedly, some ammonia diffuses back from brain to venous blood, but the underestimation of the unidirectional uptake of ammonia, introduced by neglecting this back-diffusion, probably does not exceed 8% (Raichle and Larson, 1981; Cooper et al., 1981). (Modified from Lockwood et al., 1979).

metabolite of ammonia, because the cerebral uptake of radioactivity is maximal when the specific activity of [^{13}N]ammonia in arterial blood is greatest, and the amount of metabolized ^{13}N activity in blood is very low (data not shown). However, when the specific activity of [^{13}N]-ammonia in blood declines toward baseline, the activity in brain remains virtually constant, suggesting that most of the [^{13}N]ammonia that enters brain becomes metabolically trapped in a less readily diffusible form (Phelps et al., 1977; Lockwood et al., 1979; Cooper et al., 1979). From measurements of the specific activity of [^{13}N]ammonia in arterial blood and the accumulation of ^{13}N activity in the brain in 5 normal human volunteers and 13 patients with mild-to-severe hepatic encephalopathy, it was possible to calculate the rate of uptake (and "trapping") of ammonia by the brain (Fig. 3). In this group of subjects, the cerebral uptake of ammonia was found to be linear over a 5-fold range of blood ammonia concentrations (50-250 µM), suggesting that in man, as in the rat, ammonia crosses the blood-brain barrier by simple diffusion.

In order to investigate the cerebral metabolism of blood-borne ammonia in greater detail, tracer quantities of [^{13}N]ammonia were infused into the carotid circulation of normal, awake rats; the animals were decapitated and their brains were analyzed for the distribution of ^{13}N activity among several brain metabolites. This experiment repro-duced, at physiological concentrations of ammonia in arter-ial blood, an earlier study by Berl et al. (1962a) in which coma-producing doses of [^{15}N]ammonia were infused into the carotid arteries of cats and yielded the first evidence, with a nitrogen label, that ammonia metabolism was compart-mented in brain. Most of the ^{13}N activity in the brains of control rats that were infused for 10 min with [^{13}N]ammonia was recovered in the amide nitrogen of glutamine (Table 3). Very little ^{13}N activity was recovered in glutamate or in the α-amino group of glutamine, indicating that under normal physiological conditions, the glutamate dehydrogen-ase reaction plays a minor role in the cerebral detoxifica-tion of blood-borne ammonia. The incorporation of ^{13}N into the α-amino group of glutamine was greater than that in glutamate; this finding supports the concept, advanced by Berl et al. (1962a), that the ammonia entering the brain from the blood was incorporated into glutamine in a small pool of glutamate that did not exchange readily with the bulk of brain glutamate. However, a different ^{13}N labeling

pattern in brain was observed in rats that were pretreated
with L-methionine-SR-sulfoximine (MSO, 1 mmol/kg i.p.) and
3 h later were infused through the carotid circulation
with [^{13}N]ammonia for 10 min. In these MSO-treated animals
in which the activity of brain glutamine synthetase was
inhibited by 86%: (1) less [^{13}N]ammonia was recovered in
a metabolized form; (2) more label was recovered in glutamate; and (3) the specific activity of [^{13}N]glutamate was
higher than the specific activity of the α-amino group of
glutamine (i.e., the normal precursor-product relationship
for the α-amino groups of glutamate and glutamine was obtained). This last observation indicates that after MSO
treatment, the two pools of cerebral ammonia/glutamate
metabolism were no longer metabolically distinct.

TABLE 3

DISTRIBUTION OF ^{13}N ACTIVITY IN BRAIN METABOLITES AFTER
INFUSION OF [^{13}N]AMMONIA INTO THE INTERNAL CAROTID ARTERIES
OF CONTROL AND METHIONINE SULFOXIMINE (MSO)-TREATED RATS

	% of Total ^{13}N Activity in Brain	Relative Specific Activity*
CONTROL RATS		
Ammonium ion	15.7 ± 2.2	-
Glutamine, amide N	80.4 ± 1.9	[100 ± 29]†
Glutamine, amino N	1.0 ± 0.2	1.2 ± 0.4†
Glutamate	0.3 ± 0.1	0.3 ± 0.1
MSO-TREATED RATS		
Ammonium ion	33.1 ± 5.3	-
Glutamine, amide N	40.6 ± 9.3	8.0 ± 2.3†
Glutamine, amino N	2.0 ± 0.6	0.6 ± 0.2†
Glutamate	9.8 ± 1.3	1.4 ± 0.2

*The specific activities were calculated from the normal-
ized recovery of ^{13}N activity per brain. The average total
recovery of activity in each brain metabolite (± SEM) was
divided by the concentration of that metabolite in the
brain sample; the glutamine (amide) value for the control
group was assigned a value of 100.
†Different from glutamate value in the same column, p <
0.05.
Data of Cooper et al. (1979).

In order to assess how rapidly blood-borne ammonia was incorporated into brain glutamine in vivo, rats received a bolus injection of [^{13}N]ammonia into the right common carotid artery, and 5 s later the animals were killed by a freeze-blowing technique that virtually instantaneously extrudes the brain from the skull and freezes it against a precooled aluminum block. With this approach, it was found that approximately 57% of the total ^{13}N activity recovered in the brain was in glutamine (Cooper et al., 1979). From these data, one can estimate that the $t_{\frac{1}{2}}$ for the metabolism of blood-borne ammonia to brain glutamine (amide) is 3 s or less. Despite this efficient trapping, it is probable that the brain glutamine synthetase can only handle moderate increases in ammonia load. Thus, high levels of blood ammonia lead to correspondingly higher levels of brain ammonia (e.g., Hindfelt et al., 1977) and prolonged exposure to high brain ammonia concentrations produces characteristic astrocytic pathology (Cole et al., 1972; Cavanagh, 1974).

A model that attempts to account for the cerebral metabolism of blood-borne ammonia in normal rats and in animals in which brain glutamine synthetase activity has been inhibited by methionine sulfoximine is depicted in Figure 4. [^{13}N]Ammonia is thought to cross the blood-brain barrier as the free base and to enter a small compartment (presumably astrocytic) in which it rapidly combines with glutamate to yield amide-labeled [^{13}N]glutamine. Much smaller amounts of [^{13}N]ammonia may cross into the large (mainly neuronal) compartment, diffuse back into the blood, or become incorporated into glutamate in the small compartment. In the MSO-treated animals, less [^{13}N]ammonia is retained in brain in a metabolized form. Furthermore, of the fraction that is retained, more is incorporated into [^{13}N]glutamate because the large compartment, which normally does not have ready access to [^{13}N]ammonia, now receives more of the [^{13}N]ammonia that is no longer "trapped" in the small compartment.

AMMONIA-MEDIATED INHIBITION OF THE MALATE-ASPARTATE SHUTTLE IN ASTROCYTES.

High concentrations of ammonia impair energy metabolism in brain, decrease tissue concentrations of high-energy phosphates, and raise the cytoplasmic NADH/NAD radio (Schenker et al., 1967; Hindfelt and Siesjö, 1971; Hindfelt

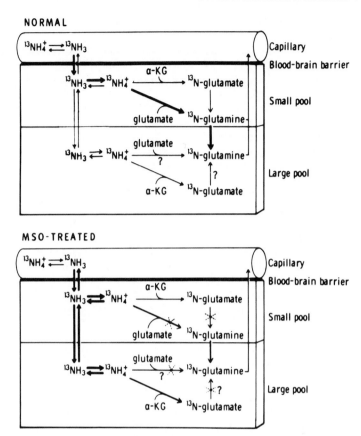

Fig. 4. Routes of arterial blood-borne [^{13}N]ammonia meta-bolism in the brains of control and methionine sulfoximine (MSO)-treated rats. The relative importance of the various pathways is indicated by the thickness of the arrows. The question marks on the figure denote uncertainty about the presence of glutamine synthetase activity in the large compartment of brain ammonia/glutamate metabolism. (Reproduced from Cooper et al., 1979).

et al., 1977; McCandless and Schenker, 1981). Interference by ammonia with the malate-aspartate shuttle, which is involved in the transport of cytoplasmically-generated reduced equivalents into the mitochondria for oxidative energy production, could underly these neurochemical abnormalities. Carrier-mediated exchange of glutamate for aspartate across the mitochondrial membrane is a key process of this shuttle system, and high concentrations of ammonia could inhibit the shuttle by depleting cytoplasmic concentrations of glutamate through the increased synthesis of glutamine (Hindfelt et al., 1977). Since glutamine synthetase is primarily an astrocytic enzyme (Norenberg and Martinez-Hernandez, 1979), ammonia-mediated inhibition of the malate-aspartate shuttle, if it occurs, may be prominent in the very cells that are thought to comprise the small compartment of cerebral ammonia/glutamate metabolism. Recent studies in our laboratory indicate that inhibition of the malate-aspartate shuttle can impair the oxidative energy metabolism of brain tissue in vitro. When rat brain cortex slices were incubated (Krebs-Ringer phosphate medium containing 10 mM glucose; 37°) with 2 mM β-methyleneaspartate to irreversibly inactivate aspartate aminotransferase, a constituent enzyme of the malate-aspartate shuttle, the oxygen consumption of the tissues declined by more than 60% [control, 420 ± 10 μmol/g dry wt/h; β-methyleneaspartate-treated, 140 ± 10 μmol/g dry wt/h (Fitzpatrick et al., 1983)].

AMINO ACIDS AS SOURCE OF SMALL-COMPARTMENT GLUTAMATE NITROGEN.

Tracer data, obtained with [^{13}N]ammonia, indicate that very little glutamate is normally synthesized from ammonia in the small (astrocytic) compartment of the brain (Table 3). However, measurements of the incorporation of [^{13}N]-ammonia into brain glutamine and of the net efflux of glutamine from brain (Table 2) suggest that glutamine is synthesized and released by the brain, and that the amount of glutamine released increases under conditions of hyper-ammonemia (e.g., portacaval shunt). Accordingly, a question arises about the origins of the small-compartment glutamate that is used for the synthesis of this brain glutamine. Berl et al. (1962b) and Waelsch et al. (1964) have demonstrated significant incorporation of CO_2 into cerebral glutamate, both in the control state and during systemic administration of ammonium acetate. We believe that blood-borne amino acids, principally the branched-chain amino acids, may be an important additional source of glutamate carbon as well as of glutamate nitrogen (Figure 5). Brain possesses branched-chain aminotransferase acti-

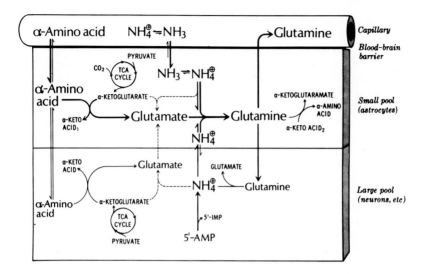

Fig. 5. Proposed mechanism by which blood-borne branched-chain amino acids may facilitate detoxification of ammonia in brain. The relative importance of the various pathways is indicated by the thickness of the arrows. (Reproduced from Duffy and Plum, 1982).

vity (Benuck et al., 1972), and brain slices incubated with L-[1-^{14}C]leucine rapidly liberate $^{14}CO_2$ (Chaplin et al., 1976), presumably following transamination with α-ketoglutarate as the obligatory first step in the degradative pathway (Meister, 1965). Administration of amino acid mixtures, enriched with branched-chain amino acids, to hyperammonemic patients with portal-systemic encephalopathy has been reported to improve neurological function in some circumstances (Fischer et al., 1976; Freund et al., 1979; Rakette et al., 1981). A possible mechanism for the beneficial effects of such treatment is that the branched-chain amino acids reduce the neurotoxicity of ammonia by promoting the synthesis of glutamate in the small (astrocytic) compartment of cerebral ammonia metabolism. Increasing the synthesis of glutamate in this metabolic compartment could have two beneficial effects: (1) incorporation of ammonia into glutamine would be facilitated by the increased availability of precursor glutamate; and (2) the presumed inhibition of the malate-aspartate shuttle, secondary to a deficiency of cytoplasmic glutamate, would be relieved.

COMMENTS AND A HYPOTHESIS ON THE NEUROCHEMISTRY OF AMMONIA.

Ammonia is potentially neurotoxic, yet it is constantly being generated in the brain and is taken up by the brain from the blood and CSF. Normally, blood-borne ammonia enters brain by diffusion, but the astrocytes, which contain most of the brain's glutamine synthetase activity, comprise an effective metabolic blood-brain barrier to this ammonia by rapidly incorporating it into glutamine (amide). The neurotoxicity of elevated concentrations of ammonia in brain may arise, in part, from depletion of cytoplasmic concentrations of glutamate in astrocytes which, in turn, could impair cerebral oxidative energy production by inhibiting intra-astrocytic transport of reduced equivalents via the malate-aspartate shuttle. If branched-chain amino acids improve neurological function in conditions of hyperammonemic encephalopathy, they may act by promoting the synthesis of glutamate in the astrocytic pool of cerebral ammonia metabolism.

ACKNOWLEDGMENT

Part of the work cited from the authors' laboratory was supported by U.S. Public Health Service Grant AM-16739.

Abdul-Ghani A-S, Marton M, Dobkin J (1978). Studies on the transport of glutamine in vivo between the brain and blood in the resting state and during afferent electrical stimulation. J Neurochem 31:541.

Benuck M, Stern F, Lajtha A (1972). Regional and subcellular distribution of aminotransferases in rat brain. J Neurochem 19:949.

Berl S, Takagaki G, Clarke DD, Waelsch H (1962a). Metabolic compartments in vivo. Ammonia and glutamic acid metabolism in brain and liver. J Biol Chem 237:2562.

Berl S, Takagaki G, Clarke DD, Waelsch H (1962b). Carbon dioxide fixation in the brain. J Biol Chem 237:2570.

Carter CC, Lifton JF, Welch MJ (1973). Organ uptake and blood pH and concentration effects of ammonia in dogs determined with ammonia labeled with 10 minute half-lived nitrogen 13. Neurology 23:204.

Cavanagh JB (1974). Liver bypass and the glia. Res Publ Assoc Nerv Ment Dis 53:14.

Chaplin ER, Goldberg AL, Diamond I (1976). Leucine oxidation in brain slices and nerve endings. J Neurochem 26: 701.

Cole M, Rutherford RB, Smith FO (1972). Experimental ammonia encephalopathy in the primate. Arch Neurol 26: 130.

Cooper AJL, Duffy TE, McDonald JM, Gelbard AS (1981). ^{13}N as a tracer for studying ammonia uptake and metabolism in the brain. Adv Chem Se 197:369.

Cooper AJL, Gross M (1977). The glutamine transaminase-ω-amidase system in rat and human brain. J Neurochem 28: 771.

Cooper AJL, McDonald JM, Gelbard AS, Gledhill RF, Duffy TE (1979). The metabolic fate of ^{13}N-labeled ammonia in rat brain. J Biol Chem 254:4982.

Cruz NF, Duffy TE (1983). Local cerebral glucose metabolism in rats with chronic portacaval shunts. J CBF Metabol 3:311.

Duda GD, Handler P (1958). Kinetics of ammonia metabolism in vivo. J Biol Chem 232:303.

Duffy TE, Plum F (1975). α-Ketoglutaramate in the CSF: clinical implications in hepatic encephalopathy. In Ingvar DH, Lassen NA (eds): "Brain Work. The Coupling of Function, Metabolism and Blood Flow in the Brain. Copenhagen: Munksgaard, p 280.

Duffy TE, Plum F (1981). Seizures, coma, and major metabolic encephalopathies. In Siegel GJ, Albers RW, Agranoff BW, Katzman R (eds): "Basic Neurochemistry." 3rd edition. Boston: Little, Brown and Company, p 693.

Duffy TE, Plum F (1982). Hepatic encephalopathy. In Arias I, Popper H, Schachter D, Shafritz DA (eds): "The Liver: Biology and Pathobiology." New York: Raven Press, p 693.

Fischer JE, Rosen HM, Ebeid AM, James JH, Keane JM, Soeters PB (1976). The effect of normalization of plasma amino acids on hepatic encephalopathy in man. Surgery 80:77.

Fitzpatrick SM, Cooper AJL, Duffy TE (1983). Use of β-methylene-D,L-aspartate to assess the role of aspartate aminotransferase in cerebral oxidative metabolism. J Neurochem 41, in press.

Freund H, Yoshimura N, Fischer JE (1979). Chronic hepatic encephalopathy. Long-term therapy with a branched-chain amino-acid-enriched elemental diet. JAMA 242:347.

Ganda OP, Ruderman NB (1976). Muscle nitrogen metabolism in chronic hepatic insufficiency. Metabolism 25:427.

Gjedde A, Lockwood AH, Duffy TE, Plum F (1978). Cerebral blood flow and metabolism in chronically hyperammonemic rats: effect of an acute ammonia challenge. Ann Neurol 3:325.

Hills AG, Reid EL, Kerr WD (1972). Circulatory transport of L-glutamine in fasted mammals: cellular sources of urine ammonia. Am J Physiol 223:1470.

Hindfelt B, Plum F, Duffy TE (1977). Effect of acute ammonia intoxication on cerebral metabolism in rats with portacaval shunts. J Clin Invest 59:386.

Hindfelt B, Siesjö BK (1971). Cerebral effects of acute ammonia intoxication. I. The influence on intracellular and extracellular acid-base parameters. Scand J Clin Lab Invest 28:353.

Howse DC, Duffy TE (1975). Control of the redox state of the pyridine nucleotides in the rat cerebral cortex. Effect of electroshock-induced seizures. J Neurochem 24:935.

Jones ME, Anderson AD, Anderson C, Hodes S (1961). Citrulline synthesis in rat tissues. Arch Biochem Biophys 95:499.

Krebs HA, Hems R, Lund P, Halliday D, Read WWC (1978). Sources of ammonia for mammalian urea synthesis. Biochem J 176:733.

Lockwood AH, Finn RD, Campbell JA, Richman TB (1980). Factors that affect the uptake of ammonia by the brain: the blood-brain pH gradient. Brain Res 181:259.

Lockwood AH, McDonald JM, Reiman RE, Gelbard AS, Laughlin JS, Duffy TE, Plum F (1979). The dynamics of ammonia metabolism in man. Effects of liver disease and hyperammonemia. J Clin Invest 63:449.

McCandless DW, Schenker S (1981). Effect of acute ammonia intoxication on energy stores in the cerebral reticular activating system. Exp Brain Res 44:325.

McDermott WV Jr, Adams RD (1954). Episodic stupor associated with an Eck fistula in the human with particular reference to the metabolism of ammonia. J Clin Invest 33:1.

Meister A (1965). "Biochemistry of the Amino Acids." 2nd edition, Vol II. New York: Academic Press, p 729.

Norenberg MD, Martinez-Hernandez A (1979). Fine structural localization of glutamine synthetase in astrocytes of rat brain. Brain Res 161:303.

Phelps ME, Hoffman EJ, Raybaud C (1977). Factors which affect cerebral uptake and retention of $^{13}NH_3$. Stroke 8:694.

Phillips GB, Schwartz R, Gabuzda GJ Jr, Davidson CS (1952). The syndrome of impending hepatic coma in patients with cirrhosis of the liver given certain nitrogenous substances. N Engl J Med 247:239.

Pitts RF (1964). Renal production and excretion of ammonia. Am J Med 36:720.

Raichle ME, Larson KB (1981). The significance of the NH_3-NH_4 equilibrium on the passage of ^{13}N-ammonia from blood to brain. A new regional residue detection model. Circ Res 48:913.

Rakette S, Fischer M, Reimann H-J, Von Sommoggy S (1981). Effects of special amino acid solutions in patients with liver cirrhosis and hepatic encephalopathy. In Walser M, Williamson JR (eds): "Metabolism and Clinical Implications of Branched Chain Amino and Ketoacids." New York: Elsevier/North-Holland, p 419.

Richter D, Dawson RMC (1948). The ammonia and glutamine content of the brain. J Biol Chem 176:1199.

Schenker S, McCandless DW, Brophy E, Lewis MS (1967). Studies on the intracerebral toxicity of ammonia. J Clin Invest 46:838.

Schultz V, Lowenstein JM (1978). The purine nucleotide cycle. Studies of ammonia production and interconversions of adenine and hypoxanthine nucleotides and nucleosides by rat brain in situ. J Biol Chem 253:1938.

Singh ID, Barclay JA, Cooke WT (1954). Blood-ammonia levels in relation to hepatic coma and the administration of glutamic acid. Lancet 1:1004.

Summerskill WHJ, Wolpert E (1970). Ammonia metabolism in the gut. Am J Clin Nutr 23:633.

Torda C (1953). Ammonium ion content and electrical activity of the brain during the preconvulsive and convulsive phases induced by various convulsants. J Pharmacol Exp Ther 107:197.

Tsukada Y, Takagaki G, Sugimoto S, Hirano S (1958). Changes in the ammonia and glutamine content of the rat brain induced by electric shock. J Neurochem 2:295.

Waelsch H, Berl S, Rossi CA, Clarke DD, Purpura DP (1964). Quantitative aspects of CO_2 fixation in mammalian brain in vivo. J Neurochem 11:717.

Walser M, Bodenlos LJ (1959). Urea metabolism in man. J Clin Invest 38:1617.

Weber FL Jr, Veach GL (1979). The importance of the small intestine in gut ammonium production in the fasting dog. Gastroenterology 77:235.

Weil-Malherbe H (1975). Further studies on ammonia formation in brain slices: The effect of hadacidin. Neuropharmacology 14:175.

Weil-Malherbe H, Gordon J (1971). Amino acid metabolism and ammonia formation in brain slices. J Neurochem 18: 1659.

White LP, Phear EA, Summerskill WHJ, Sherlock S (1955). Ammonium tolerance in liver disease: observations based on catheterization of the hepatic veins. J Clin Invest 34:158.

Windmueller HG, Spaeth AE (1974). Uptake and metabolism of plasma glutamine by the small intestine. J Biol Chem 249:5070.

**Glutamine, Glutamate, and GABA
in the Central Nervous System, pages 389–398
© 1983 Alan R. Liss, Inc., 150 Fifth Avenue, New York, NY 10011**

AMMONIA AND AMINO ACID INTERACTION IN CULTURED BRAIN CELLS:
STUDIES WITH $^{15}NH_3$

M. Yudkoff, I. Nissim, D. Pleasure, S. Kim,
K. Hummeler, S. Segal
The Division of Biochemical Development and
Molecular Diseases, The Children's Hospital of
Philadelphia, Philadelphia, PA   19104

Nitrogen-15 has been used as an isotopic tracer in
biologic research for almost 50 years. An important
example of the application of ^{15}N to the investigation of
cerebral ammonia metabolism is the work of Berl and co-
workers (1962) who infused relatively large amounts of
$^{15}NH_4Cl$ into cats and subsequently measured isotopic abundance of ^{15}N in brain amino acids with isotope ratio mass
spectrometry (IR-MS). The development of gas chromatography-mass spectrometry (GC-MS) in recent years, especially the ability for computer-controlled single ion monitoring of the gas chromatographic effluent, has augmented the
utility of mass spectrometry in biomedical research. A
particular advantage of GC-MS is the extreme sensitivity
of the technique with respect to the sample size necessary
for accurate determination of isotopic enrichment. Whereas IR-MS requires several micromoles of sample to determine
isotopic abundance, a comparable experiment with GC-MS may
require only a few picomoles (Bier, Matthews 1982).

We have used GC-MS to study $^{15}NH_3$ metabolism in organotypic cerebellar explants and cultured astrocytes (Yudkoff,
Nissim et al., 1983). Detailed accounts of our methods
for ^{15}N analysis (Nissim et al. 1981; Yudkoff et al. 1982)
and cell culture (Pleasure, Kim 1976; Kim et al. 1983)
have been published elsewhere. An example of such a study
is given in Figure 1, which illustrates isotopic abundance
in ammonia, the amide nitrogen of glutamine, glutamate,
alanine and aspartate after incubation of either organotypic cerebellar explants or cultured astrocytes in the
presence of 300 µM $^{15}NH_4Cl$. It is evident in both culture

systems that a steady-state with respect to intracellular
$^{15}NH_3$ is attained almost immediately after addition of
isotope and that this is maintained throughout the incubation. The most prominent observed response of either system to $^{15}NH_4Cl$ exposure is formation of [amide ^{15}N] glutamine. Steady-state in this compound is attained somewhat
more rapidly in the organotypic system than in the astroglia, probably because the endogenous glutamine concentration in astroglia is several times greater than that of
the astrocytes (74.1 vs. 220.1 nmol/mg protein). Incorporation of ^{15}N into glutamate, in this instance representing both the alpha nitrogen of glutamine and that of
glutamate itself, also occurred rapidly. Enrichment of
^{15}N in alanine closely paralleled that in glutamate,
suggesting rapid transamination between these two nitrogen
carriers. Of interest is the fact that we did not observe
any ^{15}N in either glycine or serine, although our method
would have detected as little as 0.1 atom % excess with a
high degree of reliability. In contrast, we have noted
$^{15}NH_3$ formation after incubation of organotypic explants
with [^{15}N] glycine, indicating that in this system the flux
of the glycine cleavage enzyme complex tends toward glycine
deamination rather than glycine synthesis.

The data in Figure 1 suggest strongly that reductive
amination of alpha-ketoglutarate to form glutamic acid
occurs in either system. Because glutamate and glutamine
were not separated from one another prior to analysis, the
^{15}N enrichment of glutamate in Figure 1 represents the
alpha nitrogen of both amino acids and it is not possible
to determine whether the enrichment of [alpha ^{15}N] glutamine would exceed that of its precursor, [^{15}N] glutamate,
as described in the in vivo studies of Berl et al. (1962)
and Cooper et al. (1979). We therefore incubated organotypic cultures in the presence of 150 µM $^{15}NH_4Cl$. The
results, illustrated in Figure 2, are significant for three
reasons. First, enrichment of [alpha ^{15}N] glutamine is
greater than that of its apparent precursor, [^{15}N] glutamate. This observation is similar to those made in vivo
(Berl et al.1962; Cooper et al. 1979), and suggests that
the metabolic compartmentation of ammonia handling noted
in the intact animal is operant also in the organotypic
explants. Second, if the incubation period is continued
long enough, it appears that intracellular enrichment in
the alpha nitrogen of both glutamate and glutamine
approaches a similar steady-state value, suggesting that

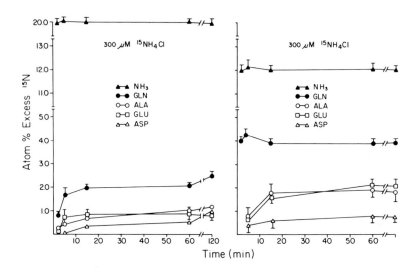

Figure 1. Intracellular isotopic abundance in ammonia, glutamine (amide N), glutamate (alpha N of both glutamate and glutamine), alanine, and aspartate after incubation at 37°C of cultured astrocytes (left) and organotypic cerebellar explants (right) in presence of MEM to which 300 μM $^{15}NH_4Cl$ (KOR isotopes) was added. At indicated times medium was removed, cells washed with saline and then frozen and thawed three times in 2 ml 0.01N HCl to liberate intracellular amino acids. Isotopic abundance in $^{15}NH_3$ and [amide ^{15}N] glutamine was determined in the supernatant according to methods we have described elsewhere (Nissim et al.1981; Yudkoff et al.1982; Yudkoff et al. 1983). Isotopic abundance in glutamate (including alpha N of glutamine), alanine and aspartate was determined by taking supernatant to dryness under N_2 and forming n-butyl-N-trifluoroacetyl derivative which was injected into the GC-MS.

although compartmentation of $^{15}NH_3$ metabolism into "small" and "large" pools does occur (Berl et al. 1962), these pools evidently articulate with one another, albeit rather slowly. A third salient feature is that the actual values of ^{15}N enrichment in this experiment, performed at 150 μM $^{15}NH_4Cl$, are higher than they were in the prior study involving incubation in 300 μM $^{15}NH_4Cl$. This was unexpected, since incubation in the presence of a higher $^{15}NH_4Cl$ concentration should increase the enrichment of both labelled ammonia and the products formed from it, i.e. [^{15}N] glutamate and [alpha ^{15}N] glutamine. The fact that this did not occur suggested the possibility that transfer of ammonia nitrogen in the organotypic explants to the alpha nitrogen of glutamate and glutamine for some reason is inhibited by the presence of relatively high ammonia concentrations. In effect, ammonia appeared to be inhibiting its own "detoxification".

To study this phenomenon further, we incubated the organotypic explants in the presence of either 150 μM, 500 μM or 1000 μM $^{15}NH_4Cl$ in MEM and determined intracellular isotopic abundance in ammonia, glutamine (alpha and amide N), and GABA. The results are illustrated in Figure 3. When the explants were incubated with 150 μM $^{15}NH_4Cl$ for a two hour period, isotopic abundance in [amide ^{15}N] glutamine, [alpha ^{15}N] glutamine and [^{15}N] glutamate was 9-10 atom % excess, or about 75% of the enrichment in $^{15}NH_3$. Enrichment in [^{15}N] GABA was only about 50% that noted in ammonia. In contrast, incubation of the explants with either 500 μM or 1000 μM $^{15}NH_4Cl$ caused a drastic reduction in the amount of ^{15}N transferred from ammonia to either glutamine, glutamate or GABA. To determine if this effect was referable to a marked expansion of the endogenous, unlabelled amino acid pool by high ammonia concentrations, perhaps through enhancement of protein breakdown, we quantitated amino acid pools, as indicated in Table 1. Some increase of glutamine was noted, but not nearly enough to account for the marked reduction of [amide ^{15}N] glutamine and [alpha ^{15}N] glutamine. No change at all was observed in the intracellular concentration of glutamate or GABA. Interference with cerebral energy metabolism by the elevated ammonia concentration might well explain the diminished ^{15}N transfer to amino acids, since glutamine synthesis requires ATP, and glutamate synthesis via the glutamate dehydrogenase reaction would require alpha-ketoglutarate, a tricarboxylic acid cycle intermediate. It may be noteworthy in the latter

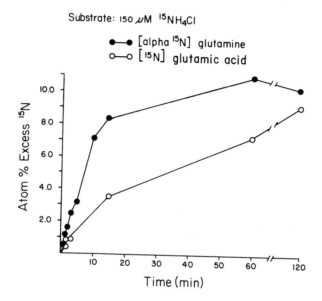

Figure 2. Intracellular isotopic abundance in [alpha 15N] glutamine and [15N]glutamate after incubation of organo-typic explants with 150 μM 15NH4Cl in MEM. Cells were handled as described in legend to Figure 1. Glutamine and glutamate were separated from one another on AG-1 (chloride) resin. After taking glutamine and glutamate fractions to dryness under N2, the n-butyl-N-trifluoroacetyl derivatives were prepared and injected into the GC-MS for measurement of isotopic abundance.

regard that the prognosis of patients with neurologic dysfunction secondary to hyperammonemia appears to be a function
of the alpha-ketoglutarate concentration in the jugular
blood (Batshaw et al. 1980). A plausible inference from
this experiment is that above a certain intracerebral concentration ammonia appears to inhibit certain crucial biochemical pathways abetting ammonia detoxification.

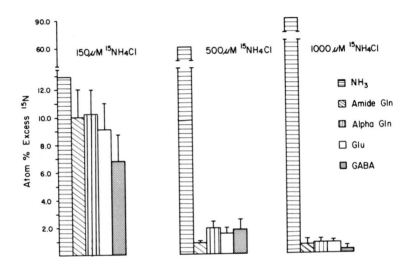

Fig. 3. Intracellular isotopic abundance in ammonia, glutamine (alpha and amide N), glutamate and GABA after incubation
of organotypic cerebellar explants for 2 hours at 37°C in
presence of indicated concentration of either 150 μM, 500 μM
or 1000 μM $^{15}NH_4Cl$ in MEM. Cells handled and derivatives
formed as described in legends to Figures 1 and 2.

Table 1
EFFECT OF AMMONIA ON AMINO ACIDS (nmol/mg protein) IN
ORGANOTYPIC EXPLANTS

	Control	0.3 mM*	1.0 mM*
Aspartic	23.1	22.8	31.6
Glutamic	78.4	67.6	80.8
Glutamine	102.0	112.4	124.4
GABA	12.6	6.6	11.5

* Ammonia concentration in medium.

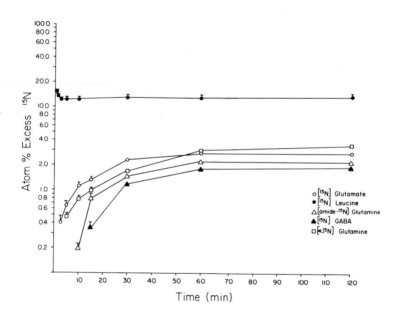

Figure 4. Intracellular isotopic abundance in glutamine
(alpha and amide N), glutamate, ammonia and GABA after
incubation of organotypic cerebellar explants for times
indicated at 37°C in MEM to which was added 15 microliters
of 7.63 mM [^{15}N] leucine. Cells handled and derivatives
formed as described in legends to Figures 1 and 2. Final
concentration of leucine 0.4 mM.

Clearly, glutamate plays a central role in ammonia
detoxification, since the synthesis of glutamate in the
GLDH reaction consumes ammonia and the formation of glutamine
in the glutamine synthetase reaction utilizes still more
ammonia. We therefore were interested in the source of
glutamate nitrogen in our culture system. Presumably,
glutamate carbon derives in large part from glucose and
glutamine (Hamberger et al. 1979) and at least some glutamate nitrogen derives from ammonia (Figure 2), but reductive
amination of alpha-ketoglutarate probably accounts for only
a fraction of glutamate nitrogen, with the remainder provided
by transamination reactions. In skeletal muscle, transamination of alpha-ketoglutarate with branched-chain amino
acids appears to be a prominent pathway of glutamate synthesis (Odessey et al. 1974). To determine whether this pathway also is operant in our culture system, we incubated the
organotypic explants in Eagle's MEM to which [^{15}N] leucine
had been added. As shown in Figure 4, a steady-state in
intracellular ^{15}N is established very quickly in leucine and
by approximately 1 hour in glutamine (amide and alpha N),
glutamate, and GABA. If we neglect for the moment the possibility of compartmentation, we can calculate the fraction of
a particular product which is synthesized from [^{15}N] leucine
from the ratio of isotopic enrichment at steady-state between
the product and leucine. The results are given in Table 2,
together with the results of a similar experiment in which
[^{15}N] valine was incubated with the organotypic cultures at
the same concentration (0.398 mM) as [^{15}N] leucine. Approximately 25% of glutamate nitrogen appeared to have been derived from leucine and about 5% more from valine. We did
not have available [^{15}N] isoleucine for testing, but even
if the isoleucine contribution were no greater than that of
valine, it would mean that approximately one-third of glutamate nitrogen in this culture system had been derived from
the branched-chain amino acids. This observation may be
of clinical relevance, since these compounds, especially
leucine, are known to cross the blood-brain barrier readily
(Oldendorf, 1971), and plasma leucine therefore might play
an important role in furnishing amino groups to the brain
for glutamate synthesis. It is of interest in this regard
that infusions of branched-chain amino acids to patients
with hepatic encephalopathy, a hyperammonemic condition,
have been reported to have a salutary effect (Fischer
et al. 1975).

Table 2

PERCENTAGE OF [15N] PRODUCT FORMED FROM [15N] LEU OR [15N] VAL

Product	[15N] Leu (± SD)	[15N] Val (± SD)
[15N] Glu	26.3 ± 4.5	4.3 ± 1.4
[alpha 15N] Gln	25.8 ± 3.7	3.7 ± 1.1
[amide 15N] Gln	13.8 ± 1.8	3.4 ± 1.2
[15N] Ala	6.8 ± 1.6	Tr
[15N] Asp	10.2 ± 2.3	Tr
15NH$_3$	13.5 ± 2.6	2.4 ± 0.6

In summary we have found that 15NH$_3$ metabolism in cultured brain cells can be studied with gas chromatography-mass spectrometry. The compartmentation of ammonia metabolism in the brain of the intact animal appears operant also in these cultured cells. Furthermore, the extent to which the 15N label is distributed to glutamine, glutamate and GABA appears to be a function of the 15NH$_4$Cl concentration in the incubation medium. At relatively high ammonia concentrations, less 15N is transferred to these important repositories of ammonia nitrogen than is true at physiologic concentrations. Finally, leucine and the other branched-chain amino acids may play an important role in brain ammonia metabolism by donating nitrogen via transamination with alpha-ketoglutarate to form glutamate. The glutamate so derived is then available for reaction with ammonia to form glutamine in the glutamine synthase pathway, which we have found to be a primary route of ammonia disposition in these cultured brain cells.

Acknowledgement:

Supported by NIH grant HD08536 and NS17752.

References:

Batshaw ML, Walser M, Brusilow SW (1980). Plasma α-ketoglutarate in urea cycle enzymopathies and its role as a harbinger of hyperammonemic coma. Pediatr Res 14:1316.
Berl S, Takagaki G, Clark, DD, Waelsch H (1962). Metabolic compartments in vivo. Ammonia and glutamic acid metabolism in brain and liver. J Biol Chem 237:2562.
Bier DM, Matthews DE (1982). Stable isotope tracer methods for in vivo investigations. Fed Proc 41:2679.

Cooper AJL, McDonald JM, Gelbard AS, Gledhill RF, Duffy TE (1979). The metabolic fate of ^{13}N-labelled ammonia in rat brain. J Biol Chem 254:4982.

Fischer JE, Funovics JM, Aguirre A et al. (1975). The role of plasma amino acids in hepatic encephalopathy. Surgery 78:276.

Hamberger AC, Chiang GH, Nyler ES, Scheff SW, Cotman CW (1979). Glutamate as a CNS Transmitter. I. Evaluation of glucose and glutamine as precursors for the synthesis of preferentially released glutamate. Brain Res 168:513.

Kim SU, Stern J, Kim MW, Pleasure DE (1983). Culture of purified rat astrocytes in serum-free medium supplemented with nitrogen. Brain Res, in press.

Nissim I, Yudkoff M, Yang W, Terwilliger T, Segal S. (1981). Gas chromatography mass spectrometry determination of [^{15}N] ammonia enrichment in blood and urine. Anal Biochem 114:125.

Odessey R, Khairallah EA, Goldberg AL (1974). Origin and possible significance of alanine production by skeletal muscle. J Biol Chem 249:7623.

Oldendorf WM (1971). Brain uptake of radiolabelled amino acids, amines, and hexoses after arterial injection. Amer J Physiol 221:1629.

Pleasure D, Kim SU (1976). Enzyme markers for myelination of mouse cerebellum in vivo and in tissue culture. Brain Res 104:193.

Yudkoff M, Nissim I, Segal S (1982) Determination of [amide ^{15}N] glutamine in plasma with gas chromatography-mass spectrometry. Clin Chim Acta 118:159.

Yudkoff M, Nissim I, Kim SU, Pleasure D, Segal S (1983). Metabolism of ^{15}NH$_3$ in Organotypic Cerebellar Explants and Cultured Astrocytes: Studies with gas chromatography-mass spectrometry. J Neurochem, in press.

**Glutamine, Glutamate, and GABA
in the Central Nervous System, pages 399–414**
© 1983 Alan R. Liss, Inc., 150 Fifth Avenue, New York, NY 10011

AMMONIA IN METABOLIC INTERACTIONS BETWEEN NEURONS AND GLIA

A. M. Benjamin

Department of Pharmacology
The University of British Columbia
Vancouver, B. C., V6T 1W5, Canada

1. INTRODUCTION

The liberation of ammonia (NH_3 + NH_4^+) in the brain is known to be altered under conditions of altered functional activity. Indeed, whereas electrical stimulation and convulsive agents enhance ammonia liberation in the brain, sleep, hibernation and anesthesia suppress it (see Benjamin 1982). Prolonged exercise leads to a reversible fall in the amide content of glutamate residues of proteins (Vrba 1957). Electrical shocks administered to rats cause reversible diminutions of adenosine and total adenylic nucleotide levels with corresponding increases of hypoxanthine derivatives (Schultz, Lowenstein 1978). The increased ammonia liberation accompanying enhanced functional activity is often associated with enhanced glutamine formation (Vrba 1957; Schultz, Lowenstein 1978), unless, of course, the synthesis of glutamine is suppressed, e.g., by methionine sulfoximine (MSO) or fluoroacetate (Tews, Stone 1965). The "burst" of ammonia in brain post-mortem probably results partly from a suppressed glutamine synthesis caused by anoxia. Cerebral amino acids, particularly glutamate and glutamine, are known to serve as excellent sources of ammonia in vitro and presumably also in vivo (Weil-Malherbe, Gordon 1971; Benjamin, Quastel 1975).

There are a number of enzymes which can act to release ammonia in the brain. These include NAD, adenosine and adenylic deaminases, guanine and guanosine deaminases, amine oxidase, glucosamine-6-phosphate deaminase, glutami-

nase, and glutamic dehydrogenase (GDH). There are, however, only two enzymes of major importance known to incor-
porate free ammonia in the brain; these are GDH and glutamine synthetase.

In keeping with the subject matter of this Symposium,
my article will be concerned mainly with ammonia, its
relationship to the amino acids of the glutamate-system
(viz. glutamate, aspartate, GABA and glutamine), its metabolic interaction between neuron and glia as revealed by
the use of certain pharmacological agents and metabolic
inhibitors, some of its toxic effects and its role in the
operation of the glutamate-glutamine cycle. This cycle
may be defined as a series of metabolic and transport
events in the brain, apparently linking neurons and glia
in the metabolism and function of amino acids of the glutamate-system.

2. LOCATION OF AMINO ACIDS OF THE GLUTAMATE-SYSTEM IN THE BRAIN

Localization of amino acids in the brain is necessary
in order to ascertain the sites of ammonia formation and
utilization. Our approach to this problem has been to use
pharmacological agents (known to affect ionic permeabili-
ties of neuronal membranes) and metabolic inhibitors as
investigational tools (Benjamin, Quastel 1972). Tetrodotoxin (TTX, 2 μM) suppresses the release of amino acid
transmitters of the glutamate-system (i.e., glutamate,
aspartate and GABA) caused by the joint action of protoveratrine (5 μM, added to cause excitation and neuronal
release of amino acids) and ouabain (0.1 mM, added to prevent re-uptake). The magnitude of the suppressions led to
the conclusion that the major pools (minima 55%) of glutamate and aspartate and probably GABA lie in the neuron.

On the other hand, TTX does not affect the release of
glutamine nor does protoveratrine accelerate it (Benjamin,
Quastel 1972). In yet unpublished experiments we have
found that enhanced [Na^+] and diminished [K^+] suppress
glutamine synthesis in brain cortex slices. It is also
known that TTX (1) blocks the inhibition of ^{14}C-acetate
oxidation to $^{14}CO_2$ brought about by electrical stimulation as a result of altered neuronal contents of Na^+
and K^+ (Chan, Quastel 1970), and (2) suppresses partially

the enhanced Na^+ influx and K^+ efflux due to ouabain (Okamoto, Quastel, 1970). However, TTX has no influence on the ouabain-induced suppression of glutamine synthesis (Benjamin, Quastel 1972). These results suggest that glutamine synthesis does not occur to any large extent in the neurons.

Using metabolic inhibitors we have found that, whereas malonate (2 mM) suppresses the TTX-sensitive protoveratrine-stimulated brain slice respiration with little concomitant effect on ATP-dependent glutamine synthesis, fluoroacetate suppresses glutamine synthesis with little effect on respiration (Benjamin, Quastel 1972). Apparently, there is no direct correlation between ATP concentrations and rates of glutamine synthesis (Benjamin, Verjee 1980). This anomaly becomes explicable if the neurons contain much of the tissue ATP and glutamine synthesis occurs in the glia. This view is supported by the fact that TTX suppresses the protoveratrine-induced fall of tissue ATP with no apparent effect on the glutamine content (Benjamin, Verjee 1980). These results, together with other observations (see section 4) support the conclusions that the major pool and site of synthesis of glutamine lie in the glia (Benjamin, Quastel 1972; Balázs et al 1973).

In our studies of glutamate transport, we have found that when rat brain cortex slices are incubated with labelled glutamate (5 mM) in a physiological glucose saline medium, the tissue/medium concentration ratio of radioactive glutamate reaches 3.1 after 30 min and 3.7 after 60 min incubation. On the other hand, if the tissue and medium glutamate is quantitated by use of an amino acid analyzer, the tissue/medium concentration ratio becomes 5.1 and 5.7 after 30 and 60 min incubation, respectively; however, these values fall to 2.8 and 3.7, respectively, if the tissue content of glutamate in the absence of added exogenous glutamate is subtracted from that in its presence. It is, thus, evident that exogenous L-glutamate taken up by brain slices is largely segregated from the endogenous (neuronal) glutamate pool. Further experiments (Okamoto, Quastel 1972) have shown that, whereas labelled glutamate derived from labelled glucose in brain slices exchanges poorly (< 10% in 30 min) with exogenous L-glutamate, labelled L-glutamate preloaded in slices exchanges quite readily (about 70% in 30 min). Thus, glucose labels the major pool of glutamate in the brain (Okamoto, Quastel

1972); on the other hand, external glutamate labels the minor pool ($\not{>}$ 20% of total glutamate; Berl et al 1961) which is predisposed to synthesize glutamine (Berl et al 1961; 1962).

3. AMMONIA FORMATION: INVOLVEMENT OF THE GLUTAMATE-SYSTEM

Brain cortex slices liberate large quantities of ammonia (14-17 μ mol/g) when they are incubated in glucose-free physiological saline medium for 1 h at 37°C. Diminutions of their glutamate and glutamine contents account for about 60% of the ammonia liberated. This value will be somewhat higher if protein-derived amino acids are taken into account. There is a rise in the aspartate content which can be accounted for by accumulation of oxaloacetate and transamination with glutamate. The bulk of the rise of aspartate occurs in the first 15 min of incubation, whereas the fall of glutamate occurs continuously and especially after the first 15 min incubation period when the rate of respiration begins to drop. With a fall in the glutamate level, liberation of ammonia from glutamine appears to be accelerated (Benjamin, Quastel 1975; Benjamin 1982). Similar changes in the levels of cerebral amino acids occur in vivo in rats with insulin-induced hypoglycemia (for references see Benjamin, Quastel 1972).

A block of cerebral endogenous glutamate oxidation results in suppression of ammonia liberation (Benjamin 1982). This block may be achieved by anoxia and by the presence of amobarbital, both of which block the regeneration of NAD(P) from NAD(P)H; by ouabain, which causes efflux of glutamate into the medium; by 5-bromofuroic acid, which suppresses GDH (Weil-Malherbe, Gordon 1971); and by glucose which suppresses oxidative deamination of glutamate by supplying the products of the reaction, α-ketoglutarate and NAD(P)H, thereby favoring the reverse reaction.

As the major pool of endogenous glutamate in the brain is neuronal, it is reasonable to conclude that ammonia liberation from endogenous glutamate is also neuronal. This view is supported by the fact that TTX blocks the protoveratrine-induced suppression of ammonia formation in brain cortex slices incubated in glucose-free medium (Table 1), presumably by allowing oxidative deamination of neuronally-retained glutamate to proceed. Moreover, exogenous glutamate, which is taken up largely into glia (Okamoto Quastel 1972; Benjamin, Quastel 1976; McLennan 1976), is a poor source of ammonia in the brain (Benjamin, Quastel 1974). Aminooxyacetic acid (5 mM, AOAA) blocks the rise of aspartate from added glutamate (2.5 mM) in glucose-free medium and concomitantly suppresses the consumption of O_2 and the liberation of CO_2; it has no effect on glutamine synthesis. (This concentration of glutamate has been used to maintain the glial content of glutamate). On the other hand, AOAA blocks glucose oxidation and thereby enhances endogenous glutamate oxidation with liberation of ammonia; aspartate and glutamine levels are not diminished (Benjamin, Quastel 1974).

Table 1. Effects of TTX (2 µM) and protoveratrine (5 µM) on the glutamate, glutamine and ammonia levels (µmol/g,± SD) of brain cortex slices incubated in Ringer-phosphate-glucose-free medium for 1 hr at 37°C

Additions	Glutamate	Glutamine	Ammonia	Σ-N
No addition	2.9 ± 0.2	2.2 ± 0.2	17.1 ± 0.6	24.4
TTX	3.6 ± 0.2	1.8 ± 0.1	16.8 ± 0.4	24.0
Protoveratrine	3.5 ± 0.2	3.9 ± 0.1	11.9 ± 0.3	23.2
Protoveratrine + TTX	3.1 ± 0.1	2.0 ± 0.1	18.0 ± 0.3	25.1

These results have led to the conclusion that, whereas endogenous (neuronal) glutamate is largely oxidized by an initial reaction with GDH with release of ammonia, exogenous (glial) glutamate, besides being converted to glutamine, undergoes initial transamination with oxaloacetate to aspartate and α-ketoglutarate before oxidation by the citric acid cycle and regeneration of oxaloacetate occurs (Benjamin, Quastel 1974). The rates of these reactions will doubtless be influenced by glucose.

Despite these conclusions, it is not suggested that glia are devoid of GDH activity nor that neurons are low in glutamate-oxaloacetate transaminase (GOT) activity. GDH must be present in glial mitochondria to account for the incorporation of labelled acetate into labelled glutamine (Berl, Clarke 1969). It must be present in the neuron to account for the liberation of ammonia from endogenous glutamate in a glucose-saline medium containing AOAA (Benjamin, Quastel 1974). This conclusion is supported by the fact that intrastriatal injection of kainic acid which destroys intrinsic neurons diminishes the activity of GDH and enhances that of glutamine synthetase in the gliotic tissue (Nicklas et al 1979). These changes are accompanied by a fall in the GOT acitivity indicating a neuronal location of the enzyme, while the suppression by AOAA of the conversion of labelled glutamate to labelled aspartate in astrocytes demonstrates its presence in glia (Yu et al 1982).

Glutaminase is another important ammonia-producing enzyme of the glutamate system. This enzyme appears to be present in neurons as well as glia (Utley 1964), although it is found to be concentrated in nerve terminals (Ward, Bradford 1979). Phosphate-activated glutaminase in rat brain homogenates (Km for glutamine, 1.6 mM) is inhibited competitively by ammonia and non-competitively by L-glutamate (Ki about 0.5 mM) (Benjamin 1981). Ca^{2+} ions (1 mM) stimulate the enzyme activity of brain homogenates prepared in isotonic Ringer's solution, but have little effect on the enhanced enzyme activity of homogenates made in distilled water (unpublished observation). It appears that stimulation by Ca^{2+} ions may occur partly due to release of glutamate from synaptosomes and partly by a Ca^{2+}-induced rise of mitochondrial pH where the enzyme is located (Benjamin 1981; see also Kvamme, Olsen 1981).

4. AMMONIA UTILIZATION IN THE BRAIN

The utilization of ammonia in the brain, as mentioned earlier, proceeds largely by the actions of GDH and glutamine synthetase. When N-labelled ammonia is introduced in the brain in vivo in tracer amounts (i.e., at normal, 0.2 mM; Cooper et al 1979) or at high concentrations (about 5 mM, Berl et al 1962), the label isotope enters the amide group of glutamine preferentially while a relatively smaller percentage (< 22% of glutamine-N) enters the α-amino group. However, a higher proportion of the labelled N atom is incorporated, presumably by GDH, into the α-amino moiety of glutamine at high concentrations of ammonia than at normal concentrations (20-22% vs. about 1%). GDH is known to be activated by high concentrations of ammonia (Norenberg 1976; Sadasivudu et al 1977; Moroni et al

1983) (Km for ammonia, 8 mM; Garcia-Bunuel et al 1962). Normally, glutamine synthetase (Km for ammonia, 0.18 mM; Pamiljans et al 1962) appears not to be saturated with respect to ammonia, and presumably therefore the glutamate concentration in the small pool (glia) is not rate-limiting (Km for glutamine synthetase, 2.5 mM; Pamiljans et al 1962). Glutamate becomes rate-limiting with the approaching saturation of glutamine synthetase, as the ammonia concentration increases. Conceivably, activation of GDH will occur to replenish the falling glutamate.

That glutamine synthetase is confined largely to the glia (astrocytes) has been revealed by pharmacological, metabolic, and ontogenic studies (Benjamin, Quastel 1972, 1975; Balázs et al 1973), by ultrastructural (Zamora et al 1973; Norenberg, Lapham 1974), and immunocytochemical (Martinez-Hernandez et al 1977) studies, and by studies with cell-cultured glia (Schousboe et al 1977; Lacoste et al 1982) or with gliotic tissue (Utley 1964; Nicklas et al 1979). Nerve terminal preparations, unlike brain slices, are unable to synthesize glutamine from glucose or glutamate (Bradford, Thomas 1969; Benjamin, Quastel 1975). Thus, whereas glucose suppresses ammonia liberation from brain slices by about 65%, it has a smaller (about 30%) suppressive effect with synaptosomal preparations, and the latter occurs, wholly by suppression of endogenous glutamate oxidation (Benjamin, Quastel 1975). These results are supported by the immunocytochemical demonstration of the absence of glutamine synthetase within nerve terminals (Norenberg, Martinez-Hernandez 1979).

Recent studies using neuroblastoma and primary cultures of glial cells (Lacoste et al 1982) suggest that, whereas the synthesis of glutamine synthetase of glia (which contain the major pool of glutamine synthetase and of glutamine) is little affected by high (2 mM) glutamine concentrations, that of neurons (if one may extrapolate from the results with neuroblastoma cells) appears to be effectively suppressed. Conceivably, the high extraneuronal glutamine normally present will repress the synthesis of the neuronal enzyme. These phenomena will account for the development of metabolic compartmentation and will require glia to serve partly as reservoirs of neuronal glutamine.

The utilization of ammonia in the presence of glucose is suppressed when uptake of neuronally released glutamate

Table 2. Effects of Ca^{2+} (2.8 mM) on ammonia utilization in rat brain cortex slices incubated in Ca^{2+}-free Ringer-phosphate medium containing L-glutamate (2.5 mM)

Additions	Glutamate[*]	Glutamine	Aspartate	Ammonia
	(μmol/g initial wet weight)[**]			
No addition	1.6 ± 0.1	1.5 ± 0.1	10.0 ± 0.2	17.2 ± 0.4
L-Glutamate	4.5 ± 0.1	3.2 ± 0.5	20.3 ± 0.5	19.2 ± 0.6
Ca^{2+}	2.0 ± 0.2	2.3 ± 0.1	9.1 ± 1.0	17.2 ± 0.3
Ca^{2+} + L-Glutamate	6.4 ± 0.2	8.3 ± 0.4	20.0 ± 0.3	12.7 ± 0.3

[*]Tissue values only. Incubation for 1 hr at 37°C. [**] ± SD.

into glia is suppressed by ouabain (see Benjamin 1982), when glial energetics are suppressed by metabolic inhibitors such as fluoroacetate (Benjamin, Quastel, 1972), and when glutamine synthetase is blocked by MSO (Benjamin, Quastel 1975). Glutamine synthesis in the presence of glucose (Benjamin, Quastel 1972) or of glutamate (Table 2) is diminished in the absence of added Ca^{2+}. This observation is especially puzzling because Ca^{2+} inhibits the isolated (Mg^{2+}-dependent) sheep brain glutamine synthetase (Elliot 1955). Part of the fall of glutamine synthesis could be due to (TTX-insensitive) diminution of tissue ATP levels in a medium devoid of Ca^{2+} (Benjamin, Verjee 1980). A diminished Ca^{2+}-ATPase activity may cause an enhanced cytosolic concentration of free Ca^{2+} released from intracellular stores. Part of the Ca^{2+}-sensitive suppression of glutamine synthesis in presence of glucose may be explained by the fact that neuronal release of glutamate (for subsequent synthesis of glutamine in the glia) is a Ca^{2+}-dependent process (see Potashner 1978).

5. TRANSPORT OF AMMONIA IN THE BRAIN

Despite the fact that glia have the capacity to produce ammonia (e.g., by glutaminase or GDH), the overriding fact that they are the major site of ammonia utilization (Section 4) makes it likely that neurons are the "net" liberators of ammonia in the brain (i.e., more ammonia leaves the neuron normally than enters it). Part of this free ammonia will diffuse out of the neuron as uncharged NH_3 and across the glial membrane. Diffusion of NH_3

across membranes apparently occurs very rapidly (Robin et al 1959); therefore, there appears to be little need for a high-affinity carrier-mediated energy-dependent transport process for ammonia. In the glioplasm NH_3 will form the NH_4^+ ion which will then be trapped by glutamine synthetase. Inhibition of the synthesis of glutamine in incubating brain slices by metabolic inhibitors occurs with liberation of ammonia, the bulk of which accumulates in the incubation medium (Table 3). Thus, ATP-dependent glutamine synthesis may be looked upon partly as an ammonia-retaining and a nitrogen-conserving mechanism in the brain.

There is no evidence of a large tissue/medium concentration ratio of free ammonia in the brain. The ratio in vivo (using total tissue ammonia values) is about 2, presumably partly because of the lower intracellular pH. Part of the tissue ammonia may be bound to cellular components. The tissue content of ammonia in vitro is approximately the same (about 2 mM; Table 3), whether or not glucose, ouabain or metabolic inhibitors are present in the incubation medium. It is suggested that ammonia above a limiting concentration largely diffuses down its concentration gradient from the neuron (the major site of its formation) into glia where it reappears largely as the amide moiety of glutamine.

Table 3. Ammonia liberation by rat brain cortex slices

Additions	Tissue		Medium
	μmol/g	μmol/ml	μmol/g
No addition	2.7	2.1	14.6
Glucose (10 mM)	1.9	2.0	4.1
" + ouabain (10 μM)	2.2	2.0	7.6
" + MSO (5 mM)	2.1	2.1	9.4
" + AOAA (5 mM)	2.3	1.9	9.3
" + fluoroacetate (1 mM)	2.2	2.3	8.6

Incubation for 1 hr at 37°C in Ringer-phosphate medium.

6. AMMONIA AND THE GLUTAMATE-GLUTAMINE CYCLE

Protoveratrine activates the TTX-sensitive sodium

current system in brain slices and thereby enhances the
release of neuronal glutamate, which, in turn, enhances
the glial synthesis of glutamine (Benjamin, Quastel 1972)
and suppresses the liberation of ammonia (Table 1) in the
absence of glucose. Protoveratrine also reduces, in a TTX-
sensitive manner, the specific radioactivity of glutamine
relative to that of glutamate in the presence of labelled
glucose (Table 4). This result may be taken to mean that

Table 4. Effects of protoveratrine (5 μM) and TTX (2 μM)
on the specific radioactivities of glutamine, GABA
and aspartate relative to that of glutamate derived
from labelled glucose in rat brain cortex slices

| | Specific radioactivities | | |
	GLN/GLU	GABA/GLU	ASP/GLU
Control	0.63	0.63	0.65
Protoveratrine	0.36	0.65	0.61
Protoveratrine + TTX	0.61	0.64	0.65

Incubation for 1 hr at 37°C in oxygenated Ringer-phos-
phate-glucose medium.

protoveratrine enhances the rate of translocation of (unlabelled, endogenous) glutamate from neuron to glia where
glutamine synthesis occurs, thereby reducing the specific
activity of glutamine in the glia and enhancing that of
glutamate in the neuron.

Studies with brain slices and nerve terminal preparations have clearly shown that neurotransmitters of the
glutamate-system are released from neurons by depolarizing
stimuli (Benjamin, Quastel 1972; Potashner 1978; Reubi
et al 1978; Bradford et al 1978; Hamberger et al 1979a,b;
Kemel et al 1979; Gauchy et al 1980). These amino acids
are known to be taken up by high-affinity uptake systems
into glia (Henn et al 1974; Benjamin, Quastel 1976;
Schousboe et al 1977). Once in the glia, they may serve
partly as precursors of glutamine (see Benjamin, Quastel
1972; 1975) which is pharmacologically inactive. That
exogenous radioactive glutamine can label releasable pools
of glutamate and GABA has been amply demonstrated in a

variety of brain areas in both <u>in vitro</u> and <u>in vivo</u> experiments (Berl et al 1961; Benjamin, Quastel 1972; Shank, Aprison 1977; Bradford et al 1978; Reubi et al 1978; Voaden et al 1978; Hamberger et al 1979ab; McGeer, McGeer 1979; Kemel et al 1979; Gauchy et al 1980; Dolphin et al 1982; Ward et al 1983).

These observations are in accord with the operation of the glutamate-glutamine cycle in the brain (Benjamin, Quastel 1972). K^+ and Ca^{2+} ions appear to play important roles in the dynamics of the glutamate-glutamine cycle. Depolarization of nerve terminals by increasing $[K^+]$ causes influx of Ca^{2+} into the synaptoplasm which then triggers the release of glutamate (for references, see Potashner 1978; Benjamin 1981). Enhanced Ca^{2+} and diminished glutamate will cause the activation of glutaminase and thereby the regeneration of glutamate (Benjamin 1981). On the other hand, the high concentration of extraneuronal glutamine linked with the high K_m of glutamine for glutaminase makes it unlikely that a high affinity uptake system for glutamine (see Shank, Campbell 1980) is of major importance in determining the rate of regeneration of glutamate from glutamine. In any event, part of the released glutamate (Section 6) and ammonia (Section 5) will enter surrounding glia. Glutamine synthesis will be facilitated and, in order to re-establish its steady-state concentration, glutamine may then flow out of the glia. Extracellular glutamate, possibly following uptake is known to cause the release of glutamine from brain slices (Benjamin, Quastel 1972), presumably from the glia. On the other hand, increasing external $[K^+]$ causes a Ca^{2+}-dependent retention of glutamine in the tissue (Benjamin, Quastel 1972). It is not certain, at present, whether this retention takes place in the glia and/or whether K^+ is directly involved in the translocation of glutamine into the neuron. High $[K^+]$ is well-known to enhance the incorporation of ^{14}C from ^{14}C-glucose into all amino acids of the glutamate-system, including neuronal glutamate and glial glutamine. Hamberger et al (1979b) have inferred from their studies that glutamine influx is enhanced following Ca^{2+}-dependent K^+-stimulated release of glutamine-derived glutamate.

The above observations need not imply that hydrolysis of glutamine is the sole pathway for the synthesis of glutamate and its derived neurotransmitters. Glutamate may arise from glucose metabolism via α-ketoglutarate (e.g., Shank, Campbell 1982) by reductive amination or by transamination with other amino acids, from ornithine (Wong et al 1981), or from proteins or peptides following hydrolysis. It may reappear in the nerve terminal following high affinity re-uptake (Logan, Snyder 1972) from the synaptic cleft. However, since glutamine is present at high concentrations, both internally (5 mM) and also externally (about 0.5 mM) and, since there is normally little   or no measurable arterio-venous difference in the concentration of glutamine, glutamate or ammonia (e.g., Hawkins et al 1973; Cooper et al 1979) despite the facts that ammonia liberation and glutamine formation are intensely and constantly taking place, it is not unreasonable to suggest that glutamine is the prime precursor of glutamate in the brain.

In conclusion, it is evident that ammonia is intimately involved in the metabolic coupling of neurons and glia in the operation of the glutamate-glutamine cycle. It should be noted, however, that metabolic uncoupling of neurons and glia may take place with increasing concentrations of ammonia (Benjamin 1982). This may occur partly by suppression of glutaminase (Benjamin 1981) and, thereby, of the synthesis and release of neuronal glutamate (Hamberger et al 1979c) and partly by depletion of α-ketoglutarate (Bessman, Bessman 1955) in glia, by activation of GDH. This latter effect may result subsequently in a diminished rate of ATP production, a decline in the enhanced rate of ATP-dependent glutamine synthesis and a concomitant rise of glutamate in the glia. The diminished rate of glutamine synthesis (Tyce et al 1981) and the enhanced neosynthesis of glutamate (Moroni et al 1983) seen in experimental models of hepatic encephalopathy may account for the increased release of glutamate (Moroni et al 1983) probably from these ATP-depleted glia (see Benjamin 1982).

7. REFERENCES

Baláⁱzs R, Patel AJ, Richter D (1973). Metabolic compartments in the brain: Their properties and relation to morphological structures. In Balazs R, Cremer JE (eds): "Metabolic Compartmentation in the Brain", London: Macmillan Press, p 167.

Benjamin AM (1981). Control of glutaminase activity in rat brain cortex in vitro: Influence of glutamate, phosphate, ammonium, calcium and hydrogen ions. Brain Res 208:363.

Benjamin AM (1982). Ammonia. In Lajtha A (ed): "Handbook of Neurochemistry", 2nd ed., Vol 1, New York, Plenum Press, p 117.

Benjamin AM, Quastel JH (1972). Locations of amino acids in brain cortex slices from the rat. Tetrodotoxin sensitive release of amino acids. Biochem J 128:631.

Benjamin AM, Quastel JH (1974). Fate of L-glutamate in the brain. J Neurochem 23:457.

Benjamin AM, Quastel JH (1975). Metabolism of amino acids and ammonia in rat brain cortex slices in vitro: A possible role of ammonia in brain function. J Neurochem 25:197.

Benjamin AM, Quastel JH (1976). Cerebral uptakes and exchange diffusion of L- and D-glutamates. J Neurochem 26:431.

Benjamin AM, Verjee ZH (1980). Control of aerobic glycolysis in the brain in vitro. Neurochem Res 5:921.

Berl S, Clarke DD (1969). Compartmentation of amino acid metabolism. In Lajtha A (ed): "Handbook of Neurochemistry", Vol 2, New York: Plenum Press, p. 447.

Berl S, Lajtha A, Waelsch H (1961). Amino acid and protein metabolism. VI. Cerebral compartments of glutamic acid metabolism. J Neurochem 7:186.

Berl S, Takagaki G, Clarke DD, Waelsch, H (1962). Metabolic compartments in vivo: Ammonia and glutamic acid metabolism in brain and liver. J Biol Chem 237:2562.

Bessman SP, Bessman AN (1955). The cerebral and peripheral uptake of ammonia in liver disease with an hypothesis for the mechanism of hepatic coma. J Clin Invest 34:622.

Bradford HF, Thomas AJ (1969). Metabolism of glucose and glutamate by synaptosomes from mammalian cerebral cortex. J Neurochem 16:1495.

Bradford HF, Ward HK, Thomas AJ (1978). Glutamine: A major substrate for nerve endings. J Neurochem 30:1453.

Chan SL, Quastel JH (1970). Effects of neurotropic drugs on sodium influx into rat brain cortex in vitro. Biochem Pharmacol 19:1071.

Cooper AJL, McDonald JM, Gelbard, AS, Gledhill RF, Duffy, TE (1979). The metabolic fate of ^{13}N-labelled ammonia in rat brain. J Biol Chem 254:4982.

Dolphin AC, Errington, ML, Bliss TVP (1982). Long-term potentiation of the perforant path in vivo is associated with increased glutamate release. Nature 297:496.

Elliot WH (1955). Glutamine synthetase. In Colowick SP, Kaplan NO (eds). Methods in Enzymol 2:337.

Garcia-Bunuel L, McDougal DB, Burch HB, Jones EM, Touhill E (1962). Oxidized and reduced pyridine nucleotide levels and enzyme activities in brain and liver of niacin deficient rats. J Neurochem 9:589.

Gauchy C, Kemel ML, Glowinski J, Besson MJ (1980). In vivo release of endogenously synthesised ^{3}H-GABA from the cat substantia nigra and the pallido entopeduncular nuclei. Brain Res 193:129.

Hamberger A Chiang GH, Nylen ES, Scheff SW, Cotman CW (1979a). Glutamate as CNS transmitter. I. Evaluation of glucose and glutamine as precursors for the synthesis of preferentially released glutamate. Brain Res 168:513.

Hamberger A Chiang GH, Sandoval E, Cotman CW (1979b). Glutamate as CNS transmitter. II. Regulation of synthesis in the releasable pool. Brain Res 168:531.

Hamberger A, Hedqvist B, Nystrom B (1979c). Ammonium ion inhibition of evoked release of endogenous glutamate from hippocampal slices. J Neurochem 33:1295.

Hawkins RA, Miller AL, Nielsen RC, Veech RL (1973). The acute action of ammonia on rat brain metabolism in vivo. Biochem J 134:1001.

Henn FA, Goldstein MN, Hamberger A (1974). Uptake of neurotransmitter candidate glutamate by glia. Nature (London) 249:663.

Kemel ML, Guachy C, Glowinski J (1979). Spontaneous and K$^+$-evoked release of ^{3}H-GABA newly synthesized from ^{3}H-glutamine in slices of rat substantia nigra. Life Sci 24:2139.

Kvamme E, Olsen BE (1981). Evidence for compartmentation of synaptosomal phosphate-activated glutaminase. J Neurochem 36:1916.

Lacoste L, Chaudary KD, Lapointe, J (1982). De-repression of the glutamine synthetase in neuroblastoma cells at low concentrations of glutamine. J Neurochem 39:78.

Logan WJ, Snyder SH (1972). High affinity uptake systems for glycine, glutamic and aspartic acids in synaptosomes of rat central nervous system. Brain Res 42:413.

Martinez-Hernandez A, Bell KP, Norenberg MD (1977). Glutamine synthetase: Glial localization in brain. Science 195:1356.

McGeer EG, McGeer PL (1979). Localisation of glutaminase in the rat neostriatum. J. Neurochem. 32:1071.

McLennan H (1976). The autoradiographic localization of L-[^{3}H]glutamate in rat brain tissue. Brain Res 115:139.

Moroni F, Lombardi G, Moneti G, Cortesini C (1983). The release and neosynthesis of glutamic acid are increased in experimental models of hepatic encephalopathy. J Neurochem 40:850.

Nicklas WJ, Nunez R, Berl S, Duvoisin R (1979). Neuronal-glial contributions to transmitter amino acid metabolism: Studies with kainic acid-induced lesions of rat striatum. J Neurochem 33:839.

Norenberg, MD (1976). Histochemical studies in experimental portal-systemic encephalopathy. I. Glutamic dehydrogenase. Arch Neurol 33:265.

Norenberg, MD, Lapham, LW (1974). The astrocyte response in experimental portal-systemic encephalopathy: An electron microscopic study. J Path Exp Neurol 33:422.

Norenberg MD, Martinez-Hernandez A (1979). Fine structure of glutamine synthetase in astrocytes of rat brain 161:303.

Okamoto K, Quastel JH (1970). Tetrodotoxin sensitive uptake of ions and water by slices of rat brain in vitro. Biochem J 120:37.

Okamoto K, Quastel JH (1972). Uptake and release of glutamate in cerebral cortex slices from the rat. Biochem J 128:1117.

Pamiljans V. Krishnaswamy DP, Dumville GD, Meister, A (1962). Studies on the mechanism of glutamine synthetase, isolation and properties of the enzyme from sheep brain. Biochemistry 1:153.

Potashner SJ (1978). Effects of tetrodotoxin, calcium and magnesium on the release of amino acids from slices of guinea pig cerebral cortex. J. Neurochem 31:187.

Reubi JC, Van Den Berg C, Cuenod M (1978). Glutamine as precursors for the GABA and glutamate transmitter pools. Neurosci Lett 10:171.

Robin ED, Travis DM, Bromberg PA, Forkner CE Jr, Tyler JM (1959). Ammonia excretion by mammalian lung. Science 129:270.

Sadasivudu B, Indira Rao T, Murthy CR (1977). Acute metabolic effect of ammonia in mouse brain. J Neurochem 2:639.

Schousboe A, Svenneby G, Hertz L (1977). Uptake and metabolism of glutamate in astrocytes cultured from mouse brain hemispheres. J Neurochem 29:999.

Schultz V, Lowenstein JM (1978). The purine nucleotide cycle: Studies of ammonia production and interconversions of adenine and hypoxanthine nucleotides and nucleosides by rat brain in situ. J Biol Chem 253:1938.

Shank RP, Aprison MH (1977). Glutamine uptake and metabolism by the isolated toad brain: Evidence pertaining to its proposed role as a transmitter precursor. J. Neurochem. 28:1189.

Shank, RP, Campbell, GL (1982). Glutamine and α-ketoglutarate uptake and metabolism by nerve terminal enriched material from mouse cerebellum. Neurochem Res 7:601.

Tews, JL, Stone WE (1965). Free amino acids and related compounds in brain and other tissues: Effects of convulsant drugs. Progr Brain Res 16:135.

Tyce GM, Ogg, J, Owen CA Jr (1981). Metabolism of acetate to amino acids in brain of rats after complete hepatectomy. J Neurochem 36:640.

Utley JD (1964). Glutamine synthetase, glutamotransferase and glutaminase in nervous and non-neural tissue in the medial geniculate body of the cat. Biochem Pharmacol 15:1383.

Voaden MJ, Lake N, Marshall J, Morjaria B (1978). The utilisation of glutamine by the retina: An autoradiographic and metabolic study. J Neurochem 31:1069.

Vrba R (1957). On the participation of ammonia in cerebral metabolism and function. Rev Czech Med 3:1.

Ward, HK, Bradford HF (1979). Relative activities of glutamine synthetase and glutaminase in synaptosomes. J Neurochem 33:339.

Ward, HK, Thanki CM, Bradford, HF (1983). Glutamine and glucose as precursors of transmitter amino acids: Ex vivo studies. J Neurochem 40:855.

Weil-Malherbe H, Gordon J (1971). Amino acid metabolism and ammonia formation in brain slices. J Neurochem 18:1659.

Wong P T-H, McGeer EG, McGeer PL (1981). A sensitive radiometric assay for ornithine amino transferase: Regional and subcellular distribution in rat brain. J Neurochem 36:501.

Yu A-C, Schousboe, A, Hertz L (1982). Metabolic fate of ^{14}C-labeled glutamate in astrocytes in primary cultures. J Neurochem 39:954.

Zamora, AJ, Cavanagh JB, Kyu MH (1973). Ultrastructural responses of the astrocytes to portocaval anastomosis in the rat. J Neurol Sci 18:25.

Support from the Division of Neurological Sciences, University of British Columbia is gratefully acknowledged.

Glutamine, Glutamate, and GABA
in the Central Nervous System, pages 415–429

GLUTAMINE: A POSSIBLE ENERGY SOURCE FOR THE BRAIN

J. Tyson Tildon

Department of Pediatrics, University
of Maryland School of Medicine,
Baltimore, Maryland 21201

Introduction

Exogenous substrates, after being taken up by the brain, can be used for three general purposes: (1) They can be used as fuel for energy, (2) they can be used as precursors for neurotransmitters and/or neurohumoral factors, and (3) they can be used for various structural components of the cell.

Since it is well documented that extreme hypoglycemia results in rapid central nervous symptoms, the role of glucose in the brain has been assumed to be absolute. However, recent studies have shown that other substrates may serve as fuel for brain. Examples of these include the two ketone bodies, acetoacetate and 3-hydroxybutyrate, which are used very extensively by the brain during early development and after long periods of starvation. (For reviews see Sokoloff (1973) and Robinson and Williamson (1980)). Other studies suggest that glutamine and its immediate metabolite glutamate may also be used as energy sources for the brain and it is the purpose of this report to attempt to codify some studies which support that proposal.

Glutamine is present in relatively high concentrations in blood (0.6 - 0.8 mM) and studies by Schwerin et al. (1948), as well as Oldendorf (1971 and 1981) have demonstrated that there is a net uptake of this amino acid by brain. It therefore seems reasonable that in its overall economy the brain might use glutamine for all three purposes. It is well established that glutamine can be incorporated into structural components such as protein and glutamine also donates nitrogen for the synthesis of nucleotides. Glutamine has also been reported as a major precursor for two neurotransmitters, γ-aminobutyric acid and glutamate (Bradford et al., 1978; Hamberger et al. 1979; Shank, Aprison 1979; Ward et al. 1983). Whether glutamine can serve as an energy source for the brain has not been firmly established, although early work by Waelsch and his colleagues (1955) strongly suggested that glutamine together with glucose provide the main nutrients for the brain. In addition, recent studies have shown that a significant amount of glutamate, the initial metabolite of glutamine, is oxidized through glutamate dehydrogenase (Benjamin, Quastel 1974) and in report by Yu et al. (1982) it was concluded that glutamate could substitute for glucose as a metabolic substrate for astrocytes in primary culture.

Nature of the Experimental System

One of the major considerations in examining the hypothesis that glutamine may be an energy source for the brain is the need to determine what kind of system provides the most appropriate information. In general most studies have focused on the uptake (transport) of glutamine and these investigations have used a variety of systems including isolated brain mitochondria (Minn 1982), nerve endings (Bradford et al. 1978; Weiler et al. 1979) and brain cortex slices (Benjamin et al. 1980). In addition the transport of glutamine in cultured neuronal and glial cells has also been described (Ramaharobandro et al. 1982).

In a recent series of experiments we compared substrate utilization by whole brain homogenates and by dissociated brain cells (Tildon et al. 1983). The value of using these two systems is that they allow for a broad range of in vitro manipulations, and the results revealed striking differences in the rates of oxidation of several substrates by the brain during development. An extension of these studies also compared the kinetics of glutamine oxidation by homogenates and intact cells and the results showed very different characteristics for glutamine oxidation by these two preparations (Tildon, Roeder 1983). The conservative inference from these studies was that a significant amount of glutamine can be oxidized via the TCA cycle and that it is a potential source of energy for the brain.

Comparison of Glutamine and Glucose Oxidation

One of the most compelling arguments for the role of glutamine as an energy source for the brain is the relative _in vitro_ rates of oxidation of glutamine as compared to that of glucose. The oxidation of [U-^{14}C] glutamine by two preparations (dissociated brain cells and whole brain homogenates) was determined at several different substrate concentrations. The results in Table 1 reveal that the rate of oxidation of [U-^{14}C] glutamine by dissociated brain cells is 3 to 4 fold greater than the rate of oxidation of [6-^{14}C] glucose. Using whole brain homogenates the difference was even greater. It should be noted that using homogenates the rates for glutamine oxidation doubled when the initial substrate concentration was increased ten-fold over the range of 0.5 to 5.0 mM. A similar increase was observed for glucose. By analogy with studies of substrate oxidation by fibroblasts from our laboratory which demonstrated that glutamine was a major source of energy for these cells (Zielke et al. 1976 and 1978), it seems reasonable to suggest that the higher rates of oxidation for glutamine may reflect, to some degree, the role of this amino acid in providing energy for the cell.

Comparison of $^{14}CO_2$ Production from Specifically Labeled Carbon Atoms in Glutamine

A major consideration in measurements of _in vitro_ substrate oxidation is the relative rates of $^{14}CO_2$ production from different specifically labeled substrates. In several experiments we compared the rates of $^{14}CO_2$ production from [U-^{14}C] glutamine with the rates obtained using [1-^{14}C] glutamine and [5-^{14}C] glutamine. The comparison of these latter two would permit the differentiation between (1) the combined $^{14}CO_2$ produced by glutamic acid decarboxylase reaction and the initial entry of glutamine products into the tricarboxylic acid cycle (TCA) with (2) the $^{14}CO_2$ produced by the repetitive cycling of glutamine products in the TCA cycle, respectively. The results are shown in Table 2. The rates using [U-^{14}C] or [5-^{14}C] glutamine were approximately the same when compared using dissociated cells and only slightly different using

Table 1. Comparison of the Rates of Glucose and Glutamine Oxidation by Whole Homogenates of Brain and Dissociated Brain Cells

Substrate Concentration (mM)	DISSOCIATED BRAIN CELLS		WHOLE BRAIN HOMOGENATES	
	Glucose	Glutamine	Glucose	Glutamine
0.5	4.02 + 0.43	12.5 + 1.6	2.7 + 0.36	15.5 + 1.33
1.0	4.35 + 0.56	14.5 + 1.5	4.09 + 0.37	22.5 + 1.06
2.0	4.36 + 0.31	16.7 + 1.0	6.07 + 0.46	27.5 + 1.12
5.0	4.45 + 0.45	19.3 + 1.2	5.18 + 0.42	30.6 + 1.35

Rates of oxidation (Mean + SEM) are expressed as nmoles/hr/mg protein of substrates converted to $^{14}CO_2$ at 37°C using methods previously described (Roeder et al., 1982). [U-14C] glutamine and [6-14C] glucose were used in these experiments. For glucose (n=4); for glutamine (n=3). The values for glucose were derived from data by Tildon et al. (1983).

whole brain homogenates. However, the rate of $[1-^{14}C]$ glutamine oxidation was consistently greater than that of either uniformly labeled glutamine or $[5-^{14}C]$ glutamine and this was true using either whole homogenates or dissociated brain cells. This differential apparently reflects the more rapid utilization of C-1 from this substrate for synthesis of the neurotransmitter GABA plus its initial passage through the TCA cycle.

Table 2. Comparison of $^{14}CO_2$ Production
From Specifically Labeled Carbon Atoms
of Glutamine and Glutamate

	Brain Whole Homogenates	Dissociated Brain Cells
	(N=5)	(N=5)
$[U-^{14}C]$ Glutamine (2 mM)	19.4 + 0.91	* 8.7 + 0.27
$[1-^{14}C]$ Glutamine (2 mM)	65.1 + 3.23	#24.2 + 0.77
$[5-^{14}C]$ Glutamine (2 mM)	13.1 + 1.10	9.4 + 0.59
$[U-^{14}C]$ Glutamate (2 mM)	19.3 + 0.59	*14.6 + 0.65
$[1-^{14}C]$ Glutamate (2 mM)	71.1 + 3.10	#41.4 + 2.45

These experiments measured the rates of $^{14}CO_2$ production from the labeled substrates and the data (Mean + SEM) are expressed as nmoles/hr/mg protein. The methods are similar to those described by Tildon et al. (1983). There is a significant difference (P < 0.01) between the glutamine and glutamate values indicated by the * and #.

To further explore the relative rates of oxidation using differentially labeled substrates, the rate of $^{14}CO_2$ production from glutamine was compared to that of glutamate labeled on the same carbon (Table 2). Using whole homogenates, the rates of $^{14}CO_2$ produced from $[1-^{14}C]$ glutamine was essentially the same as that obtained using $[1-^{14}C]$ glutamate. Similarly the rate using $[U-^{14}C]$ glutamine was identical to that using $U-^{14}C$ glutamate. In contrast, using dissociated brain cells the rate of $^{14}CO_2$ production from $[1-^{14}C]$ glutamate or $[U-^{14}C]$ glutamate was significantly higher than the rates obtained using comparably labeled glutamine compounds. These results tend to suggest a difference in the transport (uptake) of these compounds across the plasma membrane. However, it should be noted that the techniques for preparing dissociated brain cells and brain homogenates could possibly result in the selection of different cellular and subcellular components in the two preparations. If this occurred, the reduced rate of $^{14}CO_2$ production from glutamine as compared to glutamate by dissociated cells may indicate that the enzyme glutaminase is rate limiting in this preparation but not in the homogenate.

Glucose and Glutamine Compartmentation

In an attempt to determine the degree to which glucose and glutamine were oxidized in the same or different metabolic compartments, the effects of adding the unlabeled form of one of these substrates on the $^{14}CO_2$ produced from the ^{14}C-labeled alternative substrate was examined in both whole homogenates and dissociated brain cells (Roeder, Tildon 1983). In these experiments the addition of 1 or 5 mM glucose significantly reduced the rate of $[U-^{14}C]$ glutamine oxidation to $^{14}CO_2$ by dissociated brain cells, but had no effect on the rates of glutamine oxidation by homogenates prepared from the contralateral brain hemisphere of the same animals. In the reciprocal situation, when unlabeled glutamine was added to either the homogenate or to dissociated brain cells, there was a significant decrease in the rate of $^{14}CO_2$ produced from $[6-^{14}C]$ glucose by both systems, and the decrement was proportional to the amount of glutamine added. This "dilution/inhibition" of glucose oxidation by glutamine, as well as the effect of glucose on glutamine oxidation, were also observed in suckling animals as well as adults. These data indicate that although some compartmentation is present, there is some mixing of glucose and glutamine in the same pool and that they both can be substrates for energy production. This seems particularly relevant in view of the finding by Hertz and Hertz (unpublished data) that glutamate can substitute for glucose in the support of astrocyte maintenance in culture.

Table 3. Comparison of the Effects of Metabolic
Inhibitors On Substrate Oxidation
by Whole Homogenates of Brain

	GLUTAMINE $(U-^{14}C)$	GLUCOSE $(6-^{14}C)$
No Additions	100	100
Rotenone (1 µM)	14 $\pm$ 2.0%	8 $\pm$ 1.3%
Antimycin A (2 µM)	22 $\pm$ 1.7%	14 $\pm$ 0.7%
Aminooxyacetate (2 mM)	61 $\pm$ 4.5%	153 $\pm$ 20%
Ouabain (20 mM)	94 $\pm$ 1.0%	84 $\pm$ 3.9%

Rates of oxidation expressed as nmole/hr/mg protein for the individual substrates were normalized to 100%. The results listed for the various inhibitors reflect the rate of oxidation expressed as percentages of the control values (Mean $\pm$ SEM) and are all significantly different from controls (P < 0.01) except for ouabain. These data are from Tildon and Roeder (1983).

Effect of Metabolic Inhibitors

To further elucidate the metabolic fate of glutamine, we examined the effect of adding several metabolic inhibitors on the oxidation of this substrate (Tildon, Roeder 1983). In the presence of either rotenone or antimycin A, the rates of oxidation of both glucose and glutamine were inhibited 80 to 85% (Table 3); whereas the addition of ouabain (20 mM) had little or no effect on the oxidation of either substrate. In contrast, the presence of aminooxyacetate (2 mM) reduced the amount of glutamine oxidation by about 40% but increased the rate of glucose oxidation by more than 50%, suggesting that inhibition of aminotransferase activity decreases the competition between glucose and substrates utilizing that pathway. Once again these results indicate that a significant fraction of glutamine is oxidized via the TCA cycle. In addition, the effects with metabolic inhibitors are compatible with the data obtained comparing rates of $^{14}CO_2$ production from specifically labeled carbon atoms of glutamine. A recent examination of the kinetics of glutamine oxidation has revealed biphasic kinetics yielding two apparent K_m values (Tildon, Roeder 1983). In the presence of aminooxyacetate, however, there was only one K_m suggesting that at high concentrations glutamine is partially metabolized via the transaminase and glutamate decarboxylase pathway, but at low concentrations it is primarily oxidized via the TCA cycle mediated by glutamate dehydrogenase.

Table 4. The Oxidation of Glutamine and Glutamate by Whole Brain Homogenates in the Presence of γ-Aminobutyric Acid (GABA) and Ammonium Acetate (NH$_4$Ac)

	[U-^{14}C] Glutamine (N=4)	[U-^{14}C] Glutamate (N=4)
No Addition	21.6 ± 2.03	17.9 ± 2.33
NH$_4$Ac 0.2 mM	18.77 ± 2.02	21.1 ± 1.76
2.0mM	18.45 ± 2.08	18.1 ± 1.67
GABA 0.2 mM	23.2 ± 2.19	19.9 ± 1.46
2.0 mM	19.68 ± 1.27	21.4 ± 1.93

Rates of oxidation (Mean ± SEM) are expressed as nmoles/ hr/mg protein for the conversion of substrate to $^{14}CO_2$. The methods are the same as described previously (see Table 2) by Tildon et al. (1983).

GABA and Ammonia

Glutamine serves as a precursor for γ-aminobutyric acid and the subsequent degradation of this neurotransmitter proceeds via its transamination with α-ketoglutarate to succinic semialdehyde which is rapidly converted to succinate. It therefore seemed reasonable to determine whether adddition of GABA would alter the rate of $^{14}CO_2$ production from [U-^{14}C] glutamine. The results shown in Table 4 revealed that the addition of GABA at 0.2 or 2.0 mM had no effect on the rate of $^{14}CO_2$ production from either glutamine or glutamate suggesting that the bulk of glutamine oxidation in the homogenate system does not proceed via its conversion to GABA. Ammonia is also a product of glutamine metabolism and the results shown in Table 4 reveal that this cation had essentially no effect on the rate of glutamine oxidation. This latter result seems somewhat surprising since Benjamin and Quastel (1974) have proposed that ammonium ion may play a basic role in the control of the glutamate/glutamine system in the brain.

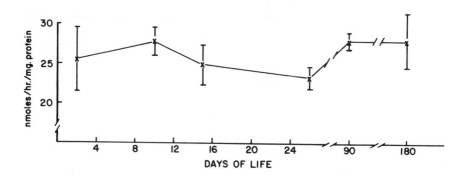

Fig. 1. Rates of oxidation of [U-^{14}C] glutamine by brain homogenates from rats of different ages. Each point represents the Mean + SEM for five or more rats. The assay method was the same as has been previously described (Tildon et al., 1983).

Glutamine Metabolism in the Developing Brain

Because of the unique sequence of events in cell maturation, an important approach to understanding the metabolic characteristics of brain is to study substrate utilization, oxidation and enzyme composition at various stages during development. This has been a useful tool in the elucidation of ketone body utilization by the neonatal rat brain (Page et al. 1971; Tildon et al. 1971; Klee, Sokoloff 1967; and Tildon et al. 1983). The results in Figure 1 show that using the homogenate system, the rate of glutamine oxidation is essentially the same throughout the entire developmental period. This relatively constant pattern of glutamine oxidation was somewhat surprising since there are striking changes in the developmental pattern of activities of the enzymes of glutamine/glutamate metabolism.

The results in Figure 2a & 2b reveal a dramatic change in the activities of all the enzymes measured. The most striking change was for glutamine synthetase which increased more than eight-fold. Glutamic acid dehydrogenase also increases during early neonatal life but falls dramatically after 15 days such that the value in the adult is essentially the same as those found in the newborn rat brain. None of these developmental profiles fit the oxidation pattern of glutamine by rat brain. However, it should be noted that glutamic acid dehydrogenase has been implicated as the key enzyme in the oxidation of glutamate in the brain of guinea pigs (Hotta, Levinson 1970). Since the specific activity of glutaminase was more than ten-fold the activities for the other enzymes, it seems reasonable to suggest that glutaminase is not the rate-limiting enzyme in the oxidation of glutamine. However, a role for glutaminase cannot be completely eliminated since Ozand et al. (1975) have shown that the amount of glutamate in the brain is highly correlated with the activity of glutaminase in the brain.

It should also be noted that glutaminase and glutamic dehydrogenase are both subject to dietary manipulations during early development. Studies from this laboratory (Ozand et al. 1975; Tildon et al. 1975) revealed that early exposure to hyperketonemia caused an alteration in glutamine and glutamate metabolism in the brain. The change was found to be associated with a suppression of the developmental pattern of the specific activities of both glutaminase and glutamate dehydrogenase without affecting that for glutamine synthetase.

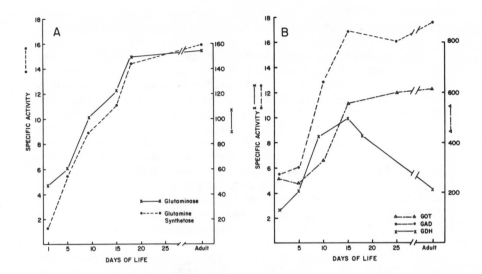

Fig. 2. The developmental pattern of the specific activity
of (a) enzymes of glutamine metabolism (glutaminase x——x
and glutamine synthetase ●---●) and (b) enzymes of glutamate
metabolism (glutamic acid dehydrogenase x——x, glutamic acid
decarboxylase ●---●, and glutamic acid, oxaloacetic
transaminase ▲ ——— ▲). The specific activities are
nmoles/min/mg protein. The data for glutaminase, glutamic
dehydrogenase and glutamine synthetase are from Tildon et
al. (1975) and Ozand et al. (1975). Glutamic oxaloacetic
transaminase was assayed by the method of Braunstein (1973)
Watanabe and Wada (1971) in brain homogenates containing 1%
triton and glutamic acid decarboxylase was assayed by the
method of Wu and Roberts (1974). Each value represents the
mean for 4 to 8 animals.

General Considerations

The proposal that glutamine may serve as fuel for the
brain is not a new concept. Quastel and Wheatley (1932) and
Weil-Malherbe (1936) showed that glutamate provided energy
for the brain in the absence of glucose. Subsequently,
Gonda and Quastel (1962) showed that labeled glutamate is
converted to CO_2 in the presence of glucose as well. It
should be noted, however, that glutamine but not glutamate
is readily taken up by the brain (Waelsch 1955; Schwerin et

al. 1948) and this difference is also reflected in the brain uptake index for these two amino acids (Oldendorf 1971).

Collectively, these facts support the proposal that glutamine may be an important energy source for the brain. Additional evidence for this proposal has been recently supplied by Yu et al. (1982). These workers demonstrated that substantial amounts of glutamate are metabolized to CO_2 by isolated astrocytes in culture. They also noted that this conversion was not sensitive to aminooxyacetate. This latter observation is in keeping with our own study (Tildon, Roeder 1983) and the data presented above which show that a substantial amount of glutamine oxidation by dissociated brain cells or whole brain homogenates was not sensitive to this metabolic inhibitor even though the oxidation of glutamine was sensitive to both rotenone and antimycin A.

Although the data provide cogent evidence that glutamine is oxidized by the brain, additional questions related to the metabolic compartmentation of these reactions are yet to be answered. Substantial evidence indicates that in many instances glutamate is converted to glutamine (Hamberger et al. 1978; Hertz 1977) and this is supported by the finding of high rates of incorporation of ammonia into glutamine (Cooper et al. 1979) and the presence of a high amount of glutamine synthetase in the brain (Shousboe et al. 1977; Norenberg, Martinez-Hernandez 1979). This would suggest that in some metabolic compartments the net flux may be toward glutamine synthesis, while in other compartments the flux is in the direction of glutamine oxidation. Studies by Roeder and Tildon (1983) and those described above indicate that the metabolic compartment for the oxidation of glutamine in some instances is different from that of glucose, and this is consistent with the observations of many workers (Berl et al. 1975). Needless to say, the demonstration that synaptosomes (Bradford et al. 1978), isolated non-synaptosomal mitochondria (Minn 1982), as well as cultured neuronal and glial (Ramaharobandro et al. 1982) cells can utilize glutamine suggest that glutamine may be metabolized via a variety of routes. However, further investigation is essential to delineate which of the specific brain regions, cell types and/or subcellular organelles use glutamine as an energy source.

Acknowledgements
    I gratefully acknowledge the able technical assistance
of Joseph Stevenson in performing the experiments included
in this report and the expert typing of Janet Coleman in the
preparation of the manuscript. I thank Drs. Lois M. Roeder
and Stephen R. Max for their helpful comments. This work
was supported in part by NIH grant # HD16596.

References

Benjamin AM, Quastel, JH (1974). Fate of L-glutamate in the
    brain. J Neurochem 23:457.

Benjamin AM, Verjee ZH, Quastel JH (1980). Kinetics of
    cerebral uptake processes in vitro of L-glutamine,
    branched-chain L-amino acids, and 1-phenylalanine:
    Effects ouabain. J Neurochem 35:67.

Berl S, Clarke DD, Schneider D, eds (1975). "Metabolic
    Compartmentation and Neurotransmission: Relation to Brain
    Structure and Function." New York: Plenum Press.

Bradford HF, Ward HK, Thomas AJ (1978). Glutamine, a major
    substrate for nerve endings. J Neurochem 30:1453.

Braunstein AE (1973). "The Enzymes IX Pt B (Boyer, PD, ed.)
    New York: Academic Press, p 379.

Cooper AJL, McDonald JM, Gelbard AS, Gledhill RF, Duffy DE
    (1979). The metabolic fate of ^{13}N-labelled ammonia in rat
    brain. J Biol Chem 254:4982.

Gonda O, Quastel JH (1962). Effects of Ouabain on cerebral
    metabolism and transport mechanisms in vitro. Biochem J
    84:394.

Hamberger A, Chiang GH, Sandoval E, Cotman CW (1979).
    Glutamate as a CNS transmitter. Regulation of synthesis
    in the releasable pool. Brain Research 168:531.

Hamberger A, Cotman CW, Sellstron A, Weiler CT (1978).
    Glutamine, glial cells and their relationship to
    transmitter glutamate. In Schoffeniels E, Franck G, Hertz
    L, Tower DB (eds): "Dynamic Properties of Glial Cells,"
    New York: Pergamon Press, p 163.

Hertz L (1977). Biochemistry of glial cells. In Fedoroff
    S, Hertz L (eds): "Cell, Tissue and Organ Cultures in
    Neurobiology" New York: Academic Press, p 39.

Hotta SS, Levinson BS (1970). The effects of
    aminooxyacetate on the metabolism of glucose and glutamate
    by homogenates of guinea pig cerebral hemispheres. Toxic
    Appl. Pharmac 16:154.

Klee CB, Sokoloff L (1967). Changes in D(-)-beta-
    hydroxybutyric acid dehydrogenase activity during brain
    maturation in rat. J Biol Chem 242:3880.

Minn A (1982). Glutamine uptake by isolated rat brain mitochondria. Neuroscience 7:2859.

Norenberg MD, Martinez-Hernandez A (1979). Fine structural localization of glutamine synthetase in astrocytes of rat brain. Brain Rev 161:303.

Oldendorf WH (1971). Brain uptake of radiolabeled amino acids, amines and hexoses after arterial injection. Amer J Physiol 221:1629.

Oldendorf WH (1981). Clearance of radiolabeled substances by brain after arterial injection using a diffusible internal standard. In Marks N, Rodnight R (eds): "Research Methods in Neurochemistry," New York: Plenum Publishing Corp, p 91.

Ozand PT, Stevenson JH, Tildon JT, Cornblath M (1975). Effects of hyperketonemia on glutamate and glutamine metabolism in developing rat brain. J Neurochem 25:67.

Page MA, Krebs HA, Williamson DH (1971). Activities of Enzymes of ketone body utilization in brain and other tissues of suckling rats. Biochem J 121:49.

Quastel JH, Wheatley AHM (1932). Oxidation by the brain. Biochem J 26:725.

Ramaharobandro N, Borg J, Mandel P, Mark J (1982). Glutamine and glutamate transport in cultured neuronal and glial cells. Brain Research 244:113.

Robinson AM, Williamson DH (1980). Physiological roles of ketone bodies as substrates and signals in mammalian tissues. Physiol Rev 60:143.

Roeder LM, Poduslo SE, Tildon JT (1982). Utilization of ketone bodies and glucose by established neural cell lines. J Neurosci Res 8:671.

Roeder LM, Tildon JT (1983). Competition among oxidizable substrates in brains of young and adult rats. Trans Amer Soc Neurochem 14:113.

Schousboe A, Svenneby G, Hertz L (1977). Uptake and metabolism of glutamate in astrocytes cultured from dissociated mouse brain hemispheres. J Neurochem 29:999.

Shank RP, Aprison MH (1979). Biochemical aspects of the neurotransmitter function of glutamate. In Filer LJ, Garattini S, Kare MR, Reynolds WA, Wurtman RJ (eds): "Glutamic Acid: Advances in Biochemistry and Physiology," New York: Raven Press, p 139.

Schwerin P, Bessman SP, Waelsch H (1948). The uptake of glutamic acid and glutamine by brain and other tissues of the rat and mouse. J Biol Chem 184:37.

Sokoloff L (1973). Metabolism of ketone bodies by the brain. Ann Rev Med 24:271.

Tildon JT, Cone AL, Cornblath M (1971). Coenzyme A transferase activity in rat brain. Biochem Biophys Res Comm 43:225.

Tildon JT, Merrill S, Roeder LM (1983). Differential substrate oxidations by dissociated brain cells and homogenates during development. Biochem J (In press).

Tildon JT, Ozand PT, Cornblath M (1975). The effects of hyperketonemia on neonatal brain and metabolism. In Hommes FA, Van den Berg CJ (eds): "Normal and Pathological Development of Energy Metabolism," New York: Academic Press, p 143.

Tildon JT, Roeder LM (1983). Glutamine oxidation by rat brain: A possible source of energy. Trans of Amer Soc for Neurochem 14:114.

Waelsch H (1955). The turnover of components of the developing brain; the blood brain barrier. In Waelsch H (ed): "Biochemistry of the Developing Nervous System, "New York: Academic Press.

Ward HK, Thanki CM, Bradford HF (1983). Glutamine and glucose as precursors of transmitter amino acids: Ex vivo studies. J Neurochem 40:855.

Watanabe T, Wada H (1971). Comparative studies on the primary structure of soluble and mitochondrial glutamic oxalacetic transaminase isoenzymes (I) Similar peptides isolated by cyanogen bromide cleavage. Biochem Biophys Res Comm 43:1310.

Weiler CT, Nystrom B, Hamberger A (1979). Characteristics of glutamine vs. glutamate transport in isolated glia and synaptosomes. J Neurochem 32:559.

Weil-Malherbe H (1936). Studies on brain metabolism . I. The metabolism of glutamic acid in brain. Biochem J 30:665.

Wu J-Y, Roberts E (1974). Properties of brain L-glutamate decarboxylase: Inhibitor studies. J Neurochem 23:759.

Yu AC, Schousboe A, Hertz L (1982). Metabolic fate of ^{14}C-labeled glutamate in astrocytes in primary cultures. J Neurochem 39:958.

Zielke HR, Ozand PT, Tildon JT, Sevdalian DA, Cornblath M (1976). Growth of human diploid fibroblasts in the absence of glucose utilization. Proc Nat Acad Sci USA 73:4110.

Zielke HR, Ozand PT, Tildon JT, Sevdalian DA, Cornblath M (1978). Reciprocal regulation of glucose and glutamine utilization by cultured human diploid fibroblasts. J Cell Physiol 95:41.

Glutamine, Glutamate, and GABA
in the Central Nervous System, pages 431–438
© **1983 Alan R. Liss, Inc., 150 Fifth Avenue, New York, NY 10011**

METABOLIC SOURCES OF ENERGY IN ASTROCYTES

Albert C.H. Yu and Leif Hertz

Dept. of Pharmacology, University of
Saskatchewan, Saskatoon, S7N OWO
Canada

INTRODUCTION

It is now well established that primary cultures of
astrocytes to a considerable extent can convert glutamate
and glutamine by an oxidative deamination to α-ketoglutarate and a subsequent oxidative decarboxylation to CO_2 and
succinyl CoA (Hertz et al. this volume). In the present
chapter we will investigate this process in more detail by
studying whether glutamate is further metabolized in the
tricarboxylic acid (TCA) cycle, a question which obviously
is of importance for the interpretation of the quantitative role of glutamate and glutamine oxidation. We will
also discuss the importance of this metabolic degradation
compared to that of other substrates (e.g., glucose) and
to the rate of oxygen uptake by the cells, as well as the
ability of glutamate or glutamine to substitute for
glucose in the maintenance of oxygen consumption. Finally,
we will present evidence that a similar oxidative degradation of glutamate also can occur in non-cultured CNS
tissue.

SUBSTRATE UTILIZATION

Glutamate and Glutamine. The production of labeled
CO_2 from $[1-^{14}C]$-labeled glutamate (50 μM) amounts in the
presence of 7.5 mM glucose to 7.4 nmol/min per mg protein
(Fig. 1), calculated on the basis of the specific activity
of glutamate in the tissue. This corresponds by itself to
a sizeable fraction of the oxygen consumption (see below)
and it raises the question whether the succinyl CoA which

is formed, is further metabolized. To answer this question, we compared production of labeled CO_2 from $[1-^{14}C]-$ and $[U-^{14}C]$-labeled glutamate. If the reaction stopped at succinyl CoA, only the C_1 carbon atom in glutamate would be split off. In the uniformly labeled compound this carbon can be expected to have an activity which is approximately one-fifth of that in $[1-^{14}C]$-labeled glutamate of the same activity. Therefore, the amount of radioactivity released from uniformly labeled glutamate would be one-fifth of that observed when the $[1-^{14}C]$-labeled compound is used. Fig. 1 shows that, although the amount of labeled CO_2 produced from uniformly labeled glutamate is lower than that from $[1-^{14}C]$-labeled glutamate, it is only reduced by a factor of 2.7, suggesting that, on the average, 1.85 (5/2.7) carbon atom of each molecule of glutamate has been metabolized. This means that the total CO_2 production from glutamate probably is almost two times higher than that observed from $[1-^{14}C]$-labeled glutamate, i.e., about 14 nmol/min per mg protein. (Table 1).

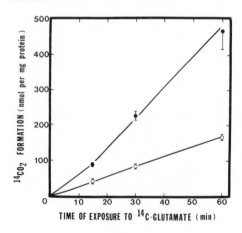

Fig. 1 Formation of $^{14}CO_2$ from $[1-^{14}C]-$ (●) and $[U-^{14}C]$-glutamate (O) by primary cultures of astrocytes as a function of the length of the incubation period. S.E.M. are indicated by vertical bars. Results are averages of 6 individual experiments.

Glutamine is metabolized in a similar fashion after initial conversion to glutamate (Hertz et al. this volume). The rate of CO_2 production from $[1-^{14}C]$-glutamine (0.5 mM) is somewhat lower than that from glutamate, i.e., 2.0 nmol/min per mg protein. The ratio between CO_2 production from the compound labeled specifically in the C_1 position and that labeled uniformly in all carbon atoms is again about 2.7, indicating that succinyl CoA is further metabolized and thus that the complete oxidation of glutamine gives rise to a CO_2 production of about 4 nmol/min per mg protein (Table 1).

   The CO_2 production from glutamate (Yu et al. 1982) or glutamine is not inhibited by AOAA, a transaminase inhibitor. This indicates that the formation of α-ketoglutarate does not involve a transamination. Due to the high activity of glutamate-oxaloacetic transaminase (GOT) and the equilibrium of this reaction, such a transamination might easily have led to an isotope exchange between α-ketoglutarate and glutamate, a reaction which would be of no functional importance. The reaction must, instead, occur as an oxidative deamination catalyzed by the glutamate dehydrogenase (GLDH). The risk of an isotope exchange is probably less in the case of this enzyme which has a much lower activity (Hertz et al. this volume). The ability of glutamine to maintain a high rate of oxygen consumption in the absence of glucose (see below) confirms that a net synthesis of α-ketoglutarate must occur from glutamate.

   Glucose. Glucose metabolism was studied in a similar manner, using [U-^{14}C]-glucose or [2-^{14}C]-glucose (7.5 mM) which both were found to be utilized at a rate of about 1 nmol glucose/min per mg protein (Fig. 2), suggesting that glucose is completely metabolized. On the assumption that the specific activity of glucose in the tissue is the same as in the medium, this corresponds to 6 nmol CO_2/min per mg protein (Table 1). Although this value is low, compared to the oxidation of glutamate, it is considerably higher than the CO_2 formation from glucose observed by Edmond et al. (1983). Conceivably, it could be an underestimate on account of the well known delay in appearance of labeled CO_2 from radioactive glucose. Experiments were therefore also carried out in cultures which had been exposed to the radioactive glucose for 18 hours, i.e., presumably long enough to label all intermediates. However, this caused only a slight increase of the CO_2 production rates (Fig. 2). Possible interactions between glucose and glutamate were studied in Ringer's solution. Replacement of the medium with Ringer's solution reduced the glucose consumption by more than 50% (Fig. 2). Addition of glutamate to this medium caused a further significant (P < 0.005) decrease, suggesting that the two substrates can partly replace each other.

A high concentration of potassium (e.g., 50 mM) is known to enhance oxidative metabolism in astrocytes (see below). It is in agreement with this that excess potassium significantly (p < 0.01) increased the rate of CO_2 production by 30% (Fig. 2). This phenomenon was consistently observed after exposure to labeled glucose for 18 hours whereas it was more variable in cultures which had not been preincubated.

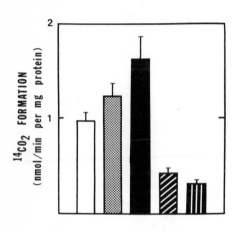

Fig. 2 Rate of CO_2 production from $[U-^{14}C]$-glucose by primary cultures of astrocytes in a normal culture medium (□); in a similar medium after pre-incubation for 18 hrs (◨); in potassium rich (55 mM K^+) medium after preincubation for 18 hrs (■); in Ringer's solution (▨) and in Ringer's solution plus 50 μM glutamate (▥). S.E.M. are indicated by vertical bars. Results are averages of 6-23 experiments.

Table 1

CO_2 production from different substrates, measured in the presence of 7.5 mM glucose.

	Concentration	CO_2 production
glutamate	0.05 mM	13.7 nmol/min per mg protein
glutamine	0.5 mM	3.7 "
glucose	7.5 mM	5.9 "
L-lactate	5.0 mM	12.3 "
alanine	1.0 mM	0.7 "
malate	0.01 mM	0.4 "
GABA	0.05 mM	0.1 "

Lactate. It has been suggested by Larrabee (1983) that lactate may be utilized as an energetic fuel transferred between different cell types, and the lactate concentration in the medium is known to increase during the culturing of astrocytes (E. Hertz, L. Hertz unpublished;

A. Schousboe personal communication). Metabolism of uniformly labeled lactate was therefore measured (in the presence of 7.5 mM glucose) and found to be 4.1 nmol lactate/min per mg protein. Provided all three carbon atoms in the lactate are utilized, this corresponds to a total production of CO_2 of about 12 nmol/min per mg protein (Table 1).

Other substrates. Alanine, malate and GABA were all utilized at a rate of at most 0.2 nmol/min per mg protein which, even on the assumption that all carbon atoms are metabolized to CO_2, at most contributed 0.7 nmol CO_2/min per mg protein (Table 1). These substrates are thus, with the possible exception of alanine (Larrabee 1983), of minor importance as metabolic fuels in astrocytes. However, acetoacetate can be utilized by primary cultures of astrocytes at a considerable rate (M Lopez-Cardozo, OM Larsson, A Schousboe personal communication; Edmond et al. 1983).

OXYGEN CONSUMPTION

Astrocytes in primary cultures show a rate of oxygen uptake ranging between 15 and 50 nmol/min per mg protein (e.g., Hertz 1978; Roth-Schechter et al. 1979; Hertz, Hertz 1979; Olson, Holtzman 1981). It tends to be higher during incubation in a tissue culture medium than during incubation in buffered saline solutions, possibly reflecting the decreased glucose utilization in Ringer's solution (Fig. 2). In our hands, it has consistently been found that 50 mM potassium causes an immediate but transient increase of the rate of respiration in astrocytes but not in neurons (Hertz 1978, 1981; Hertz, Hertz 1979). Along similar lines, Holtzman and Olson (1983) have found that astrocytic metabolism is stimulated by dinitrophenol to a much larger extent than neuronal oxygen uptake. In the absence of glucose, astrocytes in primary cultures are able to maintain a reasonably high rate of oxygen uptake with glutamine as the substrate, whereas the oxygen uptake rapidly declines in the absence of any substrate (Fig. 3). It has similarly been found that glial cells prepared by microdissection can utilize glutamate as a metabolic fuel (Hamberger 1961).

The values for oxygen consumption and for substrate utilization cannot easily be compared in an exact manner because the concentrations of compounds like lactate and

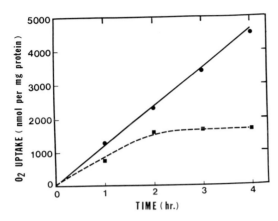

Fig. 3 Oxygen consumption by primary cultures of astrocytes as a function of the length of the incubation period in medium without any substrate (--) and with glutamine (2 mM) as the only substrate (—). Results are averages of 3 individual experiments.

glutamate in the extracellular space in vivo are unknown and in cultured cells may vary according to the feeding status of the cells. During most of the culturing period, the glutamate concentration is at least as high as the one (50 μM) used in the present study, and the glutamine concentration becomes only slightly lower than the 2 mM employed here. The glucose concentration may be lower during most of the culturing period (Cummins et al. 1983) but, in that case, the lactate concentration will be high enough that lactate might contribute substantially as a metabolic fuel. The CO_2 production from these four substrates together amounts to 35-40 nmol/min per mg protein (Table 1) and omission of either glucose or lactate will only reduce it by 6-12 nmol/min, leaving a CO_2 production of at least 25 nmol/min per mg protein. If an average R.Q. of 1.00 is assumed and, even if the oxygen consumption due to the oxidative deamination of glutamate is neglected, this corresponds to an oxygen consumption of at least 25 nmol/min per mg protein which is well within the metabolic rates which have been observed. The contribution by glutamate plus glutamine is substantial, i.e., respectively 35-50% and 15%, indicating that these 2 substrates are of major importance for energy metabolism in cultured astrocytes.

CONCLUDING REMARKS

The results presented here have shown that glutamine and especially glutamate to a major extent function as metabolic substrates for cultured astrocytes. The crucial question is to what extent similar metabolic processes

occur in the brain in vivo. Preliminary experiments have
shown that brain slices do, indeed, convert glutamate to
CO_2 (in the presence of AOAA) although a higher concentration (5 mM) was used in order to achieve a reasonable
glutamate uptake in the slices. At this concentration,
the CO_2 production from [U-^{14}C]-labeled glutamate, with
glucose (7.5 mM) present, was 6.75 nmol/min per mg protein
(calculated from the specific activity in the slices).
This value is close to one-half of that observed in the
astrocytes (Table 1) and suggests that glutamate may be an
important substrate also for the brain in vivo.
Corresponding experiments with glutamine (0.5 mM) have
shown that this substrate is also utilized by brain
slices, although to a lesser extent, as might be expected
from Table 1. This confirms observations by Tildon and
coworkers (J.T. Tildon this volume) that dissociated brain
cells and homogenates metabolize glutamine to CO_2 even in
the presence of AOAA. In the in vivo situation, the
availability of glutamine and glutamate, which seem to
function not only as metabolic substrates but also as
precursors for transmitter glutamate and GABA (see Hertz
et al. as well as Shank, Campbell this volume), might be a
problem. However, indications are found that CO_2 formation
from glutamate is a mainly astrocytic phenomenon whereas
neurons produce much less $^{14}CO_2$ from labeled glutamate
(Hertz et al. this volume). There is, furthermore, no doubt
that glutamate is released from neurons in large amounts
(Schousboe et al. this volume) and by far the major part of
this glutamate is probably accumulated into astrocytes where
the oxidative degradation is several times more intense than
glutamine formation (Hertz et al. this volume). This
glutamate might function as a major metabolic fuel. Such a
transfer of glutamate from one cell type to another, and its
utilization here, would not be in disagreement with the
fact that no net utilization of glutamate and glutamine
occurs in the whole brain (Lund 1977; Abdul-Ghani et al.
1978).

ACKNOWLEDGEMENTS

The support by the Medical Research Council of Canada
and the Saskatchewan Health Research Board (Training
Fellowship to ACH Yu) is gratefully acknowledged.

REFERENCES

Abdul-Ghani A-S, Marton M, Dobkin J (1978). Studies on the transport of glutamine in vivo between the brain and blood in the resting state and during afferent electrical stimulation. J Neurochem 31: 541.

Cummins CJ, Lust WD, Passonneau JV (1983). Regulation of glycogen metabolism in primary and transformed astrocytes in vitro. J Neurochem 40: 128.

Edmond J, Bergstrom JD, Robbins RA, Cole RA and de Vellis J (1983). Substrate utilization by glial cells from developing brain in primary culture. J Neurochem 41: S38A.

Hamberger A (1961). Oxidation of tricarboxylic acid cycle intermediates by nerve cell bodies and glial cells. J Neurochem 8: 31.

Hertz E, Hertz L (1979). Polarographic measurement of oxygen uptake by astrocytes in primary cultures using the tissue culture flask as the respirometer chamber. In Vitro 15: 429.

Hertz L (1978). Energy metabolism of glial cells. In Schoffeniels E, Franck G, Hertz L, Tower DB (eds): "Dynamic Properties of Glia Cells," Oxford: Pergamon Press, p 121.

Hertz L (1981) Features of astrocytic function apparently involved in the response of central nervous tissue to ischemia-hypoxia. J Cerebr Blood Flow Metab 1: 143.

Holtzman D, Olson JE (in press). Developmental changes in brain cellular energy metabolism in relation to seizures and their sequelae. In van Gelder N, Jasper HH (eds): "Basic Mechanisms of Neuronal Hyperexcit- ability," New York: Alan R. Liss.

Larrabee MG (1983). Lactate uptake and release in the presence of glucose by sympathetic ganglia of chicken embryos and by neuronal and nonneuronal cultures prepared from these ganglia. J Neurochem 40: 1237.

Lund P (1971). Control of glutamine synthesis in rat liver. Biochem J 124: 653.

Olson JE, Holtzman D (1980). Respiration in rat cerebral astrocytes from primary culture. J Neurosci Res 5: 497.

Roth-Schechter BF, Tholey G, Mandel P (1979). Development and mechanism of barbiturate tolerance in glial cell cultures. Neurochem Res 4: 83.

Yu ACH, Schousboe A, Hertz L (1982). Metabolic fate of [^{14}C]-labeled glutamate in astrocytes. J Neurochem 39: 954.

PHYSIOLOGY AND PATHOLOGY OF GLUTAMATE AND GABA

Glutamine, Glutamate, and GABA
in the Central Nervous System, pages 441–455
© 1983 Alan R. Liss, Inc., 150 Fifth Avenue, New York, NY 10011

ELECTROPHYSIOLOGICAL AND AUTORADIOGRAPHIC STUDIES ON GABA
AND GLUTAMATE NEUROTRANSMISSION AT THE CELLULAR LEVEL

Leo Hösli and Elisabeth Hösli

Department of Physiology
University of Basel
Vesalgasse 1, CH-4051 Basel, Switzerland

From biochemical and electrophysiological investigations, there is strong evidence that GABA and glycine act as
inhibitory transmitters, whereas glutamate and aspartate are
excitatory transmitter substances in the mammalian central
nervous system (CNS). The hyperpolarizations by GABA and
glycine are associated with an increase in Cl^-- and K^+-con-
ductance, while excitations by glutamate and aspartate are
mainly due to an increase in Na^+-conductance (Curtis, Johnston 1974; Hösli, Hösli 1978; Krnjević 1974; Nistri, Constanti 1979). On the basis of electrophysiological studies
with antagonists, it has been suggested that these amino
acid transmitters exert their effects by activating specific
types of receptors. Thus, inhibition of CNS neurones by GABA
is blocked by the convulsants bicuculline and picrotoxin,
whereas that by glycine is antagonized by strychnine (Curtis,
Johnston 1974). Receptors for the excitatory amino acids
have been classified into three types: the glutamate/quis-
qualate-preferring, the N-methyl-D-aspartate (NMDA)-prefer-
ring and the kainate-preferring receptors (Davies et al.
1982; McLennan, Liu 1982). Binding studies provide further
evidence for different types of amino acid receptors (DeFeudis 1979; Honoré et al. 1982).

Using electrophysiological and autoradiographic techniques, we have investigated physiological and pharmacological properties of amino acid receptors on neurones in organotypic cultures of rat CNS.

ELECTROPHYSIOLOGICAL STUDIES OF THE ACTION OF INHIBITORY
AND EXCITATORY AMINO ACIDS ON CULTURED NEURONES

a. Effects of GABA and Glycine

The effects of GABA and glycine on the membrane potential and conductance of cultured spinal, brain stem and cerebellar neurones were studied by adding the amino acids to
the bathing fluid at concentrations of 10^{-5} to 10^{-3}M. Both
amino acids caused hyperpolarizations (Fig. 1A) which were
associated with an increase in membrane conductance (Hösli,
Hösli 1978; Hösli et al. 1981a, 1983c). When the intracellular Cl⁻-concentration was raised by recording with a KCl-
electrode or when Cl⁻ was removed from the bathing solution,
the GABA and glycine hyperpolarizations could be reversed to
depolarizations (Fig. 1B) (Barker, Ransom 1978; Hösli, Hösli
1978; Hösli et al. 1981a, 1983c), suggesting that the hyperpolarizations by these amino acids are associated with an
increased Cl⁻-permeability of the neuronal membrane. This is
consistent with studies on spinal motoneurones in situ (Curtis et al. 1968).

Similar observations have been made with taurine, another inhibitory amino acid (Hösli, Hösli 1978) and γ-hydroxybutyrate (GHB), a reductive catabolite of GABA (Fig. 1A,B)
(Hösli et al. 1983c). Bicuculline which is known to antagonize the inhibitory actions of GABA on central neurones in
situ (Curtis, Johnston 1974; Krnjević 1974) reversibly
blocked both the hyperpolarizations and the depolarizations
by GABA and GHB of cultured CNS neurones (Fig. 1B-D) (Hösli,
Hösli 1978; Hösli et al. 1983c). The convulsant strychnine
selectively antagonized the depressant action of glycine and
taurine on spinal neurones in culture (Hösli, Hösli 1978)
and in situ (Curtis et al. 1968).

b. Effects of Glutamate, the Glutamate Analogue AMPA and
   Aspartate

Addition of glutamate, AMPA ((RS)-α-amino-3-hydroxy-5-
methyl-4-isoxazole propionic acid) and aspartate to the bathing fluid (10^{-5} to 10^{-3}M) caused a depolarization of almost all spinal and brain stem neurones tested. These depo-

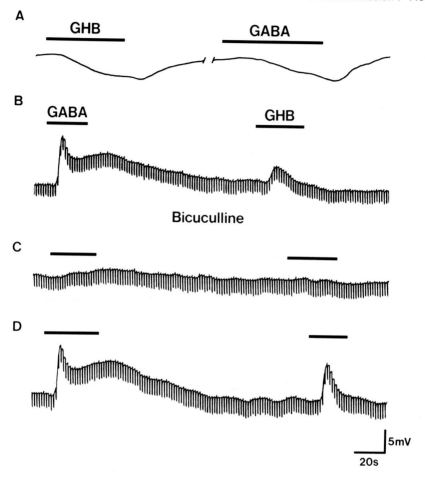

Fig. 1. A: Hyperpolarization of a spinal neurone (29 days
in vitro) by γ-hydroxybutyrate (GHB, 10^{-4}M) and GABA (10^{-4}M)
recorded with a K-acetate electrode. B: Depolarizations of
a spinal neurone (46 days in vitro) by GABA (10^{-4}M) and GHB
(10^{-4}M) recorded with a KCl-electrode. C: After perfusion
with bicuculline-methiodide (10^{-5}M), the depolarizations by
both compounds were blocked after 30 s and 2 min respectively. D: Recovery of the GABA- and GHB-depolarizations was
observed 2 and 4 min after wash-out of bicuculline. The membrane resistance (B-D) was measured by injecting hyperpolarizing current pulses of a constant intensity and duration
(1 nA, 400 ms) (membrane potentials: A: -60 mV, B-D: -55 mV)
(from Hösli et al. 1983 c).

larizations were accompanied by an increase in membrane conductance which was, however, smaller than that observed with
inhibitory amino acids (Hösli, Hösli 1978; Hösli et al.
1983b; Nistri, Constanti 1979; Ransom, Nelson 1975). On
some neurones the depolarizations were followed by small hyperpolarizations (Hösli et al., unpublished observations).
This is consistent with microelectrophoretic investigations
on spinal neurones in situ showing that the excitations by
glutamate and aspartate were often followed by postexcitato-
ry depressions (Peet et al. 1983). The depolarizations by
both amino acids were markedly reduced or abolished in Na$^+$-
free bathing solution (Hösli, Hösli 1978), suggesting that
the effects of the excitatory amino acids are mainly due to
an increase in Na$^+$-conductance.

As has been found in the mammalian spinal cord in situ
(Davies et al. 1982; Krogsgaard-Larsen et al. 1982; McLennan,
Liu 1982), the depolarizations of cultured neurones by glutamate and AMPA were blocked by the glutamate antagonist
glutamic acid diethylester (GDEE) (Fig. 2) but not by 2-ami-
no-5-phosphonovalerate (APV), an antagonist at aspartate-
preferring receptors (Fig. 3). In contrast, depolarizations
by N-methyl-D-aspartate (NMDA) were antagonized by APV (Fig.
3) but not by GDEE (Hösli et al. 1983b). This suggests that
glutamate and AMPA exert their depolarizing effects by activating glutamate/quisqualate receptors without affecting
NMDA-receptors.

INDIRECT EFFECTS OF AMINO ACID TRANSMITTERS ON CULTURED
GLIAL CELLS

Testing the amino acid transmitters on cultured glial
cells located in the vicinity of neurones, both the inhibitory (GABA, glycine) and excitatory amino acids (glutamate,
aspartate) caused depolarizations of the glial membrane. In
contrast to the action of these amino acids on neurones, the
glial depolarizations were not associated with changes in
membrane conductance. The actions of the amino acids were
clearly dependent on the location of the glial cells in the
culture. Only glial cells which were lying in the vicinity
of neurones were depolarized by the amino acids, whereas isolated glial cells in the outgrowth zone of the culture were
not affected (Hösli et al. 1981a,b,c).

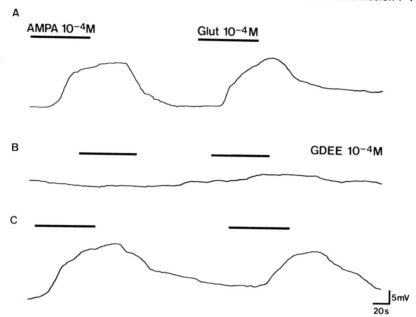

A

AMPA 10⁻⁴M

Glut 10⁻⁴M

B

GDEE 10⁻⁴M

C

5mV

20s

Fig. 2. Effect of the glutamate antagonist GDEE on the depolarizations of a spinal neurone by AMPA and glutamate
(culture 28 days in vitro, membrane potential -75 mV).
A: Depolarizations by AMPA (10^{-4}M) and glutamate (10^{-4}M).
B: After perfusion with bathing solution containing GDEE
(10^{-4}M) the depolarizations by AMPA and glutamate were
blocked. C: Recovery was observed 6 min after wash-out of
GDEE. Duration of perfusion with AMPA and glutamate is indicated by horizontal bars.

Simultaneous recordings of the glial membrane potential
and measurements of extracellular K^+-concentration ($[K^+]_0$)
revealed that the amino acid-induced depolarization of glial
cells correlates well in amplitude and time course with an
increase of $[K^+]_0$ measured in close vicinity of the impaled
glial cell (Fig. 4A,B) (Hösli et al. 1981a,b,c). 4-Aminopy-
ridine, a blocker of K^+-channels, reversibly abolished the
glial depolarization and the increase of $[K^+]_0$ caused by the
amino acid transmitters (Hösli et al. 1981a). This suggests
that the glial depolarization is an indirect effect due to
the efflux of K^+ from adjacent neurones and that the glial
cells, unlike neurones, do not possess receptors for these
amino acid transmitters.

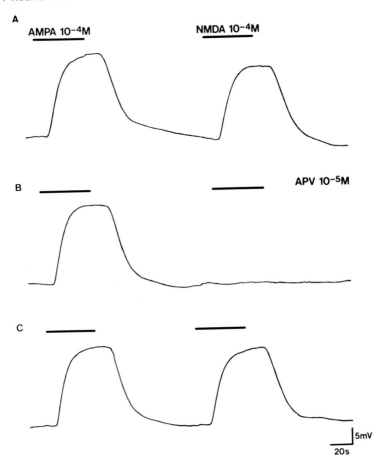

Fig. 3. Action of the NMDA antagonist APV on the depolarizations of a spinal neurone produced by AMPA and NMDA (culture 13 days in vitro, membrane potential -72 mV). A: Depolarizations by AMPA (10^{-4}M) and NMDA (10^{-4}M). B: Perfusion of the culture with APV (10^{-5}M) did not affect the depolarization by AMPA, but completely blocked the action of NMDA after 4 min. C: Recovery was observed 4 min after wash-out of APV. Duration of perfusion with AMPA and NMDA is indicated by horizontal bars (from Hösli et al. 1983b).

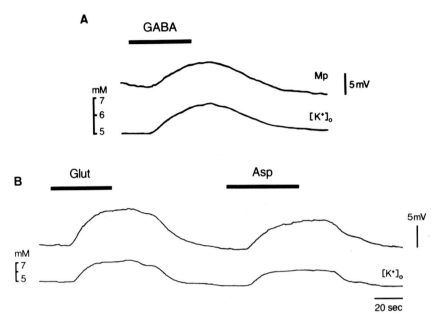

Fig. 4. Simultaneous recordings of the effects of GABA (A), glutamate and aspartate (B) on the membrane potential (upper traces) of cultured glial cells and on $[K^+]_0$ (lower traces). The resting potentials of the glial cells in A were -65 mV and in B -73 mV (spinal cord culture, 30 and 15 days in vitro respectively). Duration of perfusion with the amino acids (concentrations 10^{-4}M) is indicated by horizontal bars above tracings (A: from Hösli et al. 1981b; B: from Hösli et al. 1981c).

AUTORADIOGRAPHIC LOCALIZATION OF BINDING SITES FOR INHIBITORY AND EXCITATORY AMINO ACIDS ON CULTURED NEURONES

a. Binding of ^{3}H-GABA and ^{3}H-Glycine

Binding of ^{3}H-GABA, ^{3}H-glycine and their antagonists ^{3}H-bicuculline-methiodide (^{3}H-BCM) and ^{3}H-strychnine was studied in Na^+-containing (0 ^{0}C) and in Na^+-free incubation media (35 ^{0}C) at concentrations of 10^{-9} to 10^{-8}M. In cerebellar cultures, ^{3}H-GABA, its agonist ^{3}H-muscimol as well as ^{3}H-BCM were bound to many neurones such as Purkinje cells

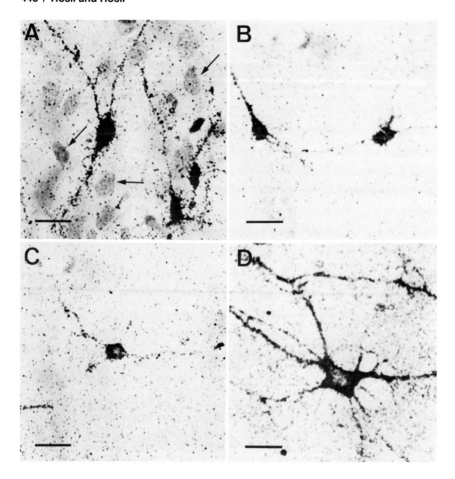

Fig. 5. A,B: Binding of ^{3}H-GABA (10^{-8}M, A) and ^{3}H-bicucul-
line-methiodide (10^{-8}M, B) to large cerebellar neurones,
probably Purkinje cells (culture 26 and 12 days in vitro
respectively). Note that glial cells (A, arrows) are almost
free of label (culture in A was counterstained with cresyl
violet). C: Medium-sized spinal neurone revealing binding
sites for ^{3}H-GABA (10^{-8}M, culture 18 days in vitro).
D: Large spinal neurone, probably a motoneurone, which is
intensely labelled by ^{3}H-glycine (10^{-8}M, culture 30 days in
vitro). Bars: 30 µm (A: from Hösli et al. 1981a; B,C: from
Hösli et al. 1980; D: from Hösli, Hösli 1981).

(Fig. 5A,B) and interneurones. The cell bodies of small neu-rones, presumably granule cells, were unlabelled but their processes and a great number of surrounding fibres showed intense labelling of ^{3}H-GABA and ^{3}H-BCM (Hösli et al. 1980). These findings are consistent with autoradiographic studies in cerebellar slices demonstrating a high density of label-ling with ^{3}H-GABA and ^{3}H-muscimol in the Purkinje cell layer and in the granule cell layer (Chan-Palay 1978; Palacios et al. 1980). ^{3}H-Flunitrazepam, a benzodiazepine known to inter-act with GABA mediated neurotransmission was also bound to many cerebellar Purkinje cells and interneurones (Hösli et al. 1980). In contrast, almost no binding of ^{3}H-glycine and ^{3}H-strychnine was observed. In spinal cord and brain stem cultures, however, a large number of neurones showed binding sites for both ^{3}H-glycine, ^{3}H-GABA and their antagonists. It appeared that in the spinal cord, mainly small to medium-sized neurones, presumably interneurones, were labelled by ^{3}H-GABA (Fig. 5C), ^{3}H-BCM and ^{3}H-flunitrazepam, whereas bin-ding sites for ^{3}H-glycine (Fig. 5D) and ^{3}H-strychnine were predominantly localized on large neurones, probably motoneu-rones (Hösli et al. 1980; Hösli, Hösli 1981). Binding of ^{3}H-GABA and ^{3}H-BCM was inhibited by adding unlabelled GABA and bicuculline (10^{-3}M); binding of ^{3}H-glycine and ^{3}H-strychnine was blocked by unlabelled glycine and strychnine (10^{-3}M).

b. Binding of the Glutamate Analogue ^{3}H-AMPA

Biochemical studies have shown that ^{3}H-AMPA binds to glutamate receptors without affecting the glutamate trans-port mechanism (Honoré et al. 1982). Our autoradiographic studies have demonstrated that in spinal cord and brain stem cultures, a large number of neurones of varying size and shape revealed binding of ^{3}H-AMPA. Binding sites could be localized on the cell bodies and processes of the neurones (Fig. 6A,B) (Hösli et al. 1983a). Our findings are consi-stent with biochemical binding studies which also show a high density of AMPA binding sites on membranes from rat pons and medulla (Honoré et al. 1982) and with electrophy-siological investigations demonstrating that AMPA is a po-tent excitant of spinal neurones (Krogsgaard-Larsen et al. 1982; Hösli et al. 1983b). Addition of unlabelled AMPA or L-glutamate (10^{-3}M) inhibited binding of ^{3}H-AMPA, whereas

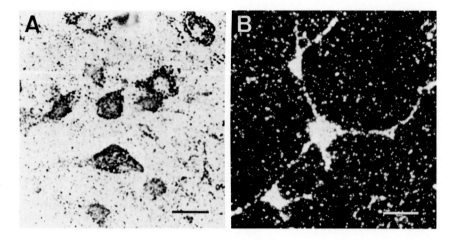

Fig. 6. A: Binding of ³H-AMPA (10⁻⁸M) to spinal neurones (culture 20 days in vitro). B: Dark field illumination micrograph of labelled brain stem neurones after incubation with ³H-AMPA (10⁻⁸M, culture 18 days in vitro). Bars: 30 µm (from Hösli et al. 1983a).

the glutamate antagonist GDEE markedly reduced but did not completely block binding of the radio-ligand. Our data suggest that ³H-AMPA binding sites have properties expected for glutamate receptors.

No binding sites for any of the amino acids and their antagonists studied were found on glial elements (Fig. 5A, arrows) (Hösli et al. 1980, 1981a, 1983a; Hösli, Hösli 1981). This finding is in agreement with biochemical binding studies demonstrating that ³H-GABA and ³H-muscimol were not bound to cultured astroblasts (Ossola et al. 1980). The lack of binding sites for the amino acid transmitters on glial cells agrees well with our electrophysiological findings (Hösli et al. 1981a,b,c).

UPTAKE OF ^{3}H-GABA AND L-^{3}H-GLUTAMIC ACID BY NEURONES AND
GLIAL CELLS

There is considerable evidence that specific high-affinity uptake systems are involved in terminating the action
of amino acid transmitters at central synapses (Hösli, Hösli
1978). By means of autoradiographic techniques we have studied the cellular localization of the uptake of ^{3}H-GABA and
L-^{3}H-glutamic acid in cultures of rat CNS. In cerebellar
cultures, many neurones showing morphological features of
Purkinje cells (Fig. 7A) but also interneurones were intensely labelled by ^{3}H-GABA (Hösli, Hösli 1976a). In brain stem
and spinal cord cultures, ^{3}H-GABA and L-^{3}H-glutamic acid
were accumulated by many neurones of all sizes (Hösli, Hösli
1976b, 1978). Some neurones showed a heavy accumulation of
the amino acids, whereas others seemed to be almost free of
label (Fig. 7B). Similar uptake patterns were observed with
glycine, β-alanine, taurine and aspartic acid (Hösli, Hösli
1976b, 1978). The uptake of the amino acids was Na$^+$- and
temperature-dependent, being considerably reduced after removal of Na$^+$ from the incubation medium or after incubation
at 0 ^{0}C (Hösli, Hösli 1976a,b, 1978).

Biochemical studies have shown that glial cells, too,
are able to accumulate amino acid transmitters by a high-
affinity transport mechanism (Schousboe 1981; Sellström,
Hamberger 1975). These findings as well as our autoradiographic investigations demonstrating that amino acid transmitters are taken up to a great extent by glial cells (Fig. 7C,
D) suggest that glial elements might also be involved in the
inactivation of these amino acids (Hertz 1979; Hösli, Hösli
1976a,b, 1978; Schousboe 1981).

SUMMARY

The effects of the amino acid transmitters GABA, glycine, glutamate and aspartate and their interactions with
antagonists have been studied on the membrane potential and
conductance of neurones of cultured rat CNS. GABA and glycine caused a hyperpolarization, whereas glutamate, aspartate and the glutamate analogue AMPA depolarized the neuronal
membrane, both effects being associated with an increase in
membrane conductance. Studies on ionic mechanisms underlying
the action of these amino acids were made by altering the

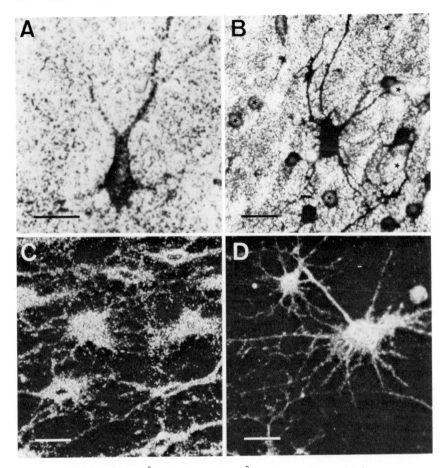

Fig. 7.   Uptake of ^{3}H-GABA and L-^{3}H-glutamic acid by neurones and glial cells.   A: Cerebellar culture after incubation
with ^{3}H-GABA (10^{-6}M). The soma and dendrites of the Purkinje
cell are intensely labelled (culture 17 days in vitro).
B: Spinal cord culture after incubation with L-^{3}H-glutamic
acid (10^{-6}M). Some neurones show a heavy accumulation of
silver grains over the cell bodies and processes; other neurones (*) are almost free of label (culture 18 days in vitro).
C,D: Dark field illumination micrograph of intensely labelled glial cells after incubation with ^{3}H-GABA (10^{-6}M, C) and
L-^{3}H-glutamic acid (10^{-6}M, D)   (C: cerebellar culture, 18
days in vitro; D: spinal cord culture, 28 days in vitro).
Bars: A: 20 µm; B,C,D: 30 µm (A and C: from Hösli, Hösli
1976a; B and D: from Hösli, Hösli 1976b).

ionic composition of the extracellular fluid (removal of Cl^- or Na^+) or by injecting Cl^- into the cells. Our findings suggest that the hyperpolarization by GABA and glycine is accompanied by an increase in Cl^--conductance, while the depolarization by glutamate and aspartate is mainly dependent on an increased Na^+-conductance. The inhibitory effects by GABA were antagonized by bicuculline, whereas the hyperpolarization by glycine was reversibly blocked by strychnine. The depolarizations by glutamate and AMPA were reversibly antagonized by the glutamate-antagonist GDEE but not by APV, a NMDA-antagonist, indicating that both compounds exert their effects by activating glutamate/quisqualate-preferring receptors.

Autoradiographic studies have shown binding of ^{3}H-AMPA, ^{3}H-GABA, ^{3}H-glycine and the antagonists ^{3}H-bicuculline and ^{3}H-strychnine to the soma and processes of many neurones in cultured rat CNS. However, no binding sites for these amino acid transmitters and their antagonists were found on glial cells. This is consistent with our electrophysiological observations indicating that unlike neurones, glial cells do not possess receptors for amino acid transmitters and that the glial depolarization by amino acids is an indirect effect due to the efflux of K^+ from adjacent neurones. Uptake of amino acids was observed into neurones as well as into glial cells, suggesting that glial elements might also be involved in the inactivation of amino acid transmitters.

REFERENCES

Barker JL, Ransom BR (1978). Amino acid pharmacology of mammalian central neurones grown in tissue culture. J Physiol (Lond) 280:331.

Chan-Palay V (1978). Autoradiographic localization of γ-aminobutyric acid receptors in the rat central nervous system by using [^{3}H]muscimol. Proc Natl Acad Sci USA 75:1024.

Curtis DR, Hösli L, Johnston GAR, Johnston IH (1968). The hyperpolarization of spinal motoneurones by glycine and related amino acids. Exp Brain Res 5:235.

Curtis DR, Johnston GAR (1974). Amino acid transmitters in the mammalian central nervous system. In Reviews of Physiology Vol LXIX, Berlin-Heidelberg-New York: Springer-Verlag, p 97.

Davies J, Evans RH, Jones AW, Smith DAS, Watkins JC (1982).
Differential activation and blockade of excitatory amino
acid receptors in the mammalian and amphibian central nervous systems. Comp Biochem Physiol 72C:211.

DeFeudis FV (1979). Binding and iontophoretic studies on
centrally active amino acids - a search for physiological
receptors. Int Rev Neurobiol 21:129.

Hertz L (1979). Functional interactions between neurons and
astrocytes. I. Turnover and metabolism of putative amino
acid transmitters. Progr Neurobiol 13:277.

Honoré T, Lauridsen J, Krogsgaard-Larsen P (1982).
The binding of (^{3}H)AMPA, a structural analogue of glutamic
acid, to rat brain membranes. J Neurochem 38:173.

Hösli E, Hösli L (1976a). Autoradiographic studies on the
uptake of ^{3}H-noradrenaline and ^{3}H-GABA in cultured rat
cerebellum. Exp Brain Res 26:319.

Hösli E, Hösli L (1976b). Uptake of L-glutamate and
L-aspartate in neurones and glial cells of cultured human
and rat spinal cord. Experientia 32:219.

Hösli E, Hösli L (1981). Binding of (^{3}H)glycine, (^{3}H)β-
alanine and (^{3}H)strychnine in cultured rat spinal cord
and brain stem. Brain Res 213:242.

Hösli E, Krogsgaard-Larsen P, Hösli L (1983a). Binding
sites for the glutamate-analogue ^{3}H-AMPA in cultured rat
brain stem and spinal cord. Brain Res 268:177.

Hösli E, Möhler H, Richards JG, Hösli L (1980).
Autoradiographic localization of binding sites for (^{3}H)γ-
aminobutyrate, (^{3}H)muscimol, (+)(^{3}H)bicuculline methiodide
and (^{3}H)flunitrazepam in cultures of rat cerebellum and
spinal cord. Neuroscience 5:1657.

Hösli L, Hösli E (1978). Action and uptake of neurotransmitters in CNS tissue culture. Rev Physiol Biochem Pharmacol 81:135.

Hösli L, Hösli E, Andrès PF, Landolt H (1981a). GABA and
glycine receptors in CNS cultures: autoradiographic
binding and electrophysiological studies. In DeFeudis FV
and Mandel P (eds): "Amino Acid Neurotransmitters",
New York: Raven Press, p 437.

Hösli L, Hösli E, Andrès PF, Landolt H (1981b). Evidence
that the depolarization of glial cells by inhibitory
amino acids is caused by an efflux of K$^+$ from neurones.
Exp Brain Res 42:43.

Hösli L, Hösli E, Landolt H, Zehntner C (1981c). Efflux of potassium from neurones excited by glutamate and aspartate causes a depolarization of cultured glial cells. Neurosci Lett 21:83.

Hösli L, Hösli E, Lehmann R, Eng P (1983b). Effects of the glutamate analogue AMPA and its interaction with antagonists on cultured rat spinal and brain stem neurones. Neurosci Lett 36:59.

Hösli L, Hösli E, Lehmann R, Schneider J, Borner M (1983c). Action of γ-hydroxybutyrate and GABA on neurones of cultured rat CNS. Neurosci Lett in press.

Krnjević K (1974). Chemical nature of synaptic transmission in vertebrates. Physiol Rev 54:418.

Krogsgaard-Larsen P, Hansen JJ, Lauridsen J, Peet MJ, Leah JD, Curtis DR (1982). Glutamic acid agonists. Stereochemical and conformational studies of DL-α-amino-3-hydroxy-5-methyl-4-isoxazolepropionic acid (AMPA) and related compounds. Neurosci Lett 31:313.

McLennan H, Liu J-R (1982). The action of six antagonists of the excitatory amino acids on neurones of the rat spinal cord. Exp Brain Res 45:151.

Nistri A, Constanti A (1979). Pharmacological characterization of different types of GABA and glutamate receptors in vertebrates and invertebrates. Progr Neurobiol 13:117.

Ossola L, DeFeudis FV, Mandel P (1980). Lack of Na^{+}-independent binding of (^{3}H)GABA or (^{3}H)muscimol to particulate fractions of cultured astroblasts. J Neurochem 34:1026.

Palacios JM, Young WS III, Kuhar MJ (1980). Autoradiographic localization of γ-aminobutyric acid (GABA) receptors in the rat cerebellum. Proc Natl Acad Sci USA 77:670.

Peet MJ, Malik R, Curtis DR (1983). Post-excitatory depression of neuronal firing by acidic amino acids and acetylcholine in the cat spinal cord. Brain Res 263:162.

Ransom BR, Nelson PG (1975). Neuropharmacological responses from nerve cells in tissue culture. In Iversen LL, Iversen SD, Snyder SH (eds): "Handbook of Psychopharmacology", Vol 2 Principles of Receptor Research, New York/London: Plenum Press, p 101.

Schousboe A (1981). Transport and metabolism of glutamate and GABA in neurons and glial cells. Int Rev Neurobiol 22:1.

Sellström Å, Hamberger A (1975). Neuronal and glial systems for γ-aminobutyric acid transport. J Neurochem 24:847.

Glutamine, Glutamate, and GABA
in the Central Nervous System, pages 457–472
© 1983 Alan R. Liss, Inc., 150 Fifth Avenue, New York, NY 10011

MECHANISMS OF GABA RELEASE

John C. Szerb

Department of Physiology and Biophysics
Dalhousie University
Halifax, N.S., Canada B3H 4H7

In the 1960's, as increasing evidence supporting the role of GABA as the main central inhibitory transmitter was gradually accumulating, several groups were looking for one of the essential requirements for demonstrating the transmitter role of GABA, namely for a depolarization induced Ca^{2+}-dependent release. In these experiments the then well known transmitters, acetylcholine and noradrenaline were used as models but it soon became apparent that the release of GABA induced under certain conditions behaved unlike that of acetylcholine or noradrenaline. For instance, release of GABA evoked by electrical stimulation (Srinivasan et al. 1969) or protoveratrine (Benjamin, Quastel 1972) was not dependent on extracellular Ca^{2+}; labelled GABA taken up not only by neurons but also by glia was released by elevated K^+ (Minchin, Iversen 1974) therefore questioning the source of GABA released from the whole brain or from brain slices. Furthermore, although a Na^+-dependent, high-affinity uptake of labelled GABA into neurons and glia could be demonstrated there was doubt whether this represented a net uptake or only a homoexchange of GABA (Levi, Raiteri 1974). The purpose of this article is to review more recent developments relating to the above controversies and to see whether they have been resolved. Since the methods of measuring released GABA have some bearing on the interpretation of data they will be first reviewed briefly.

A. METHODS OF MEASURING GABA RELEASE

In early studies the release of labelled GABA accumulated during preliminary incubation was measured by most workers (Srinivasan et al. 1969; Hammerstad et al. 1971; Okada, Hassler 1973; Orrego, Miranda 1976) and they all agreed that the high K^+-induced release of this exogenous labelled GABA was to a large extent Ca^{2+}-dependent. However, since exogenous labelled GABA is rapidly metabolized (Machiyama et al. 1970; Szerb 1982a) amino-oxyacetic acid (AOAA), an inhibitor of GABA-T, had to be present both during incubation with labelled GABA and while measuring release. The use of AOAA in these experiments introduced some uncertainty as to the origin of released labelled GABA because AOAA preserves accumulated labelled GABA not only in terminals, where GABA normally is formed, but also in glia whose GABA content is derived almost exclusively from the uptake of GABA (Hertz 1979).

To assure that released labelled GABA originated from terminals and not glia, a number of investigators measured the release of endogenously formed labelled GABA which should be stored preferentially at the site of its formation, namely in GABA-ergic terminals. In general, the Ca^{2+}-dependent, high K^+-induced release of labelled GABA taken up or synthesized endogenously were similar, regardless whether the precursor was [U-^{14}C] glucose (Minchin 1977; Potashner 1978b), glutamate (Minchin 1977; Szerb 1983), glutamine (Tapia, Gonzalez 1978; Reubi et al. 1978; Kemel et al. 1979) or pyruvate (Gauchy et al. 1977), although it was apparent that glutamine and pyruvate labelled releasable GABA stores more selectively than the other two precursors. In contrast, labelled acetate was a poorer precursor of GABA released by high K^+ and was ineffective in labelling GABA that was released by protoveratrine (Minchin 1977).

Neither was the Ca^{2+} dependence of high K^+-induced release markedly different when, instead of labelled GABA, the release of endogenous GABA was measured (Nadler et al. 1977; Szerb et al. 1981; Fan et al. 1982). However, high K^+ released somewhat larger fraction of exogenous labelled than of endogenous GABA from synaptosomes in the absence of Ca^{2+} (Haycock et al. 1978). Release of endogenous, unlike that of exogenous GABA evoked by electrical stimulation was reported by Valdes, Orrego (1978) to be Ca^{2+}-dependent in a biphasic way: it was reduced when the Ca^{2+} content was decreased from 1 to 0.1 mM but increased again when Ca^{2+} was totally eliminated. However, similar biphasic Ca^{2+}-dependence of electrically evoked release of exogenous labelled GABA can be seen (Birsel, Szerb 1980) or, when the stimulus parameters are carefully chosen, even total omission of Ca^{2+} can reduce electrically evoked release of exogenous labelled GABA by more than 60 per cent (Szerb 1979; Birsel, Szerb 1980). Thus, there does not appear to be a great deal of difference between the Ca^{2+}-dependence of electrically induced release of exogenous labelled or endogenous GABA. Similarly, the veratrum alkaloid-evoked Ca^{2+}-independent release of exogenous labelled GABA (Szerb 1979; Neal, Bowery 1979; Minchin 1980b; Cunningham, Neal 1981), of labelled GABA formed endogenously from glutamate (Szerb 1983) and of endogenous GABA (Benjamin, Quastel 1972; Szerb et al. 1981; Szerb 1983) is nearly indistinguishable.

As the above summary suggests that there is little difference between the compartments from which released GABA measured by different methods originates and other experimental strategies were required for the elucidation of the role of Ca^{2+} in GABA release. However, the method of measuring GABA release was important in demonstrating the role of uptake in limiting the overflow of released GABA. This will be discussed in Section D.

B. RELEASE INDUCED IN THE ABSENCE OF EXTRACELLULAR Ca^{2+}

a. Veratrum Alkaloids

Veratrum alkaloids are not the only agents that increase the release of GABA at least as much in the absence of Ca^{2+} as in its presence (Minchin 1980a) but so do ouabain (Benjamin, Quastel 1972; Sandoval 1980), K^+-free solution and quinidine (Sandoval 1980). Nor is GABA the only amino acid transmitter released by veratrum alkaloids and by the other conditions listed above in the absence of Ca^{2+}: the release of glutamate and aspartate behaves similarly (Benjamin, Quastel 1972; Nadler et al. 1977). Furthermore, in the absence of Ca^{2+} veratrum alkaloids cause a prolonged release of exogenous labelled noradrenaline from cortical slices (Schoffelmeer, Mulder

1983) and acetylcholine is released in the absence of Ca^{2+} by ouabain or by K^+-free media from cortical slices (Vizi 1972) and neuromuscular junction (Vizi, Vyskocil 1979).

In apparent contradiction to the above, there are a number of reports on the Ca^{2+} dependence of veratrum alkaloid-induced transmitter release. The likely reason for these different findings is the slower rate of release of transmitters evoked by veratrum alkaloids in the absence than in the presence of Ca^{2+}. For instance, the release of [^{3}H] noradrenaline induced by 10 min exposure to 5 µM veratrine reached its peak during the application of the drug in the presence of Ca^{2+}. In the absence of Ca^{2+} release was reduced to less than half during the same period but then doubled again during the following 10 min period when veratrine was no longer present (Schoffelmeer, Mulder 1983). Therefore measuring noradrenaline release only during the 10 min application of veratrine would show a partially Ca^{2+}-dependent, while over a longer period a Ca^{2+}-independent release. Indeed, a Ca^{2+}-dependent veratridine-induced release of noradrenaline measured over a 10 min period was reported by Blaustein et al. (1972) and for noradrenaline and acetylcholine by Cunningham, Neal (1981) who measured during a 4 min period. However, in the latter report labelled GABA release induced by veratridine measured during the same short time period was enhanced by an absence of Ca^{2+}, indicating that GABA was more readily released by veratridine in the absence of Ca^{2+} than the other transmitters.

There is a general agreement that the primary event in transmitter release induced by agents other than elevated K^+ is an increase in intracellular Na^+ either by the opening of regenerative Na^+ channels, in case of veratrum alkaloids, or by inhibition of the Na^+-pump in case of ouabain or K^+-free medium. There is, however, disagreement as to the mechanism whereby this elevated intracellular Na^+ leads to GABA release in the absence of extracellular Ca^{2+}. Sandoval (1980), Cunningham, Neal (1981) and Schoffelmeer, Mulder (1983) proposed that the elevation of intracellular Na^+ results in the release of Ca^{2+} and this internally released Ca^{2+} is responsible for transmitter release. This conclusion is based on the following observations: since preincubation with the neuronal GABA transport inhibitor DABA does not reduce veratrum alkaloid-induced release in the absence of Ca^{2+} but inhibits GABA homoexchange, carrier mediated outward transport is not involved in veratrum alkaloid-induced release in the absence of Ca^{2+} (Sandoval 1980; Cunningham, Neal 1981); ruthenium red, an inhibitor of mitochondrial Ca^{2+} uptake, increases both the spontaneous and veratrum alkaloid-induced release of GABA in the absence of Ca^{2+} but nearly abolishes that induced by high K^+ in the presence of Ca^{2+} (Cunningham, Neal 1981; Schoffelmeer, Mulder 1983). This intracellular Ca^{2+} mobilization hypothesis therefore implies that the transmitter released in the presence or absence of extracellular Ca^{2+} originates from the same source but the Ca^{2+} required for release can either enter from the outside or can be released from intracellular sites.

On the other hand, Szerb (1979) and Szerb et al. (1981) suggested that GABA released by veratridine in the absence of Ca^{2+} originates from a different compartment than that released by high K^+ or veratridine in the presence of Ca^{2+}. This conclusion was based on the following observations: a prolonged (48 min) exposure to 50 mM K^+ in the presence of Ca^{2+} depletes the pool of exogenous [^{3}H] GABA from which the Ca^{2+}-dependent high K^+-induced release originates because a second exposure to 50 mM K^+ and Ca^{2+} releases less than 1/4 of that released by the first exposure. Release by veratridine in the presence of Ca^{2+} is reduced to the same extent by a preliminary exposure to 50 mM K^+ and Ca^{2+}. However, the same preliminary exposure decreases the release induced by veratridine in the absence of Ca^{2+} only by 30%, suggesting that the compartment of [^{3}H] GABA released in the presence of Ca^{2+} by high K^+ or veratridine and that released in the absence of Ca^{2+} by veratridine are largely different (Szerb 1979). The size of the compartments of endogenous and exogenous [^{3}H] GABA was analyzed kinetically by Szerb et al. (1981). In the presence of AOAA, which blocked both the synthesis and breakdown of GABA, 50 mM K^+ in the presence of Ca^{2+} depleted endogenous GABA from a pool which was only 10% and [^{3}H] GABA from a pool which was only 25% of the total present initially. In contrast to the release evoked by 50 mM K^+ and Ca^{2+}, which declined at a constant rate over a 48 min period, release induced by veratridine, especially in the absence of Ca^{2+}, declined at two distinct rates: an initial fast rate lasting about 20 min and a later very slow rate which lasted for at least 120 min. The specific activity of GABA released by veratridine in the absence of Ca^{2+} was initially just as high as that released by high K^+ and Ca^{2+} but during the very slow phase it was only 50% of the initial specific activity (Szerb et al. 1981).

The conclusion of Sandoval (1980), Cunningham, Neal (1981), Schoffelmeer, Mulder (1983) that veratrum alkaloids-induced Ca^{2+}-independent release is due to the mobilization of stored Ca^{2+} and that of Szerb (1979) and Szerb et al. (1981) that this release originates from a compartment different from that giving rise to a Ca^{2+}-dependent release probably refer to two phases of release. The first group of workers measured the effect of drugs such as DABA and ruthenium red on veratrum alkaloid-induced release during a short (1.5 - 10 min) stimulation period while measurement of release from different compartments involved prolonged (48 min) periods of stimulation. Indeed, the two types of experiments show a remarkable agreement when the two phases of release are considered separately. The initial fast release induced by veratridine in the absence of Ca^{2+}, but not the late slow release, was reduced by the depletion of Ca^{2+}-dependent pool by high K^+ (Szerb 1979). The specific activity of GABA released by veratridine in the absence of Ca^{2+} was initially just as high as that released by high K^+ in the presence of Ca^{2+} (Szerb et al, 1981), indicating that veratridine in the absence of Ca^{2+} could have released initially GABA from the same compartment as high K^+ in the presence of Ca^{2+}. In conclusion, therefore the release of transmitters induced by veratrum alkaloids in the absence of Ca^{2+} involves probably an initial mobilization of stored Ca^{2+} and a slow release from a compartment different from that mobilized by high K^+ in the presence of Ca^{2+}.

The physiological significance of release induced in the absence of extracellular Ca^{2+} is uncertain. However, processes involved in GABA release may not always require Ca^{2+} but may be mediated by carriers as was shown recently in the goldfish retina by Yazulla, Kleinschmidt (1983). Release of transmitters from different compartments may also have different postsynaptic effects as illustrated by the observation of Vizi, Vyskocil (1979) on the mouse phrenic nerve-diaphragm preparation in which the release of acetylcholine and its postjunctional effects on miniature end plate potentials were monitored simultaneously. Ouabain released acetylcholine both in the presence and absence of Ca^{2+} but while release evoked in the presence of

Ca^{2+} caused a large increase in end plate potential frequency, the almost identical release produced in the absence of Ca^{2+} had no postjunctional effect. This suggests that the Ca^{2+}-independent release originated at a different site from that giving rise to the Ca^{2+}-dependent release. In case of GABA, however, evidence suggests that both the Ca^{2+}-dependent and independent release induced by veratrum alkaloids come from neurons and not from glia (Minchin 1980a). Evidence derived from compartmental analysis supports this view because the presumed small GABA content of glia cannot explain the very much larger Ca^{2+}-independent pool observed.

b. Electrical Stimulation

Early reports indicated that electrical stimulation also released exogenous labelled GABA in a Ca^{2+}-independent manner (Srinivasan et al. 1969; Orrego, Miranda 1976) and that TTX did not reduce this release (Hammerstad, Cutler 1972). In these studies high frequency (80 - 100 Hz) and rather high intensity stimulation had to be employed to obtain release and no precautions were taken to avoid either the polarization of electrodes, which results in changes in pH, or the overheating of the bath (Srinivasan et al. 1969). The absence of a Ca^{2+}-requirement of the electrically induced GABA release was in contrast with the absolute Ca^{2+}-dependence of electrically evoked release of labelled acetylcholine (Somogyi, Szerb 1972; Birsel, Szerb 1980) and of noradrenaline (Taube et al. 1977) which could be obtained at low frequencies (1 - 4 Hz) of stimulation. When in later reports care was taken to avoid polarization of electrodes by applying symmetrical sine wave stimulation (Valdes, Orrego 1978) or biphasic rectangular pulses (Potashner 1978a) suppression by TTX (Potashner 1978b) and partial Ca^{2+}-dependence of electrically evoked release (Valdes, Orrego 1978; Potashner 1978b) could be obtained. Furthermore, it could be shown (Birsel, Szerb 1980) that high frequency (64 Hz) non-polarizing stimulation applied at $37^{\circ}C$ causes damage to the slices by overheating which results in an increased Ca^{2+}-independent and reduced Ca^{2+}-dependent release. This could be avoided by reducing the temperature of the bath to $32^{\circ}C$.

The Ca^{2+}-independent release induced by electrical stimulation and by veratrine alkaloids appears to be related: transmitters, such as acetylcholine and noradrenaline, which are released by electrical stimulation in a clearly Ca^{2+}-dependent manner are released by veratrine alkaloids only to a limited extent in the absence of Ca^{2+}, while GABA and other transmitter amino acids whose release by veratrine alkaloids is much more pronounced in the absence of Ca^{2+}, are released by electrical stimulation much more readily in the absence of Ca^{2+}. Indeed, as was shown by Szerb (1979), the Ca^{2+}-independent release of GABA induced by electrical stimulation is decreased much less by previous depletion of the Ca^{2+}-dependent pool than is the release in the presence of Ca^{2+}, indicating that, similarly to veratridine, electrical stimulation releases GABA from at least partly different compartments in the presence or absence of Ca^{2+}. A comparison of the kinetics of the Ca^{2+}-dependent and independent release processes of various transmitters may shed more light on the compartmentalization of transmitters in relation to their release.

C. NEURONAL VERSUS GLIAL ORIGIN OF DEPOLARIZATION-INDUCED GABA RELEASE

It is now well established that central and peripheral neuroglia possess a GABA transport mechanism which may be as effective as the neuronal uptake system (Hertz 1979). Therefore, exogenous labelled GABA will accumulate not only in neurons but also in glia, especially in larger slices (Riddall et al. 1976). Over the past number of years considerable controversy developed over the contribution of GABA located in glia to the depolarization induced release. Firstly, there was disagreement whether depolarization releases GABA at all from glia and secondly, whether such a release, when observed, is Ca^{2+}-dependent or not. Since in most preparations release occurs probably not entirely from either neurons or glia, the most useful observations are those in which release from preparations containing predominately one or the other element are compared quantitatively. Such studies show that release of GABA from glia by high K^+ proceeds at a slower rate and requires higher concentration of K^+ than release from neurons and this glial release is reduced to a much lesser extent by removing Ca^{2+} and adding Mg^{2+} than release from neurons. These conclusions were reached by Neal, Bowery (1979) from a comparison of neuronal GABA release from cortical slices and frog retina and glial release from spinal and sympathetic ganglia and rat retina; by Bowery et al. (1979) from a comparison of glial GABA and neuronal acetylcholine release in sympathetic ganglia; by Sellstrom, Hamberger (1977) from a comparison between bulk-isolated glia, neuronal perikarya and synaptosomes and by Pearce et al. (1981) by comparing release from cultured dissociated cerebellar neurons and astrocytes.

On the other hand, Minchin, Iversen (1974) found a four fold increase in the release of [^{3}H] GABA by high K^+ from glia in rat dorsal root ganglia which was depressed moderately (by 48%) in a Ca^{2+}-free, high Mg^{2+} medium. However, this release was not inhibited by the Ca^{2+} channel blockers lanthanum and D-600 (Minchin, 1975). Roberts (1974), while finding a similar Ca^{2+}-dependent high K^+-evoked release of exogenous [^{3}H] GABA from dorsal root ganglia, did not observe any increase in endogenous GABA efflux with high K^+. Minchin, Nordmann (1975) reported that the high K^+ induced release of [^{3}H] GABA from the posterior pituitary was depressed 50% by the omission of Ca^{2+} and even electrical stimulation was effective in evoking release. They assumed that, since there was no known function of GABA in the posterior pituitary, GABA must have been taken up into and released from glia. However, recent evidence (Tomiko et al. 1983) indicates that GABA acts as a transmitter in the pars intermedia and therefore some of the labelled GABA released may have come from nerve terminals.

In support of the neuronal origin of high K^+-induced release of [^{3}H] GABA Hammerstad, Lytle (1976) observed that in brain slices DABA, which releases exogenous GABA preferentially from neurons, abolished the high K^+-induced release, while β-alanine, which primarily exchanges with glial GABA, did not. In subsequent experiments on synaptosomes, however, Hammerstad et al. (1979) found that neither DABA nor β-alanine interfered with high K^+ or protoveratrine-induced GABA release. However, high K^+ increased the release of [^{3}H] GABA much less from synaptosomes than from slices and it is possible that the fraction of [^{3}H] GABA releasable by high K^+ which exchanges with DABA was not present in the synaptosomes. Recently Jaffe, Cuello (1981) compared release of [^{3}H] GABA from the microdissected olfactory nerve layer containing mostly glia and from the external plexiform layer containing GABA-ergic terminals in the denervated rat olfactory bulb. High K^+ increased release more than twice as much from the layer containing nerve terminals than from the glia layer. Release from glia was partly Ca^{2+}-dependent but not inhibited by D-600, while release from neurons was very sensitive to this Ca^{2+} channel blocker.

In summary, it appears that there is a quantitative difference between neuronal and glial GABA release induced by high K^+: neuronal release is always more vigorous and its Ca^{2+}-dependence is more pronounced than of glial release. However, there is an absolute difference between glia and neurons in their sensitivity to Ca^{2+} channel blockers which suggests that release from the two sources occurs through different mechanisms. Although in vivo glia may normally contain significant amounts of GABA (Hertz 1979) it releases GABA less readily than do neurons. Therefore it is unlikely that glial GABA release should have a neuromodulatory role (Bowery et al. 1979). However, in vivo treatment with GABA-T inhibitors may increase glial GABA content to such an extent that a Ca^{2+}-independent release of GABA from glia may become significant (Szerb 1982a).

D. INACTIVATION OF RELEASED GABA BY UPTAKE

After the initial description of high affinity labelled GABA uptake into terminals by Neal, Iversen (1969) and into glia by Bowery, Brown (1972) it was assumed that these mechanisms were responsible for the removal of released GABA from the synaptic cleft. This assumption was questioned by Levi, Raiteri (1974) who showed that synaptosomes exchange extracellular labelled GABA with endogenous GABA without a net change in extracellular GABA concentration. As summarized by Levi et al. (1978) this exchange is carrier-mediated and extracellular GABA, up to 25 μM, not only is not removed by the synaptosomes but it enhances GABA release induced by several methods, except that evoked by high K^+. Later on other workers, however, were able to demonstrate net GABA uptake by synaptosomes which were either depleted of their endogenous GABA content by prior incubation in high K^+ (Ryan, Roskoski 1977) or which were prepared by an improved method which maintained their membrane potential (Pastuszko et al. 1981).

An alternative method to show the role of uptake in terminating the effect of released GABA, namely by observing an increased overflow in the presence of a transport inhibitor, has not been successful either up to very recently. Although a number of inhibitors of neuronal and glial transport are known, all of them are taken up by the processes they inhibit and by heteroexchange they release GABA from intracellular sites (Johnston et al. 1976; Bowery et al. 1976), especially exogenous labelled GABA (Szerb 1982b). This depletion of exogenous labelled GABA by specific inhibitors of neuronal or glial transport systems has been used to identify the sources of depolarization-induced labelled GABA release (Hammerstad, Lytle 1976; Jaffe, Cuello 1981). Thus, GABA transport inhibitors have been found to inhibit, not to potentiate the depolarization-induced overflow of exogenous GABA, opposite to what one could expect if transport was involved in the inactivation of released GABA.

However, an increase in the depolarization-induced overflow of GABA from slices by a transport inhibitor, nipecotic acid, could be readily demonstrated when instead of exogenous, endogenous GABA release was measured (Szerb 1982b). In the presence of nipecotic acid high K^+-induced overflow was increased nearly four fold. This increased overflow was as Ca^{2+}-dependent as that in the absence of nipecotic acid, suggesting that under both conditions released GABA originated from nerve terminals. Similarly, overflow of endogenous GABA induced by electrical stimulation was greatly potentiated by nipecotic acid. In contrast, the overflow of exogenous [^{3}H] GABA induced by high K^+ was increased only two fold and that by electrical stimulation hardly at all. It appears therefore that measuring the release of endogenous GABA is the ideal method to demonstrate the role of uptake in the inactivation of synaptically released GABA because endogenous GABA is released less by the transport inhibitor than is exogenous GABA and released endogenous, unlike exogenous GABA, can be replaced by synthesis. The role of uptake in the termination of synaptically released GABA could also be demonstrated electrophysiologically in the hippocampal dentate gyrus (Matthews et al. 1981).

In summary, recent results suggest more strongly than the earlier ones that the mechanisms involved in GABA release are indeed those that could be expected if GABA was a transmitter: there is a compartment of GABA, although a small one, from which release is Ca^{2+}-dependent, glia contributes only little to the depolarization-induced release and uptake is the most important mechanism of inactivation of synaptically released GABA. A large compartment, comprising nearly 90% of that present, is not released in a Ca^{2+}-dependent manner. The presence of this compartment contributed probably to the early difficulties in obtaining a Ca^{2+}-dependent release. Establishing the role of the large Ca^{2+}-independent compartment is probably the greatest remaining challenge in the field of GABA release.

References

Benjamin AM, Quastel JH (1972). Location of amino acids in brain slices from the rat. Tetrodotoxin-sensitive release of amino acids. Biochem J 128:631.

Birsel S, Szerb JC (1980). Factors influencing the release of labelled γ-aminobutyric acid and acetylcholine evoked by electrical stimulation with alternating polarity from rat cortical slices. Can J Physiol Pharmac 58:1158.

Blaustein MD, Johnson EM, Needleman P (1972). Calcium-dependent norepinephrine release from presynaptic nerve endings in vitro. Proc Nat Acad Sci USA 69:2237.

Bowery NG, Brown DA (1972). γ-aminobutyric acid uptake by sympathetic ganglia. Nature New Biol 238:89.

Bowery NG, Brown DA, Marsh S (1979). γ-aminobutyric acid efflux from sympathetic glial cells: effect of "depolarizing" agents. J Physiol (Lond) 293:75.

Bowery NG, Jones GP, Neal MJ (1976). Selective inhibition of neuronal GABA uptake by cis-1,3-aminocyclohexane carboxylic acid. Nature 264:281.

Cunningham J, Neal MJ (1981). On the mechanism by which veratridine causes a calcium-independent release of γ-aminobutyric acid from brain slices. Br J Pharmac 73:655.

Fan SG, Lee CM, Assaf SY, Iversen LL (1982). Endogenous GABA release from slices of rat cerebral cortex and hippocampus in vitro. Brain Res 235:265.

Gauchy CM, Iversen LL, Jessell TM (1977). The spontaneous and evoked release of newly synthesized [^{14}C] GABA from rat cerebral cortex, in vitro. Brain Res 138:374.

Hammerstad JP, Cawthon ML, Lytle CR (1979). Release of [^{3}H] GABA from in vitro preparations: comparison of the effect of DABA and β-alanine on the K^+ and protoveratrine stimulated release of [^{3}H] GABA from brain slices and synaptosomes. J Neurochem 32:195.

Hammerstad JP, Cutler RWP (1972). Sodium ion movements and the spontaneous and electrically stimulated release of [^{3}H] GABA and [^{14}C] glutamic acid from rat cortical slices. Brain Res 47:401.

Hammerstad JP, Lytle CR (1976). Release of [^{3}H] GABA from rat cortical slices: neuronal vs glial origin. J Neurochem 27:399.

Hammerstad JP, Murray JE, Cutler RWP (1971). Efflux of amino acid neurotransmitters from rat spinal cord slices. II. Factors influencing the electrically induced efflux of [^{14}C] glycine and [^{3}H] GABA. Brain Res 35:357.

Hertz L (1979). Functional interactions between neurons and astrocytes. I. Turnover and metabolism of putative amino acid transmitters. Progr Neurobiol 13:277.

Hycock JW, Levy WB, Denner LA, Cotman CW (1978). Effects of elevated [K^+]$_o$ on the release of neurotransmitters from cortical synaptosomes: efflux or secretion? J Neurochem 30:1113.

Jaffe EH, Cuello AC (1981). Neuronal and glial release of [^{3}H] GABA from the rat olfactory bulb. J Neurochem 37:1457.

Johnston GAR, Staphanson AL, Twitchin B (1976). Uptake and release of nipecotic acid by rat brain slices. J Neurochem 26:83.

Kemel ML, Gauchy C, Glowinski J, Besson MJ (1979). Spontaneous and potassium-evoked release of ^{3}H-GABA newly synthesized from ^{3}H-glutamine in slices of the rat substantia nigra. Life Sci 24:2139.

Levi G, Banay-Schwartz M, Raiteri M (1978). Uptake, exchange and release of GABA in isolated nerve endings. In Fonnum F (ed): "Amino Acids as Chemical Transmitters", New York: Plenum Press, p 327.

Levi G, Raiteri M (1974). Exchange of neurotransmitter amino acid at nerve endings can simulate high affinity uptake. Nature 250:735.

Machiyama Y, Balazs R, Hammond BJ, Julian T, Richter D (1970). The metabolism of γ-aminobutyrate and glucose in potassium ion-stimulated brain tissue in vitro. Biochem J 116:469.

Matthews WD, McCafferty GP, Setler PE (1981). An electrophysiological model of GABA-mediated neurotransmission. Neuropharmacology 20:561.

Minchin MCW (1975). Factors influencing the efflux of [³H] gamma-aminobutyric acid from satellite glial cells in rat sensory ganglia. J Neurochem 24:571.

Minchin MCW (1977). The release of amino acids synthesised from various compartmented precursors in rat spinal cord slices. Exp Brain Res 29:515.

Minchin MCW (1980a). Veratrum alkaloids as transmitter-releasing agents. J Neurosci Meth 2:111.

Minchin MCW (1980b). The role of Ca^{2+} in the protoveratrine-induced release of γ-aminobutyrate from brain slices. Biochem J 190:333.

Minchin MCW, Iversen LL (1974). Release of [³H] gamma-aminobutyric acid from glial cells in rat dorsal root ganglia. J Neurochem. 23:533.

Minchin MCW, Nordmann JJ (1975). The release of [³H] gamma-aminobutyric acid and neurophysin from the isolated rat posterior pituitary. Brain Res 90:75.

Nadler JV, White WF, Vaca KW, Redburn DA, Cotman CW (1977). Characterization of putative amino acid transmitter release from slices of rat dentate gyrus. J Neurochem 29:279.

Neal MJ, Bowery NG (1979). Differential effects of veratridine and potassium depolarization on neuronal and glial GABA release. Brain Res 167:337.

Neal MJ, Iversen LL (1969). Subcellular distribution of endogenous and [³H] γ-aminobutyric acid in rat cerebral cortex. J Neurochem 16:1245.

Okada Y, Hassler R (1973). Uptake and release of γ-aminobutyric acid (GABA) in slices of substantia nigra of rat. Brain Res 49:214.

Orrego F, Miranda R (1976). Electrically induced release of [³H] GABA from neocortical thin slices. Effects of stimulus waveform and of amino-oxyacetic acid. J Neurochem 26:1033.

Pastuszko A, Wilson DF, Erecinska M (1981). Net uptake of γ-aminobutyric acid by a high-affinity system of rat brain synaptosomes. Proc Nat Acad Sci USA 78:1242.

Pearce BR, Currie DN, Beale R, Dutton GR (1981). Potassium stimulated, calcium dependent release of [³H] GABA from neuron- and glia-enriched cultures of cells dissociated from rat cerebellum. Brain Res 206:485.

Potashner SJ (1978a). The spontaneous and electrically evoked release, from slices of guinea-pig cerebral cortex, of endogenous amino acids labelled via metabolism of D[U-¹⁴C] glucose. J Neurochem 31:177.

Potashner SJ (1978b). Effects of tetrodotoxin, calcium and magnesium on the release of amino acids from slices of guinea-pig cerebral cortex. J Neurochem 31:187.

Reubi J-C, van der Berg C, Cuenod M (1978). Glutamine as precursor for the GABA and glutamate transmitter pools. Neurosci Lett 10:171.

Roberts PJ (1974). Amino acid release from isolated rat dorsal root ganglia. Brain Res 74:327.

Ryan LD, Roskoski R Jr (1977). Net uptake of γ-aminobutyric acid by a high affinity synaptosomal transport system. J Pharm Exp Ther 200:285.

Sandoval ME (1980). Sodium-dependent efflux of [^{3}H] GABA from synaptosomes probably related to mitochondrial calcium mobilization. J Neurochem 35:915.

Schoffelmeer ANM, Mulder AH (1983). [^{3}H] Noradrenaline release from brain slices induced by an increase in the intracellular sodium concentration: role of intracellular calcium stores. J Neurochem 40:615.

Sellstrom A, Hamberger A (1977). Potassium-stimulated γ-aminobutyric acid release from neurons and glia. Brain Res 119:189.

Somogyi GT, Szerb JC (1972). Demonstration of acetylcholine release by measuring efflux of labelled choline from cerebral cortical slices. J. Neurochem 19:2667.

Srinivasan V, Neal MJ, Mitchell JF (1969). The effect of electrical stimulation and high potassium concentrations on the efflux of [^{3}H] γ-aminobutyric acid from brain slices. J Neurochem 16:1235.

Szerb JC (1979). Relationship between Ca^{2+}-dependent and independent release of [^{3}H] GABA evoked by high K^+, veratridine or electrical stimulation from rat cortical slices. J Neurochem 32:1565.

Szerb JC (1982a). Turnover and release of GABA in rat cortical slices: effect of a GABA-T inhibitor, gabaculine. Neurochem Res 7:191.

Szerb JC (1982b). Effect of nipecotic acid, γ-aminobutyric acid transport inhibitor, on the turnover and release of γ-aminobutyric acid in rat cortical slices. J Neurochem 39:850.

Szerb JC (1983). The release of [^{3}H] GABA formed from [^{3}H] glutamate in rat hippocampal slices: comparison with endogenous and exogenous labelled GABA. Neurochem Res 8:341.

Szerb JC, Ross TE, Gurevich L (1981). Compartments of labelled and endogenous γ-aminobutyric acid giving rise to release evoked by potassium or veratridine in rat cortical slices. J Neurochem 37:1186.

Tapia R, Gonzalez RM (1978). Glutamine and glutamate as precursors of the releasable pool of GABA in brain cortex slices. Neurosci Lett 10:165.

Taube HD, Starke K, Borowski E (1977). Presynaptic receptor systems on the noradrenergic neurones of rat brain. Naunyn-Schmiederg's Arch Pharmac 299:123.

Tomiko SA, Taraskevich PS, Douglas WW (1983). GABA acts directly on cells of pituitary pars intermedia to alter hormone output. Nature 301:706.

Valdes F, Orrego F (1978). Electrically induced, calcium-dependent release of endogenous GABA from rat brain cortex slices. Brain Res 141:357.

Vizi ES (1972). Stimulation, by inhibition of $(Na^+-K^+-Mg^{2+})$-activated ATP-ase, of acetylcholine release in cortical slices from rat brain. J Physiol (Lond) 226:95.

Vizi ES, Vyskocil F (1979). Changes in total and quantal release of acetylcholine in the mouse diaphragm during activation and inhibition of membrane ATPase. J Physiol (Lond) 286:1.

Yazulla S, Kleinschmidt J (1983). Carrier-mediated release of GABA from retinal horizontal cells. Brain Res 263:63.

Glutamine, Glutamate, and GABA
in the Central Nervous System, pages 473–492
© 1983 Alan R. Liss, Inc., 150 Fifth Avenue, New York, NY 10011

EXTRACELLULAR GABA, GLUTAMATE AND GLUTAMINE IN VIVO -
PERFUSION-DIALYSIS OF THE RABBIT HIPPOCAMPUS

Anders Hamberger, Claes-Henric Berthold*, Birgitta
Karlsson, Anders Lehmann and Britta Nyström

Institute of Neurobiology and Department of Anatomy*,
University of Göteborg, P.O.B. 33 031, S-400 33
Göteborg, Sweden

The increasing orientation of neurochemistry towards
the physiology and pharmacology of the nervous system
certainly is a catalyst to the understanding of integrated
functions. Inherent drawbacks of the biochemical approach
are unfortunately often relatively low precision, poor
availability for dynamic studies and the frequent need of
elaborate models or subfractionation schemes. The communication channel between brain cells, the extracellular
space is, however, relatively atraumatically available,
and is suitable for continuous biochemical monitoring of
events from living animals.

The development of probes suitable to withdraw minute
fluid samples from and/or apply test agents to defined CNS
regions largely without interfering with the normal activities of the awake and unrestrained animal began 20-30
years ago. The recent availability of analysis techniques
having the sensitivity necessary for the small amounts of
endogenous compounds has considerably widened the potential of this approach. Such methods include, in addition
to cyclic voltammetry, the push-pull cannula (Gaddum,
1961), the cortical cup (McIntosh and Oborin, 1953; Dodd
et al., 1974), chemitrodes and dialytrodes (Delgado et
al., 1972; Myers, 1974; Kovacs et al., 1976) and dialysis
tubes (Ungerstedt et al., 1982; Hamberger et al., 1982).
The aim of this report is to gather available experience
on brain perfusion-dialysis, particularly with respect to
the metabolic relationships of glutamine, glutamate and
GABA.

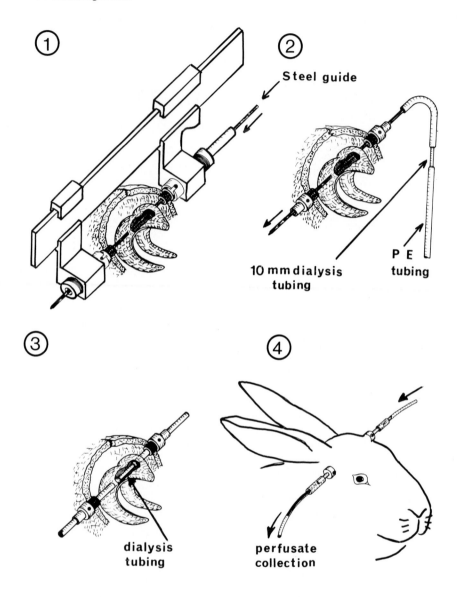

Fig. 1 Implantation of dialysis tube in the rabbit hippocampus, 1) Insertion of steel guide, 2) Attachment of tube arrangement, 3) Dialysis tube pulled into desired position within the hippocampus, 4) The animal in perfusion experiments.

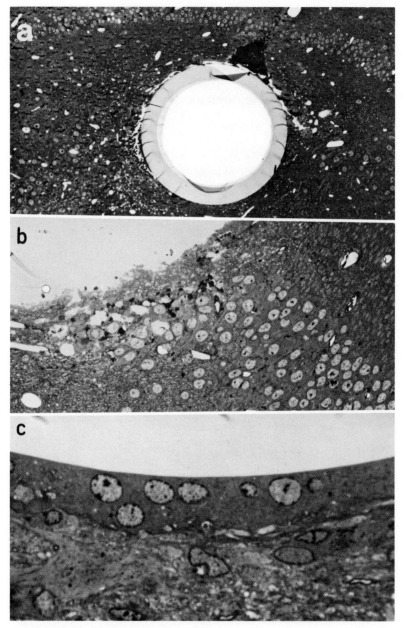

Fig. 2 Dialysis tube in hippocampus. (a) Low power survey 3 days, x140, (b) Segment of tissue lining, 1 day, x400, (c) Segment of tissue lining, 12 days, x500.

The dialysis tube

The dialysis tube technique applied to studies of the rabbit hippocampus (Hamberger et al., 1982; Lehmann et al., 1983) involves the permanent implantation (Fig. 1) of an approximately 10 mm long tube (Cuprophan B4AH, o.d. 0.34 mm, i.d. 0.28 mm, mol.weight cut off 3000). The tube is routinely perfused at 2.5 μ l/min with Krebs-Ringer bicarbonate buffer via polyethylene and silicone tube in- and outlets which are sealed between experiments. The surgery is done under sterile conditions and the animals are given chlormycetin (50 mg x 2 i.v., twice daily) which turned out to be necessary in chronic experiments, judged by routine bacteriological examinations. The tissue reaction around the tube was followed histologically for two weeks (Fig. 2). The tube was mostly lost during sectioning of the perfusion fixed hippocampus. Macroscopically, occa- sional slight bleeding could be observed. The tissue lin- ing towards the lumen was slightly uneven during the first two days, but became smooth and evenly "endothelialized" by the third day. Occasional monocytes were observed in addition to some extravasated erythrocytes during the first 2-3 days after implantation. The peritubular tissue (a 50 μm wide zone) showed intra- and extracellular oedema during the first two days but neurons and neuropil appear- ed intact otherwise. A 50-70 μm thick "collar" of mainly monocytes developed around the tube during days 3 to 7. This envelope thinned out with time and at day 12, apparently intact neuropil was seen 20 - 30 μ m from the tube. An increased vascularization was evident in the area around the tube after a few days, the vessels sometimes being lined by monocytes of the same appearance as those surrounding the tube. A several hundred μm wide region outside the non-neuronal cells exhibited pronounced gliosis at 5 and 12 days, as revealed by GFA and S-100 immunoreactivity.

To obtain an estimate of the diffusion of small mole- cules in the hippocampal tissue, the dialysis tube was perfused with radiolabelled leucine, glutamine or glucose and then rinsed with non-labelled medium. The brain was perfusion-fixed with glutaraldehyde and strips approxi- mately 1x1x10 mm were sectioned for measurements (Fig. 3). The distribution profiles showed that glucose and gluta- mine radioactivity was high in a cylinder with a radius exceeding that of the tube by 4-500 μ m , while leucine

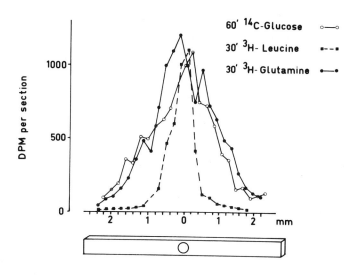

Fig. 3 Distribution of radioactivity in adjacent hippocampal tissue after perfusion with radiolabelled glucose, leucine and glutamine.

radioactivity decreased considerably 100 - 200 μm from the
tube. Although not conclusive, the results indicate that
transport properties of neuronal and glial cells influence
the extent of penetration of an applied test substance.

Some basic properties of the dialysis tube were
examined in vitro. The transport of amino acids at physiological concentrations was studied as a function of the
rate of perfusion of KRB buffer through the tube which was
immersed in a beaker containing the amino acid mixture
(Table 1). Initially, recovery (concentration in
perfusate-dialysate/concentration in outer medium x 100)
and net inflow (recovery x vol/min) was recorded. The
recovery is linearly related to the length of the tube in
the 4 - 20 mm range and independent of external amino acid
concentration in the range 10^{-6} - 10^{-3} M. In an
approximately 10 mm long tube the recovery was close to 50
per cent at a perfusion rate of one μl/min and decreased
to approximately one per cent at 200 μl/min. Net transport
increased somewhat with increasing perfusion rate. The
factors varied to some extent among amino acids. Finally,
small difference was seen when KRB buffer was compared

TABLE 1

TRANSPORT CHARACTERISTICS – CUPROPHAN B4AH DIALYSIS TUBE (o.d. 0.3 mm, length 10 mm)
Recovery (dialysate/medium x 100) and net inflow (recovery x vol/min) at different perfusion rates assayed in vitro. Net inflow at 2.5 µl/min set to 100.

AMINO ACID	RECOVERY				NET INFLOW			
	Perfusion rate (µl/min)				Perfusion rate (µl/min)			
	1	2.5	20	200	1	2.5	20	200
ASN	54	22	4	1	100	100	150	250
GLU	57	21	9	5	100	100	360	1400
GLN	52	21	3	0.4	100	100	130	100
TAU	61	33	4	0.8	80	100	120	150
ALA	59	26	5	1.6	90	100	160	370
VAL	48	20	3	0.7	100	100	150	220
PHE	39	19	3	0.5	100	100	150	170
ILEU	41	17	4	0.8	100	100	170	300
LEU	40	17	4	0.5	100	100	150	200

with CSF.

The increase of net flow with perfusion rate was used to examine whether perfusion of the hippocampus in vivo might deplete the pool of amino acids available to the tubing (Table 2). There was, however, no suggestion of such an effect; on the contrary, in vivo net flow was slightly higher than the corresponding in vitro transport which may suggest a mobilization of amino acids with increased sample withdrawal. Upon return to the 2.5 µl/min perfusion rate after one hour of perfusion at 200 µl/min, the perfusate contained very similar concentrations of amino acids as during the 2.5 µl/min period before the high-speed perfusion.

TABLE 2

NET INFLUX FROM TISSUE TO MEDIUM IN VIVO IN CUPROPHAN

B4AH DIALYSIS TUBE IMPLANTED IN THE RABBIT HIPPOCAMPUS

Influx given as net transport in vivo/in vitro x 100.

AMINO	Perfusion rate (µl/min)			
ACID	1	2.5	20	200
GLU	120	100	100	120
GLN	100	100	80	100
TAU	110	100	160	490
ALA	90	100	180	390
LEU	90	100	130	340

Amino acid concentrations in the extracellular space

In spite of the continuous removal of amino acids in the dialysis tube system, which amounts to approximately the total amino acid content in 0.5 µl of extracellular

TABLE 3

FREE AMINO ACIDS IN PLASMA, HIPPOCAMPAL EXTRA-
CELLULAR FLUID AND CEREBROSPINAL FLUID (CSF)

AMINO ACID	PLASMA (n=7)	EXTRACELL. FLUID (n=8)	CSF (n=6)
TAU	48 + 6	6.4 + 0.5	5.6 + 1.4
P-EtOH	24 + 3	6.2 + 0.7	11.8 + 0.9
SER	275 + 25	36 + 2.8	105.9 +10.7
ASN	60 + 6	2.8 + 0.2	15.9 + 1.6
GLU	56 + 9	3.4 + 0.8	9.6 + 2.2
GLN	821 + 56	225.8 +26.9	582.9 + 27.4
ALA	361 + 41	14.2 + 1.4	39.4 + 5.2
VAL	179 + 19	11.4 + 1.3	13.8 + 1.2
ILEU	112 + 12	8.2 + 0.9	7.4 + 0.7
LEU	91 + 13	8.1 + 1.0	7.3 + 0.3
PHE	46 + 5	5.4 + 0.5	7.0 + 0.6
ORN	45 + 7	3.7 + 0.4	9.2 + 2.4

Means + S.E., µmoles/ l.

fluid per min, the system is in an apparent steady state. This finding and the intact appearance of the cells in the vicinity of the tubing led to the presumption that the composition of the extracellular fluid could be determined with the dialysis-perfusion system. Further support was obtained by the fluctuations of calcium ion concentration in the dialysate (Lazarewicz, Hagberg and Hamberger, in preparation). Perfusion with veratridine (100 μM) decreased the calcium level in the perfusate by 75 % and this was completely inhibited when 2 μM tetrodotoxin was added. Finally, the effects of amino acid uptake inhibitors (see below) were in support of changes in the extracellular space.

Table 3 presents the amino acid composition of the extracellular fluid of the rabbit hippocampus, measured the day after implantation of the dialysis tube. Small difference was seen when similar measurements were done during days 2 - 3. The concentrations of taurine, valine, leucine, isoleucine and phenylalanine were similar in the extracellular fluid and rabbit CSF (Table 3) while glutamate, glutamine, alanine, asparagine and ornithine concentrations in the extracellular fluid were considerably below those in the CSF. Although the extracellular glutamine level was 40 % of that in the CSF, glutamine was the dominant amino acid representing approximately 50 % of total amino acid nitrogen in the compartment. There was no indication of blood leakage or BBB damage in the tube region as plasma amino acids are far higher than in both CSF and extracellular fluid (Table 3). Aspartate, and particularly GABA, occurred at extremely low levels in the extracellular fluid, GABA at approximately 0.3 μM. The results consequently suggest that the amino acid composition of the extracellular fluid, at least in the hippocampus, is distinctly different from that in the CSF.

The extracellular space in the brain is in the range of 10 per cent of the total volume and the concentration of free amino acids in the extracellular fluid (Table 3) is 10 per cent or less of that in the total tissue. Consequently, the contribution of extracellular amino acids to the total free pool of amino acids in the brain is less than one per cent. Because free amino acids in total tissue can be taken to represent intracellular amino acids (with an error of about one per cent) the results from Table 3 can be used (together with data on total free

amino acids) for estimate of steady state in vivo intra/
extracellular concentration ratios. Such ratios have been
calculated to be approximately 9,000 for GABA, 3,000 for
glutamate, 400 for taurine and phosphoethanolamine, 19 for
leucine and 6 for lysine, i.e. the amino acids essentially
being ranked as for tissue/medium ratios in slice incubation studies.

Evoked release of amino acid transmitters

Depolarisation of the hippocampus in the vicinity of
the dialysis tube could be achieved by perfusion with
veratridine (0.1 mM). This resulted in decreased Ca^{2+}
and increased K^+ in the dialysate (Lazarewicz, Hagberg &
Hamberger, in preparation). Elevated K^+ (56 or 80 mM) or
kainic acid (Lehmann et al., 1983) in the perfusion medium
also produced a decreased Ca^{2+} concentration. The
volume of depolarized tissue is, however, unknown.
Glutamate and GABA levels increased by a factor of 2 - 5
during depolarization (Hamberger et al., 1982). The
largest effects were observed for taurine and phosphoethanolamine which increased 5 - 10 times in the dialysate
and for glutamine which decreased to approximately 50 % of
the basal level (Lehmann et al., 1983). The concentration
of other amino acids was essentially unaffected during
depolarization. The veratridine-induced decrease in glutamine concentration was inhibited when tetrodotoxin ($2 \mu M$)
was included in the perfusing medium (Jacobsson and
Hamberger, in preparation) which supports a possible connection between the increase in extracellular glutamate
and GABA and decrease in glutamine (Van den Berg and
Garfinkel, 1971; Bradford and Ward, 1975; Cotman and
Hamberger, 1978). However, the decrease in glutamine
amounted to approximately 100 μmoles/ml, while the sum of
the increase in glutamate and GABA was close to 10 μmoles/
ml. This discrepancy probably is due to the uptake systems
for glutamate and GABA in neuronal and glial cells. Inhibitory uptake of glutamate and GABA should increase the
levels of these amino acids in the dialysate. Table 4
shows that this is the case for GABA, for example, the
addition to the medium of nipecotic acid, one of the most
potent inhibitors of GABA uptake by both neuronal and
glial cells (Krogsgaard-Larsen and Johnston, 1975;
Schousboe et al., 1978), elevated GABA levels in the
dialysate 10 - 30 times. Furthermore, both diaminobutyric
acid (DABA) and guvacin, when perfused at 2 mM in the KRB

TABLE 4

EFFECTS OF LOCAL ADMINISTRATION OF GABA UPTAKE INHIBITORS
IN VIVO ON EXTRACELLULAR AMINO ACIDS IN THE HIPPOCAMPUS

Compound	Conc. (mM)	GABA	Taurine	Phospho-ethanol-amine
KRB medium		100	100	100
+ Nipecotic acid	0.5	500	100	100
	1.0	1150	130	160
	2.0	2850	220	210
+ DABA	0.5	250	140	100
	1.0	500	150	100
	2.0	1000	190	130
+ Homo-β-proline	2.0	270	100	100
+ Guvacin	2.0	800	100	100
+ Valproate	2.0	100	100	100
+ THPO	2.0	100	100	100

The compounds were included in the medium perfusing the
dialysis tube. Perfusion rate 2.5 μl/min. Results
expressed in per cent of control (GABA = 0.3 μM, taurine
= 6.4 μM, phosphoethanolamine = 6.2 μM).

medium, increased GABA concentrations by approximately ten-fold (Table 4).

The striking elevation of taurine and phosphoethanolamine after administration of depolarizing agents exhibited some unusual features. First, the concentration increase occurred later than for glutamate and GABA, the

TABLE 5

EFFECTS OF EXCITATORY AMINO ACID AGONISTS IN VIVO ON EXTRACELLULAR TAURINE AND PHOSPHOETHANOLAMINE LEVELS IN THE RABBIT HIPPOCAMPUS

Conditions	Taurine	Phospho-ethanolamine
Control medium	100	100
+ 1 mM kainic acid	900	1000
+ 5 mM dihydro-kainic acid	400	900
+ 5 mM N-methyl-DL-aspartic acid	1200	2500
+ 5 mM cis-2,3-piperidine dicarb-oxylic acid	700	1500
+ 5 mM quinolinic acid	800	1600

100 for both taurine and phosphoethanolamine = 6 μM.

peaks being delayed by at least ten min in a typical experiment. We have accumulated data which suggest a close interrelationship between the levels of taurine and phosphoethanolamine. Perfusion with guanidinoethane sulfonic acid, a taurine uptake blocker (Hruska et al., 1978), increased the extracellular level of not only taurine, but also of phosphoethanolamine, all other amino acids being unaffected (Lehmann and Hamberger, in preparation). The enhancing effect of some GABA uptake inhibitors on taurine and phosphoethanolamine concentrations (Table 4) may be due to a direct inhibition by GABA of taurine accumulation (Lähdesmäki and Oja, 1973) and of taurine on phosphoethanolamine. Perfusion with excitatory amino acid agonists selectively increased taurine and phospho-ethanolamine levels in the extracellular space (Table 5). The agonist effects may reflect a postsynaptic release of taurine and phosphoethanolamine, although terminals and/or glial cells can not be excluded. Taurine, regarded as an unspecific, weak inhibitor with an unknown mechanism of action (Collins, 1977), probably derives from the cyto-plasmic pool in neurons and/or glia. The origin of phos-phoethanolamine is less certain. It could be phosphatidyl-ethanolamine in neuronal membranes, as well as cytoplasmic pools. Hypothetically, taurine may be released from the postsynaptic neuron in response to excitation to alter the phospholipid composition of the neuronal membranes. Then it could influence the translocation of calcium ions (Sun and Sun, 1976) and/or modulate GABA - membrane inter-actions (Giambalvo and Rosenberg, 1976).

Experimentally induced changes in glutamine and glutamate

In addition to the advantage of the dialysis technique to give direct comparisons of effects on extra- and intracellular compartments, the possibility opens to compare the effects of systemic administration of a test substance with those of local administration via the tube. Two situations are exemplified: methionine sulfoximine (MSO) intoxication and galactosamine-induced acute ful-minant hepatic failure (Miller et al., 1976).

MSO intoxication - The quantitative importance of glutamine and its reactivity during depolarization focus-sed further interest on changes in the glutamine system, particularly with respect to possible effects on the depolarization-evoked release of glutamate. MSO is a potent inhibitor of glutamine synthetase but it affects other systems (Folbergrova et al., 1969; Hevor and Gayat, 1981). It is commonly used for induction of experimental epilepsy: seizures occur a few hours after an intraperitoneal injection of MSO. However, its mechanism of action is unknown. By analogy with the astrocytic glial localization of glutamine synthetase (Norenberg and Martinez-Hernandez, 1979), the primary histological effects of MSO are on astrocytes, including swelling and glycogen accumulation (Gutierrez and Norenberg, 1979). Few studies have been reported on brain amino acids during MSO intoxication. Tews and Stone (1964) saw an increase in alanine and a decrease in glutamine and glutamate in the brains of MSO-intoxicated dogs. Fig. 4 (left part) shows the time-course of extracellular glutamine, alanine and glutamate after an intraperitoneal injection of MSO (250 mg/kg). This is compared with the changes in the same amino acids when 2 mM MSO was included in the perfusion medium for 60 min. It is apparent that the brain enzyme was affected by MSO at least to the same extent as that of other body organs, as reflected by plasma levels. Similarly, brain alanine was increased. In both cases, the effects on both basal levels of glutamate and on the K-evoked increase in glutamate (data not shown) were small. The experiments consequently did not suggest an immediate correlation between glutamine and releasable glutamate. Fig. 5 shows only the effects after an i.p. injection of MSO. The most obvious finding was the relatively stronger effect of MSO on brain alanine. There was no evidence that the brain cells accumulated alanine to provide a normalized extracellular concentration. However, such a mechanism seemed to exist for glutamate. The reduction of glutamine levels appeared as marked in brain as in plasma.

It is interesting to note that the hippocampus apparently has an interrelation of glutamine and alanine similar to that reported for rat skeletal muscle (Garber, 1980). For muscle, alanine has been suggested as part of a glucose-alanine cycle between muscle and liver which may take care of nitrogen disposal from the muscle. Alanine is, furthermore, the predominant substrate for hepatic gluconeogenesis. In the brain, however, neither the MSO-induced gluconeogenesis (Forbergrova et al., 1969; Phelps, 1975) nor the enhanced alanine levels are completely understood.

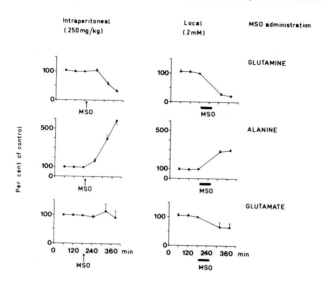

Fig. 4 Time course of changes in endogenous extracellular glutamine, alanine and glutamate. Arrow indicates the time of i.p. injection of MSO (left part). Filled bar indicates the period of local perfusion with 2 mM MSO (right part).

Experimental acute liver failure - A common disturbance of CNS glutamine metabolism is the expression of liver failure via the liver-brain axis. This is expressed as encephalopathy, astrocytosis, excitation, coma, hyperammonemia, etc (Conn and Lieberthal, 1979). In the CNS, ammonia is detoxified by glutamine formation as in skeletal muscle and, furthermore, ammonia inhibits the breakdown of CNS glutamine to transmitter glutamate (Matheson and Van den Berg, 1975). We have recently monitored the time course of amino acid changes during 45 hrs after induction of liver failure with galactosamine (Miller et al., 1976). Virtually all plasma amino acids increase 20 - 45 hours after galactosamine injection. A comparison of the changes in plasma amino acids with those in the extra- and intracellular compartments of the hippocampus is shown in Fig. 6. The alterations in hippocampal amino acids were generally more modest than in plasma. Fig. 6 also shows

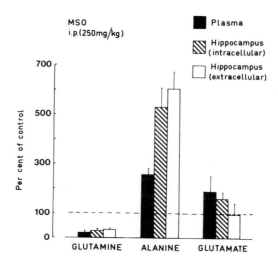

Fig. 5 Glutamine, alanine and glutamate changes in plasma, intracellular and extracellular compartments of the hippocampus at the end of the experiment described in Fig. 4 (left).

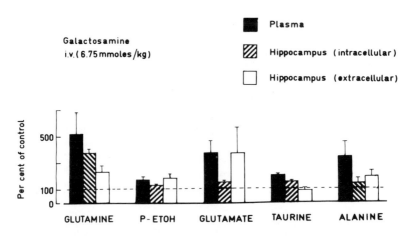

Fig. 6 Changes in glutamine, phosphoethanolamine, glutamate, taurine and alanine in plasma, intracellular and extracellular compartments of the hippocampus 45 hours after i.v. injection of galactosamine hydrochloride.

that certain amino acids increase more in the extracellular space, while others are increased mainly in the
intracellular compartment. The elevated extracellular
glutamate is in agreement with the recent results of
Moroni et al. (1983). The authors, employing the cortical
cup technique, showed that intraperitoneal administration
of ammonium ions increased the release of glutamate from
the cortical surface in vivo.

Conclusions

The dialysis tube approach has a number of unique
features as an in vivo probe for on-line monitoring of
levels of amino acids in the extracellular fluid: there is
no bulk fluid passage into the tissue, there are minimal
mechanical effects on the tissue, the probe may be calib-
rated to give exact concentrations and there is little
protein in the perfusate, so clean-up steps are not needed
for amino acid analysis. The potential of the dialysis
tube in studies of the metabolic relationship of glutamine, glutamate and GABA has been shown:
a) the accumulative capacity for "transmitter" amino
acids is considerable, while that for others, such as
glutamine and taurine, and particularly for leucine and
lysine, is much less expressed.
b) depolarization of an otherwise not uptake - inhibited
hippocampus results in a quantitative dominant increase in
taurine and phosphoethanolamine.
c) MSO-induced an 80 % reduction in glutamine levels
but had no apparent effect on the evoked release of
glutamate. Alanine was the single amino acid which
increased considerably.
d) experimental liver failure increased plasma levels of
many amino acids. Brain levels were more moderately
affected.

Acknowledgements - This work was supported by grants
from the Swedish Medical Research Council (12X-00164) and
from Axel and Margret Axelson Johnson Foundation. The
skilful secretarial work of Ms. Gull Grönstedt is gratefully acknowledged.

References

Bradford HF, Ward HK (1975) Glutamine as a metabolic substrate for isolated nerve-endings. Inhibition by ammonium ions. Biochem Soc Trans 3: 1223.

Collins GGS (1977) On the role of taurine in the mammalian central nervous system. Essays Neurochem Neuropharmacol 1: 43.

Conn HO, Lieberthal MM, (eds) (1979) "The Hepatic Coma Syndromes and Lactulose", Williams and Wilkins Company, Baltimore, U.S.A.

Cotman CW, Hamberger A (1978) Glutamate as a CNS neurotransmitter: Properties of release, inactivation and biosynthesis. In Fonnum F (ed) "Amino Acids as Chemical Transmitters", Plenum Press, p. 379.

Delgado JMR, De Feudis FV, Roth RH, Ryngo DK, Mitruka BM (1972) Dialytrode for long-term intracerebral perfusion in awake monkeys. Arch Int Pharmacodyn 198:9.

Dodd PR, Bradford HF (1972) Release of amino acids from the chronically superfused mammalian cerebral cortex. J Neurochem 23: 289.

Folbergrova J, Passonneau JV, Lowry OH, Schulz DW (1969) Glycogen, ammonia and released metabolites in the brain during seizures evoked by methionine sulphoximine. J Neurochem 16: 191.

Gaddum JH (1961) Push-pull cannulae. J Physiol 155: 1.

Garber AJ (1980) Glutamine metabolism in skeletal muscle. In Mora J, Palacios R (eds) "Glutamine: Metabolism, Enzymology and Regulation", Academic Press.

Giambalvo CT, Rosenberg P (1976) Phospholipids and the GABA receptor. Adv Exp Med Biol 72: 265.

Gutierrez JA, Norenberg MD (1977) Ultrastructural study of methionine sulfoximine-induced Alzheimer type II astrocytes. Am J Pathol 86: 285.

Hamberger A, Jacobsson I, Molin SO, Nyström B, Sandberg M, Ungerstedt U (1982) Metabolic and transmitter compartments for glutamate. In Bradford H (ed) "Neurotransmitter Interaction and Compartmentation", Plenum Press, p. 359.

Hevor T, Gayet J (1981) Stimulation of fructose-1,6-biphosphatase activity and synthesis in the cerebral cortex of rats submitted to the convulsant methionine sulfoximine. J Neurochem 36: 949.

Hruska RE, Pajden A, Bresler R, Yamamura HJ (1978) Taurine: sodium-dependent, high-affinity transport into rat brain synaptosomes. Mol Pharmacol 14: 77.

Kovacs DA, Zoll JG, Erickson CK (1976) Improved intracerebral chemitrode for chemical and electrical studies of the brain. Pharmac Biochem Behav 4: 621.

Krogsgaard-Larsen P, Johnston GAR (1975) Inhibition of GABA uptake in rat brain slices by nipecotic acid, various isoxazoles and related compounds. J Neurochem 25: 797.

Lehmann A, Isacsson H, Hamberger A (1983) Effects of in vivo administration of kainic acid on the extracellular amino acid pools in the rabbit hippocampus. J Neurochem 40: 1314.

Lähdesmäki P, Pasula M, OJA SS (1975) Effect of electrical stimulation and chlorpromazine on the uptake and release of taurine, γ-aminobutyric acid and glutamine acid in mouse brain synaptosomes. J Neurochem 25: 675.

MacIntosh FC, Oborin PE (1953) Release of acetylcholine from intact cerebral cortex. Proc XIX Int Congr Physiol, p. 580.

Matheson DF, Van den Berg CJ (1975) Ammonia and brain glutamine: inhibition of glutamine degradation by ammonia. Biochem Soc Trans 3: 525.

Miller DJ, Hickman R, Fratter R, Terblanche J, Saunders SJ (1976) An animal model of fulminant hepatic failure: a feasibility study. Gastroenterol 71: 109.

Moroni F, Lombardi G, Moneti G, Cortesini C (1983) The release and neosynthesis of glutamic acid are increased in experimental models of hepatic encephalopathy. J Neurochem 40: 850.

Myers RD (1974) "Handbook of Drug and Chemical Stimulation of The Brain. Behavioral, Pharmacological and Physiological Aspects", New York, Van Nostrand Reinhold, p. 759.

Norenberg MD, Martinez-Hernandez A (1979) Fine structural localizations of glutamine synthetase in astrocytes of rat brain. Brain Research 161: 303.

Phelps CH (1975) An ultrastructural study of methionine sulfoximine-induced glycogen accumulation in astrocytes of the mouse cerebral cortex. J Neurocytol 4: 479.

Schousboe A, Krogsgaard-Larsen P, Svenneby G, Hertz L (1978) Inhibition of high-affinity, net uptake of GABA into cultured astrocytes by β-proline, nipecotic acid and other compounds. Brain Research 153: 623.

Sun AY, Sun GY (1976) Functional roles of phospholipids of synaptosomal membrane. Adv Exp Med Biol 72: 169.

Tews JK, Stone WE (1964) Effects of methionine sulfoximine on levels of free amino acids and related substances in brain. Biochem Pharmacol 13:543.

Ungersted U, Herrera-Marschitz M, Jungelins U, Ståhle L, Tossman U, Zetterström T (1982) Dopamine synaptic mechanisms reflected in studies combining behavioural recording and brain dialysis. In Kosaka M et al. (eds) Adv Dopamine Research 37: 219.

Van den Berg CJ, Garfinkel DA (1971) A simulation study of brain compartments: metabolism of glutamate and related substances in mouse brain. Biochem J 123: 211.

Glutamine, Glutamate, and GABA
in the Central Nervous System, pages 493–508

GLUTAMATE AND GABA LOCALIZATION AND EVOKED RELEASE IN
CEREBELLAR CELLS DIFFERENTIATING IN CULTURE

GIULIO LEVI and M. TERESA CIOTTI

Istituto di Biologia Cellulare, CNR,
Via G. Romagnosi 18/A
00196 Roma, Italy

Primary cell cultures have become a powerful tool for distinguishing among the behaviors of different neural cell types and for studying differentiation-related functional parameters (Giacobini et al. 1980; Pfeiffer 1982). Using primary cultures of cells dissociated from postnatal rat cerebella, which can be greatly enriched in granule cells or in astrocytes, depending on the culture conditions (Lasher 1974; Messer 1977; Currie, Kelly 1981; Dutton et al.1981; Woodhams et al. 1981; Drejer et al. 1982; Levi et al. 1983a, 1983b; Wilkin et al. 1983), we studied in parallel the morphological differentiation of the cells, the autoradiographic localization of radioactive putative transmitter amino acids, and the development of voltage- and Ca^{2+}-dependent neurotransmitter release processes.

CULTURE CONDITIONS

Cells dissociated from 8-day-old rat cerebella (Dutton et al. 1981; Levi et al. 1983a) were resuspended in Basal Modified Eagle's Medium supplemented with 10% fetal calf serum, 25 mM KCl (only in the case of interneuron cultures), 2 mM glutamine and 0.1 mg/ml of gentamycin, and were plated (2.5 x 10^6 cells/dish) on poly-L-lysine coated 35 mm Falcon dishes containing, for the immunofluorescence and autoradiography experiments, four 12 mm glass coverslips. The cells were incubated at 37°C in 95% air/5% CO_2.After 18 hours of incubation the antimitotic cytosine arabinoside (0.01 mM) was added to the cultures to be enriched in neurons. All the other procedures are described elsewhere (Gallo et al. 1982; Levi et al. 1983a).

CELL CHARACTERIZATION BY IMMUNOFLUORESCENCE AND AUTORADIO-
GRAPHY

Primary cultures of dissociated postnatal cerebellar
cells consist essentially of granule cell neurons when an
antimitotic is added to the culture medium to prevent the re-
plication of non-neuronal cells (Messer 1977; Drejer et al.
1982; Fields et al. 1982; Patel et al. 1982; Levi et al.
1983a). At 2 DIV (days in vitro), cultured granule cells already emit processes; at 4-5 DIV initial aggregates and a
fine network of fibers are clearly apparent; at 8 and 12 DIV
most of the granule cells are grouped in large clumps, connected by bundles of fasciculated fibers (Gallo et al. 1982).

The most abundant contaminants of granule cell cultures
are astrocytes and GABAergic neurons, while other cells (fibroblasts, endothelial cells, oligodendrocytes) are present
in negligible amounts (Lasher 1974; Currie, Kelly 1981;
Messer, 1977; Pearce, Dutton 1981; Fields et al. 1982; Webb
1982; Levi et al. 1983a, 1983b). As the number of astrocytes
and GABAergic interneurons may vary substantially in relation
to relatively minor differences in the experimental conditions, it seemed important to assess the proportion of these
cell types at the stages selected for our biochemical analyses.

The morphological features and the number of astrocytes
were determined by indirect immunofluorescence staining with
rabbit anti-GFAP (glial fibrillary acidic protein; Bignami,
Dahl 1974) antibodies and anti-rabbit rhodamine conjugate,
and by ^{3}H-D-aspartate autoradiography (Levi et al. 1983b).
In fact, astrocytes are known to accumulate avidly acidic
amino acids (Currie, Kelly 1981; Levi et al. 1983a, 1983b)
and we have shown that they do so independently of their
shape, size and differentiation (Levi et al. 1983b). In interneuron cultures at 2 DIV, astroglial cells accounted for
about 5% of the total cells (Levi et al. 1983b). Most of them
were elongated, highly fluorescent and had few thick processes, while some were stellate, with thin radial processes,
and were often less fluorescent or not fluorescent at all (as
suggested by comparative counts of GFAP(+) stellate cells and
non-neuronal stellate cells labeled by ^{3}H-D-aspartate; see
Levi et al. 1983b) (Fig. 1A, 1B). At the next stage studied
(5 DIV), the number of astrocytes decreased to half or less,
while the relative proportion of stellate astrocytes (which
were now larger, more fluorescent and with more numerous and
elaborated processes) increased (Fig. 1D, 1E). The cell counts

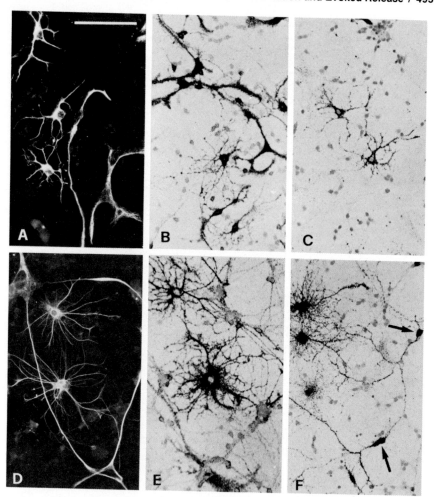

Fig. 1. Pictures of cerebellar interneuron cultures at 2 DIV (A, B, C) and 5 DIV (D, E, F). Indirect immunofluorescence staining with rabbit anti-GFAP and anti-rabbit rhodamine conjugate (A, D) and autoradiograms after exposure of the cells for 10 min to 2 μCi/ml of ^{3}H-D-aspartate (B, E) or ^{3}H-GABA (C, F). Stellate astrocytes are visualized by all 3 procedures, astrocytes with other shapes are labeled by anti-GFAP and ^{3}H-D-aspartate only. Granule cells are not labeled (2 DIV) or modestly labeled by ^{3}H-D-aspartate (5 DIV). Heavily labeled GABAergic neurons are clearly seen at 5 DIV (arrows in F). Scale bar = 80 μm (A and D) and 100 μm (B, C, E and F).

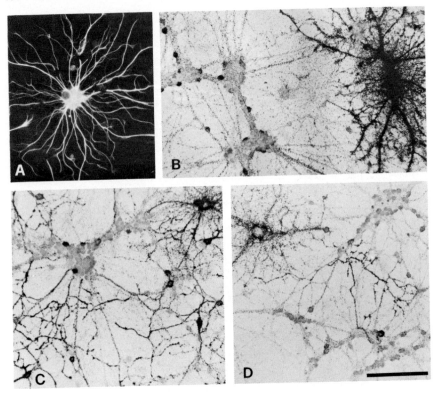

Fig. 2. Pictures of differentiated cerebellar interneuron cultures at 12 DIV. Anti-GFAP immunofluorescence (A), ^{3}H-D-aspartate (B) and ^{3}H-GABA (C, D) autoradiography. Pictures C and D are from parallel cultures; the culture medium was renewed at 2 DIV in C (note many labeled neurons) and at 2 and 7 DIV in D (only one neuron is labeled in the field shown. Scale bar = 80 μm (A) and 100 μm (B, C and D).

based on GFAP positivity and ^{3}H-D-aspartate labeling were similar (Levi et al. 1983b). The non-stellate astrocytes had heterogeneous shapes and accounted for less than half of the total astrocytes. At later stages (8 and 12 DIV)(Fig. 2A, 2B) the number of astrocytes further decreased, particularly at the expense of the non-stellate cells. At 12 DIV, astrocytes accounted for about 0.5% of the total cells, with 70-80% of them having a stellate morphology (Levi et al. 1983b). This trend was opposite to the one observed in astrocyte-enriched

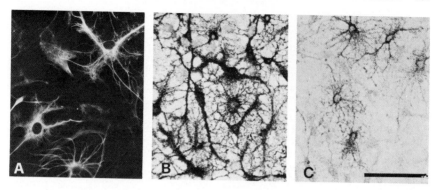

Fig. 3. Pictures of cerebellar astrocyte-enriched cultures
at 5 DIV. Of all the astrocyte types evidenced by anti-GFAP
staining (A), only those bearing a stellate shape are labeled
by ^{3}H-GABA (C), while all are heavily labeled by ^{3}H-D-asparta-
te (B). For more details, see Wilkin et al. 1983. Scale bar
= 80 μm (A) and 100 μm (B, C).

cultures, where the relative proportion of stellate astrocytes was maximal at around day 5 (Fig. 3) and then rapidly
declined to almost total disappearance at stages at which
the cells approached confluency (Wilkin et al. 1983).

In contrast to the high accumulation of ^{3}H-D-aspartate
seen in all astrocytes, the uptake of the amino acid by granule cells and their processes became substantial only at advanced stages of cell differentiation, namely in 8 DIV and
12 DIV cultures (Levi et al. 1983a). Even at these stages the
granule cells were not uniformely labeled, and only some of
them were heavily labeled (Fig. 2B). The uptake of ^{3}H-D-aspar-
tate observed in this study was more pronounced than expected
on the basis of the previous autoradiographic literature on
the subject (Currie, Kelly 1981; Wilkin et al. 1982; Levi et
al. 1982), but is consistent with previous biochemical data
(Schousboe 1981; Drejer et al. 1982; Yu, Hertz 1982).

While ^{3}H-D-aspartate was avidly taken up by all the astrocyte types found at the various stages, ^{3}H-GABA was accumulated only by the astrocytes with stellate morphology (Figs. 1C,
1E, 2C, 2D). Even within the stellate astrocyte type, the uptake of the amino acid differed greatly among the various
cells, and some cells did not appear to accumulate ^{3}H-GABA
at all, particularly in the older cultures (Levi et al. 1983b).

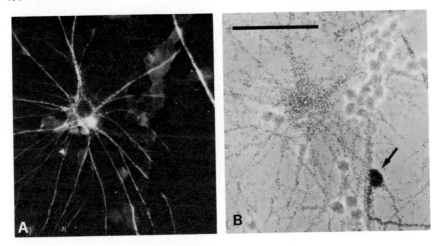

Fig. 4. Double labeling of the large stellate cells present in cerebellar interneuron cultures (12 DIV) by anti-GFAP immunofluorescence (A) and ^{3}H-GABA autoradiography (B). The two pictures show the same microscopic field under rhodamine and phase contrast optics, respectively. The stellate cell is labeled and granule cells are unlabeled in both pictures. The arrow in B points to a neuron labeled by ^{3}H-GABA. Scale bar = 50 μm.

A similar pattern of ^{3}H-D-aspartate and ^{3}H-GABA uptake was observed in astrocyte-enriched cultures (Fig. 3C), where the number of ^{3}H-GABA-labeled cells decreased drastically as the cells approached confluency and stellate astrocytes tended to disappear (Wilkin et al. 1983).

The possibility that the stellate cells labeled by ^{3}H--GABA are neurons was excluded not only by comparative cell counts (cells labeled by ^{3}H-D-aspartate, by ^{3}H-GABA and GFAP(+) cells), and by a lack of labeling with the neuronal membrane marker tetanus toxin (Levi et al. 1983b), but also by double labeling experiments (^{3}H-GABA autoradiography and GFAP staining) which showed the coexistence of ^{3}H-GABA grains and GFAP immunofluorescence in the same stellate cells (Fig.4).

^{3}H-GABA was heavily accumulated by a limited number of neurons, whose morphology differed from that of granule cells (Lasher 1974; Levi et al. 1983a). Their perikaryon was larger, they had no tendency to aggregate, and their long axon had a characteristic, branched shape, with frequent bead-like structures along it (Fig. 2C, 2D). In contrast to granule cells, the GABAergic neurons showed an intense labeling and an advanced morphological differentiation already in 5 DIV cultures. At this stage they accounted for about 2% of the total cells, and this proportion was maintained at later stages, unless the cultures were subjected to a medium change at day 7. This procedure caused, for reasons that we are currently analyzing, a loss of about 90% of the ^{3}H-GABA-accumulating cells (Fig. 2D), already detectable the next day.

^{3}H-GABA (in the presence or in the absence of amino-oxyacetic acid) was accumulated to a very modest degree also by granule cells and their processes (Fig. 2C, 2D), probably through a transport system different from that of GABAergic neurons. In fact, the accumulation by granule cells was abolished by beta-alanine (which, under the present conditions, did not prevent the autoradiographic accumulation of ^{3}H-GABA into GABAergic neurons nor that into stellate astrocytes), and was unaffected by ACHC (cis-1,3-aminocyclohexane carboxylic acid) which behaved as a strong inhibitor of ^{3}H-GABA uptake by both GABAergic neurons and stellate astrocytes (Levi et al. 1983b).

DEVELOPMENT OF STIMULUS-COUPLED RELEASE PROCESSES

I. Acidic Amino Acids

The availability of a highly purified population of granule cells undergoing a rapid differentiation in vitro seemed ideal for clarifying whether glutamate is the transmitter of these cells (see Levi et al. 1982 and Gallo et al. 1982, for bibliography). We faced the problem by studying whether endogenous and newly synthesized glutamate and exogenous ^{3}H-D-aspartate (a non-metabolized marker of glutamate "reuptake pool"; see Balcar, Johnston 1972) can be released from cultured cerebellar granule cells in a way compatible with a neurotransmitter role. Amino acid release was evoked by depolarizing the cells with a high K^+ concentration or with the alkaloid veratridine. At 2 DIV, the high K^+-induced release of glutamate (endogenous or previously synthesized from radioactive glutamine) was small and Ca^{2+}-independent. At later stages, the evoked release became progressively and steadily larger in the presence of Ca^{2+}, but did not change appreciably in its absence (Fig. 5) (Gallo et al. 1982). In a pre-

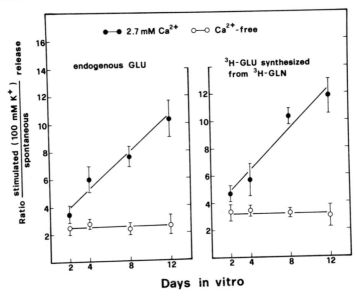

Days in vitro

Fig. 5. Development of Ca^{2+}-dependent, depolarization-induced release of endogenous and newly synthesized glutamate in cerebellar granule cell cultures. Cultures at different stages (see abcissa) were prelabeled for 45 min with 290 nM ^{3}H-glutamine in a Krebs-Ringer medium and then subjected to 5 min washes. The 3rd wash contained 100 mM KCl (replacing an equivalent amount of NaCl), and in half of the dishes Ca^{2+} was omitted from the medium starting from the 2nd wash. Endogenous glutamate and newly formed ^{3}H-glutamate were measured in the wash media and in acid extracts of the cells. The results are expressed as ratios between the release measured during a 5 min depolarization and that measured during the preceeding 5 min, in the presence or in the absence of Ca^{2+}, respectively. Data recalculated from Gallo et al. 1982.

vious study (Pearce, Dutton 1981) a small Ca^{2+}-dependent, K^{+}-evoked release of endogenous glutamate and GABA was detected in 14 DIV, but not in 7 DIV granule cell cultures. In cultures at 12 DIV, the response to high K^{+} increased gradually with increasing concentrations of K^{+}, and was similar with 50 and 100 mM KCl (unpublished data). No decrease in the fractional rate constant of evoked release of endogenous glutamate was observed when 12 DIV cultures were subjected to 3 consecutive 5 min depolarizations with 50 mM KCl, indicating a

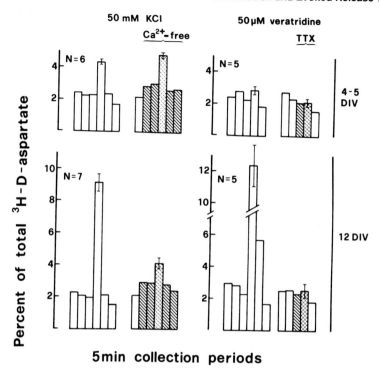

Fig. 6. Depolarization-induced release of ^{3}H-D-aspartate from cerebellar granule cell cultures. Cell cultured for 4-5 DIV or for 12 DIV were incubated in a Krebs-Ringer medium with 1 μCi/ml of ^{3}H-D-aspartate, and then subjected to 5 min washes. The medium of the 4th wash contained either 50 mM KCl or 0.05 mM veratridine. Ca^{2+}-free media were applied starting from the 2nd wash, tetrodotoxin (TTX) was added at the 3rd and 4th wash (see dashed bars). The radioactivity recovered in each wash was expressed as a percent of that present in the cells before the washes. N = number of paired experiments. SEMs are shown on the bars corresponding to the 4th collection period (stimulated release). Data from Levi et al. (1983a).

good cell viability even under drastic experimental conditions (Levi et al. 1983a). Veratridine (0.05 mM), which depolarizes excitable cells by holding open the Na^{+}-channels (Catterall 1975), did not evoke glutamate release at 2 DIV, but caused a massive release of endogenous and newly synthesized glutamate at 8 DIV, and its action was totally prevented by 0.5 uM tetrodotoxin (Gallo et al. 1982). No evidence for a

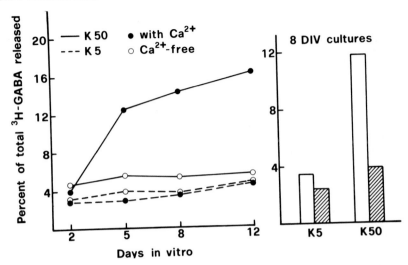

Fig. 7. Development of Ca^{2+}-dependent, depolarization-induced release of ^{3}H-GABA in cerebellar interneuron cultures. Left panel: cultures at 2, 5, 8 and 12 DIV were preincubated with 1 µCi/ml of ^{3}H-GABA in the presence of 0.01 mM amino-oxyacetic acid, and then subjected to 5 min washes. The medium of the 4th wash contained 50 mM KCl; Ca^{2+}-free media were applied starting from the 2nd wash. The radioactivity recovered in the wash with high K$^+$ and in the preceeding wash are expressed as a percentage of that present in the cells before the washes. Averages of 2-5 duplicate experiments are shown. Right panel: representative experiment in cultures at 8 DIV; the cultures were subjected to a medium change at 2 DIV (white bars) or to 2 medium changes (at 2 and 7 DIV, dashed bars). Experimental details as in the left panel. Unpublished results of Aloisi, Ciotti and Levi.

stimulus-coupled release of aspartic acid (endogenous or previously synthesized from ^{3}H-glutamine) was obtained, making it unlikely that this amino acid acts as a transmitter of granule cells (Gallo et al. 1982; see also Pearce, Dutton 1981).

    Calcium-dependent, high K$^+$-evoked release and tetrodotoxin-sensitive, veratridine-induced release of ^{3}H-D-aspartate were detectable in cultures at 8 or 12 DIV, being higher in the latter (Levi et al. 1983a), but not at earlier stages (Fig. 6). The lack of ^{3}H-D-aspartate Ca^{2+}-dependent or veratridine-induced release at 4-5 DIV (a stage at which the uptake of the amino acid was essentially confined to astrocytes, many of which had a differentiated, stellate shape) confirms previous findings obtained with confluent astrocyte cultures. These had shown that neither exogenous (Drejer et al. 1982; Levi et al. 1982) nor endogenous acidic amino acids (Pearce, Dutton 1981; Gallo et al. 1982) can be released by depolarizing stimuli in a neurotransmitter-like fashion.

II. Gamma-aminobutyric Acid (GABA)

In view of the small number of GABAergic neurons present in our cultures, the development of the evoked release of GABA was studied only with respect to the preaccumulated ^{3}H-amino acid. Similarly to what observed with glutamate, and in agreement with previous observations (Pearce, Dutton 1981; Pearce et al. 1983), no stimulus-coupled release of ^{3}H-GABA was detectable in 2 DIV cultures depolarized with either 50 mM KCl (Fig. 7) or 0.05 mM veratridine (data not shown). At this stage, ^{3}H-GABA uptake was mainly confined to astroglial cells. At 5 DIV, the morphological differentiation of GABAergic neurons, as judged by ^{3}H-GABA autoradiography (Fig. 1E), was quite advanced, and the Ca^{2+}-dependent release of the amino acid evoked by high K^+ was already 70% of that observed at 12 DIV (Fig. 7)(see also Pearce et al. 1983). Thus, the morphological and functional differentiation of GABAergic neurons appears to preceed that of granule cells. This may reflect a more advanced differentiation stage of GABAergic neurons at the time of cell dissociation and plating. It is worth noting that cultures subjected to a medium change at day 7, which caused a loss of 90% of GABAergic neurons without affecting appreciably the number of astrocytes, did no longer exhibit Ca^{2+}-dependent GABA release (Fig. 7, right panel).

AMINO ACID DEPLETION SITES UPON DEPOLARIZATION

In order to obtain further evidence that depolarization does not induce glutamate and GABA release from the differentiated, stellate astrocytes present in neuronal cultures, and also to visualize the neuronal sites from which the amino acids are released, two other sets of experiments were performed: in one set, differentiated granule cell cultures were prelabeled with ^{3}H-glutamine (in conditions in which around 70% of the radioactivity present in the cells at the time of the release experiment was accounted for by newly synthesized

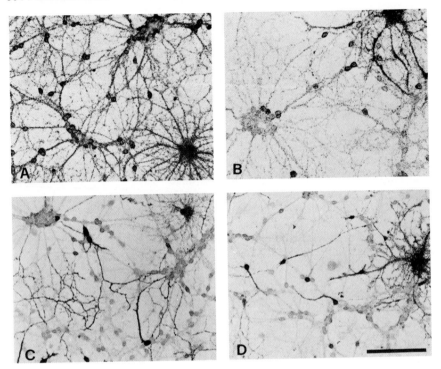

Fig. 8. Depletion of newly synthesized ^{3}H-glutamate (A, B) and of preaccumulated ^{3}H-GABA (C, D) in cerebellar interneuron cultures exposed to consecutive depolarizations. In A and B, 12 DIV cultures were incubated in the presence of ^{3}H-glutamine and then washed, in conditions in which most of the radioactivity remaining in the cells was accounted for by ^{3}H--glutamate (see Levi et al. 1983a). In C and D, the cells were incubated in the presence of ^{3}H-GABA and amino-oxyacetic acid. The cultures pictured in B and D were depolarized 3 times for 5 min at 10 min intervals, with 50 mM KCl. The control cultures were washed for the same time period without depolarization (see Levi et al.1983a, for the washing paradigm in A). Only neuronal structures are depleted of radioactivity in B and D. Scale bar = 100 μm for all pictures.

^{3}H-glutamate (Levi et al. 1983a)). In another set, the cultures were prelabeled with ^{3}H-GABA. In both instances, depolarization caused a selective loss of radioactivity from neuronal structures (Fig. 8). Interestingly, while in the case of glutamate the depletion of radioactivity occurred from the whole neuronal structure of granule cells (perikarya and processes, see Fig. 8B), in the case of ^{3}H-GABA the perikarya and the proximal part of the axons remained heavily labeled, and the loss of radioactivity was prominent in the distal part of the axon and in its branchings (Fig. 8D).

CONCLUSIONS

1. The existence of a selective stimulus-coupled release of glutamate in a highly purified population of cerebellar granule cells strongly supports the concept that glutamate is utilized as a transmitter by these cells.

2. The expression of the biochemical machinery for the neurosecretory process appears to be gradual, and coupled with that of differentiated morphological structures.

3. The existence of a substantial Ca^{2+}-dependent, depolarization-induced release of endogenous glutamate at stages at which granule cells are still unable to accumulate the exogenous amino acid suggests that evoked release and membrane transport have independent, non-coupled developmental patterns, and may indicate that reuptake does not provide a major pool for glutamate release.

4. The expression of a stimulus-coupled neurosecretory process for glutamate does not appear to require the existence of synaptic interactions between granule cells and their natural target. Electron microscopic examination of differentiated granule cell cultures revealed the existence of many presynaptic boutons filled with vesicles and of vesicle-filled structures resembling synapses "en passage" along the axonal processes; however, "classical" synapses with pre- and post-synaptic thickenings of the membrane are few in number (Woodhams and Balàzs, unpublished data), and may represent interactions with the few GABAergic cells present.

5. The fact that depolarization caused glutamate depletion from the whole neuronal structure suggests that the amino acid is not selectively released from synaptic vesicles. If the glutamate-depletion pattern described represents a genuine behavior of glutamate releasing cells, it is tempting to suggest that astrocytes, which have great avidity for the amino acid, may have a crucial role in buffering any glutamate re-

leased from non-synaptic sites.

6. Astrocytes do not exhibit stimulus-coupled release of transmitter amino acids even when they have a differentiated, stellate shape, as in our neuron-enriched cultures (see the data on ^{3}H-D-aspartate release at 4-5 DIV, or those on ^{3}H-GABA release in cultures depleted of GABAergic neurons).

7. The neuronal sites from which ^{3}H-GABA was released by depolarization (distal part of the axons) differed from the sites from which endogenously formed ^{3}H-glutamate was released (whole neuronal structure).

8. The fact that ^{3}H-GABA, but not ^{3}H-D-aspartate uptake was restricted to the astrocytes having a stellate morphology raises a number of questions: is astroglial GABA transport a differentiation-related function, or is it expressed only by a subpopulation of cerebellar astrocytes? Do astrocytes from other brain areas have a similar behavior? Is the functional role of ^{3}H-GABA uptake by astrocytes different from that of acidic amino acid uptake? Can the expression of a given transport system by astrocytes be related to the type of neurons present in the environment, in vivo as well as in culture?

ACKNOWLEDGEMENTS

The following collaborations are gratefully acknowledged: Dr. G.P. Wilkin, for the studies on astrocytes; Drs. F. Aloisi and V. Gallo, for the release experiments; Drs. R. Balàzs and P. Woodhams, for discussing their unpublished electron microscopic data. Financial support was received from NATO (Research Grant n. 58/80) and from the Italian National Research Council (Prog. Fin. MPR, Grant n. 104520/83/8209333).

REFERENCES

Balcar VJ, Johnston GAR (1972). Structural specificity of high affinity uptake of L-glutamate and L-aspartate by rat brain slices. J Neurochem 19: 2657-2666.
Bignami A, Dahl D (1974). Astrocyte specific protein and neuroglial differentiation: an immunofluorescent study with antibodies to the glial fibrillary acidic protein. J Comp Neurol 153: 27-38.
Catterall WA (1975). Activation of the action potential Na$^+$

ionophore of cultured neuroblastoma cells by veratridine and batrachotoxin. J Biol Chem 50: 4053-4059.

Currie DN, Kelly JS (1981). Glial versus neuronal uptake of glutamate. J Exp Biol 95: 181-193.

Drejer J, Larsson OM, Schousböe A (1982). Characterization of L-glutamate uptake into and release from astrocytes and neurons cultured from different brain regions. Exp Brain Res 47: 259-269.

Dutton GR, Currie DN, Tear K (1981). An improved method for the bulk isolation of viable pericarya from postnatal cerebellum. J Neurosci Methods 3: 421-427.

Fields KL, Currie DN, Dutton GR (1982). Development of Thy-1 antigen on cerebellar neurons in culture. J Neurosci 2: 663-673.

Gallo V, Ciotti MT, Coletti A, Aloisi F, Levi G (1982). Selective release of glutamate from cerebellar granule cells differentiating in culture. Proc Natl Acad Sci USA 79: 7919-7923.

Giacobini E, Vernadakis A, Shahar A (Eds)(1980)."Tissue Culture in Neurobiology." New York: Raven Press.

Lasher RS (1974). The uptake of $[^3H]$ GABA and differentiation of stellate neurons in cultures of dissociated postnatal rat cerebellum. Brain Res 69: 482-488.

Levi G, Gordon RD, Gallo V, Wilkin GP, Balàzs R (1982). Putative acidic amino acid transmitters in the cerebellum. I. Depolarization-induced release. Brain Res 239: 425-445.

Levi G, Aloisi F, Ciotti MT, Gallo V (1983a). Autoradiographic localization and depolarization-induced release of acidic amino acids in differentiating cerebellar granule cell cultures. Brain Res, in press.

Levi G, Wilkin GP, Ciotti MT, Johnstone S (1983b). Enrichment of differentiated, stellate astrocytes in cerebellar interneuron cultures as studied by GFAP immunofluorescence and autoradiographic uptake patterns with ^{3}H-D--aspartate and ^{3}H-GABA. Dev Brain Res, in press.

Messer A (1977). The maintenance and identification of cerebellar granule cells in monolayer cultures. Brain Res 130: 1-12.

Patel AJ, Hunt A, Gordon RD, Balàzs R (1982). The activities in different neural cell types of certain enzymes associated with the metabolic compartmentation of glutamate. Dev Brain Res 4: 3-11.

Pearce BR, Dutton GR (1981). K^+-stimulated release of endogenous glutamate, GABA and other amino acids from neuron- and glia-enriched cultures of the rat cerebellum. FEBS Lett 135: 215-218.

Pearce BR, Gard AL, Dutton GR (1983). Tetanus toxin inhibition of K^+-stimulated $[^3H]$ GABA release from developing cell cultures of the rat cerebellum. J Neurochem 40: 887-890.

Pfeiffer SE (1982). "Neuroscience Approached through Cell Culture", Vol. 1. Boca Raton, Florida: CRC Press.

Schousboe A (1981). Transport and metabolism of glutamate and GABA in neurons and glial cells. Internat Rev Neurobiol 22: 1-45.

Webb M (1983). Cell surface sialoglycoproteins of cultured rat cerebellar interneurons. J Neurochem 40: 769-776.

Wilkin GP, Garthwaite, Balàzs R (1982). Putative acidic amino acid transmitters in the cerebellum. II. Electron microscopic localization of transport sites. Brain Res 244: 69-80.

Wilkin GP, Levi G, Johnstone SR, Riddle PN (1983). Cerebellar astroglial cells in primary culture: expression of different morphological appearances and differential ability to take up $[^3H]$ D-aspartate and $[^3H]$ GABA. Dev Brain Res, in press.

**Glutamine, Glutamate, and GABA
in the Central Nervous System, pages 509–516**
© **1983 Alan R. Liss, Inc., 150 Fifth Avenue, New York, NY 10011**

INHIBITION BY GABA OF EVOKED GLUTAMATE RELEASE FROM CULTURED
CEREBELLAR GRANULE CELLS

E. Meier, J. Drejer & A. Schousboe

Department of Biochemistry A, Panum Institute,
University of Copenhagen
Denmark.

INTRODUCTION

The amino acids GABA, glutamate and aspartate play an
important role as neurotransmitters in the mammalian brain.
A large number of studies has established GABA as the primary inhibitory neurotransmitter (DeFeudis & Mandel, 1981)
and several lines of evidence suggest that a large number of
neurons in the CNS employs glutamate or aspartate as excitatory neurotransmitters (Hösli & Hösli, this volume).

Specific receptors for GABA are found throughout the
brain with the highest density in cerebellum (Enna & Snyder,
1975). The major part of the receptors in cerebellum seems
to be present on the granule cells (Simantov et al., 1976)
which apparently employ glutamate as neurotransmitter (Young
et al., 1974). It might be anticipated that one function of
these GABA receptors could be a modulation of evoked glutamate release from the granule cells. A modulatory effect of
GABA has recently been demonstrated by Levi & Gallo (1981)
using synaptosomes isolated from cerebellum. Such experiments
may, however, be difficult to interpret since synaptosome preparations necessarily are heterogeneous and, moreover, the
membranes are partly damaged. It might therefore be an advantage to use cultured cells since such preparations offer
functionally intact nerve endings and also represent a less
complex model system. We have therefore used cultures of
cerebellar granule cells to study the effect of GABA on
evoked glutamate release.

CEREBELLAR GRANULE CELL CULTURES

Granule cells were cultured from 7-day-old rat cerebella as previously described (Meier & Schousboe, 1982). Briefly, cells were isolated by mild trypsinization followed by trituration in a DNAse solution containing a trypsin inhibitor. The cells were plated on poly-L-lysine-coated culture flasks or dishes (5×10^5 cells/cm^2) and grown in Dulbecco's minimum essential medium containing 10% fetal calf serum and the following constituents to favor nerve cell differentiation: 24.5 mM KCl, 30 mM glucose, 7 µM p-aminobenzoic acid and 100 mU/l insulin. After 2 days in culture, 40 µM cytosine arabinoside was added and 24 hours later this medium was changed to an analogous medium without the mitotic inhibitor. The cells were maintained in culture for 1-2 weeks. Such cultures have been shown to consist of 80-90% granule cells and less than 10% astrocytes (Currie, 1980).

In accordance with the observation that the major part of the GABA-receptors in the cerebellum seems to be present on the granule cells, we found that granule cell cultures were enriched in GABA-receptors (Meier & Schousboe, 1982). However, the binding kinetics were different from that seen for whole cerebellum as granule cells in culture only exhibited one binding site for GABA of the high affinity type (Meier & Schousboe, 1982), whereas two or more binding sites are found in cerebellum as well as in other brain areas (Olsen et al., 1981; Falch & Krogsgaard-Larsen, 1982). Also in accordance with in vivo observations, it has been established that such cultured granule cells release glutamate upon stimulation in a calcium-dependent manner (Drejer et al., 1982; Gallo et al., 1982; Drejer et al., 1983). It was investigated whether this evoked glutamate release could be affected by GABA. It was found that although GABA-receptors are present on the cultured granule cells, it was not possible to demonstrate any effect of GABA on evoked release of glutamate. This, together with the observation that only high affinity GABA-receptors were present on the cultured granule cells regardless of the age of the cultures (8-21 days, Table 1), indicated that the culture system was deficient in an important endogenous regulatory factor mediating the development of functionally active GABA-receptors. The transmitter itself might represent a strong candidate for such an endogenous regulator (Giacobini et al., 1973). Since granule cell cultures lack the ability to release endogenous GABA (Gallo et al., 1982), the granule cells were cultured in the presence of 50 µM GABA.

Table 1. Kinetic constants (K_D and B_{max}) for GABA binding to membranes from cultured granule cells.

Granule cell cultures	K_D (nM)		B_{max} (pmol $\times$ mg^{-1})	
	high affinity	low affinity	high affinity	low affinity
8 D.I.V.	7.0±0.5	n.d.	0.466±0.002	n.d.
8 D.I.V. + 50 μM GABA	7.0±0.5	550±160	0.621±0.006	0.413±0.112
21 D.I.V.	5.6±0.6	n.d.	0.481±0.042	n.d.

Kinetic constants were estimated from original binding data by computer analyses according to Olsen et al. (1981). Values are averages ± S.E.M. of 3 individual experiments. D.I.V.: Days In Vitro. From Meier et al. (1983a).

IN VITRO DEVELOPMENT OF GRANULE CELLS IN THE PRESENCE OF GABA

In the presence of GABA the cells showed a more profound morphological differentiation than in the absence of GABA as the number of neurite extending cells was increased by 50% (Meier et al., 1983a). This is in agreement with reports (Wolff et al., 1978; Spoerri & Wolff, 1981) of morphological changes at the electron microscope level of neurons exposed to extracellular GABA in vivo and of neuroblastoma cells cultured in the presence of GABA. In these reports an increase was observed in presynaptic thickenings and specialized synaptic contacts after exposure of the tissue to GABA. This led to the suggestion of a dual role of GABA in neurotransmission and synaptogenesis. Lately, we have completed a study at the electron microscope level of the effect of GABA on the development of cultured granule cells (Meier et al., 1983b; G. Hansen, E. Meier & A. Schousboe, in preparation). It was demonstrated that already after one day of culture in a GABA-containing medium a variety of morphological parameters was affected. Organels such as coated vesicles, neurofilaments, rough endoplasmatic reticulum and the Golgi apparatus were significantly increased in number, whereas mitochondria and smooth endoplasmatic reticulum were apparently not affected by the presence of GABA in the culture medium.

EFFECT OF GABA ON THE EXPRESSION OF GABA-RECEPTORS

As shown in Table 1 the presence of GABA in the culture

medium led to the appearance of low affinity GABA-receptors
on the cultured cells. The kinetic property of this receptor
was found to be almost identical to that of the low affinity
receptor found in cerebellar membranes of the corresponding
in vivo age (Meier & Schousboe, 1982). The presence of both
high and low affinity GABA-receptors on the cultures treated
with GABA is in agreement with results obtained for GABA-
binding to membranes from cultures of cerebral cortical neurons maintained in culture for 3 weeks (Ticku et al., 1980).
The presence of only the high affinity site in cultures grown
under standard conditions (i.e. without GABA) agrees, however,
with analogous studies on cortical neurons cultured for only
3 days (DeFeudis et al., 1979). The difference in the expression of high and low affinity GABA-receptors on 3-day-old
and 21-day-old cultures of cerebral cortical neurons, respectively, might be explained by the absence of extracellular
GABA in the younger cultures and presence of GABA in the older ones. In cultured cortical neurons the ability to synthesize and release GABA does apparently not develop until the
second week in culture (Snodgrass et al., 1980) consistent
with the appearance of low affinity receptors in cultures of
this age. These observations strongly indicate that GABA
might play an important role in vivo as a regulatory substance for the development of GABA-receptors. In support of
this, it has been observed that injections of nipecotic acid,
a component known to increase synaptic levels of GABA (Wood
et al., 1980), into rat retina lead to an increased number of
retinal GABA-receptors (Madtes & Redburn, 1983).

INHIBITORY ACTION OF GABA ON EVOKED GLUTAMATE RELEASE

The evoked release of L-glutamate and D-aspartate, a
non-metabolizable analogue of L-glutamate, from cultured
granule cells is shown in Fig. 1. As mentioned above this
release was not affected by GABA when cells were grown in
the absence of GABA. However, when granule cells were cultured in the presence of GABA, the evoked release of L-glutamate or D-aspartate could be inhibited by exposing the cultures to GABA during the release experiment (Meier et al.,
1983a). The nature of this inhibition with respect to bicuculline sensitivity and the inhibitory potency of GABA was investigated. It proved, however, difficult to quantify these
effects since the responses varied between experiments, although GABA consistently inhibited the evoked release when
cultures had been grown in the presence of GABA. These expe-

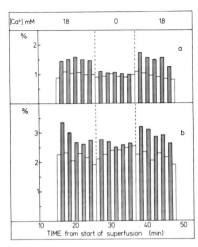

FIG. 1. Fractional release (% in fraction of total radioactivity remaining in tissue prior to the fraction in question) of D-aspartate (a) or L-glutamate (b) from cultured cerebellar granule cells preloaded with ^{3}H-D-aspartate or ^{3}H-L-glutamate. Open bars represent release into physiological (5.0 mM KCl) media and hatched bars represent release into high potassium (55 mM KCl) media. The Ca^{2+} concentration in the superfusion media is indicated at the top of the figure.
From Drejer et al. (1983).

riments indicated that the EC_{50} value for GABA was approximately 5-10 µM and that the inhibitory response was sensitive to bicuculline. A more detailed pharmacological characterization of the inhibitory action of GABA is in progress.

One explanation for the variability of the inhibitory response to GABA could rest with the presence of varying amounts of other neuronal cell types, mainly GABAergic neurons in the granule cell cultures (approximately 5-10% GABAergic neurons (Currie, 1980)). Since such GABAergic neurons in contrast to the granule cells are sensitive to the neurotoxic agent, kainic acid (Garthwaite & Wilkin, 1982) we included 50 µM kainic acid in the culture media. Such treatment of the cultures decreased the experimental variations considerably. Fig. 2 shows a release experiment performed using cultures grown in the presence of 50 µM kainic acid and varying concentrations of GABA. It is seen that GABA inhibited D-aspartate release from cultures grown in the presence of 50 µM GABA, whereas no effect of GABA could be observed in cultures grown in 10 µM GABA or without GABA.

CONCLUDING REMARKS

It has been observed that low affinity GABA receptors are present on cultured granule cells only when they have been grown in the presence of GABA at a concentration higher than 10 µM. Moreover, GABA has the ability to inhibit evoked

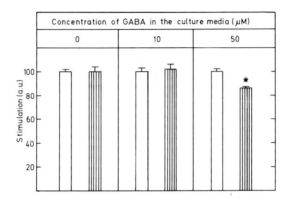

Fig. 2. Effect of external GABA on K[+]-induced stimulation of ^{3}H-D-aspartate release from granule cells grown in the presence of 50 µM kainic acid and 0, 10 or 50 µM GABA. The columns represent the average evoked release (means ± S.E.M.) from 3 successive stimulations on 3 individual cultures. For the sake of comparison the values obtained prior to the addition of 500 µM GABA to the superfusion media have been expressed as 100 a.u. in each experiment. The magnitudes of the actual evoked releases corresponded to 80-100% of the basal release regardless of the culture conditions. Open columns represent release in the presence of 100 mM KCl and hatched columns represent release in the presence of 100 mM KCl plus 500 µM GABA. The asterisk indicates a statistically significant difference from the release in the absence of GABA (P < 0.001). E. Meier, J. Drejer & A. Schousboe, unpublished.

glutamate release only in such cultures. Hence, it is likely that the inhibitory effect of GABA on glutamate release is brought about either by low affinity GABA-receptors alone or by a concerted effect of GABA on high and low affinity receptors. The observation that it is primarily the number of low affinity receptor sites which increases as a function of maturation (Meier & Schousboe, 1982) suggests that also in the in vivo situation low affinity GABA-receptors are essential for the GABA-induced activation/deactivation of the GABA-receptor ionophore complex.

ACKNOWLEDGEMENTS

The technical assistance of Miss Else Bang Larsen, Mrs. Susanne Johannessen and Mrs. Grete Rossing is gratefully acknowledged. The work has been supported financially by the following granting agencies: Danish State Medical Research Council (12-2309; 12-3229; 12-3889; 12-3419), Danish State Natural Science Research Council (511-20817), P. Carl Pedersen's Foundation, Hans Lønborg Madsen's Memorial Foundation, NOVO Foundation and King Chr. X's Foundation.

REFERENCES

Currie DN (1980). Identification of cell types by immunofluorescence in defined cell cultures of cerebellum. In Giacobini E, Vernadakis A, Shahar A (eds): "Tissue Culture in Neurobiology", New York: Raven Press, p 75.

DeFeudis FV, Ossola L, Schmitt G, Mandel P (1979). High-affinity binding of [^{3}H]muscimol to subcellular particles of neurone-enriched culture of embryonic rat brain. Neurosci Lett 14:195.

DeFeudis FV, Mandel P (eds) (1981). "Amino Acid Neurotransmitters", New York: Raven Press.

Drejer J, Larsson OM, Schousboe A (1982). Characterization of L-glutamate uptake into and release from astrocytes and neurones cultured from different brain regions. Exp Brain Res 47:259.

Drejer J, Larsson OM, Schousboe A (1983). Characterization of uptake and release processes for D- and L-aspartate in primary cultures of astrocytes and cerebellar granule cells. Neurochem Res 8:231.

Enna SJ, Snyder SH (1975). Properties of γ-aminobutyric acid (GABA) receptor binding in rat brain synaptic membrane fractions. Brain Res 100:81.

Falch E, Krogsgaard-Larsen P (1982). The binding of the specific GABA agonist [^{3}H]THIP to rat brain synaptic membranes. J Neurochem 38:1123.

Gallo V, Ciotti MT, Coletti A, Aloisi F, Levi G (1982). Selective release of glutamate from cerebellar granule cells differentiating in culture. Proc Natl Acad Sci USA 79:7919.

Garthwaite J, Wilkin GP (1982). Kainic acid receptors and neurotoxicity in adult and immature rat cerebellar slices. Neuroscience 7:2499.

Giacobini G, Filogamo G, Weber M, Bouquet P, Changeux J-P (1973). Effects of a snake alpha-neurotoxin on the development of innervated skeletal muscles in chick-embryo. Proc

Natl Acad Sci USA 70:1708.

Levi G, Gallo V (1981). Glutamate as a putative transmitter in cerebellum: stimulation by GABA of glutamic acid release from specific pools. J Neurochem 37:22.

Madtes P jr, Redburn DA (1983). Synaptic interactions of the GABA system during postnatal development in rabbit retina. J Neurosci in press.

Meier E, Schousboe A (1982). Differences between GABA receptor binding to membranes from cerebellum during postnatal development and from cultured cerebellar granule cells. Dev Neurosci 5:546.

Meier E, Drejer J, Schousboe A (1983a). Trophic actions of GABA on the development of physiologically active GABA receptors. In Mandel P, DeFeudis FV (eds): "CNS-Receptors - from Molecular Pharmacology to Behaviour", New York: Raven Press, in press.

Meier E, Hansen GH, Schousboe A (1983b). Light and electron microscopic analysis of a trophic effect of GABA on maturation of cerebellar granule cells in culture. 9th Meeting Int Soc Neurochem. J Neurochem, in press.

Olsen RW, Bergman MO, Van Ness PC, Lummis SC, Watkins AE, Napias C, Greenlee DV (1981). γ-Aminobutyric acid receptor binding in mammalian brain. Heterogeneity of binding sites. Mol Pharmacol 19:217.

Simantov R, Oster-Granite ML, Herndon RM, Snyder SH (1976). Gamma-aminobutyric acid (GABA) receptor binding selectively depleted by viral-induced granule cell loss in hamster cerebellum. Brain Res 105:365.

Snodgrass SR, White WF, Biales B, Dichter M (1980). Biochemical correlates of GABA function in rat cortical neurons in culture. Brain Res 190:123.

Spoerri PE, Wolff JR (1981). Effect of GABA-administration on murine neuroblastoma cells in culture. Cell Tissue Res 218:567.

Ticku MK, Huang A, Barker JL (1980). Characterization of GABA receptor binding in cultured brain cells. Mol Pharmacol 17:285.

Wolff JR, Joó F, Dames W (1978). Plasticity in dendrites shown by continuous GABA administration in superior cervical ganglion of adult rat. Nature (Lond) 274:72.

Wood JD, Schousboe A, Krogsgaard-Larsen P (1980). In vivo changes in the GABA content of nerve endings (synaptosomes) induced by inhibitors of GABA uptake. Neuropharmacol 19:1149.

Young AB, Oster-Granite ML, Herndon RM, Snyder SH (1974). Glutamic acid: Selective depletion by viral-induced granule cell loss in hamster cerebellum. Brain Res 73:1.

**Glutamine, Glutamate, and GABA
in the Central Nervous System, pages 517–535**
© **1983 Alan R. Liss, Inc., 150 Fifth Avenue, New York, NY 10011**

PHARMACOLOGY OF GLUTAMATE RECEPTORS

Peter J. Roberts and Steven P. Butcher

Department of Physiology and Pharmacology,
University of Southampton,
Southampton, SO9 3TU, U.K.

Approximately 100α -amino acids have been found to interact with excitatory receptors on vertebrate central neurons (Davies, Evans, Francis, Jones, Watkins 1980). The primary candidates for the endogenous ligands which activate these receptors are L-glutamate and L-aspartate. However, other endogenous excitants such as L-cysteine sulphinate, quinolinic acid, peptides containing dicarboxylic amino acid residues eg N-acetyl-asp-glu, DL- β -hydroxybutyl-asp-asp-glu, and molecules containing a polyglutamate structure (eg folates) deserve serious consideration, particularly as discrepancies have been reported between synaptic responses, and the effects of ionophoretically applied glu or asp at synapses thought to be operated by these substances (Hori, Auter, Braitman, Carpenter 1981; Shields, Falk, Naghshinch 1981).

Systematic neuropharmacological studies over the last few years, and the development of new agonists and antagonists (Krogsgaard-Larsen, Honoré, Hansen, Curtis, Lodge 1980; Watkins 1981) have suggested the existence of at least 3 distinct classes of receptors with which the neurotransmitters glu, asp and other endogenous dicarboxylic amino acids may interact. These receptors are activated preferentially by N-methyl-D-aspartate (NMDA), kainate (KA) and quisqualate (QA) (Watkins 1981). The NMDA site has been well characterised electrophysiologically, with the availability of highly potent and specific antagonists, notably: 2-amino-5-phosphonovalerate (APV) and 2-amino-7-phosphonoheptanoate (APH) (Evans, Watkins 1981; Watkins 1981; Evans, Francis, Jones Smith, Watkins 1982; Perkins, Collins, Stone 1982).

Besides the NMDA receptor category, it is uncertain how many other receptor types or subclasses exist. L-glutamate diethylester (GDEE) has been reported to antagonise QA (and glutamate)but not KA responses in cat spinal neurons (Davies, Watkins 1979; McLennan, Lodge 1979). This compound is however of low potency, and generally considered to be a rather unreliable antagonist. The most potent antagonist at QA receptors is cis-2,3-piperidine dicarboxylate, although this substance also blocks KA receptors, and may be a partial NMDA agonist. γ-D-glutamylglycine will discriminate between QA and KA receptors, depressing spinal neuronal responses elicited by the latter compound (Davies, Watkins 1981), while γ-D-glutamylaminomethylsulphonate (GAMS) antagonises responses to KA > QA > NMDA. Interestingly, GAMS frequently depressed synaptic excitation, while failing to influence responses to either L-glu or L-asp (Davies, Watkins 1982).

Neurochemical approaches to investigating excitatory amino acid receptors have focussed primarily on binding studies (see Roberts 1981 for review), and have been limited largely by the lack of suitably specific ligands of adequate specific radioactivity. However, binding sites on synaptic plasma membranes (SPM's) have been described for L-glu (Michaelis, Michaelis, Boyarsky 1974; Roberts 1974; Foster, Roberts 1978; Biziere, Thompson, Coyle 1980; Baudry, Lynch 1979a; Foster, Mena, Fagg, Cotman 1981), aspartate (Sharif, Roberts 1981; Di Lauro, Meek, Costa 1982), KA (Simon, Contrera, Kuhar 1976; London, Coyle 1979; Slevin, Collins, Coyle 1983), and the ibotenate analogue, α-amino-3-hydroxy-5-methylisoxazole-4-propionate (AMPA) (Honoré, Lauridsen, Krogsgaard-Larsen 1982). In the latter case, binding of AMPA was inhibited potently by QA and L-glu. Compounding the problems due to the lack of suitable probes, has been the finding of a number of anomalies when comparing binding sites with the receptors investigated electrophysiologically. The particular problems that may be encountered with binding studies, include the interactions of labelled ligand with non-functional receptors (eg extrajunctional sites), non-receptor binding sites eg enzymes, carrier molecules, and the investigation of binding often under highly unphysiological conditions with respect to ions and other regulatory substances to which the receptors are likely to be exposed in vivo. In this chapter, our aim is to emphasise the current state of the art with regard to excitatory amino acid binding studies, and the possible reconciliation of the differences observed between electrophysiological and binding data. In

combination with other model systems, such as the stimulation of cyclic GMP levels by glu and other excitatory amino
acids (Foster, Roberts 1980) detailed biochemical charact-
erisations of these receptors will soon be possible.

PHARMACOLOGY OF BINDING SITES FOR L-GLUTAMATE

Foster and Roberts (1978) and Sharif and Roberts (1981)
carried out detailed analyses of the structural specificity
of the binding of L-^{3}H-glutamate to rat cerebellar SPM's
utilising a Tris-HCl(pH 7.4) buffer system (Table 1).

Table 1. Inhibition of L-^{3}H-glutamate binding to cerebellar
synaptic membranes

Compound	IC_{50} (μ M)
L-Glutamate	4.8
(+) Ibotenate	8.1
DL-Quisqualate	8.4
DL-Homocysteate	10.8
cis-cyclopentylglutamate	18.5
DL-2-amino-4-phosphonobutyrate	25.6
DL- α-aminoadipic acid	26.3
D-Glutamate	28.8
L-Aspartate	42.1
D-Aspartate	138.0

L-^{3}H-glu was added at a final concentration of 0.8μ M with
a wide range of inhibitor concentrations added in 10μ l, in
a final vol of 0.5 ml. Incubations were for 10 min at 37°
and terminated by microcentrifugation.Weakly active, or
inactive compounds included KA, NMDA, GDEE, 2-APP and a
variety of other neurotransmitters.

L-glu was the most potent inhibitor, followed by QA and
ibotenate. The finding that cyclopentylglu was less active
than L-glu, suggests that glu may interact with its binding
site in an extended form. D and L-aspartate, and particularly
NMDA were poor inhibitors of binding. Binding was not affected by threo-3-hydroxyaspartate, or by DL-aspartate-β -hydrox-
amate; thus binding was not likely to be related to uptake
recognition sites.

A number of later studies using modifications of our assay system, additional pharmacological probes, and other regions of the CNS, have largely confirmed these findings in mammalian brain tissues (Biziere, Thompson, Coyle 1980; Baudry, Lynch 1981; Slevin, Collins, Lindsley, Coyle 1982; Fagg, Foster, Mena, Cotman 1982, 1983) and also in other preparations such as retina (Höckel, Müller 1982; Francis, Quitschke, Schechter 1981). The cerebellar binding sites for L-glu, appeared from saturation analysis to be homogeneous, with a Hill coefficient of unity, and a K_D =750nM and a binding capacity of approx. 70 pmol/mg membrane protein. However, a recent detailed examination of the kinetics on interaction of agonists and reputed amino acid antagonists with L-^{3}H-glu binding, indicated Hill coefficients substantially less than unity for the agonists QA and NMDA, and for the antagonists aminoadipate, and the phosphonates APB and APV (Slevin, Collins, Lindsley, Coyle 1982). These data suggest that L-glu binding is resolvable into sub-populations by means of certain selective agonists or antagonists. This is perhaps hardly surprising since in electrophysiological studies, L-glu and L-asp are mixed agonists, interacting with the several receptor types (Watkins, Evans 1981).

PHOSPHONATE ANALOGUES AND THE BINDING OF L-^{3}H-GLUTAMATE

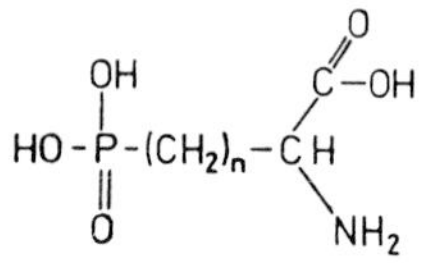

$$HO-\underset{\underset{O}{\parallel}}{\overset{\overset{OH}{|}}{P}}-(CH_2)_n-\underset{\underset{NH_2}{|}}{\overset{\overset{\displaystyle C-OH}{\overset{\parallel}{O}}}{C}}H$$

n	Compound	Abbreviations
1	2-amino-3-phosphonopropionic acid	APP
2	2-amino-4-phosphonobutyric acid	APB
3	2-amino-5-phosphonovaleric acid	APV
4	2-amino-6-phosphonohexanoic acid	APHX
5	2-amino-7-phosphonoheptanoic acid	APH

Fig. 1.   Structures of phosphonic amino acids

As seen in Table 1, DL-2-amino-4-phosphonobutyrate (APB) is a potent inhibitor of L-^{3}H-glutamate binding. In a later study (Roberts, Foster, Sharif, Collins 1982), the lower homologue 2-amino-3-phosphonopropionate (APP) was virtually devoid of activity, while the 3-carbon (APV), 4-carbon (APHX) and 5-carbon (APH) homologues were all active. Of interest was the marked inhibitory effect exerted by APHX which has also been observed by other workers (Fagg, Foster, Mena, Cotman 1983), but not however by Slevin et al (1982) using an essentially similar assay system. In contrast to APV and APH, APHX is a poor antagonist of NMDA-induced neuronal excitation (Evans, Watkins 1981), although systematic studies with other selective agonists have not been carried out.

Identification Of Subpopulations Of Glu Binding Sites From The Effects Of Ions And The Effects Of Phosphonate Analogues

Ionic effects on binding. In our original paper (Foster, Roberts 1978) and later studies, we reported that binding of L-^{3}H-glu to SPM's was increased in Tris-HCl as opposed to Tris-citrate buffer, and was further increased by performing the binding assays in a Tris-Krebs medium. We found that Na$^+$ over the concentration range 25-100 mM enhanced, while low concentrations (1-5 mM) inhibited binding. We did not however investigate other ionic effects. More recently, the binding of L-glu was shown to be capable of modification by other ions, in particular Ca^{2+} (Baudry, Lynch 1979b,1980; Fagg, Foster, Mena, Cotman 1982,1983) and chloride (Mena, Fagg, Cotman 1981; Fagg, Foster, Mena, Cotman,1983). Calcium enhances glu binding, although the presence of Cl$^-$ appears to be mandatory for this effect to be manifest.

Phosphonates. Of considerable significance, is the finding of a good correlation between the K_i for the inhibition of L-glu binding in Ca^{2+}/Cl$^-$ -containing buffer, and the K_i for synaptically-evoked responses in the rat dendate gyrus by the phosphonate series of compounds (Fagg, Mena, Cotman 1983). The presence or absence of Ca^{2+}/Cl$^-$ in the medium is crucial to the relative inhibitory potency of these substances on L-^{3}H-glu binding. In the presence of CaCl2 , the order of potency was APB >APV >APP, with L-APB being some 15 times more effective than its enantiomer (Fagg, Foster Mena, Cotman 1983). Of the total glutamate binding assayed in the presence of CaCl2, only approximately 20% was insensitive to inhibition by APB, and indeed, in the presence of 0.1 mM

L-APB, the binding of L-glu was the same, whether assayed in the presence or absence of these ions. This indicates that there is concordance between APB-sensitive, and Ca^{2+}/Cl^- - dependent binding sites.

BINDING STUDIES WITH DL-3,4-^{3}H-APB

Very recently, DL-^{3}H-APB has become available (NEN) (Monaghan, Fagg, Mena, Nieto-Sampedro, McMills, Chamberlin, Cotman 1982) and we have investigated the characteristics of L-glutamate-sensitive binding sites for this compound on rat brain SPM's. Binding assays were performed in Hepes-KOH buffer (pH 7.4) usually containing 2.5 mM $CaCl_2$. Specific binding was defined by the inclusion of 1 mM L-glu in parallel assays.

Time Course Of Association And Dissociation

Specific binding of DL-^{3}H-APB (30 nM) in the presence of $CaCl_2$ was biphasic with an initial rapid phase attaining equilibrium within 10 min. This was sustained for approx 10 min, after which there was observed a second slower phase of binding which established a new equilibrium after 50 - 60 min (Fig.). Dissociation was very rapid, with a half-life of approx 90s.

Saturability Of Binding

Studies were carried out with incubations of both 10 and 60 min duration. Untransformed specific binding data obtained over the concentration range 10-2000 nM DL-^{3}H-APB were analysed.

Table 2. Kinetic parameters of DL-^{3}H-APB binding

Time (min)	K_D (μM)	B_{max} (pmol/mg protein)	
10	1.26 $\pm$ 0.07	12.08 $\pm$ 0.51	(4)
60	1.09 $\pm$ 0.06	39.35 $\pm$ 0.95	(4)

The longer incubation period apparently resulted in an increase in the number of binding sites without significantly affecting the affinities. Hill slopes revealed values of 1.26 and 1.35 respectively. Thus there may be site heterogeneity, or binding site interactions.

Pharmacological Specificity Of DL-^{3}H-APB Binding

This was investigated by incubating SPM's with 30 nM ligand for 10 min at 37° in the presence of inhibitor (0.3 μM-1.0 mM) (Table 3).

Table 3.   Inhibition of the binding of DL-^{3}H-APB

Compound	IC_{50} (μM)
Quisqualate	0.398
L-Homocysteate	1.21
L-Glutamate	1.70
L-Cysteate	4.00
D-Homocysteate	6.30
L-Aspartate	6.97
L-Cysteine sulphinate	7.08
DL-Fluoroglutamate	7.90
(±) Ibotenate	10.00
D-Glutamate	18.10
AMPA	25.24
D-Aspartate	56.20
DL-α-Aminosuberate	1.58
L(+)-APB	2.24
L-α-Aminoadipate	3.00
DL-APB	3.61
DL-α-Aminoadipate	6.13
DL-APHX	14.40
D-α-Aminoadipate	16.18
L(+)-APH	18.96
L(+)-APV	20.00
D(-)-APB	30.06
DL-APH	32.60
DL-APV	39.80
D(-)-APH	100
D(-)-APV	126

weakly active: NMDA, quinolinate, cis-2,3-piperidine dicarboxylate, γ-D-glutamylglycine.
inactive: kainate, dihydrokainate, GABA, carbachol, glycine
and HA-966. Synaptic membranes were incubated in Hepes-KOH
buffer containing 2.5 mM $CaCl_2$.

As might be anticipated, the pharmacology corresponds
closely with that for APB-sensitive glutamate binding. In
our hands, ibotenate was less active against APB than glu
binding. The L isomer of APB was approximately 15 times
more potent than the D form in inhibiting binding. L/D
isomer ratios of 6, 11, and 9 were obtained for homocysteate,
glu and asp respectively. With each of the (NMDA receptor)
antagonist molecules that were found to be active, such as
the phosphonates APV and APH, and α-aminoadipate and α-amino-
suberate, again it was the L(+) isomers that were more potent.
Strikingly, L(+)-APB, in common with the L isomers of the
sulphur-containing amino acids, and the very potent inhibitor
QA, were able to inhibit APB binding to a substantially
greater extent than the 100 per cent defined by 1 mM L-glu.
It thus follows that notwithstanding the finding of Hill
coefficients of close to unity, the sites labelled by DL-^{3}H-
APB are not homogeneous.

Effects Of Ions On DL-^{3}H-APB Binding

In view of the report that Cl^- is the prime ionic species
in stimulating L-^{3}H-glutamate binding, and that Ca^{2+} acts
only in the presence of Cl^- to enhance this response further
(Mena, Fagg, Cotman 1981), we have investigated the effects
of a number of ionic species on APB binding (Fig.2).

In the absence of any added ions other than K^+ (50 mM
Hepes-KOH buffer, pH 7.4), the binding of DL-^{3}H-APB was
negligible. When the effect of anions as their ammonium
salts was investigated, 2.5 mM Cl^- markedly enhanced APB
binding. This effect could partially be reproduced by bromide
but not by fluoride, acetate or sulphate. Divalent cations
also influenced binding. If they were tested as their acetate
salts however, no stimulation above basal levels was observed.
In the presence of Cl^-, Ca^{2+} produced an approximate two fold
increase in binding as compared with Cl^- alone. Ca^{2+} produced
the greatest effect, although manganese, magnesium and str-
ontium possessed some activity. Neither barium, not the

monovalent cations, sodium, lithium or caesium could increase binding. Thus the effect of cations was dependent on the anion employed.

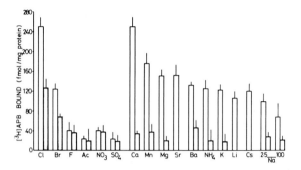

Fig.2. Ionic regulation of DL-^{3}H-APB binding. The APB binding assay was carried out in the presence of added ions (2.5 mM unless indicated). For the anions, LH column is Ca^{2+} salt, RH column, ammonium. For cations, RH column is acetate and LH column is chloride.

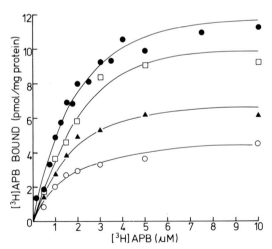

Fig. 3. Saturation of DL-^{3}H-APB binding in the presence of added ions. ^{3}H-APB binding was investigated over the range 100nM-10µM, in the presence of 1mM NH_4Cl (o), 2.5mM NH_4Cl (▲), 2.5mM NH_4Cl + 1mM calcium acetate (□), or 2.5mM $CaCl_2$ (●). Results are from quadruplicate assays.

The effects of the ions on the kinetic characteristics of DL-^{3}H-APB binding were examined in more detail by the construction of saturation curves in the presence of fixed concentrations of added ions.

Chloride ions elicited a concentration-dependent incr- ease in receptor numbers, without modifying the affinity. The further stimulation produced by calcium (added as the chloride salt) also resulted in a concentration-dependent increase in receptor density, with little effect on affinity (Table 4).

Table 4. Effects on kinetic parameters of DL-^{3}H-APB binding of added ions

Added Ions	K_D (μM)	B_{max} (pmol/mg prot)
1mM NH$_4$Cl	1.30	4.6
2.5mM NH$_4$Cl	1.48	7.6
2.5mM CaCl$_2$	1.36	12.06
1mM calcium acetate + 2.5mM NH$_4$Cl	1.44	10.17

Drug inhibition studies were also carried out in NH$_4$Cl, CaCl$_2$ -containing media, and in Krebs-Hepes. There were no significant qualitative or quantitative differences observed with any of the agonists or antagonists tested.

Reversibility of Ca^{2+}/ Cl$^-$ Effects on Binding

As seen in Table4, the presence of Ca^{2+} during a 10 min incubation period, increases APB binding, apparently by exposing additional sites, which do not differ in their pharmacological characteristics from those seen in the absence of this ion (Cl$^-$ present). It has been suggested that with L-glutamate binding to SPM's, the stimulation observed with Ca^{2+} is due to activation of a membrane-bound protease, which irreversibly unmasks additional binding sites (Baudry, Lynch 1980; Baudry, Bundman, Smith, Lynch 1981; Vargas, Greenbaum, Costa 1980). The finding of increased binding of

L-^{3}H-glutamate to synaptic membranes from hippocampal slices after high frequency electrical stimulation to the Schaffer-commissural systems (Lynch, Halpain, Baudry 1982) has led to the proposal that such a protease system may be involved in the up-regulation of receptors as in long-term synaptic potentiation in the hippocampus. In contrast, Fagg et al (1983) reported that the Ca^{2+} (Cl^- -dependent, APB-sensitive) enhancement of L-^{3}H-glu binding was wholly reversible, as evidenced by removal of ions from the medium by washing, or addition of EGTA. We have investigated this discrepancy in further detail. As described earlier, the specific binding of DL-^{3}H-APB was biphasic in the presence of $CaCl_2$. This is illustrated better in Figure 4.

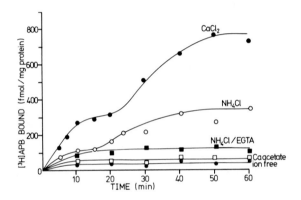

Fig. 4. Effects of ions on the time course of DL-^{3}H-APB binding. SPM's were incubated as described previously, for between 5 and 60 min in the presence or absence of added ions (2.5mM), or additionally, with EGTA (0.1mM).

The second component of binding, which is accompanied by some clumping and precipitation of membrane particles appears to be wholly Ca^{2+}- dependent, but again, is expressed only in the presence of Cl^-. The appearance of a (much reduced) second phase in the presence of NH_4Cl is almost certainly attributable to residual Ca^{2+}, since further addition of EGTA reduced the binding substantially. It is pertinent to note that Fagg et al (1983) utilised exposure times to Ca^{2+} of 20-30 min, followed by extensive washing, or addition of a high concentration of EGTA (5mM). Thus it is possible that the second phase was not being studied

under these conditions. We have used several inhibitors of
protease activity in an attempt to resolve this question of
reversibility (Fig. 5).

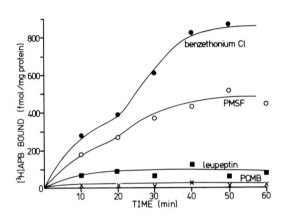

Fig. 5. Effects of protease inhibitors on the time course
of ^{3}H-APB binding. Assays were performed in 2.5mM CaCl$_2$ -
containing media, with the addition of one of the following
inhibitors: benzethonium chloride, PMSF and PCMB (all at
0.1mM) and leupeptin (0.1 mg/ml).

     Benzethonium chloride did not influence APB binding,
suggesting that arylamino- and arylimino peptidase-like
enzymes are not involved. PMSF reduced both binding components by approximately one third. This substance inhibits
enzymes possessing a serine residue at the active site
(eg AChE, trypsin). Leupeptin essentially reduced the binding
in the presence of CaCl$_2$ to that observed with Cl$^-$ alone
(cf Fig. 4). This agrees well with the findings of Baudry
and Lynch (1980) and Vargas et al (1980). Leupeptin has
been suggested to be a rather selective inhibitor of neutral
thiol proteinases (Toyo-Oka, Shimizu, Masaki 1978) and
recently, it was reported that this substance prevented the
degradation of cytoskeletal-associated proteins (eg micro-
tubule-associated proteins, and fodrin), concomitant with
abolishing the Ca^{2+} increase in ^{3}H-glu binding sites (Baudry,
Siman, Smith, Lynch 1983). Finally, the profound effect of
PCMB on both binding components is probably due to its
potent effect in alkylating thiol groups; this is likely to

interfere directly with ligand-receptor interactions.

Thus, our experiments have not provided evidence for any reversibility of the Ca^{2+}-enhanced binding occurring during either long or short incubation periods, and our data support the proposal for an involvement of a protease in this phenomenon.

CONCLUSIONS

Several studies performed within the last few years have demonstrated the binding of L-glutamate and aspartate to apparently homogeneous populations of membrane sites in the CNS, which exhibit many of the broad characteristics that are expected of physiological receptors. However, it has usually been difficult to relate the structural specif- icity of binding directly to the pharmacology as observed electrophysiologically. It would now seem likely that a major factor involved, is the effect of ions. In particular, whether or not Cl^- and Ca^{2+} are included in the incubation medium, greatly influences L-^{3}H-glu binding, both quantitat- ively and qualitatively (Fagg, Foster, Mena, Cotman 1983). Thus the data that have been generated in studies using diverse buffers such as Tris-HCl, Tris-citrate, phosphate, might be anticipated to be discrepant.

Within the framework of Watkins' categorisation of excitatory amino acid receptors into 3 primary types, viz NMDA, KA and QA -preferring, there is reasonably good correlation between ^{3}H-KA binding data and electrophysiol- ogical results, with the receptors being activated by domoate, glu and quisqualate. It is now generally considered that KA interacts with a subpopulation of excitatory amino acid receptors, possibly activated physiologically by glu itself, or some closely related substance. The bulk of the sites labelled by L-^{3}H-glu appear to be Cl^-/ Ca^{2+}-dependent, and, in the absence of these ions, binding is very substant- ially reduced and is changed in its pharmacological profile. Foster and Roberts (1978) first reported that in contrast to other receptor systems, L-^{3}H-glu binding in Tris-HCl medium was reduced by approximately 80 per cent following freezing and thawing of SPM's. In our present work, we have found that freezing virtually abolished DL-^{3}H-APB binding (Butcher, Roberts, Collins 1983a,b), and similar findings were reported for Cl^-/Ca^{2+}-dependent L-^{3}H-glu binding.

Fagg, Mena and Cotman (1983) have proposed that L-^{3}H-glu binding assays conducted in the absence of Cl^-/Ca^{2+}, or by the use of L-^{3}H-asp, permit the visualisation of NMDA sites. NMDA receptors probably occur at low density on SPM's and they persist following freezing. From data derived from electrophysiology, the most potent inhibitors of binding would therefore be anticipated to be NMDA itself, ibotenate, and the antagonists APV and APH, with little effect by APB, GAMS or GDEE. To some extent this is borne out (Fagg, Foster, Mena, Cotman (1983) with APV and APH being good inhibitors of binding. D-APH was more potent than the L-isomer, but only approximately twice as active. This contrasts sharply with the electrophysiology, where the antagonistic activity resides almost exclusively in the D isomer (Perkins, Collins, Stone 1982). D-alpha-amino adipate and cis 2,3-PDA were only very weakly active and quisqualate and ibotenate were of similar potencies. Most seriously however, NMDA was a poor inhibitor of binding (Fagg, Foster, Mena, Cotman 1982). Thus, we do not believe that Cl^-/Ca^{2+}-independent binding involves primarily an NMDA receptor. Its significance remains to be elucidated. The NMDA receptor remains problematical for study in neurochemical experiments. Investigations with ^{3}H-NMDA have not been fruitful (Roberts 1981), nor have those with DL-^{3}H-APH (Schwarcz, Foster, Roberts, unpublished). The most promising results to emerge have been from Watkins' group (Jones, Olverman, Watkins 1983) using D-^{3}H-APV, where binding was inhibited potently by APV, APH, PDA, and importantly, NMDA. Interestingly, quinolinate was relatively ineffective.

The APB (or L-glu), Cl^-/Ca^{2+}-sensitive sites show a striking pharmacological specificity. They are probably not homogeneous as discussed earlier, since QA, APB itself, and certain other amino acids were found to inhibit ^{3}H-APB binding to a greater extent than L-glu or L-asp etc. The binding site preferentially recognises L-isomers (agonists) and it is highly relevant that L(+)-APB possesses a potent and stereoselective synaptic depressant action (Koerner, Cotman 1981; Davies, Watkins 1982b). It has been proposed by the latter workers that L(+)-APB may act by specifically inhibiting the release of an excitatory amino acid transmitter (eg glu) acting at non-NMDA receptors, or alternatively, by antagonising the postsynaptic effects of an unidentified transmitter. In contrast to the L isomer, D-APB appears to be a rather weak antagonist at NMDA receptors.

It is tempting to suggest that DL-^{3}H-APB is labelling
an agonist-preferring, possibly QA type binding site. It
should be noted however, that AMPA (a proposed selective
QA receptor agonist) was much weaker in inhibiting APB
binding than expected. However, the specificity of this
agonist for QA receptors is not clearly defined. Electrophysiologically, the effect of AMPA is antagonised by
GDEE (Krogsgaard-Larsen, Honore, Hansen, Curtis, Lodge 1980)
while its binding is not (Honore, Lauridsen, Krogsgaard-
Larsen 1982). A further interesting finding with regard to
the binding of APB, was the greater potency of APHX than
either APV or APH in inhibiting binding. The pharmacological
profile of this phosphonate is not defined, except that it
is a poor antagonist of NMDA responses.

At present, it is clear that Cl^-/Ca^{2+}-dependent APB
binding sites, and those for APB-sensitive L-glu interactions,
are present on synaptic membranes in high density. They may
be localised postsynaptically and play a major physiological
role, or may occur presynaptically also eg at presynaptic
autoreceptors (McBean, Roberts 1981).

These studies, coupled with autoradiography, and
further binding experiments utilising selective lesioning
procedures in different regions of the CNS will help to
build up a more detailed picture of the localisation and
types of excitatory amino acid receptors occurring in the
nervous system.

ACKNOWLEDGEMENTS

We should like to thank Jim Collins for his involvement
in this work, and Drs J.F. Watkins and C.H. Eugster for
the very generous gifts of compounds. This work was supported
by an S.E.R.C. Project Grant to P.J.R.

Baudry M, Bundman M, Smith E, Lynch G (1981). Micromolar
   levels of calcium stimulate proteolytic activity and
   glutamate receptor binding in rat brain synaptic membranes.
   Science 212:937.
Baudry M, Lynch G (1979a). Two glutamate binding sites in
   rat hippocampal membranes. Eur J Pharmacol 57:283.
Baudry M, Lynch G (1979b). Regulation of glutamate receptors
   by cations. Nature 282:748.

Baudry M, Lynch G (1980). Regulation of hippocampal glutamate receptors: evidence for the involvement of a calcium-activated protease. Proc Natl Acad Sci USA 77:2298.

Baudry M, Siman R, Smith EK, Lynch G (1983). Regulation by calcium ions of glutamate receptor binding in hippocampal slices. Eur J Pharmacol 90:161.

Biziere K, Thompson H, Coyle JT (1980). Characterisation of specific high-affinity binding sites for L-^{3}H-glutamic acid in rat brain membranes. Brain Res 183:421.

Butcher SP, Roberts PJ, Collins JF (1983a). DL-^{3}H-2-amino-4-phosphonobutyrate binding to L-glutamate-sensitive sites on rat brain synaptic membranes. IRCS Med Sci 11:4.

Butcher SP, Roberts PJ, Collins JF (1983b). Characterisation of DL-^{3}H-2-amino-4-phosphonobutyrate binding to L-glutamate sensitive sites on rat brain synaptic membranes. Br J Pharmacol (in press).

Davies J, Evans RH, Francis AA, Jones AW, Watkins JC (1980). Excitatory amino acid receptors in the vertebrate central nervous system. In Littauer UZ, Dudai Y, Silman I, Teichberg VI, Vogel Z (eds): " Neurotransmitters and their Receptors", Chichester: John Wiley and sons Ltd, p 333.

Davies J, Watkins JC (1979). Selective antagonism of amino acid-induced and synaptic excitation in the cat spinal cord. J Physiol Lond 297:621.

Davies J, Watkins JC (1981). Differentiation of kainate and quisqualate receptors in the cat spinal cord by selective antagonism with gamma-D (and L)-glutamylglycine. Brain Res 206:172.

Davies J, Watkins JC (1982a). Selective excitatory amino acid antagonist action of gamma-D-glutamyl-aminomethyl-sulphonate (GAMS) on cat spinal neurones. J Physiol Lond 332:108P.

Davies J, Watkins JC (1982b). Actions of D and L forms of 2-amino-5-phosphonovalerate and 2-amino-4-phosphonobutyrate in the cat spinal cord. Brain Res 235:378.

Di Lauro A, Meek JL, Costa E (1982). Specific high-affinity binding of L-^{3}H-aspartate in rat brain membranes. J Neurochem 38:1261.

Evans RH, Francis AA, Jones AW, Smith DAS, Watkins JC (1982). The effects of a series of ω-phosphonic-α-carboxylic amino acids on electrically evoked and excitant amino acid-induced responses in isolated spinal cord preparations. Br J Pharmacol 75:65.

Evans RH, Watkins JC (1981). Pharmacological antagonists of excitatory amino acids. Life Sci 28:1303.

Fagg GE, Foster AC, Mena EE, Cotman CW (1982). Chloride

and calcium ions reveal a pharmacologically-distinct population of L-glutamate binding sites in synaptic membranes:
correspondence between biochemical and electrophysiological
data. J Neurosci 2:958.

Fagg GE, Foster AC, Mena EE, Cotman CW (1983). Chloride
and calcium ions separate L-glutamate receptor populations
in synaptic membranes. Eur J Pharmacol 88:105.

Fagg GE, Mena EE, Cotman CW (1983). L-glutamate receptor
populations in synaptic membranes: effects of ions and
pharmacological characteristics. In DeFeudis FV, Mandel P
(eds): "Receptors - Behaviour to Molecular Aspects" New
York: Raven Press, in press.

Foster AC, Mena EE, Fagg GE, Cotman CW (1981). Glutamate
and aspartate binding sites are enriched in synaptic
junctions isolated from rat brain. J Neurosci L:620.

Foster AC, Roberts PJ (1978). High-affinity L-^{3}H-glutamate
binding to postsynaptic receptor sites on rat cerebellar
synaptic membranes. J Neurochem 31:1467.

Foster GA, Roberts PJ (1980). Pharmacology of excitatory
amino acid receptors mediating the stimulation of rat
cerebellar cyclic GMP levels in vitro. Life Sci 27:215.

Francis A, Quitschke W, Schechter N (1981). Glutamic acid
binding in goldfish brain and denervated optic tectum.
Brain Res 216:375.

Höckel SHJ, Müller WE (1982). L-glutamate receptor binding
in bovine retina. Exp Eye Res 35:55.

Honoré, T, Lauridsen J, Krogsgaard-Larsen P (1982). The
binding of ^{3}H-AMPA, a structural analogue of glutamic
acid to rat brain membranes. J Neurochem 38:173.

Hori NC, Auter CR, Braitman DJ, Carpenter DO (1981).
Lateral olfactory tract transmitter: glutamate,aspartate
or neither ? Cell Mol Neurobiol 1:115.

Jones AW, Olverman HJ, Watkins JC (1983). A study of N-
methyl-D-aspartate receptor sites on rat brain membranes
using ^{3}H-D-(-)-2-amino-5-phosphonovalerate as a labelled
ligand. J Physiol Lond (in press).

Koerner JF, Cotman CW (1981). Micromolar L-2-amino-4-phos-
phonobutyric acid selectively inhibits perforant path
synapses from lateral entorhinal cortex. Brain Res 216:
192.

Krogsgaard-Larsen P, Honoré T, Hansen JJ, Curtis DR, Lodge
D (1980). New class of glutamate agonist structurally
related to ibotenic acid. Nature 284:64.

London ED, Coyle JT (1979). Specific binding of ^{3}H-kainic
acid to receptor sites in rat brain. Mol Pharmacol 15:492.

Lynch G, Halpain S, Baudry M (1982). Effects of high-frequency synaptic stimulation on glutamate receptor binding studied with a modified in vitro hippocampal slice preparation. Brain Res 244:101.

McBean GJ, Roberts PJ (1981). Glutamate-preferring receptors regulate the release of D-^{3}H-aspartate from rat hippocampal slices. Nature 291:593.

McLennan H, Lodge D (1979). The antagonism of amino acid-induced excitation of spinal neurones in the cat. Brain Res 169:83.

Mena EE, Fagg GE, Cotman CW (1981). Chloride ions enhance L-glutamate binding to rat brain synaptic membranes. Brain Res 243:378.

Michaelis EK, Michaelis ML, Boyarsky LL (1974) High-affinity glutamic acid binding to brain synaptic membranes. Biochim Biophys Acta 367:338.

Monaghan DT, Fagg GE, Mena EE, Nieto Sampedro MC, McMills AR, Chamberlin AR, Cotman CW (1982). New ligands for studying acidic amino acid receptors: ^{3}H-APB and ^{3}H-L-serine-o-sulphate. Soc Neurosci Abst 8:403.

Perkins MN, Collins JF, Stone TW (1982). Isomers of 2-amino-7-phosphonoheptanoic acid as antagonists of neuronal excitation. Neurosci Lett 32:65.

Roberts PJ (1974). Glutamate receptors in the rat central nervous system. Nature 252:399.

Roberts PJ (1981). Binding studies for the investigation of receptors for L-glutamate and other excitatory amino acids. InRoberts PJ, Storm-Mathisen J, Johnston GAR (eds): "Glutamate:Transmitter in the Central Nervous System", Chichester: John Wiley and Sons Ltd, p 35.

Roberts PJ, Foster GA, Sharif NA, Collins JF (1982). Phosphonate analogues of acidic amino acids: inhibition of excitatory amino acid transmitter binding to cerebellar membranes and of the stimulation of cerebellar cyclic GMP levels. Brain Res 238:475.

Sharif NA, Roberts PJ (1981). L-aspartate binding sites in rat cerebellum: a comparison of the binding of L-^{3}H-glutamate and L-^{3}H-aspartate to synaptic membranes. Brain Res 211:293.

Shields RA, Falk G, Naghshinch S (1981). Action of glutamate and aspartate analogues on rod horizontal and bipolar cells. Nature 294:592.

Simon JR, Contrera JF, Kuhar MJ (1976). Binding of ^{3}H-kainic acid, an analogue of L-glutamate, to brain membranes. J Neurochem 26:141.

Slevin JT, Collins JF, Coyle JT (1983). Analogue interactions with the brain receptor labelled with ^{3}H-kainic acid.

Brain Res 265:169.
Slevin JT, Collins J, Lindsley K, Coyle JT (1982). Specific
    binding of ^{3}H-L-glutamate to cerebellar membranes:evidence
    for recognition site heterogeneity. Brain Res 249:353.
Toyo-Oka T, Shimizu T, Masaki T (1978). Inhibition of
    proteolytic calcium-activated neutral protease by leupeptin
    and antipain. Biochem Biophys Res Comm 82:484
Vargas F, Greenbaum L, Costa E (1980). Participation of
    cystein proteinase in the high affinity Ca^{2+}-dependent
    binding of glutamate to hippocampal synaptic membranes.
    Neuropharmacol 19:791.
Watkins JC (1981). Pharmacology of excitatory amino acid
    transmitters. In DeFeudis FV, Mandel P (eds): "Amino Acid
    Neurotransmitters", Chichester: John Wiley and Sons Ltd,
    p 205.
Watkins JC, Evans RH (1981). Excitatory amino acid trans-
    mitters. Ann Rev Pharmacol Toxicol 21:165.

**Glutamine, Glutamate, and GABA
in the Central Nervous System, pages 537–557**
© 1983 Alan R. Liss, Inc., 150 Fifth Avenue, New York, NY 10011

GABA AGONISTS: STRUCTURAL, PHARMACOLOGICAL AND CLINICAL
ASPECTS

Povl Krogsgaard-Larsen

Department of Chemistry
Royal Danish School of Pharmacy
DK-2100 Copenhagen, Denmark

Mapping of the role of 4-aminobutyric acid (GABA) in
the central regulation of physiological processes and in the
pathophysiology of certain neurological and psychiatric disorders has become a very active multidisciplinary research
field. GABA has been shown to be involved in the regulation
of cardiovascular mechanisms (DiMicco et al. 1979; DeFeudis
1981), the secretion of hormones (Enna 1981), and the sensa-
tion of pain (Hill et al. 1981) and anxiety (Hoehn-Saric
1983). GABA appears to have a complicity in epilepsy (Meldrum 1982), Huntington's chorea (Roberts et al. 1976; Di
Chiara, Gessa 1981), and spasticity (Naftchi et al. 1979),
although our knowledge of the nature and cause of the GABA
dysfunctions in these diseases is still very incomplete.
Circumstantial evidence of imbalances of unknown nature between GABA and dopamine in Parkinson's disease and schizophrenia (Roberts et al. 1976; Krogsgaard-Larsen et al.
1979b) has further stimulated interests in the pharmacology
of GABA.

GABA neurones are ubiquitous in the mammalian central
nervous system (CNS), and if GABA-operated synapses throughout the CNS were to contain identical receptors, enzymes and
transport systems, pharmacological manipulation of GABA synapses would appear to be impracticable in diseases with re-
gioselective degeneration of GABA neurones. Furthermore,
cardiovascular functions (DiMicco et al. 1979), seizure processes (Iadarola, Gale 1982), anxiety (Scheel-Krüger, Petersen 1982), and aggressive behaviour (Mandel et al. 1979) appear to be subject to control by GABA neurones in discrete
brain areas. If only one type of GABA synapse were to exist

in the CNS, GABA therapies might not be suitable for the regulation of dysfunctions of these functions.

In the light of the fundamental role of GABA in the CNS the existence of only one population of GABA receptors seems unlikely, and accumulating evidence actually does indicate that GABA receptors with dissimilar agonist specificities exist. In this chapter the development of selective GABA agonists will be discussed.

SELECTIVE PHARMACOLOGICAL MANIPULATION OF GABA SYNAPTIC MECHANISMS

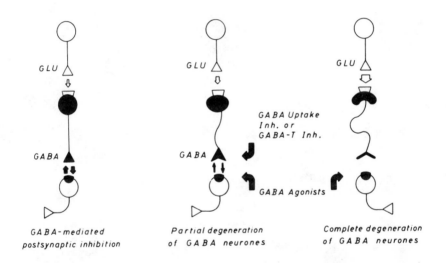

Fig. 1. A schematic illustration of GABA-mediated postsynaptic inhibition and the potential pharmacological sites of attack after partial or total degeneration of GABA neurones.

In diseases, where GABA neurones are still functioning but at an abnormally low level, presynaptic mechanisms as well as postsynaptic receptors are potential pharmacological sites of attack, whereas in the case of extensive neuronal degeneration GABA agonist therapies seem to be of primary interest (Fig. 1) (Krogsgaard-Larsen 1981). A prerequisite

for studies of the susceptibility of the GABA synaptic mechanisms to pharmacological manipulation is the availability
of specific tools and drugs. The discovery of irreversible
inhibitors of GABA:2-oxoglutarate aminotransferase (GABA-T)
such as gabaculine and 4-aminohex-5-enoic acid (γ-vinyl-
GABA) (Palfreyman et al. 1981) and the characterization of
the structural specificities of the postsynaptic receptors
and uptake systems (Schousboe et al. 1979; Krogsgaard-Larsen
1980; Krogsgaard-Larsen, Falch 1981) represent important
steps in the development of the pharmacology of GABA.

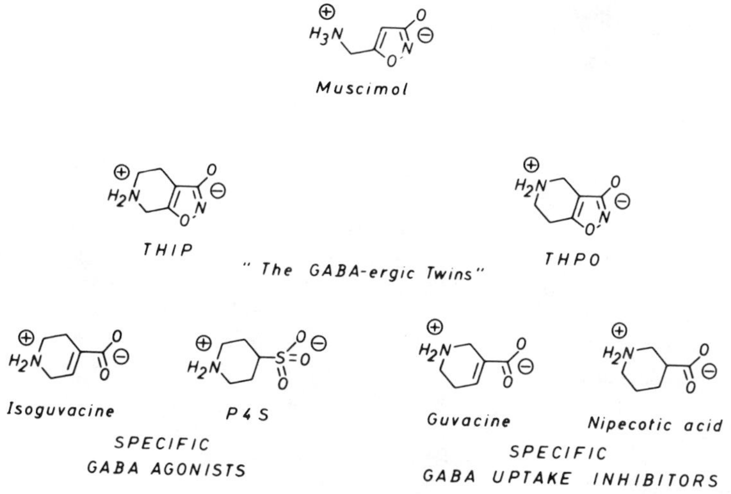

Fig. 2. The structures of muscimol, of THIP and related GABA
agonists, and of THPO and related GABA uptake inhibitors.

    The naturally occurring heterocyclic GABA analogue mus-
cimol has been an important lead structure for the design of
specific GABA agonists and uptake inhibitors (Krogsgaard-
Larsen et al. 1981a) (Fig. 2). While muscimol interacts with
the GABA receptors (Krogsgaard-Larsen et al. 1979a) as well
as with the GABA uptake systems (Schousboe et al. 1979) and
GABA-T (LJ Fowler, unpublished), the "GABA-ergic twins"
4,5,6,7-tetrahydroisoxazolo[5,4-c]pyridin-3-ol (THIP) and
4,5,6,7-tetrahydroisoxazolo[4,5-c]pyridin-3-ol (THPO) have

specific actions. THIP is a specific GABA agonist (Krogsgaard-Larsen et al. 1977) whereas THPO is an inhibitor of
GABA uptake (Krogsgaard-Larsen 1980) with selective effect
on the glial uptake system (Schousboe et al. 1981), and neither compound interacts with GABA-T. These findings led to
the design of a series of specific GABA agonists related to
THIP, such as isoguvacine and piperidine-4-sulphonic acid
(P4S) (Krogsgaard-Larsen, Falch 1981), and some amino acid
analogues of THPO with potent and specific effects on GABA
uptake (Krogsgaard-Larsen 1980) (Fig. 2).

BICUCULLINE, A SELECTIVE GABA ANTAGONIST

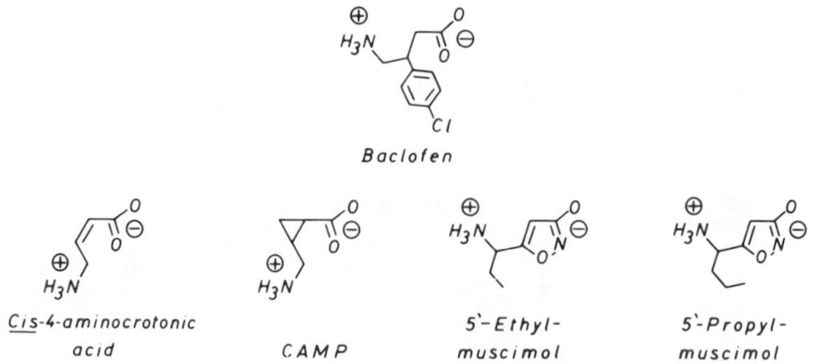

Fig. 3. The structures of baclofen and a number of other bicuculline-insensitive neuronal depressants structurally related to GABA.

The discovery of the GABA antagonist actions of the alkaloid (+)-bicuculline (BIC) (Fig. 4) and bicuculline methochloride (BMC) represents a milestone in the studies of the
GABA receptors (Curtis et al. 1971a; Johnston et al. 1972).
Based on electrophysiological and receptor binding studies
the GABA receptors are at present most conveniently subdivided
into two apparently heterogeneous classes:
  1) Receptors at which the depressant effect of GABA can
     be competitively antagonized by BIC or BMC and
  2) receptors insensitive to BIC or BMC.

The GABA analogue baclofen (Fig. 3) is a BIC-insensitive depressant of neuronal firing (Curtis et al. 1974), and baclofen interacts with a population of receptors (GABA-B receptors), which bind GABA but not BIC or various BIC-sensitive GABA agonists including isoguvacine and THIP (Hill, Bowery 1981). These receptors seem to modulate the release of monoamines in the CNS (Bowery et al. 1980), but the mechanism(s) underlying the therapeutic effects of baclofen in spastic patients are still unknown (Curtis et al. 1981).

Other groups of BIC-insensitive GABA receptors may exist in the mammalian CNS, although the evidence is still indirect and very scanty. Thus, 5'-ethyl- and 5'-propylmuscimol (Fig. 3) are moderately potent BMC-insensitive depressants of neuronal firing (Krogsgaard-Larsen et al. 1975), but these compounds do not interact significantly with the GABA-B receptor sites (NG Bowery, unpublished) or other BIC-insensitive GABA receptor sites in vitro (FV DeFeudis, unpublished). Similarly, the mechanism of action of the BMC- and strychnine-insensitive neuronal depressants cis-4-aminocrotonic acid (Johnston et al. 1975) and cis-2-(aminomethyl)-cyclopropanecarboxylic acid (CAMP) (Allan et al. 1980a) is not known.

BIC-sensitive GABA receptors include <u>presynaptic</u> as well as <u>postsynaptic</u> receptors (Curtis 1978; Curtis, Johnston, 1974). While these receptors, which are located on postsynaptic membranes on different neuronal structures, have similar agonist specificities, <u>extrasynaptic</u> BIC-sensitive GABA receptors (Curtis 1978; Brown 1979) apparently have different characteristics (Allan et al. 1980b; Alger, Nicoll 1982).

PHARMACOLOGICAL CHARACTERISTICS OF SPINAL AND SUPRASPINAL BICUCULLINE-SENSITIVE GABA RECEPTORS

There is an increasing amount of evidence supporting the view that BIC-sensitive GABA receptors can be subdivided into groups with different agonist/antagonist specificities. The development of a number of BIC-sensitive GABA agonists (Table 1) have made detailed studies of these aspects possible. The ability of the compounds listed in Table 1 to displace radioactive GABA from GABA receptor sites was studied using rat brain membranes and their relative potencies in vivo were studied on cat spinal neurones. In spite of the positive correlation between the results of these two series of experiments there is evidence for differences between spinal and supraspinal GABA receptors.

Table 1. Structures, in vitro and in vivo potencies, and protolytic properties of some BIC-sensitive GABA agonists.

COMPOUND	STRUCTURE	INHIBITION of GABA Binding $IC_{50}, \mu M$	GABA AGONIST Activity Rel. Potency	PK_A VALUES	I/U RATIO
GABA		0.033	— — —	4.0 ; 10.7	800,000
P 4 S		0.034	— — — —	<1 ; 10.3	>1,000,000
Isoguvacine		0.037	— — — —	3.6 ; 9.8	200,000
Muscimol		0.006	— — — —	4.8 ; 8.4	900
N-Methyl-muscimol		4.2	— —	4.5 ; 8.7	1,000
THIP		0.13	— — — (—)	4.4 ; 8.5	1,500
Thiomuscimol		0.019	— — — —	6.1 ; 8.9	13
N-Methyl-thiomuscimol		8.3	— —	5.4 ; 8.5	62
Thio-THIP		4 2	—	6.1 ; 8.5	16

The GABA binding studies using rat brain membranes (Falch, Krogsgaard-Larsen 1982), the microelectrophoretic studies on cat spinal neurones (Krogsgaard-Larsen et al. 1979a), and the calculation of I/U ratios (Krogsgaard-Larsen, Falch 1981) were accomplished as described earlier in detail.

While pre- and postsynaptic GABA receptors on cat spinal neurones have very similar agonist specificities (Curtis et al. 1980), earlier electrophysiological studies have disclosed different relative sensitivity of GABA receptors in the cat spinal cord and cerebral cortex to GABA and muscimol (Curtis et al. 1971a; Curtis et al. 1971b). These pharmacological differences between spinal and supraspinal GABA receptors have recently been further elucidated. While muscimol and thiomuscimol are approximately equipotent as agonists at cat spinal neurones (Krogsgaard-Larsen et al. 1979a) thiomuscimol is more than two orders of magnitude weaker than muscimol in inducing circling behaviour in rats, an effect which appears to be mediated by BIC-sensitive GABA receptors in the substantia nigra pars reticulata (Arnt et al. 1979). Similar differences between muscimol and thiomuscimol have been observed after local injection into regions of rat brains known to be rich in GABA receptors (J Scheel-Krüger, unpublished) suggesting that thiomuscimol is a selective agonist at GABA receptors in the spinal cord. Muscimol, isoguvacine, and GABA are agonists with a decreasing order of potency at BIC-sensitive GABA receptors in the cat spinal cord (Krogsgaard-Larsen et al. 1979a) (Table 1), but these compounds seem to activate BIC-sensitive GABA receptors in rat brains which regulate the release of glutamic acid with a different order of potency (Mitchell 1982). At these receptors, apparently of presynaptic nature, muscimol is only a moderately potent agonist weaker than GABA, whereas isoguvacine is more potent than GABA.

As exemplified in Table 2 even minor alterations of the structure of THIP result in complete loss of GABA agonist activity (Krogsgaard-Larsen et al. 1982a). All of these analogues of THIP do, however, antagonize glycine-induced depression of the firing of cat spinal neurones (Krogsgaard-Larsen et al. 1982a). While neither 5,6,7,8-tetrahydro-4H-isoxazolo[3,4-d]azepin-3-ol (iso-THAZ) nor 5,6,7,8-tetrahydro-4H-isoxazolo[4,5-d]azepin-3-ol (THAZ) affects the GABA receptors in the cat spinal cord (Krogsgaard-Larsen et al. 1982a), iso-THAZ, but not THAZ, has a GABA antagonist profile after local injection into the substantia nigra of rats (Arnt, Krogsgaard-Larsen 1979). 5-(3-Pyrrolidinyl)-3-isoxazolol (3-PYOL), on the other hand, is an antagonist at both GABA and glycine receptors in the cat spinal cord (Krogsgaard-Larsen et al. 1982a). Thus, the structure-activity studies summarized in Table 2 seem to suggest different pharmacological characteristics of spinal and supraspinal GABA

Table 2. Structures and biological effects of GABA, THIP and
some THIP analogues

COMPOUND	STRUCTURE	GABA AGONIST ACTIVITY Spinal cord (Rel. potency)	GABA ANTAGONIST ACTIVITY		GLYCINE ANTAGONIST ACTIVITY Spinal cord
			Spinal cord	Substantia nigra	
GABA		— — —			
THIP		— — — (—)			
N-Methyl-THIP		0	No	N.t.	Yes
3-PYOL		0	Yes	N.t.	Yes
THAZ		0	No	No	Yes
Iso-THAZ		0	No	Yes	Yes

The GABA agonist, GABA antagonist, and glycine antagonist
activities on cat spinal neurones were measured microelec-
trophoretically (Krogsgaard-Larsen et al. 1982a). The GABA
antagonist activities in the substantia nigra pars reticulata of rats were measured after local injection of the compounds (Arnt, Krogsgaard-Larsen 1979). N.t., not tested.

receptors.

Recent binding studies have shown that the ratio of low-
to high-affinity GABA binding sites is much higher in the
spinal cord than in the brain of rats and mice (Frere et al.
1982). These findings, supported by electrophysiological
studies (Nowak et al. 1982) led these authors to suggest
that the high-affinity GABA binding sites represent the phy-

siologically relevant postsynaptic receptors, whereas low-affinity sites represent presynaptic receptors. This hypothesis does, however, not readily explain the, apparently different, pharmacological specificities of GABA receptors in the brain and the spinal cord described above.

INTERACTION OF GABA AGONISTS WITH THE POSTSYNAPTIC GABA
RECEPTOR COMPLEX

In Fig. 4 our present knowledge of the structure of the postsynaptic GABA receptor complex is summarized (Olsen 1981; Skolnick, Paul 1981). The chloride channel is regulated by the GABA receptor consisting of two (Olsen et al. 1981) or possibly three GABA binding sites (Falch, Krogsgaard-Larsen

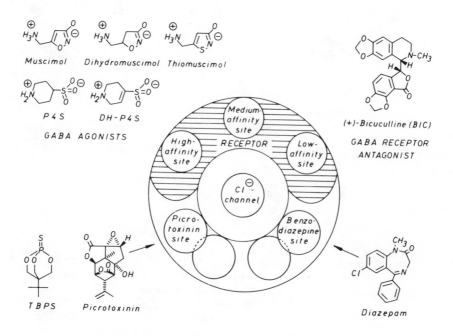

Fig. 4. A schematic illustration of the postsynaptic GABA receptor complex and of the sites of action of some GABA agonists, the GABA receptor antagonist bicuculline, and various other compounds.

Table 3. GABA agonist activities and effects on benzodiazepine binding of some GABA analogues

COMPOUND	STRUCTURE	GABA AGONIST Activity Rel. Potency	INHIBITION of GABA Binding $IC_{50}, \mu M$	ACTIVATION of Diazepam Binding Max. Activation (%)	$EC_{50}, \mu M$
GABA	$H_3N^{\oplus}$ ... $^{\ominus}$	— — —	0.033	100	3.8
$\underline{N}$-Methyl-GABA	$H_2N^{\oplus}/$ ...	0	67	18	
Isonipecotic acid	$H_2N^{\oplus}$ ...	— — —	0.33	78	
$\underline{t}$-ACA	$H_3N^{\oplus}$ ...	— — —	0.080	100	7.4
$\underline{N}$-Methyl-$\underline{t}$-ACA	$H_2N^{\oplus}/$ ...	—	28	33	
Isoguvacine	$H_2N^{\oplus}$ ...	— — — —	0.037	42	
Mus-cimol	$H_3N^{\oplus}$ ...	— — — —	0.006	100	0.6
$\underline{N}$-Methyl-muscimol	$H_2N^{\oplus}/$ ...	— —	4.2	90	
THIP	$H_2N^{\oplus}$ ...	— — — (—)	0.13	11	

The GABA agonist activities were measured microelectrophore-
tically (Krogsgaard-Larsen et al. 1977; Krogsgaard-Larsen et
al. 1979a; DR Curtis and P Krogsgaard-Larsen, unpublished).
The GABA binding studies (Falch, Krogsgaard-Larsen 1982) and
the studies on the stimulation of diazepam binding at 0°C
and in the absence of chloride ions (Braestrup et al. 1979)
were performed as described earlier.

1982), although the physiological relevance of these multiple
binding sites, which can be detected in vitro under different
experimental conditions, is unclear. The GABA receptor func-

tion appears to be modulated by various additional units, which can be detected in vitro as distinct binding sites for the benzodiazepines (BZ) (Squires, Braestrup 1977) and picrotoxinin (Ticku et al. 1978). There is some evidence of heterogeneity of both the BZ and the picrotoxinin binding sites (Olsen 1981) (Fig. 4) and of the existence of a distinct binding site at the receptor complex for the avermectines (Supavilai, Karobath 1981).

The physiological relevance of these additional sites of the GABA receptor complex is unknown, but the intimate contact and allosteric interactions between these sites as detected in vitro may reflect certain aspects of the dynamic properties of the GABA receptors (Olsen 1981, Pong, Wang 1982). At present these sites are most conveniently described as the pharmacological receptors for a variety of therapeutic agents and pharmacological tools as exemplified in Fig. 4 (Olsen 1981; Squires et al. 1983).

The interaction of GABA agonists with the GABA receptor complex in vitro has been extensively studied (Braestrup et al. 1979; Karobath et al. 1979; Krogsgaard-Larsen, Falch 1981). These studies have disclosed striking differences between the effects on BZ binding of different "structural classes" of GABA agonists and pronounced effects of temperature and chloride ions on the degree of GABA agonist-induced stimulation of BZ binding (Supavilai, Karobath 1980). GABA and the GABA-agonists trans-4-aminocrotonic acid (t-ACA), muscimol, dihydromuscimol, and thiomuscimol (Fig 4 and Table 3) quite effectively activate BZ binding at 0°C and in the absence of chloride ions, but even minor alterations of the structures of these "parent compounds" normally have substantial effects on the effectiveness of the compounds in this test system. While there generally is a positive correlation between the potency of these GABA analogues as GABA agonists and as inhibitors of GABA receptor binding, there obviously is no simple correlation between the potency of GABA agonists and their ability to stimulate BZ binding (Table 3). Comprehensive structure-activity studies on this latter effect of GABA agonists indicate that three structural parameters of GABA agonists are of major importance (Krogsgaard-Larsen 1981; Krogsgaard-Larsen, Falch 1981):

1) The structure of the acid moiety of the agonists,
2) the degree of substitution at the basic nitrogen atom, and
3) the conformational mobility of the entire molecule.

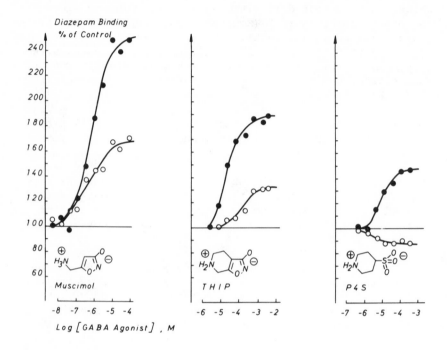

Fig. 5. Effects of some GABA agonists on the binding of 3H-diazepam at 30°C in the presence ● or absence ○ of 150 mM sodium chloride. Experiments were performed in analogy with published procedures (Braestrup et al. 1979; P Krogsgaard-Larsen, E Falch, P Jacobsen, unpublished).

In Fig. 5 the effects of muscimol, THIP, and P4S on BZ binding at 30°C and in the absence or presence of chloride ions are illustrated. The presence of chloride ions in the incubation media substantially enhances the ability of these GABA agonists to stimulate BZ binding, and the addition of chloride actually converts P4S from a deactivator to an activator of BZ binding. Very similar effects of chloride were observed for the specific GABA agonist 1,2,3,6-tetrahydropyridine-4-sulphonic acid (DH-P4S) an unsaturated analogue of P4S (Fig. 4) (P Krogsgaard-Larsen, E Falch, P. Jacobsen, unpublished).

The pharmacological relevance of these conspicuously dissimilar effects of different "structural classes" of GABA agonist on BZ binding in vitro is unclear. The results illustrated in Fig. 5 are reminiscent of partial GABA agonist effects of THIP and P4S, but so far electrophysiological studies have not disclosed partial agonist profiles of for example THIP or P4S.

Further studies along these lines may eventually elucidate some of the mechanisms underlying the apparently complex function of the postsynaptic GABA receptor machinery. In any case, the test systems concerned appear to be useful in the evaluation and characterization of GABA agonists. On the basis of the results summarized in Table 3 and Fig. 5 it is tempting to assume that it is possible to develop specific BIC-sensitive GABA agonists with different behavioural pharmacological profiles.

Our studies on the molecular pharmacology of GABA agonists have embraced labelling of THIP and P4S (Krogsgaard-Larsen et al. 1982b) and comparative studies on the binding of radioactive GABA, THIP, and P4S (Krogsgaard-Larsen et al. 1981b; Falch, Krogsgaard-Larsen 1982) (Table 4).

While the K_D values for these ligands are comparable, considerable differences between the B_M values were measured. The density of the high-affinity binding sites for THIP was low compared with those measured for GABA and P4S. There is, however, no obvious correlation between these data and the effects of the GABA agonists concerned on BZ binding, and the pharmacological relevance of the observed differences is unclear as yet.

PHARMACOKINETIC ASPECTS OF BICUCULLINE-SENSITIVE GABA AGONISTS

All compounds so far known with specific GABA agonist actions have zwitterionic structures. Small, and frequently negligible, fractions of amino acids exist as unionized molecules in solution, the ratio between the concentrations of ionized and unionized molecules (I/U ratio) being a function of the difference between the pKA I and II values (Krogsgaard-Larsen, Falch 1981). A great difference between the two pKA values of neutral amino acids is tantamount to high I/U ratios for the compounds.

Table 4. Binding data and kinetic constants for radioactive GABA, THIP and P4S

Binding and kinetic parameters		Radioactive ligand		
		$[^3H]GABA$	$[^3H]THIP$	$[^3H]P4S$
K_{D1}	(nM)	6 ± 3	4 ± 2	6 ± 2
B_{M1}	(pmol/mg)	0.31 ± 0.1	0.05 ± 0.03	0.55 ± 0.15
K_{D2}	(nM)	175 ± 35	80 ± 23	56 ± 15
B_{M2}	(pmol/mg)	1.7 ± 0.4	0.5 ± 0.1	0.96 ± 0.35
K_{D3}	(nM)	$>5,000$	$>10,000$	$>1,500$
k_{on} (high-aff.)	$M^{-1}min^{-1}$	$2\cdot10^7$	$-$	$7\cdot10^7$
k_{off} $-$	min^{-1}	0.2	$-$	0.8

Since amino acids are likely to penetrate the blood-brain barrier (BBB) in the unionized form, it is of pharmacological interest to develop analogues of GABA with small differences in the pKA values, and thus low I/U ratios, compared to GABA. From the data given in Table 1 it is understandable that neither GABA, P4S, nor isoguvacine are capable of penetrating the BBB to any significant extent. On the other hand, approximately 0.1% of doses of THIP or muscimol exist as unionized molecules in aqueous solution, and this value can readily explain, why THIP and muscimol enter the brain after peripheral administration in animals and man (Moroni et al. 1982; Schultz et al. 1981; Christensen et al. 1982). The low I/U ratios of thiomuscimol, N-methylthiomuscimol, and thio-THIP (Table 1) suggest that these compounds are capable of penetrating the BBB very easily. These aspects are under investigation at present.

The low I/U ratios of the thio analogues of muscimol, N-methylmuscimol, and THIP have been obtained at the expense of their GABA agonist activities (Table 1). While thiomuscimol appears to be a selective agonist at spinal GABA receptors (see earlier section of this chapter), N-methylthiomuscimol and in particular thio-THIP are weak GABA agonists (Krogsgaard-Larsen et al. 1981a; Krogsgaard-Larsen 1981). In the light of the very similar structures of THIP and thio-THIP (Fig. 6) these observations emphasize the pronounced structural specificity of the GABA receptors.

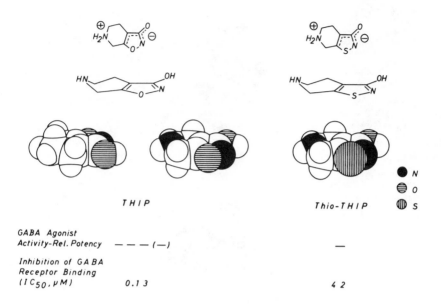

GABA Agonist
Activity-Rel. Potency — — — (—)   —

Inhibition of GABA
Receptor Binding
$(IC_{50}, \mu M)$ 0.13   42

Fig. 6. A comparison of the structures and GABA agonist activities of THIP and thio-THIP. The low-energy conformations
of these compounds were derived from computer analyses (JS
New, P Krogsgaard-Larsen, unpublished).

As discussed in an earlier section of this chapter, muscimol is a non-specific GABA agonist, and the toxicity and
metabolic instability of muscimol (Moroni et al. 1982) further reduce the pharmacological importance of this compound.
THIP, on the other hand, is well tolerated by various animal
species (Christensen et al. 1982). It is active after oral
administration and excreted unchanged, and to some extent in
a conjugated form, in the urine from animals and humans
(Schultz et al. 1981; Christensen et al. 1982). The major
metabolite of THIP has not been isolated in a pure form yet,
but it has chromatographic properties identical with those
of synthetic THIP-N-glucuronide (Fig. 7) (B Schultz, H Mik-
kelsen, P Krogsgaard-Larsen, unpublished).

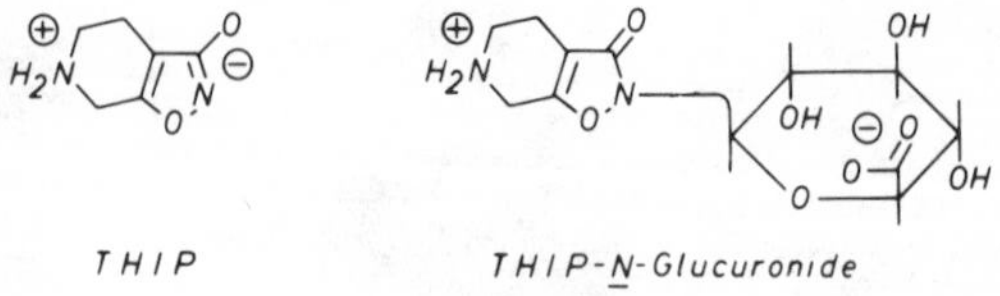

THIP   THIP-N-Glucuronide

Fig. 7. The structures of THIP and THIP-N-glucuronide.

PHARMACOLOGICAL AND CLINICAL STUDIES ON THIP

Among various pharmacological effects of THIP, its anticonvulsant properties in animals (Meldrum, Horton 1980; Löscher 1982), its inhibition of food intake in the rat (Blavet et al. 1982), and the decreases in blood pressure observed after injection of THIP into the brain ventricles of
cats (Gillis et al. 1982) may have therapeutic interest.

In the human clinic the positive effects of THIP in
spastic patients (Mondrup, Pedersen 1983) and in chronic anxiety patients (Hoehn-Saric 1983) are encouraging. So far,
the analgesic effects of THIP in humans have been most extensively studied (Christensen et al. 1982). The inability of
naloxone to reverse THIP-induced analgesia in animals (Hill
et al. 1981; Kendall et al. 1982) indicates that THIP does
not interact directly with the opiate receptors. The lack of
effect of BIC on THIP analgesia may indicate that a distinct
sub-type of GABA receptor mediates this effect of THIP,
which in most animal models and in man is comparable in potency with that of morphine (Christensen et al. 1982). This
combination of anxiolytic and analgesic effects combined
with the observation that THIP, in contrast to morphine, does
not cause respiratory depression (Christensen et al. 1982)
has stimulated the interest in THIP, and GABA agonists in
general, as analgesic drugs.

ACKNOWLEDGEMENTS

This work was supported by grants from the Danish Medical Research Council. The secretarial and technical assistance of Mrs. B. Hare and Mr. S. Stilling are acknowledged.

REFERENCES

Alger BE, Nicoll RA (1982). Pharmacological evidence for two kinds of GABA receptors on rat hippocampal pyramidal cells studied in vitro. J Physiol (London) 328:125.

Allan RD, Curtis DR, Headley PM, Johnston GAR, Lodge D, Twitchin B (1980a). The synthesis and activity of cis- and trans-2-(aminomethyl)cyclopropanecarboxylic acids as conformationally restricted analogues of GABA. J Neurochem 34:652.

Allan RD, Evans RH, Johnston GAR (1980b). 4-Aminobutyric acid agonists: an in vitro comparison between depression of spinal synaptic activity and depolarization of spinal root fibres in the rat. Br J Pharmacol 70:609.

Arnt J, Krogsgaard-Larsen P (1979). GABA agonists and potential antagonists related to muscimol. Brain Res 177:395.

Arnt J, Scheel-Krüger J, Magelund G, Krogsgaard-Larsen P (1979). Muscimol and related GABA receptor agonists: the potency of GABA-ergic drugs in vivo determined after intranigral injection. J Pharm Pharmacol 31:306.

Blavet N, DeFeudis FV, Clostre F (1982). THIP inhibits feeding behaviour in fasted rats. Psychopharmacology 76:75.

Bowery NG, Hill DR, Hudson AL, Doble A, Middlemiss DN, Shaw J, Turnbull M (1980). (-)-Baclofen decreases neurotransmitter release in the mammalian CNS by an action at a novel GABA receptor. Nature 283:92.

Braestrup C, Nielsen M, Krogsgaard-Larsen P, Falch E (1979). Partial agonists for brain GABA-benzodiazepine receptor complex. Nature 280:331.

Brown DA (1979). Extrasynaptic GABA systems. Trends Neurosci. 2:271.

Christensen AV, Svendsen O, Krogsgaard-Larsen P (1982). Pharmacodynamic effects and possible therapeutic uses of THIP, a specific GABA agonist. Pharm Weekbl Sci Ed 4:145.

Curtis DR (1978). Pre- and non-synaptic activities of GABA and related amino acids in the mammalian nervous system. In Fonnum F (ed): "Amino Acids as Chemical Transmitters", New York: Plenum Press, p 55.

Curtis DR, Bornstein JC, Lodge D (1980). In vivo analysis of GABA receptors on primary afferent terminations in the cat. Brain Res 194:255.

Curtis DR, Duggan AW, Felix D, Johnston GAR (1971a). Bicuculline, an antagonist of GABA and synaptic inhibition in the spinal cord of the cat. Brain Res 32:69.

Curtis DR, Duggan AW, Felix D, Johnston GAR, McLennan H (1971b). Antagonism between bicuculline and GABA in the cat brain. Brain Res 33:57.

Curtis DR, Game CJA, Johnston GAR, McCulloch RM (1974).
Central effects of β-(p-chlorophenyl)-γ-aminobutyric acid.
Brain Res 70:493.

Curtis DR, Johnston GAR (1974). Amino acid transmitters in
the mammalian central nervous system. Ergebn Physiol 69:97.

Curtis DR, Lodge D, Bornstein JC, Peet MJ (1981). Selective
effects of (-)baclofen on spinal synaptic transmission in
the cat. Exp Brain Res 42:158.

DeFeudis FV (1981). GABA and "neuro-cardiovascular" mechanisms. Neurochem Int 3:113.

Di Chiara G, Gessa GL (1981). "GABA and the Basal Ganglia".
New York: Raven.

DiMicco JA, Gale K, Hamilton B, Gillis RA (1979). GABA receptor control of parasympathetic outflow to heart: characterization and brainstem localization. Science 204:1106.

Enna SJ (1981). GABA receptor pharmacology. Functional considerations. Biochem Pharmacol 30:907.

Falch E, Krogsgaard-Larsen P (1982). The binding of the GABA
agonist [3H]THIP to rat brain synaptic membranes. J
Neurochem 38:1123.

Frere RC, MacDonald RL, Young AB (1982). GABA binding and
bicuculline in spinal cord and cortical membranes from
adult rat and from mouse neurons in culture. Brain Res
244:145.

Gillis RA, Williford DJ, Souza JD, Quest JA (1982). Central
cardiovascular effects produced by the GABA receptor agonist drug, THIP. Neuropharmacology 21:545.

Hill DR, Bowery NG (1981). 3H-Baclofen and 3H-GABA bind to
bicuculline-insensitive GABA-B sites in rat brain. Nature
290:149.

Hill RC, Maurer R, Buescher HH, Roemer D (1981). Analgesic
properties of the GABA-mimetic THIP. Eur J Pharmacol
69:221.

Hoehn-Saric R (1983). Effects of the GABA agonist THIP on
chronic anxiety patients. Psychopharmacol Bull 19:114.

Iadarola MJ, Gale K (1982). Substantia nigra: site of anticonvulsant activity mediated by 4-aminobutyric acid.
Science 218:1237.

Johnston GAR, Beart PM, Curtis DR, Game CJA, McCulloch RM,
Maclachlan RM (1972). Bicuculline methochloride as a GABA
antagonist. Nature New Biology 240:219.

Johnston GAR, Curtis DR, Beart PM, Game CJA, McCulloch RM,
Twitchin B (1975). Cis- and trans-4-aminocrotonic acid as
GABA analogues of restricted conformation. J Neurochem
24:157.

Karobath M, Placheta P, Lippitsch M, Krogsgaard-Larsen P
(1979). Is stimulation of benzodiazepine receptor binding
mediated by a novel GABA receptor? Nature 278:748.
Kendall DA, Browner M, Enna SJ (1982). Comparison of the an-
tinociceptive effect of GABA agonists: evidence for a cholinergic involvement. J Pharmacol Exp Ther 220:482.
Krogsgaard-Larsen P (1980). Inhibitors of the GABA uptake
systems. Mol Cell Biochem 31:105.
Krogsgaard-Larsen P (1981). γ-Aminobutyric acid agonists,
antagonists, and uptake inhibitors. Design and therapeutic
aspects. J Med Chem 24:1377.
Krogsgaard-Larsen P, Brehm L, Schaumburg K (1981a). Muscimol,
a psychoactive constituent of amanita muscaria, as a medici-
nal chemical model structure. Acta Chem Scand B35:311.
Krogsgaard-Larsen P, Falch E (1981). GABA agonists. Development and interactions with the GABA receptor complex. Mol
Cell Biochem 38:129.
Krogsgaard-Larsen P, Hjeds H, Curtis DR, Leah JD, Peet MJ
(1982a). Glycine antagonists structurally related to muscimol, THIP, or isoguvacine. J Neurochem 39:1319.
Krogsgaard-Larsen P, Hjeds H, Curtis DR, Lodge D, Johnston
GAR (1979a). Dihydromuscimol, thiomuscimol, and related
heterocyclic compounds as GABA analogues. J Neurochem
32:1717.
Krogsgaard-Larsen P, Johansen JS, Falch E (1982b). Deuterium
labelling of the GABA agonists THIP, piperidine-4-sulphonic
acid and the GABA uptake inhibitor THPO. J labelled
Compd 19:689.
Krogsgaard-Larsen P, Johnston GAR, Curtis DR, Game CJA, McCul-
loch RM (1975). Structure and biological activity of a
series of conformationally restricted analogues of GABA.
J Neurochem. 25:803.
Krogsgaard-Larsen P, Johnston GAR, Lodge D, Curtis DR (1977).
A new class of GABA agonist. Nature 268:53.
Krogsgaard-Larsen P, Scheel-Krüger J, Kofod H (1979b).
"GABA-Neurotransmitters". Copenhagen: Munksgaard.
Krogsgaard-Larsen P, Snowman A, Lummis SC, Olsen RW (1981b).
Characterization of the binding of the GABA agonist [3H]-
piperidine-4-sulphonic acid to bovine brain synaptic mem-
branes. J Neurochem 37:401.
Löscher W (1982). Comparative assay of anticonvulsant and
toxic potencies of sixteen GABAmimetic drugs. Neurophar-
macology 21:803.
Mandel P, Ciesielski L, Maitre M, Simler S, Mack G, Kempf E
(1979). Involvement of central GABA-ergic systems in convulsions and aggressive behaviour. In Mandel P, DeFeudis

FV (eds): "GABA-Biochemistry and CNS Functions", New York: Plenum, p 475.

Meldrum B (1982). Pharmacology of GABA. Clin Neuropharmacol 5:293.

Meldrum B, Horton R (1980). Effects of the bicyclic GABA agonist, THIP, on myoclonic and seizure responses in mice and baboons with reflex epilepsy. Eur J Pharmacol 61:231.

Mitchell R (1982). Interactions of agonists and antagonists with a novel type of GABA receptor. Biochem Pharmacol 31:2684.

Mondrup K, Pedersen E (1983). The acute effect of the GABA-agonist, THIP, on proprioceptive and flexor reflexes in spastic patients. Acta Neurol Scand 67:48.

Moroni F, Forchetti MC, Krogsgaard-Larsen P, Guidotti A (1982). Relative disposition of the GABA agonists THIP and muscimol in the brain of the rat. J Pharm Pharmacol 34:676.

Naftchi NE, Schlosser W, Horst WD (1979). Correlation of changes in the GABA-ergic system with the development of spasticity in paraplegic cats. Adv Exp Med Biol 123:431.

Nowak LM, Young AB, MacDonald RL (1982). GABA and bicuculline actions on mouse spinal cord and cortical neurons in cell culture. Brain Res 244:155.

Olsen RW (1981). GABA-benzodiazepine-barbiturate receptor interactions. J Neurochem 37:1.

Olsen RW, Bergman MO, Van Ness PC, Lummis SC, Watkins AE Napias C, Greenlee DV (1981). Gamma-aminobutyric acid receptor binding in mammalian brain: Heterogeneity of binding sites. Mol Pharmacol 19:217.

Palfreyman MG, Schechter PJ, Buckett WR, Tell GP, Koch-Weser J (1981). The pharmacology of GABA-transaminase inhibitors. Biochem Pharmacol 30:817.

Pong SS, Wang CC (1982). Avermectin B1a modulation of γ-aminobutyric acid receptors in rat brain membranes. J Neurochem 38:375.

Roberts E, Chase TN, Tower DB (1976). "GABA in Nervous System Function". New York: Raven.

Scheel-Krüger J, Petersen EN (1982). Anticonflict effect of the benzodiazepines mediated by a GABAergic mechanism in the amygdala. Eur J Pharmacol 82:115.

Schousboe A, Larsson OM, Hertz L, Krogsgaard-Larsen P (1981). Heterocyclic GABA analogues as new selective inhibitors of astroglial GABA transport. Drug Dev Res 1:115.

Schousboe A, Thorbek P, Hertz L, Krogsgaard-Larsen P (1979). Effects of GABA analogues of restricted conformation on GABA transport in astrocytes and brain cortex slices and on

GABA receptor binding. J Neurochem 33:181.

Schultz B, Aaes-Jørgensen T, Bøgesø KP, Jørgensen A (1981). Preliminary studies on the absorption, distribution, metabolism, and excretion of THIP in animal and man using 14C-labelled compound. Acta Pharmacol Toxicol 49:116.

Skolnick P, Paul SM (1981). Benzodiazepine receptors. Ann Rep Med Chem 16:21.

Squires RF, Braestrup C (1977). Benzodiazepine receptors in rat brain. Nature 266:732.

Squires RF, Casida JE, Richardson M, Saederup E (1983). 35S-t-Butyl-bicyclophosphothionate binds with high affinity to brain specific sites coupled to GABA-A and ion recognition sites. Mol Pharmacol 23:326.

Supavilai P, Karobath M (1980). The effect of temperature and chloride ions on the stimulation of [3H]flunitrazepam binding by the muscimol analogues THIP and piperidine-4-sulphonic acid. Neurosci Lett 19:337.

Supavilai P, Karobath M (1981). In vitro modulation by avermectin Bla of the GABA/benzodiazepine receptor complex of rat cerebellum. J Neurochem 36:798.

Ticku MK, Van Ness PC, Haycock JW, Levy WB, Olsen RW (1978). Dihydropicrotoxinin binding sites in rat brain: comparison to GABA receptors. Brain Res 150:642.

**Glutamine, Glutamate, and GABA
in the Central Nervous System, pages 559–569**
© **1983 Alan R. Liss, Inc., 150 Fifth Avenue, New York, NY 10011**

FUNCTIONAL ALTERATIONS IN CENTRAL GABA NEURONS INDUCED BY
STRESS

Kinya Kuriyama, Kouiji Kanmori and Yukio Yoneda

Department of Pharmacology, Kyoto Prefectural
University of Medicine, Kamikyo-ku, Kyoto 602
Japan.

INTRODUCTION

It has been well established that a variety of stressors induce significant alterations in the metabolism and/or
function of various putative neurotransmitters in the
mammalian central nervous system (CNS). For example, various environmental stressors induce a significant reduction
of the endogenous steady-state levels of catecholamines (CA)
such as noradrenaline (NA), adrenaline (Ad) and dopamine
(DA), with a concomitant acceleration of their in vivo turnover (Thierry et al. 1968; Lidbrink et al. 1972).

On the other hand, relatively little attention has been
paid to functional alterations in cerebral γ-aminobutyric
acid (GABA) systems following the application of various
experimental stresses; GABA is an established inhibitory
neurotransmitter in the mammalian CNS. In this study, we
have attempted to determine whether or not stress affects
the function and metabolism of cerebral GABA neurons. In
addition, we have also examined the effect of various central depressants, including ethanol, on stress-induced
alterations in cerebral GABA system.

RESULTS

Stress and GABA Metabolism

Adult male Wistar rats weighing 180-220 g were individually confined for 3 h in a metallic restraint stress-cage

which was kept in a water bath maintained at 25°C so that
the xiphoid process of the animal was immersed (Nakagawa,
Kuriyama 1975; Yoneda et al. 1983). We have termed this
treatment as "cold and immobilization stress." Animals were
sacrificed between 11:00 a.m. and 12:00 p.m. to avoid
possible circadian variations in the cerebral GABA systems.

Fig. 1 shows the stress-induced alterations in the cerebral metabolism of GABA. The application of stress resulted
in a significant elevation of the striatal as well as hypothalamic GABA contents with a concomitant reduction of its
metabolic precursor, L-glutamic acid (GLU). No significant
alteration was, however, detected in the endogenous levels
of GABA and GLU in the substantia nigra. These alterations
were restored at 12 h after the termination of stress treatment. It was also found that the stress significantly elevated the activity of L-glutamic acid decarboxylase (GAD),
which was responsible for the formation of GABA from GLU, in
central structures such as the striatum and hypothalamus.
These results indicate that the elevation of GAD activity
contributes to the increase of GABA content and the decrease
of GLU content under the stressful situations employed.

Stress and GABA Turnover

To evaluate the functional state of GABA neurons in the
brain, the in vivo turnover of cerebral GABA was estimated
using two different methods (Kuriyama et al. 1983; Yoneda et
al. 1983). The stress treatment, however, failed to induce
a significant alteration in the in vivo turnover rate of
GABA in the striatum, hypothalamus and cerebellum when
measured by either method (Yoneda et al. 1983).

Stress and GABA Transport

Since the stress application induced a more significant
alteration in the metabolism of GABA in the striatum than in
the hypothalamus, we have employed the striatum to investigate possible neurochemical alterations in cerebral GABA
neurons induced by stress. The stress treatment, however,
failed to affect either the high affinity or the low affinity
uptake system for [^{3}H]GABA. Similarly no profound change
was detected in the net accumulation of GABA into striatal
slices following the stress application.

On the other hand, the release of preloaded [³H]GABA from the striatal slices was found to consist of an initial rapid phase followed by a slow phase. Application of a high

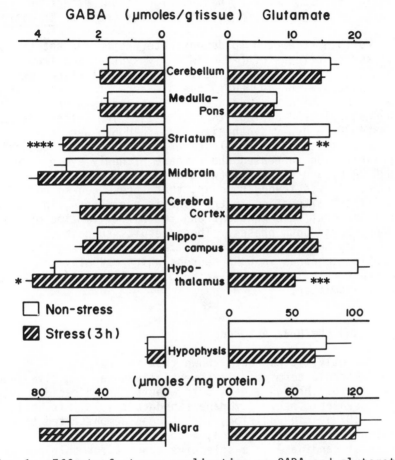

Fig. 1. Effect of stress application on GABA and glutamate contents in rat brain. Following the application of cold and immobilization stress for 3 h, animals were sacrificed by focused microwave irradiation (5 KW for 0.7 sec) between 11:00 a.m. and 12:00 p.m. Each value represents the mean ± S.E.M. obtained from 3-6 separate experiments. *P<0.05, **P<0.02,***P<0.01,****P<0.001, compared with each non-stress control value. (Modified from Kuriyama et al. 1983)

potassium stimulation induced a significant elevation of the release of [3H]GABA which was dependent on the presence of external Ca^{2+}. The in vivo application of cold and immobilization stress, however, had no significant effect on the release of [3H]GABA from striatal slices measured in vitro.

We then attempted to demonstrate whether or not stress affects the release of [3H]GABA newly synthesized from [3H]GLU in the striatal slices. The striatal slices were preincubated with [3H]GLU in the presence of nipecotic acid (5×10^{-5} M), which was added to prevent possible reuptake of [3H]GABA released during its synthesis. The slices loaded with [3H]GABA newly synthesized from [3H]GLU were then subjected to subsequent release experiments. High potassium depolarization increased the release of newly synthesized [3H]GABA by approximately twofold in a Ca^{2+} dependent manner. It was found, however, that stress caused no significant alteration in the kinetic parameters, including the fractional rate constant and the half-life time of the component for both phases. These results suggest that stress may have no significant effect on the integrity of synaptic membranes in GABA neurons which may play an important role in the regulation of in vitro release of the neurotransmitter.

Stress and the GABA Autoreceptor

Recently, it has been shown that the release of GABA from GABAergic terminals is potentially under negative feedback control through a GABA autoreceptor which resides on the presynaptic nerve membrane (Snodgrass 1978; Mitchell, Martin 1978). In addition, it has been demonstrated that δ-aminolevulinic acid (DALA), a porphyrin precursor, is a potential candidate as a selective agonist for this presynaptic GABA autoreceptor (Brennan, Cantrill 1979). In vitro addition (10^{-5} M) of DALA, as well as GABA agonists such as muscimol (MUS) and imidazoleacetic acid, caused a significant suppression of the evoked release of [3H]GABA by 30 mM KCl from striatal slices without affecting the spontaneous non-stimulated release. These suppressive actions were invariably antagonized by the addition (10^{-5} M) of GABA antagonists, including bicuculline and picrotoxin, but not strychnine. As shown in Fig. 2(A), in striatal tissue from animals stressed in vivo there was a significantly greater suppression of the KCl-evoked release of [3H]GABA by

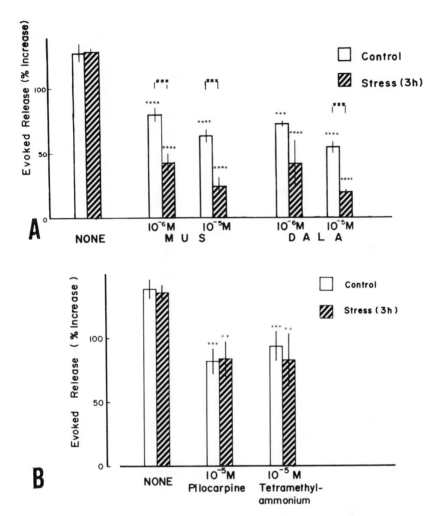

Fig. 2. Effect of premortem stress on suppressive action of (A) GABA agonists and (B) cholinergic agonists on [3H]GABA release from striatal slices preloaded by incubation with 133 nM [3H]GABA (28.2 Ci/mmole) at 25°C for 30 minutes. The release evoked by 30 mM KCl was calculated as a percentage increase of the radioactivity released over that found immediately before the high potassium stimulation. Each value represents the mean ± S.E.M. obtained from 3-9 separate experiments. **P<0.02,***P<0.01,****P<0.001, compared with the value with no addition. ###P<0.01, compared with each non-stress control value.

MUS and DALA than was found in tissue from control, non-stressed animals. In contrast, the stress had no significant effect on the suppression of KCl-evoked release of [^{3}H]-GABA from the slices by pilocarpine and tetramethylammonium, although these cholinergic agonists exhibited a significant inhibition of the release (Fig. 2(B)). These results suggest that stress may enhance the negative feedback control on the release of GABA from its nerve terminals by a presynaptic GABA autoreceptor in preference to the suppression by cholinergic neurons in the striatum.

Preventive Effect by Ethanol

Since several lines of evidence indicate a cross relationship between ethanol and stress (Kahn et al. 1964; Pohorecky et al. 1980; Kuriyama et al. 1983), we have also examined the effect of ethanol administration on the stress-induced alterations in cerebral GABA systems described above in order to evaluate further such a relationship.

Sedative doses of ethanol were given orally to animals concurrently with the initiation of stress application and the same doses were again administered at a half period of the treatment (1.5 h). It was found that relatively high doses of ethanol (2-3 g/kg) not only prevented the stress-induced elevation of the endogenous levels of GABA in the striatum and hypothalamus, but also eliminated the significant declines of striatal and hypothalamic GLU contents induced by stress. Sedative doses (2-5 mg/kg, i.p.) of diazepam, a benzodiazepine (BZP) minor tranquilizer, also exerted a similar preventive action against the stress-induced alterations in cerebral GABA metabolism. It was found that the preventive action of ethanol was abolished by the pretreatment of animals with pyrazole, an inhibitor of alcohol dehydrogenase, and was enhanced by pre-treatment with an inhibitor of aldehyde dehydrogenase (disulfiram). These results suggest that ethanol may exhibit its preventive action on the stress-induced alterations in cerebral GABA metabolism after being metabolized to acetaldehyde in the body. Acetaldehyde has been reported to condense with aromatic amines including 5-hydroxytryptamine to yield β-carboline derivatives (Cohen 1976), which are putative endogenous ligands for the BZP receptor (Braestrup et al. 1980). Considering these previous reports, along with the fact that diazepam also exerted a profound, protective action similar to that of ethanol, it seems possible that ethanol may exhibit its preventive action through an inter- action with a cerebral BZP receptor after yielding condensa- tion products, including β-carbolines, of acetaldehyde with aromatic amines.

To examine such a possibility, the effect of the BZP antagonist, Ro15-1788 (Hunkeler et al. 1981; Mohler, Richards 1981), on the preventive action of ethanol was investigated. Simultaneous administration of Ro15-1788 (10 mg/kg, i.p.) with ethanol was found to eliminate completely the preventive action of ethanol against the stress-induced alterations in the metabolism of GABA in the striatum and hypothalamus (Fig. 3).

DISCUSSION

Application of a cold and immobilization stress to ani- mals for 3 h induced a significant elevation of the steady- state level of GABA accompanied by a reduction of that of GLU, with a concomitant enhancement of GAD activity. The increase in GAD activity seems to be due to the induction of the enzyme protein, since the stress-induced elevation of the activity was prevented by pretreatment of animals with an inhibitor of protein synthesis such as cycloheximide. Similar rapid augmentation of GAD activity has been shown to occur in the thalamus and spinal cord following acute admin- istration of an analgesic dose of morphine (Kuriyama, Yoneda 1978). The possible involvement of cerebral GABA neurons in the occurrence of analgesia has been suggested by several lines of evidence, including the pain-induced increase in cortical GABA content (Sherman, Gebhart 1974), modulation of morphine induced analgesia by GABAergic drugs (Yoneda et al. 1976), and morphine-induced alterations of the microdistri- bution of GABA in the thalamus and spinal cord (Yoneda et al. 1977; Kuriyama, Yoneda 1978). These previous findings, together with the results obtained in the present study, seem to support the proposal that the stress causes the above described alterations in the metabolism of GABA through the generation of analgesic and/or painful stimuli.

It is noteworthy that stress induces a significant en- hancement of the suppression of KCl-evoked release of [^{3}H]GABA from striatal slices by GABAmimetics without affect- ing that by cholinomimetics. This suppression by GABA

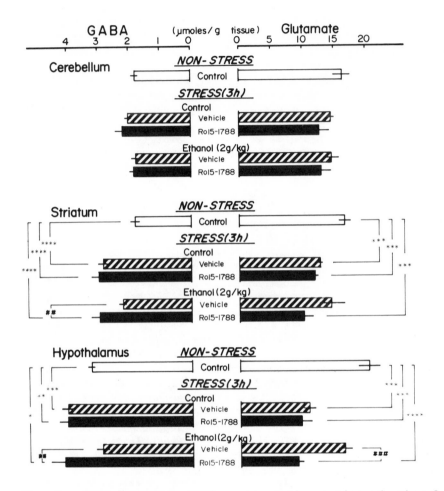

Fig. 3. Effect of Ro15-1788 on preventive action of ethanol against stress-induced alterations of GABA and glutamate contents in rat brain. A benzodiazepine antagonist, Ro15-1788 (10 mg/kg), was administered intraperitoneally to rats simultaneously with the administration of ethanol at the beginning of the stress treatment and again at a half period of the treatment. Each value represents the mean ± S.E.M. obtained from 5-6 separate experiments. *P<0.05,**P<0.02, ***P<0.01,****P<0.001, compared with each non-stress control value. ##P<0.02,###P<0.01, compared with each value obtained from stressed animals treated with ethanol alone.

agonists has been considered to be attributable to a negative feedback control by a GABA receptor which resides on GABAergic nerve terminals (Snodgrass 1978; Mitchell, Martin 1978). Since these GABA agonists had no significant effect on the non-stimulated and Ca^{2+}-independent spontaneous release of [^{3}H]GABA from the striatal slices, it seems possible that stress may enhance the alteration, induced by MUS and DALA, in the concentration of intracellular free Ca^{2+} available for neurotransmitter release. Another interpretation of these results is that stress may cause a significant facilitation of the association of MUS and DALA with presynaptic GABAergic auto-receptors in the striatum. DALA is proposed as a potential and selective agonist for the presynaptic GABAergic auto-receptor (Brennan, Cantrill 1979).

It should be emphasized that ethanol had a significant preventive action on the stress-induced alterations in cerebral GABA metabolism. This preventive action of ethanol seems to be related to the activation of cerebral BZP receptors. Possible reasons for proposing such a hypothesis include: (1) the effect was abolished by pyrazole (an inhibitor of alcohol dehydrogenase); (2) it was enhanced by disulfiram (an inhibitor of aldehyde dehydrogenase); (3) acetaldehyde has been reported to form condensation products with aromatic amines such as β-carbolines in the brain (Cohen 1976); (4) β-carbolines have been shown to be endogenous ligands for the BZP receptor (Braestrup et al. 1980); (5) a BZP tranquilizer, diazepam, exhibited a similar preventive action to ethanol; and (6) a BZP antagonist, Ro15-1788, completely eliminated the preventive action of ethanol. The exact molecular mechanisms underlying these phenomena, as well as the pharmacological and/or physiological significances of the preventive action of ethanol, however, remain to be elucidated.

CONCLUSION

There is no doubt that stress not only induces profound alterations in the metabolism and function of cerebral monoamines such as NA, Ad, DA and 5-HT, but also causes significant changes in those of γ-aminobutyric acid (GABA) in the brain. It is quite conceivable that these functional alterations in cerebral GABA neurons may play an important physiological role in the production of various neuropsychiatric symptoms induced by stress in rodents, such as short-lived analgesia and/or depressive psychosis. Ethanol, as well as diazepam, had a significant preventive effect on the stress-induced alterations in cerebral GABA metabolism. The preventive action by ethanol seems to be attributable to the formation of β-carbolines, which are condensation products of acetaldehyde with aromatic amines in the brain and are considered to be endogenous ligands for cerebral BZP receptors.

Acknowledgements: Authors wish to thank Nippon Roche K.K., Tokyo, Japan, for providing us with Ro15-1788. This work was supported in part by Grants-in-Aid for Scientific Research (Nos. 56480104 and 57870019) from the Ministry of Education, Science and Culture, Japan.

REFERENCES

Braestrup C, Nielsen M, Olsen CE (1980). Urinary and brain carboline-3-carboxylates as potent inhibitors on brain benzodiazepine receptor. Proc Natl Acad Sci USA 77:2288.
Brennan MJW, Cantrill RC (1979). δ-Aminolevulinic acid is a potent agonist for GABA autoreceptor. Nature 280:514.
Cohen G (1976). Alkaloid products in the metabolism of alcohol and biogenic amines. Biochem Pharmacol 25:1123.
Hunkeler W, Mohler H, Pieri L, Polc P, Bonetti EP, Cumin R, Schaffner R, Haefely W (1981). Selective antagonists of benzodiazepines. Nature 290:514.
Kahn AU, Forney RB, Hughes FW (1964). Plasma free fatty acids in rats after shock as modified by centrally active drugs. Arch Int Pharmacodyn Ther 151:466.
Kuriyama K, Yoneda Y (1978). Morphine induced alterations of γ-aminobutyric acid and taurine contents and L-glutamate decarboxylase activity in rat spinal cord and thalamus: Possible correlates with analgesic action of morphine. Brain Res 148:163.
Kuriyama K, Kanmori K, Yoneda Y (1983). Preventive effect of alcohol on stress-induced alterations in metabolism and function of biogenic amines and gamma-aminobutyric acid (GABA) in neuroendocrine system. In Pohorecky LA, Brick J (eds): "Stress and Alcohol Use, " New York: Elsevier Biomedical, p 403.
Lidbrink P, Corrodi H, Fuxe K, Olson L (1972). Barbiturates and meprobamate: Decrease in catecholamine turnover of

central dopamine and noradrenaline neuronal system and the influence of immobilization stress. Brain Res 45:597.

Mitchell PR, Martin IL (1978). Is GABA release modulated by presynaptic receptors? Nature 274:904.

Mohler H, Richards JG (1981). Agonist and antagonist benzodiazepine interaction in vitro. Nature 294:763.

Nakagawa K, Kuriyama K (1975). Effect of taurine on alteration in adrenal functions induced by stress. Japan J Pharmacol 25:737.

Pohorecky LA, Rassi E, Weiss JM, Michalak V (1980). Biochemical evidence for an interaction of ethanol and stress: Preliminary studies. Alcohol Clin Exp Res 4:423.

Sherman A, Gebhart GF (1974). Regional levels of GABA and glutamate in mouse brain following exposure to pain. Neuropharmacol 13:673.

Snodgrass SR (1978). Use of ^{3}H-muscimol for GABA receptor studies. Nature 273:392.

Thierry AM, Javoy F, Glowinski J, Kety SS (1968). Effect of stress on the metabolism of norepinephrine, dopamine and serotonin in the central nervous system of the rat. I. Modification of norepinephrine turnover. J Pharmacol Exp Ther 163:163.

Yoneda Y, Takashima S, Kuriyama K (1976). Possible involvement of GABA in morphine analgesia. Biochem Pharmacol 25:2669.

Yoneda Y, Kuriyama K, Kurihara E (1977). Morphine alters distribution of GABA in thalamus. Brain Res 124:373.

Yoneda Y, Kanmori K, Ida S, Kuriyama K (1983). Stress-induced alterations in metabolism of γ-aminobutyric acid in rat brain. J Neurochem 40:350.

Glutamine, Glutamate, and GABA
in the Central Nervous System, pages 571–580
© 1983 Alan R. Liss, Inc., 150 Fifth Avenue, New York, NY 10011

GABA AND PIPECOLIC ACID, A POSSIBLE RECIPROCAL MODULATION IN
THE CNS

Ezio Giacobini and Maria del Carmen Gutierrez

Department of Pharmacology
Southern Illinois University School of Medicine
Springfield, IL 62708

Pipecolic acid (PA), one of the three cyclic secondary
amino acids or imino acids present in the brain, along with
proline and hydroxyproline, represents the major metabolite
of lysine in the CNS (Giacobini et al. 1980; Giacobini 1983).
Its presence in the vertebrate brain has been demonstrated
only recently (Schmidt-Glenewinkel et al. 1977, 1978). Its
concentration in whole brain is relatively low (18 ± 4 nmol/
g, mouse brain); however, it is not lower than that of several cerebral amino acids. We have shown that, in brain, as
in bacteria and plants, the biosynthetic pathway which leads
to the piperidine nucleus of pipecolic acid originates from
lysine via one of the intermediates of lysine metabolism
(Schmidt-Glenewinkel et al. 1977, 1978). The conversion of
lysine into pipecolic acid, cadaverine and piperidine is
possible under in vitro conditions in brain and various
other organs of the mouse (Schmidt-Glenewinkel et al. 1977,
1978), as well as in the rat brain (Chang 1976, 1978).

The description of a severe metabolic disorder of the
nervous system related to abnormally elevated amounts of
pipecolic acid in brain, serum and urine of newborn patients
(Gatfield et al. 1968; Gatfield, Taller 1971; Thomas et al.
1975) has drawn new attention to some aspects of lysine metabolism (Giacobini et al. 1980). As a result of our limited
knowledge about the role and metabolism of pipecolic acid in
the brain, the etiology of this neurological disturbance is
presently unknown.

We have demonstrated saturable uptake of PA in brain
synaptosomes, Ca^{++}-dependent release from brain slices,

saturable transport across the blood-brain barrier (BBB) and a high affinity binding of ^{3}H-PA in the mouse CNS that is associated with the GABA system (Giacobini et al. 1980; Giacobini 1983). This evidence suggests that PA containing neurons or terminals may exist in brain.

Others have shown that PA depresses the firing of cortical neurons (Kase et al. 1980) and that this response is blocked by bicuculline (Takahama et al. 1982). It has therefore been suggested that PA may be taken up into terminals of GABA neurons (Kase et al. 1980) and its inhibitory effect may be related to GABAergic transmission.

a. Uptake of ^{3}H-PA in Brain Slices, Synaptosomal Preparations and Glial Cells

We have demonstrated that ^{3}H-PA (4 x 10^{-7}M) is taken up by mouse synaptosomal preparations by means of a Na$^+$-dependent, temperature-sensitive mechanism (Nomura et al. 1980). The uptake is strongly affected by ouabain (10^{-4}M). Kinetic studies indicated that the uptake is saturable at higher substrate concentrations. A two-component system is present with K_m(s) of 3.9 x 10^{-6}M and 90.2 x 10^{-6}M, which suggests that PA is transported by both a high and a low affinity transport system. Table 1 compares reported data on brain concentration and kinetic properties of synaptosomal uptake for three neurotransmitter amino acids (glutamate, aspartate and GABA) with those we find for PA. The K_m found for PA is of the same order of magnitude as those for the other high affinity systems reported. The V_{max} value for the high affinity uptake of PA is 25-fold lower than that reported for GABA (Table 1). However, taking into consideration the vast differences in brain concentrations and the high level of GABA terminals in the cerebral cortex of the rat, this is not surprising.

Compounds structurally related to PA, such as glycine, L-proline, 4-amino-n-butyric acid (GABA) and 5-aminovaleric acid, show an inhibitory effect on PA uptake at a concentration of 10^{-4}M or less. A mutual inhibition of PA and L-proline was shown, favoring the hypothesis of a common transport system for these two imino acids. L-Proline also inhibits the transport of PA in vivo (Nishio, Giacobini 1981).

Pipecolic acid significantly inhibits the initial GABA

Table 1. Comparison of Concentrations and Uptake Kinetics of Amino Acids in Rodent Brain

Amino Acid	Brain Concn. (μmol/g)*	K_m (μM)	V_{max} (pmol/mg protein-min)
Glutamate	11.7	4.3**	125**
Aspartate	3.75	4.1**	105**
GABA	2.37	4.0**	1100***
Pipecolic acid	0.02	3.9****	43****

*Mouse brain (Lajtha, Toth 1973). **Rat whole brain synaptosomes (Plaitakis et al. 1981). ***Rat cerebral cortex synaptosomes (Martin 1973). ****Mouse whole brain synaptosomes (Nomura et al. 1980).

uptake into synaptosomal fractions in the rat (Nomura et al. 1978) and increases high K^+-induced release of GABA (Okuma et al. 1979; cf Table 2). We compared the uptake and release of GABA and PA in synaptosomal fractions, brain slices and glial cell enriched fractions of rat brain (Nomura et al. 1981). Our results show that the synaptosomal uptake of ^{3}H-PA is much less than that of GABA. Pipecolic acid and GABA mutually inhibit the other's uptake into synaptosomes, but GABA and nipecotic acid produce a greater inhibition of synaptosomal ^{14}C-GABA uptake than of synaptosomal ^{3}H-PA uptake (Table 2).

The fact that nipecotic acid, a potent inhibitor of GABA uptake (Johnston et al. 1976), does not inhibit PA uptake as strongly indicates that PA and GABA are not taken up into synaptosomal fractions via the same carrier-mediated transport system. PA may be taken up into different sites than GABA-containing neurons (or glial cells) in the CNS. In addition, since GABA (10^{-4}M) affected neither the spontaneous nor the K^+-induced release of PA (Table 2), the latter may not be displaced by GABA at its storage site.

Only a small amount of ^{3}H-PA was taken up in glial cell fractions. This contrasted with the marked uptake (and the different time course of uptake) of ^{14}C-GABA into glial cell fractions. However, PA inhibited the initial ^{14}C-GABA uptake into such fractions (Table 2).

Table 2. Effect of Pipecolic Acid (PA), GABA and Nipecotic Acid on the Uptake, Release and/or Binding of ^{3}H-GABA and ^{3}H-PA

	SLICES	SYNAPTOSOMES	GLIA	MEMBRANES
PIPECOLIC ACID (10^{-4}M)	GABA RELEASE ↑	PA UPTAKE ↓		
		GABA UPTAKE ↓	GABA UPTAKE ↓↓↓	
PIPECOLIC ACID (5×10^{-3}M)				[1]GABA BINDING O
GABA (10^{-4}M)	PA RELEASE O	GABA UPTAKE ↓↓↓	GABA UPTAKE ↓↓↓	
		PA UPTAKE ↓		[2]PA BINDING O
NIPECOTIC ACID (10^{-4}M)		GABA UPTAKE ↓↓↓	GABA UPTAKE ↓↓↓	
		PA UPTAKE ↓		[3]PA BINDING O

↑ = increase   ↓ = decrease   O = no effect

In conclusion, it is possible that PA plays a physiological regulatory role on GABAergic neurotransmission by controlling GABA concentrations at the synaptic cleft, either by inhibiting its reuptake in both glial cells and nerve endings or by increasing its release.

b. Release of Pipecolic Acid from Rat Brain Slices and Synaptosomal Preparations

In our study (Nomura et al. 1979), we investigated whether or not a high concentration of K$^+$ could induce the release of PA from brain slices preloaded with radioactive PA.

The K$^+$-induced depolarization of rat brain slices was accompanied by the release of radioactive PA. Since the K$^+$-induced release of this imino acid was significantly inhibited when the preparation was perfused with Ca^{++}-free medium in the presence of EGTA for 15 minutes, it seems probable that this release is Ca^{++}-dependent, as reported for other putative neurotransmitters. Verapamil, at the concentration of 10^{-5}M which is known to inhibit Ca++ influx, significantly inhibited the K$^+$-induced release of labelled PA. This might be taken as evidence that the influx of Ca^{++} into nerve terminals containing PA is a necessary event in the release mechanism. GABA (10^{-4}M) affected neither the spontaneous

nor the high K^+-induced release of ^{3}H-PA from brain slices
(Nomura et al. 1981) although, as previously mentioned, PA
enhances K^+-induced release of ^{14}C-GABA. In both crude
mitochondrial P_2 fractions and glial-enriched fractions of
rat brain, K^+-induced depolarization evoked a release of
preloaded ^{3}H-PA (Nomura et al. 1981).

c. Blood-Brain Barrier for Pipecolic Acid

We have miniaturized the procedure of Oldendorf (1971)
to fit the particular vascular requirements of the mouse.
Using this technique, we have extended our investigation of
PA uptake to a comparative study of amino acids, imino acids
and amines in the mouse brain (Nishio, Giacobini 1981). We
have shown that the Brain Uptake Index (BUI) of all these
substances is generally lower in the mouse brain than in the
rat brain, with the sole exception of proline. However, the
characteristics and classes of transport are basically similar in the two species, although the BBB is comparatively
stronger in the mouse. Our results show, for the first time,
that appreciable amounts of PA can cross the BBB and enter
the brain. Using ^{3}H-water as reference, the BUI for ^{3}H-D,L-
PA was established at 3.4% (at 0.114 mM).

Kinetic analysis of the BUI of PA shows that this is
saturable between the concentrations of 0.114 and 0.344 mM
and suggests the presence of two kinds of transport systems
with $K_m(s)$ of 0.283 and 4.54 mM, respectively (Nishio, Giacobini 1981). Compounds structurally related to PA show an inhibitory effect on PA uptake. These include compounds with
a piperidil or pyrrolidil structure, such as nipecotic acid,
isonipecotic acid, piperidine and L-proline. Among several
amino acids tested, only GABA shows an inhibitory effect.

d. Receptor Binding of Pipecolic Acid and Modulatory Effect
   of GABA

A high affinity, Na^+-dependent specific binding of ^{3}H-
PA has been determined (K_D = 33.2 nM) in mouse brain (Fig. 1).
The binding was shown to be saturable at 70 nM of ^{3}H-PA.

Unlabeled PA displaced specific binding of ^{3}H-PA in a
concentration-dependent manner (Table 3); proline showed the
same pattern of displacement. Under these conditions, GABA

did not displace the specific binding of ³H-PA at the concentrations tested (10⁻¹¹ to 10⁻³M). When, however the tissue

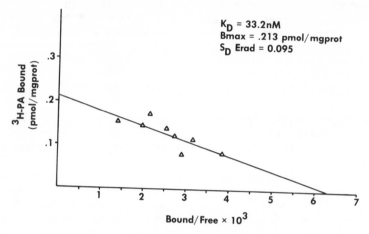

Fig. 1.   Eadie-Hofstee Plot of Specific ³H-PA Binding to
          Crude P₂ Fraction Membranes
Crude P₂ fraction membranes were incubated for 2 hrs at 4ºC
in Tris-Cl (50 mM), NaCl (100 mM) and MgCl₂ (1 mM) buffer,
pH 7.6, with different concentrations of ³H-PA in the nM
range. Non-specific binding was determined in the presence
of unlabeled PA (1 mM). S_D Erad = Coefficient of goodness
of fit (Zivine, Waud 1982).

Table 3.   Percent Specific Binding of ³H-PA* in the Presence
           of Various Concentrations of Unlabeled Ligands.

		Ligand	
Molarity	GABA	Pipecolic Acid	Proline
10⁻³	92.7	0	0.8
10⁻⁵	101.2	65.2	64.6
10⁻⁷	116.2	84.3	93.1
10⁻⁹	103.1	91.2	100.6
10⁻¹¹	104.5	96.2	98.2

*Non-specific binding was determined in the presence of 10⁻³M
unlabeled PA. This was considered to displace 100% of the
specific binding and all other values were determined as
percentages of this displacement.

is incubated with different concentrations of GABA prior to the assay, the effect on ^{3}H-PA binding varies depending on both PA and GABA concentrations (Table 4). At high concentrations of unlabeled PA (10^{-3}M) there is no effect of GABA; however, at lower concentrations (10^{-5} and 10^{-6}M), GABA can increase or decrease the ^{3}H-PA binding observed. Higher concentrations (10^{-3} - 10^{-5}M) of GABA seem to decrease the inhibition of ^{3}H-PA binding by the cold PA while, more interestingly, lower concentrations (10^{-11}M) seem to facilitate the inhibition. These results suggest a modulatory action of GABA on PA receptor sites, and a possible increase in specific binding in the presence of low GABA levels.

At concentrations of 5 x 10^{-3}M and 10^{-3}M, PA does not displace ^{3}H-GABA binding (Table 2).

Table 4. Percent Inhibition of Specific Binding of ^{3}H-PA after Preincubation with GABA*

[PA](M)	Molar Concentration of GABA					
	0	10^{-3}	10^{-5}	10^{-7}	10^{-9}	10^{-11}
10^{-3}	100	97.1	93.3	120.3	104.2	101.9
10^{-5}	41	25.0	16.9	36.7	34.8	64.0
10^{-6}	10	0	0	0	11.0	37.5

*Crude P_2 fraction membranes (2.5 mg/ml) were preincubated 10 minutes with different concentrations of GABA. ^{3}H-PA (40 nM) was then added and binding was determined in the presence of three concentrations of unlabeled PA. 10^{-3}M PA without GABA is assumed to displace all specific binding; other values are calculated relative to this figure.

CONCLUDING REMARKS

Two possibilities are suggested by our findings of PA uptake, release and binding in the CNS. The first is that a PA-containing neuronal system is present. The second is that PA is a co-transmitter in GABA-containing neurons.

Our results, taken together with the evidence for the presence, localization and metabolism of PA in the brain (Giacobini et al. 1980; Giacobini 1983), support the possibility that PA-containing neurons exist in the brain. Such neurons may be able to synthesize and transport PA to terminals located in proximity to GABAergic neurons. The PA released could then act as a modulator of GABA action. Alternatively, PA could coexist in GABAergic terminals and be released simultaneously with GABA. The possibility of a direct action of PA on its own separate receptor sites should also be considered.

Table 2 summarizes the relationship between the effects of GABA and PA in the rodent CNS. This schematic represent-ation is based on studies (Giacobini et al. 1980; Giacobini 1983) performed on three different kinds of nerve preparat-ions: brain slices, synaptosomes and fraction membranes. Pipecolic acid has been shown to exert a dual action, i.e. to increase GABA release from brain slices and to decrease its uptake in synaptosomes. GABA, which does not have any effect on PA release, does decrease PA uptake. GABA uptake into glia is strongly inhibited by PA. This uptake is one of the major mechanisms for regulating the concentration of GABA in the synaptic cleft. Therefore, the action of PA could result in an amplification of GABA action by increas-ing its concentration in the cleft. Such an hypothesis is supported by electrophysiological results in which PA, when applied electrophoretically, produced a bicuculline-sensit-ive inhibitory response in cortical neurons (Kase et al. 1980; Takahama et al. 1982). Moreover, the binding studies suggest that GABA itself could influence the effect of the released PA by modulating, in a concentration-dependent manner, its binding properties to a receptor site. This second mechanism implies the presence of GABA-releasing ter-minals located near to PA receptive sites. The demonstra-tion of a close anatomical relationship between PA and GABA systems in the CNS would provide the basis for a new modulatory form of interaction between two brain endogenous neuroactive substances as suggested by our results.

ACKNOWLEDGMENT

This study was supported by U.S. Public Health Service Grants NS 11430 and NS 14086 to E. Giacobini.

REFERENCES

Chang YF (1976). Pipecolic pathway: The major lysine meta-bolic route in the rat brain. Biophys Res Commun 69:174.
Chang YF (1978). Lysine metabolism in the rat brain: The

pipecolic acid-forming pathway. J Neurochem 30:347.
Gatfield PD, Taller E, Hinton GG, Wallace AC, Abdelnour GM, Haust MD (1968). Hyperpipecolatemia: A new metabolic disorder associated with neuropathy and hepatomegaly (A case study). Can Med Assoc J 99:1215.
Gatfield PD, Taller E (1971). Accumulation of lysine dipeptides in the brain in hyperpipecolatemia. Brain Res 29:170.
Giacobini E, Nomura Y, Schmidt-Glenewinkel T (1980). Pipecolic acid: Origin, biosynthesis and metabolism in the brain. Cell Mol Biol 26:135.
Giacobini E (1983). Imino acids of the brain. In Lajtha A (ed): "Handbook of Neurochemistry," Vol 3(2) Plenum 563.
Johnston GAR, Stephanson AL, Twitchen B (1976). Uptake and release of nipecotic acid by rat brain slices. J Neurochem 26:83.
Kase Y, Takahama K, Hashimoto T, Kaisaku J, Okano Y, Miyata T (1980). Electrophoretic study of pipecolic acid, a biogenic imino acid, in the mammalian brain. Brain Res 193:608.
Lajtha A, Toth J (1973). Perinatal changes in the free amino acid pool of the brain in mice. Brain Res. 55:238-241.
Martin DL (1973). Kinetics of the sodium-dependent transport of gamma-aminobutyric acid by synaptosomes. J Neurochem 21:345.
Nishio H, Giacobini E (1981). Brain uptake of pipecolic acid, amino acids, and amines following intracarotid injection in the mouse. Neurochem Res 6:835.
Nomura Y, Okuma Y, Segawa T (1978). Influence of piperidine and pipecolic acid on the uptake of monoamines, GABA and glycine into P_2 fractions of the rat brain and spinal cord. J Pharmacobio-Dyn 1:251.
Nomura Y, Okuma Y, Segawa T, Schmidt-Glenewinkel T, Giacobini E (1979). A calcium-dependent, high potassium-induced release of pipecolic acid from rat brain slices. J Neurochem 33:803.
Nomura Y, Schmidt-Glenewinkel T, Giacobini E (1980). Uptake of piperidine and pipecolic acid by synaptosomes from mouse brain. Neurochem Res 5:1163.
Nomura Y, Okuma Y, Segawa T, Schmidt-Glenewinkel T, Giacobini E (1981). Comparison of synaptosomal and glial uptake of pipecolic acid and GABA in rat brain. Neurochem Res 6:391.
Okuma Y, Nomura Y, Segawa T (1979). The effect of piperidine and pipecolic acid on high potassium-induced release

of noradrenaline, serotonin and GABA from rat brain slices. J Pharm Dyn 2:261.

Oldendorf WH (1971). Brain uptake of radiolabeled amino acids, amines and hexoses after arterial injection. Amer J Physiol 221:1629.

Plaitakis et al. (1981). In Haber B et al. (eds): "Serotonin," Adv Exp Med and Biol 133, Plenum Press: p 540.

Schmidt-Glenewinkel T, Nomura Y, Giacobini E (1977). The conversion of lysine into piperidine, cadaverine and pipecolic acid. Neurochem Res 2:619.

Schmidt-Glenewinkel T, Giacobini E, Nomura Y, Okuma Y and Segawa T (1978). Presence, metabolism and uptake of pipecolic acid in the mouse brain. 2nd Meet Eur Soc Neurochem Abst 618.

Takahama K, Miyata T, Hashimoto T, Yoshiro O, Hitoshi T, Kase Y (1982). Pipecolic acid: a new type of α-amino acid possessing bicuculline-sensitive action in the mammalian brain. Brain Res 239:294.

Thomas GH, Haslam RH, Batshjaw ML, Capute AJ, Nedengard L, Ransom JL (1975). Hyperpipecolic acidemia associated with hepatomegaly, mental retardation, optic nerve dysplasia and progressive neurological disease. Clin Gen 8:376.

Zivine JA, Waud DR (1982). How to analyze binding, enzyme and uptake data: the simplest case, a single phase. Life Sci 30:1407.

Glutamine, Glutamate, and GABA
in the Central Nervous System, pages 581–594
© 1983 Alan R. Liss, Inc., 150 Fifth Avenue, New York, NY 10011

LEVELS OF GLUTAMINE, GLUTAMATE AND GABA IN
CSF AND BRAIN UNDER PATHOLOGICAL CONDITIONS

Thomas L. Perry, M.D.

Department of Pharmacology
The University of British Columbia
Vancouver, B. C., Canada, V6T 1W5

Conventional automatic amino acid analysis of cerebrospinal fluid (CSF), using ninhydrin detection, has for
some time been useful in providing clues to amino acid
abnormalities of brain in various metabolic and neurological disorders. Direct measurement of amino acid contents
in autopsied and biopsied human brain by this technique
has more recently supplied valuable information in a number
of diseases, but studies of this sort have yet to be
undertaken for many important brain disorders. Finally,
the development of greatly increased sensitivity in detection of amino compounds, using the fluorescence produced
by their reaction with o-phthalaldehyde, has made it possible to measure γ-aminobutyric acid (GABA) accurately in
CSF. This chapter briefly describes some conditions in
which abnormal levels of glutamine (Gln), glutamic acid
(Glu), or GABA are found in human CSF and brain.

GLUTAMINE

Gln concentrations in CSF and brain are usually elevated, and sometimes very markedly so, in conditions where
ammonia fails to be converted into urea, either as a result
of structural or biochemical failure in the liver, or as a
result of any of the 6 genetically-determined urea cycle
metabolic defects (Walser 1983). Some conditions in which
Gln levels are elevated in CSF and brain are listed in
Table 1.

Table 1. Abnormal Glutamine Levels in Human CSF and Brain

Condition	CSF	Brain
Control subjects	587 ± 86 µmol/l (lower in infants)	4.55 ± 1.34 µmol/g (autopsied frontal cortex)
Hepatic encephalopathy	↑↑	↑↑
Urea cycle disorders	↑↑	↑↑
Anticonvulsant drugs:		
phenobarbital, primidone	↑	?
valproate	↑	?

↑ = increased; ↑↑ = markedly increased.

Concentrations of Gln in CSF in urea cycle disorders and hepatic encephalopathy are often higher than they are in specimens of plasma obtained simultaneously, and can be elevated as much as 2-5 times the normal values of about 600 µmol/l (adults) and 500 µmol/l (infants). Gln content in autopsied brain, which is similar to that found in living human brain (Perry et al. 1981a), varies between 4 and 6 µmol/g wet weight in different brain regions in control patients. In autopsied brain from patients dying with hepatic encephalopathy due to hepatitis or alcoholic cirrhosis, and in brain of infants dying with ornithine carbamoyl transferase deficiency or argininosuccinate lyase deficiency (Perry et al. 1980), Gln content in different brain regions varies from 10 to 28 µmol/g wet weight.

Brain "detoxifies" ammonia, which has not already been disposed of in the urea cycle, by Gln formation. The first step reacts ammonia with α-ketoglutarate, derived from the tricarboxylic acid cycle, and is catalyzed by glutamate dehydrogenase. The second step reacts further ammonia with Glu and is catalyzed by glutamine synthetase. Elevated Gln levels in plasma, CSF and brain regularly accompany hyperammonemia due to any cause.

Gln concentrations are sometimes found elevated in CSF in patients given certain anticonvulsant drugs (Table 1),

especially infants and children receiving phenobarbitone
and primidone (Perry et al. 1976). Valproic acid may also
produce moderate hyperammonemia and can raise Gln levels,
possibly by inhibiting carbamoyl phosphate synthetase, the
first enzyme in the urea cycle, or by blocking the synthesis of N-acetylglutamate, the essential activator of this
enzyme (Batshaw, Brusilow 1982; Murphy, Marquardt 1982).
Table 2 illustrates the effects of valproate administration
on Gln concentrations in CSF and plasma of an epileptic
adult, and shows that Gln concentrations may be normal in
plasma even while significantly elevated in CSF. Whether
or not Gln content is elevated in brain (Table 1), and
whether significant ammonia accumulates there to produce
harmful effects when these anticonvulsant drugs are used
is not known, but this phenomenon might explain some of
these drugs' untoward central effects.

Table 2. Valproate Effects on Glutamine Concentrations

	Plasma	CSF
	(μmol/l; mean $\pm$ SD)	
Control adults	624 $\pm$ 118	587 $\pm$ 86
Epileptic man,	Receiving valproic acid, 30 mg/kg daily	
age 35	580	962
	632	869
	560	833
		978
	After valproate discontinued	
	571	437

GLUTAMIC ACID

Most published values for the normal concentration of
Glu in CSF are at least an order of magnitude higher than
the true values. In my laboratory, 140 adults with various
neurological disorders have shown a CSF Glu level of 1.0 $\pm$
0.7 (mean $\pm$ SD) μmol/l. If excessive amounts of sulfosal-

icylic acid are added to CSF specimens to deproteinize
them, as is often the case, and the specimens are then
applied to very small cation exchange columns which are
operated at high temperature during chromatography, some
compounds such as homocarnosine or γ-aminobutyryl choline
can be hydrolyzed to yield free GABA (Perry et al. 1982b).
Under such conditions, Gln too can be partially hydrolyzed
to Glu. Thus, unless the lowest amount of sulfosalicylic
acid necessary for deproteinization is employed, and unless
the amino acid analyzer column is operated at low temperature until Gln has been eluted (Perry et al. 1968), arte-
factually high Glu values are apt to be obtained in CSF.
We have not found clearly abnormal Glu levels in any of
approximately 400 patients whose CSF has been submitted to
quantitative amino acid analysis.

Glu is usually the most abundant free amino acid in
human brain. In autopsied brain, the highest Glu contents
(10 to 12 μmol/g wet weight) are found in the putamen and
caudate, with relatively high contents (in decreasing
order) also present in the cerebellar cortex, thalamus,
and frontal and occipital cortex (Table 3). Contents of
Glu are similar in biopsied and autopsied brain, somewhat
surprisingly regardless of increasing intervals between
death and freezing of the brain (Perry et al. 1981a).
Mean Glu contents of biopsied cerebral and cerebellar
cortex from a number of nonepileptic patients were found
to be about 7.6 μmol/g wet weight (Perry 1982a).

Several conditions in which Glu contents are altered
in human brain are shown in Table 3. In some forms of
dominantly-inherited olivopontocerebellar atrophy, type I
(OPCA I) (Konigsmark, Weiner 1970), Glu and aspartate
contents are markedly reduced in the cerebellar cortex
(Perry et al. 1981b). However, in affected patients from
at least one pedigree clinically diagnosed as OPCA I, Glu
contents in the cerebellar cortex were normal (Perry et al.
1981b). Several different dominantly-inherited diseases
clearly are included in what is currently described as
OPCA I. In patients clinically characterized as OPCA IV,
we found Glu contents not only markedly decreased in the
cerebellar cortex, but also in the frontal cortex and caudate nucleus (Perry et al. 1981b). The Glu deficiency in
cerebellar cortex in those forms of OPCA where it occurs is
presumably due to loss of granule cells, whose excitatory

Table 3. Glutamate Levels in CSF and Brain
in Several Disorders

Disorder	CSF	Brain
Control subjects	1.0± 0.7 μmol/l	Highest (8-12 μmol/g) in autopsied putamen> caudate > cerebellum > thalamus> cerebral cortex
Olivopontocerebellar atrophies (OPCA)	N	N to ↓↓ (cerebellar cortex) (and other regions in OPCA IV)
Focal epilepsies	N	N or ↑ (biopsied foci)
Huntington's chorea	N	↓ (caudate, putamen, occipital cortex)
Schizophrenias	N	N

N = normal; ↑, ↓ = moderately increased, decreased;
↓↓ = markedly decreased

neurotransmitter is believed to be Glu (McBride et al. 1973; Guidotti et al. 1975; Roffler-Tarlov, Sidman 1978).

When epileptogenic brain tissue is removed neurosurgically from patients with temporal lobe focal epilepsy, the content of Glu is found to be unusually high in a minority of these biopsied foci (Perry, Hansen 1981). Excessive amounts of Glu, acting locally as an excitatory neurotransmitter, might be responsible for initiating focal seizures.

Mean contents of Glu are significantly reduced in the caudate nucleus, putamen, and occipital cortex of autopsied brain from patients dying with Huntington's chorea, but not in frontal cortex and many other brain regions (Table 4). This Glu deficiency in the striatum in Huntington's chorea may simply reflect the marked cell loss characteristic for this region. However, it may be of more importance. Coyle et al. (1978) hypothesized that Huntington's chorea might

Table 4. Brain Glutamate Content in Huntington's Chorea

Patients	Frontal Cortex	Occipital Cortex	Caudate Nucleus	Putamen
Controls	8.34 ± 0.31 (26)	8.41 ± 0.24 (25)	10.47 ± 0.33 (32)	11.69 ± 0.54 (18)
Huntington's Chorea	8.40 ± 0.74 (20)	$6.70 \pm 0.54^{\dagger}$ (21)	$7.37 \pm 0.61^{*}$ (23)	$7.86 \pm 1.19^{\dagger}$ (8)

Glu content (mean ± SEM) in μmol/g wet weight. Number of patients in brackets. *P < 0.001; †P < 0.005.

involve a genetically-inherited abnormality of neurotransmission mediated by Glu in which increased amounts of Glu are released by corticostriatal glutamatergic neurons to cause excessive depolarization and eventual destruction of postsynaptic striatal neurons. Could the low levels of Glu in caudate and putamen of Huntington's chorea brain at autopsy reflect increased local release of Glu?

Glu levels have been reported by one group (Kim et al. 1980) as being low in schizophrenic patients, and these investigators suggested that there might be either impaired function or degeneration of glutamatergic neurons in schizophrenia. In our laboratory, we have found no reductions in Glu levels in either CSF or autopsied brain from schizophrenic patients (Perry 1982b). We have recently found the CSF Glu concentration of 140 adults with a variety of neurological diseases to be 1.0 ± 0.1 μmol/l (mean ±SEM), of 23 adult schizophrenics to be 0.8 ± 0.2 μmol/l, and of 46 Huntington's chorea patients to be 1.1 ± 0.1 μmol/l. None of these mean CSF Glu values differ significantly.

GABA

GABA levels have been studied in CSF and brain in a number of neurological and psychiatric disorders. Findings for some of these are summarized in Table 5.

Table 5. Gaba Levels in CSF and Brain in Various Disorders

Disorder	CSF	Brain	Remarks
Control subjects	86 ± 42 nmol/l		Highest (4 to 7 μmol/g) in autopsied globus pallidus ❯ substantia nigra > dentate nucleus > nucleus accumbens
Huntington's chorea	N	↓↓ or ↓	(caudate, putamen, globus pallidus, substantia nigra, occipital cortex)
Dialysis encephalopathy	↓ or N	↓↓ or ↓	(cerebral and cerebellar cortex, thalamus, caudate)
Olivopontocere-bellar atrophies	N	↓ or ↓↓	(cerebellar cortex, dentate nucleus)
Parkinson's disease	N	↑	(putamen)
Schizophrenias	N	N or ↓	(nucleus accumbens, thalamus)
Focal epilepsies	?	N	(biopsied foci)
Mutiple sclerosis, action tremor	N or ↓	?	
Torsion dystonias	N	?	
GABA-T inhibiting drugs (hydrazine, γ-vinyl GABA)	↑↑	?	

N = normal; ↑ , ↓ = moderately,
↑↑, ↓↓ = markedly increased, decreased

Mean GABA concentrations in lumbar CSF from normal adult subjects have been widely reported as averaging between 220 and 240 nmol/l (Böhlen et al. 1978; Wood et al. 1979; Manyam et al. 1980; Hare, Manyam 1980), when CSF has been subjected to ion-exchange column chromatography, and the eluted GABA then detected by its fluorescence after reaction with o-phthalaldehyde. In my laboratory, however, we find considerably lower CSF GABA levels, using a modification of the ion-exchange fluorometric method which includes improved resolution of GABA from unknown compounds eluted from the column close to it, and which minimizes on-column hydrolysis of bound GABA by excessive sulfosalicylic acid (Perry et al. 1982b). Our current CSF value (mean ± SD) for adult controls is 86 ± 42 nmol/l.

GABA content in human brain rises very rapidly after death, reaching a maximum level within 1-2 hr of death under typical mortuary conditions (Perry et al. 1981a). This maximum GABA level is stable for death-to-freezing intervals up to 96 hr. Thus it is reasonable to compare brain GABA values between control subjects and patients with specific disorders, since autopsies are seldom done and brain is rarely frozen sooner than 2 hr after patients die. The highest regional GABA contents in autopsied brain (4-7 μmol/g wet weight) are found (in descending order) in globus pallidus, substantia nigra, dentate nucleus, and nucleus accumbens (Perry 1982a).

Huntington's chorea was the first disorder in which brain GABA content was found to be significantly reduced (Perry et al. 1973). GABA content is low (Table 6) in the

Table 6. Brain GABA Deficiency in Huntington's Chorea

Patients	Caudate Nucleus	Putamen	Globus Pallidus	Substantia Nigra
Controls	2.90 ± 0.14 (32)	2.91 ± 0.20 (19)	7.32 ± 0.40 (16)	6.05 ± 0.26 (28)
Huntington's Chorea	1.37 ± 0.16* (23)	1.30 ± 0.15* (8)	2.75 ± 0.34* (9)	2.59 ± 0.18* (23)

GABA content (mean ± SEM) in μ mol/g wet weight. Number of patients in brackets. *$P < 0.001$.

caudate nucleus, putamen, globus pallidus, substantia nigra and occipital cortex in Huntington's chorea, but not in frontal or cerebellar cortex, and not in a region such as the dentate nucleus where its content is normally very high. The reduced GABA contents in the basal ganglia in Huntington's chorea are almost certainly due to selective loss of intrinsic GABAergic interneurons and of striatonigral GABAergic neurons. GABA concentrations do <u>not</u> appear significantly reduced in the CSF of Huntington's chorea patients (Perry et al. 1982b), despite published reports to the contrary (Glaeser et al. 1975; Enna et al. 1977). Current figures from my laboratory are shown in Table 7. CSF obtained at lumbar puncture may or may not accurately reflect biochemical changes in the brain. From the medical point of view, it is unfortunate that measurement of CSF GABA levels is valueless in the diagnosis or preclinical detection of Huntington's chorea.

Table 7. GABA Concentrations in CSF of Controls
and Huntington's Chorea Patients

Neurologically normal controls	Neurologically abnormal controls	Huntington's chorea	Chorea: other forms
86 ± 7 (35)	81 ± 5 (43)	80 ± 8 (40)	90 ± 17 (10)

Values (mean ± SEM) are expressed in nmol/l. Figures in brackets indicate number of subjects examined. None of the means differ significantly.

GABA content is moderately reduced in the cerebellar cortex, and often markedly reduced in the dentate nucleus in the dominantly-inherited OPCAs (Perry et al. 1981b) (Table 5). Here too the GABA deficiency probably represents specific loss of Purkinje neurons and of cerebellar cortical inhibitory interneurons. GABA is almost certainly the inhibitory neurotransmitter of many of the efferent Purkinje cells (Obata 1976; Storm-Mathisen 1976; Roberts 1979), and it may be the neurotransmitter of one or more of the 3 types of inhibitory interneurons in the cerebellar cortex -- the basket, stellate and Golgi cells (Storm-Mathisen 1976; Roberts 1979).

Other disorders in which low levels of brain GABA are found include the schizophrenias (Table 5), some forms of which appear to have unusually low GABA contents in the nucleus accumbens and thalamus (Perry et al. 1979). We have not found CSF GABA levels reduced in the small group of schizophrenic patients we have studied. Recently, we found that GABA contents are markedly reduced in autopsied brain from patients dying with dialysis encephalopathy (Alfrey 1978). Here GABA deficiency is most marked in frontal and occipital cortex, cerebellar cortex, thalamus and caudate nucleus, while regions such as the putamen, globus pallidus and substantia nigra have normal GABA contents, in contrast to the situation in Huntington's chorea. GABA concentrations are often reduced in the CSF of patients with dialysis encephalopathy, as well as in patients having severe action tremor complicating multiple sclerosis. We have not found GABA content reduced in biopsies of temporal cortex removed from patients with focal epilepsy (Perry, Hansen 1981), nor have we found abnormal GABA levels in the CSF of patients with torsion dystonias (Perry et al. 1982a).

Finally, GABA levels are raised in brain in at least 2 conditions (Table 5). In Parkinson's disease, GABA content of the putamen is significantly elevated as compared to age-matched controls (Perry et al. 1983). Whether this indicates increased GABAergic neuronal activity in the striatum in Parkinson's disease as we postulated, or decreased GABAergic activity as suggested earlier by Hornykiewicz et al. (1976), remains to be determined. GABA concentrations can be markedly elevated in CSF by drugs that inhibit GABA aminotransferase (GABA-T), such as hydrazine, a terminal metabolite of isoniazid (Perry et al. 1981c), γ-vinyl GABA (Grove et al. 1981) and γ-acetylenic GABA (Tell et al. 1981). There is every reason to believe that these GABA-T inhibitors also increase GABA levels in human brain, just as they have been shown to in the brains of experimental animals. Although measurement of CSF GABA concentration is not useful in the diagnosis of Huntington's chorea, CSF GABA determinations can be valuable in monitoring biochemical responses to drugs designed to increase brain GABA content.

CONCLUSION

Measurements of Gln, Glu and GABA in brain and CSF have contributed important information to our knowledge of underlying biochemical abnormalities in human brain disorders, and it is likely that careful measurement of these compounds in various regions of brain in heretofore unstudied diseases will lead to further advances. Ability to manipulate brain GABA levels with drugs may eventually lead to useful therapies for presently untreatable neurological disorders, including Huntington's chorea, multiple sclerosis, and dialysis encephalopathy.

ACKNOWLEDGEMENTS

Much of the research summarized here was supported by the Medical Research Council of Canada, and by the Huntington Society of Canada. I thank Mrs. Shirley Hansen for help both with preparation of this chapter, and for much of the original research.

REFERENCES

Alfrey AC (1978). Dialysis encephalopathy syndrome. Ann Rev Med 29:93.

Batshaw ML, Brusilow SW (1982). Valproate-induced hyperammonemia. Ann Neurol 11:319.

Böhlen P, Schechter PJ, van Damme W, Coquillat G, Dosch J-C, Koch-Weser J (1978). Automated assay of γ-aminobutyric acid in human cerebrospinal fluid. Clin Chem 24:256.

Coyle JT, McGeer EG, McGeer PL, Schwarcz R (1978). Neostriatal injections: A model for Huntington's chorea. In McGeer EG, Olney JW, McGeer PL (eds): "Kainic Acid as a Tool in Neurobiology", New York: Raven Press, p. 139.

Enna SJ, Stern LZ, Wastek GJ, Yamamura HI (1977). Cerebrospinal fluid γ-aminobutyric acid variations in neurological disorders. Arch Neurol 34:684.

Glaeser BS, Vogel WH, Oleweiler DB, Hare TA (1975). GABA levels in cerebrospinal fluid of patients with Huntington's chorea: A preliminary report. Biochem Med 12:380.

Grove J, Schechter PJ, Tell G, Koch-Weser J, Sjoerdsma A, Warter JM, Marescaux C, Rumbach L (1981). Increased gamma-aminobutyric acid (GABA), homocarnosine and β-alanine in cerebrospinal fluid of patients treated with γ-vinyl GABA (4-amino-hex-5-enoic acid). Life Sci 28:2431.

Guidotti A, Biggio G, Costa E (1975). 3-Acetylpyridine: A tool to inhibit the tremor and the increase of cGMP content in cerebellar cortex elicited by harmaline. Brain Res 96:201.

Hare TA, Manyam NVB (1980). Rapid and sensitive ion-exchange fluorometric measurement of γ-aminobutyric acid in physiological fluids. Anal Biochem 101:349.

Hornykiewicz O, Lloyd KG, Davidson L (1976). The GABA system, function of the basal ganglia, and Parkinson's disease. In Roberts E, Chase T, Tower DB (eds): "GABA in Nervous System Functions", New York: Raven Press, p. 479.

Kim JS, Kornhuber HH, Schmid-Burgk W, Holzmüller B (1980). Low cerebrospinal fluid glutamate in schizophrenia and a new hypothesis of schizophrenia. Neurosci Lett 20:379.

Konigsmark BW, Weiner LP (1970). The olivopontocerebellar atrophies: A review. Medicine 49:227.

McBride WJ, Nadi NS, Altman J, Aprison MH (1973). Effects of selective doses of X-irradiation on the levels of several amino acids in the cerebellum of the rat. Neurochem Res 1:141.

Manyam NVB, Katz L, Hare TA, Gerber JC III, Grossman MH (1980). Levels of γ-aminobutyric acid in cerebrospinal fluid in various neurological disorders. Arch Neurol 37:352.

Murphy JV, Marquardt K (1982). Asymptomatic hyperammonemia in patients receiving valproic acid. Arch Neurol 39:591.

Obata K (1976). Association of GABA with cerebellar Purkinje cells: Single cell analysis. In Roberts E, Chase T, Tower DB (eds): "GABA in Nervous System Function", New York: Raven Press, p. 217.

Perry TL, (1982a). Cerebral amino acid pools. In Lajtha A (ed): "Handbook of Neurochemistry", Vol. 1, 2nd ed, New York: Plenum Press, p. 151.

Perry TL (1982b). Normal cerebrospinal fluid and brain glutamate levels in schizophrenia do not support the hypothesis of glutamatergic neuronal dysfunction. Neurosci Lett 28:81.

Perry TL, Hansen S (1981). Amino acid abnormalities in epileptogenic foci. Neurology 31:872.

Perry TL, Hansen S, Gandham SS (1981a). Postmortem changes of amino compounds in human and rat brain. J Neurochem 36:406.

Perry TL, Hansen S, Kloster M (1973). Huntington's chorea: Deficiency of γ-aminobutyric acid in brain. N Engl J Med 288:337.

Perry TL, Hansen S, MacLean J (1976). Cerebrospinal fluid and plasma glutamine elevation by anticonvulsant drugs: A potential diagnostic and therapeutic trap. Clin Chim Acta 69:441.

Perry TL, Hansen S, Quinn N, Marsden CD (1982a). Concentrations of GABA and other amino acids in CSF from torsion dystonia patients. J Neurochem 39:1188.

Perry TL, Hansen S, Wall RA, Gauthier SG (1982b). Human CSF GABA concentrations: Revised downward for controls, but not decreased in Huntington's chorea. J Neurochem 38:766.

Perry TL, Javoy-Agid F, Agid Y, Fibiger HC (1983). Striatal GABAergic neuronal activity is not reduced in Parkinson's disease. J Neurochem 40:1120.

Perry TL, Kish SJ, Buchanan J, Hansen S (1979). γ-Aminobutyric-acid deficiency in brain of schizoprenic patients. Lancet I:237.

Perry TL, Kish SJ, Hansen S, Currier RD (1981b). Neurotransmitter amino acids in dominantly inherited cerebellar disorders. Neurology 31:237.

Perry TL, Kish SJ, Hansen S, Wright JM, Wall RA, Dunn WL, Bellward GD (1981c). Elevation of brain GABA content by chronic low-dosage administration of hydrazine, a metabolite of isoniazid. J Neurochem 37:32.

Perry TL, Stedman D, Hansen S (1968). A versatile lithium buffer elution system for single column automatic amino acid chromatography. J Chromatog 38:460.

Perry TL, Wirtz MLK, Kennaway NG, Hsia YE, Atienza FC, Uemura HS (1980). Amino acid and enzyme studies of brain and other tissues in an infant with argininosuccinic aciduria. Clin Chim Acta 105:257.

Roberts E (1979). New directions in GABA research: I. Immunocytochemical studies of GABA neurons. In Krogsgaard-Larsen P, Scheel-Krüger J, Kofod H (eds): "GABA-Neurotransmitters: Pharmacochemical, Biochemical, and Pharmacological Aspects," New York, Academic Press, p. 28.

Roffler-Tarlov S, Sidman RL (1978). Concentrations of glutamic acid in cerebellar cortex and deep nuclei of normal mice and weaver, staggerer and nervous mutants. Brain Res 142:269.

Storm-Mathisen J (1976). Distribution of the components of the GABA system in neuronal tissue: Cerebellum and hippocampus -- effects of axotomy. In Roberts E, Chase T, Tower DB (eds): "GABA in Nervous System Function", New York: Raven Press, p. 149.

Tell G, Böhlen P, Schechter PJ, Koch-Weser J, Agid Y, Bonnet AM, Coquillat G, Chazot G, Fischer C (1981). Treatment of Huntington disease with γ-acetylenic GABA, an irreversible inhibitor of GABA-transaminase: Increased CSF GABA and homocarnosine without clinical amelioration. Neurology 31:207.

Walser M (1983). Urea cycle disorders and other hereditary hyperammonemic syndromes. In Stanbury JB, Wyngaarden JB, Fredrickson DS, Goldstein JL, Brown MS (eds): "The Metabolic Basis of Inherited Disease," 5th Ed., New York: McGraw-Hill, p. 402.

Wood JH, Hare TA, Glaeser BS, Ballenger JC, Post RM (1979). Low cerebrospinal fluid γ-aminobutyric acid content in seizure patients. Neurology 29:1203.

**Glutamine, Glutamate, and GABA
in the Central Nervous System, pages 595–608**
© 1983 Alan R. Liss, Inc., 150 Fifth Avenue, New York, NY 10011

METABOLISM OF GLUTAMATE AND RELATED AMINO ACIDS IN INSULIN
HYPOGLYCAEMIA.

Roger F. Butterworth, Ph.D.

Laboratory of Neurochemistry,
Clinical Research Center,
Hôpital Saint-Luc (University of Montreal)
1058 St-Denis St., Montreal, Quebec   H2X 3J4

INTRODUCTION

Severe hypoglycaemia is accompanied by gross functional
impairment resulting ultimately in cessation of spontaneous
electroencephalographic (EEG) potentials and coma. Prolonged hypoglycaemia may lead to irreversible brain damage.

Since most of the glucose entering the CNS is utilised
for the production of high energy phosphate compounds, many
previous studies have focussed on the effect of hypoglycaemia on cerebral energy metabolism. Results of some early
studies suggested that energy failure in the CNS was responsible for the neurological manifestations of hypoglycaemia (Chesler and Himwich, 1944; Tews et al., 1965). More
recent work, however, has provided evidence to support the
now widely-held view that severe neurological dysfunction
and accompanying EEG abnormalities are observed in hypoglycaemia at times when cerebral energy reserves are intact
(Lewis et al., 1974; Ratcheson et al., 1981; Ghajar et al.,
1982).

REGIONAL CEREBRAL NEUROTRANSMITTER FUNCTION IN HYPOGLYCAEMIA

Clinically, hypoglycaemia leads to depression of CNS
function with rostral brain regions being more affected than
caudal ones (Himwich 1951). Thus, in severe hypoglycaemia
associated with an isoelectric EEG trace, cortical function
is absent but medullary function persists as indicated by
maintenance of effective respiratory and cardiovascular activity. Neuropathological studies provide further evidence

for the selective vulnerability of certain brain structures
to hypoglycaemic insult. Following prolonged severe hypoglycaemia, cellular damage is observed in caudate nucleus
and cerebral cortex while brain stem appears to be spared
(Hicks 1950; Brierley et al., 1971). In addition, many neurons are found to display only minor morphological alterations while nearby neurons show extensive changes. It has
been suggested that this phenomenon may depend on the functional activity of the neurons or on their metabolic characteristics (Agardh et al., 1980). Regional susceptibility to
hypoglycaemia does not appear to be reflected in selective
regional changes in glucose, glycogen, glycolytic intermediates, pyruvate, lactate, ATP or phosphocreatine (Ratcheson et
al., 1981). However, glucose oxidation by brain functions
not only to provide energy in the form of the anhydride bonds
of ATP, but is also required for the synthesis, under normal
physiological conditions, of certain intermediates essential
for neuronal function. Such substances include the neurotransmitters acetylcholine, GABA, glutamate and aspartate
and it has been suggested that the neurological disturbances
associated with hypoglycaemia (prior to the isoelectric EEG
stage, at least) might be the result of "transmission failure"
involving one or more of these neurotransmitter systems
(Siesjo 1978).

Pyruvate derived from glucose appears to be the major
precursor of the acetyl group of acetylcholine and recent
studies have demonstrated that inhibition of pyruvate oxidation caused a proportionate reduction of acetylcholine
synthesis in brain slices (Gibson et al., 1975). Incorporation of ^{14}C-choline into acetylcholine in brain *in vivo* was
subsequently found to be decreased in insulin-hypoglycaemia
(Gibson and Blass 1976). Several lines of evidence support
the contention that impairment of glucose oxidation leads to
a decrease in the synthesis of a physiologically important
pool of acetylcholine. Physostigmine, the central cholines-
terase inhibitor, was found to delay the appearance of hypoglycaemic seizures (Gibson and Blass 1976) and it has been
demonstrated that transmission across the cholinergic synapse
of superior cervical ganglion is more sensitive to a lack of
glucose than is axonal conduction (Dolivo 1974).

In addition, there is a growing body of evidence to suggest that modification of GABA neurotransmission may be responsible for some of the neurological manifestations of hypoglycaemia. In 1961, De Ropp and Snedeker observed decreased

GABA levels during hypoglycaemia, a finding later confirmed
in studies from several laboratories (Tews et al., 1965;
Butterworth et al., 1982). In one study, it was noted that
cerebral cortical GABA levels were progressively reduced in
hypoglycaemic animals as EEG activity became depressed (Lewis
et al., 1974). In subsequent studies, cerebellar GABA was
found to be selectively decreased at early stages of insulin-
hypoglycaemia in mice (Gorell et al., 1976) and rats
(Butterworth et al., 1982). Certain drugs whose mechanism
of action is reportedly mediated via the GABA system prevent
hypoglycaemic convulsions. Such drugs include aminoxyacetic
acid, mesantoin (Saad 1972) and phenytoin (Butterworth 1982).
A recent electrophysiological study has provided evidence to
suggest that hypoglycaemia may produce, in the early stages,
selective dysfunction of GABA neurons (Raabe 1981). Furthermore, histologically defined damage to certain GABAergic
cells has been described following insulin-hypoglycaemia of
sufficient severity of abolish spontaneous EEG in rats
(Agardh et al., 1981).

Dysfunction of GABA and glutamate-mediated neuronal
systems may result from diminished synthesis of the neurotransmitter pool of these amino acids resulting from the utilisation of their respective precursor amino acids (glutamate and glutamine) as alternative energy substrates in hypoglycaemia, as outlined in the following section.

CEREBRAL AMINO ACIDS AS ALTERNATIVE ENERGY SOURCES IN HYPO-
GLYCAEMIA.

In insulin hypoglycaemia, as blood glucose concentrations
fall below 3mM, cerebral metabolic rate for glucose (CMR_{gl})
declines at a faster rate than does the cerebral metabolic
rate for oxygen (CMR_{O_2}) indicating oxidation of endogenous
substrates other than glucose (Lewis et al., 1974; Ghajar et
al., 1982). Possible endogenous substrates include carbohydrate reserves, amino acids and phospholipids. When fasted
adult male rats are treated with insulin (100 I.U./kg), a
sequence of neurobehavioral abnormalities occurs progressing
from disturbances of motor coordination to convulsions, followed by deep coma (Butterworth et al., 1982). The relationship between the neurological impairment, blood glucose and
the accompanying EEG abnormalities in insulin treated rats is
summarised in Figure 1.

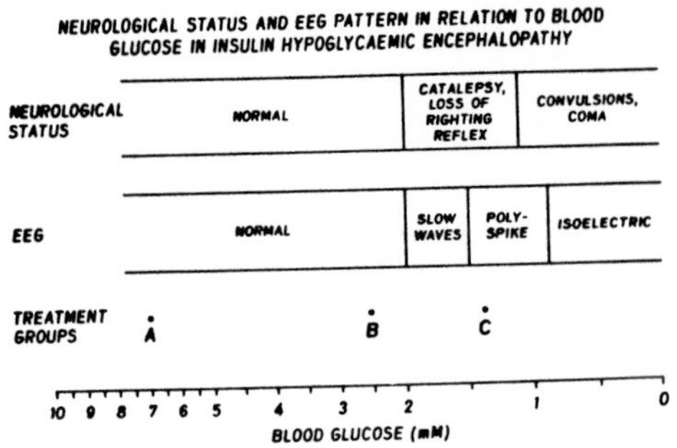

Fig. 1. Neurological status and EEG pattern in relation to blood glucose in insulin hypoglycaemic encephalopathy.

Thus, as blood glucose falls below 2mM, animals show marked catalepsy and loss of righting reflex accompanied by EEG traces characterised predominantly by slow wave activity (Norberg et al., 1975). Convulsions and polyspike traces follow as blood glucose concentrations fall below 1.5mM. A recent study showed that at blood glucose levels below this, glucose transport into brain becomes rate-limiting and insufficient to support cerebral energy metabolism (Ghajar et al., 1982). Below blood glucose levels of approximately 1mM, EEG traces are isoelectric, a state of deep coma exists and ATP levels start to decline (Siesjo 1978).

As part of a series of studies of cerebral metabolism in metabolic encephalopathy, we recently completed an investigation of regional amino acid changes in relation to function in insulin hypoglycaemia. Concentrations of the cerebral amino acids glutamate, glutamine, GABA and aspartate were measured during the early stages of insulin hypoglycaemic encephalopathy (ie: prior to the onset of convulsions or coma associated with isoelectric EEG and diminished cerebral ATP Levels). Treatment groups A, B and C, as defined in Figure 1 were chosen, corresponding to groups of animals treated as follows:

Group A: 24 hr. fasted, saline-treated (controls)
Group B: insulin-hypoglycaemic, presymptomatic
Group C: insulin-hypoglycaemic, symptomatic but preconvulsive

Cerebral amino acids were determined using a sensitive dou-
ble-isotope dansyl microassay (Butterworth et al., 1982) in
the following regions of brain: cerebral cortex (CO), hippocampus (HI), caudate nucleus (CN), hypothalamus (HT), midbrain (MB), cerebellum (CE) and medulla-pons (MO). Regional
changes in concentrations of glutamate, glutamine, GABA and
aspartate are summarised in Figures 2-5 (expressed as per
cent of saline-treated control values) as a function of blood
glucose concentrations. In a previous report, whole brain
concentrations of glutamate, glutamine and GABA were found to
be unchanged prior to the convulsive stage of insulin hypoglycaemia (Butterworth et al., 1982). However, as can clearly be seen from Figs. 2-5, certain region-selective amino
acid changes were apparent as blood glucose few below 3mM.
For example, glutamate and glutamine levels declined significantly in caudate nucleus whilst showing little net change
in medulla-pons (Figs. 2 and 3).

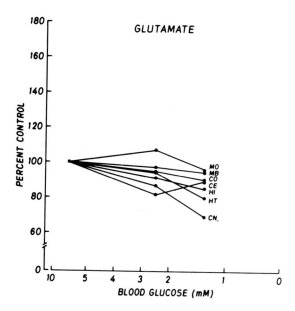

Fig. 2. Regional changes in cerebral glutamate as a
function of blood glucose in insulin hypoglycaemia. Values
are expressed as a function of saline-treated 24h. fasted
(control) values. MO: medulla-pons, MB: midbrain, CO: cerebral cortex, CE: cerebellum, HI: hippocampus, HT: hypothalamus, CN: caudate nucleus.

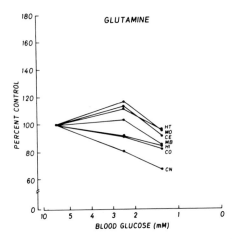

Fig. 3. Regional changes in cerebral glutamine as a function of blood glucose in insulin hypoglycaemia. Legend as for Figure 2.

Significantly decreased GABA levels were observed in cerebral cortex and cerebellum (Fig. 4). Aspartate concentrations, on the other hand, were significantly increased as hypoglycaemia progressed (Fig. 5) in confirmation of previous findings (Lewis et al., 1974; Gorell et al., 1976).

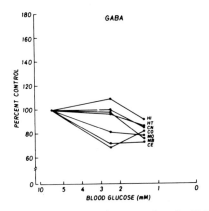

Fig. 4. Regional changes in cerebral GABA as a function of blood glucose in insulin hypoglycaemia. Legend as for Figure 2.

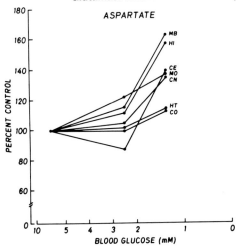

Fig. 5. Regional changes in cerebral aspartate as a function of blood glucose in insulin hypoglycaemia. Legend as for Figure 2.

Reports of decreased cerebral glutamate and increased aspartate have led to the suggestion that carbon atoms from glutamate are fed into the tricarboxylic acid cycle via the aspartate aminotransferase reaction (Lewis et al., 1974), prior to oxidation as alternative energy substrates. However, in order to fulfil such a role, amino acids must first cross the mitochondrial membrane. Glutamate appears to have limited access to mitochondria, being transport by a specific translocase system coupled to the extrusion of aspartate (Brand and Chappell 1974). Glutamine, on the other hand, readily crosses the mitochondrial membrane where, as a first step to being oxidised, it is deaminated by the mitochondrial enzyme, glutaminase:

$$GLUTAMINE \rightarrow GLUTAMATE + NH_3 \qquad [1]$$

The glutamate thus formed is then available for transamination by aspartate aminotransferate (AAT):

$$GLUTAMATE + OXALOACETATE \rightleftharpoons \alpha\text{-}KETOGLUTARATE + ASPARTATE \qquad [2]$$

Previous studies have shown that glutaminase and the mito-chondrial type of AAT have the same intracellular distribu-tion (Van den Berg 1970).

Thus, α-ketoglutarate is formed (from reaction [2]) from which oxidative energy is released following conversion to oxaloacetate in the tricarboxylic acid cycle:

$$\alpha\text{-KETOGLUTARATE} \rightarrow \text{OXALOACETATE} + \text{ENERGY} \qquad\qquad [3]$$

The net effect of reactions 1,2 and 3 would then be:

$$\text{GLUTAMINE} \rightarrow \text{ASPARTATE} + NH_3 + \text{ENERGY}$$

In this way, a molecule of glutamine is converted into as-partate with formation of ammonia and energy (in the form of 8 molecules of ATP). Moreover, accumulating intramitochon-drial aspartate is made available for translocation with glutamate which may than be further oxidised according to reactions 2 and 3.

If reactions 1, 2 and 3 were the only ones occurring during hypoglycaemia, the decreased glutamate and glutamine would be equal to the increase in aspartate (ie: mobilisa-tion of substrate from amino acids would occur by deamida-tion of glutamine and transamination reactions). However, as blood glucose concentrations fall below 2mM, the sum of the amino acids (glutamate, glutamine, GABA and aspartate) decreases by 2.2 and 3.5 μmole g^{-1} in cerebral cortex and caudate nucleus respectively (Figure 6), suggesting (at least in these brain regions) that oxidative deamination took place according to the reaction catalysed by glutamate dehydrogenase (GDH):

$$\text{GLUTAMATE} \rightleftharpoons \alpha\text{-KETOGLUTARATE} + NH_4^+$$

$$[4]$$

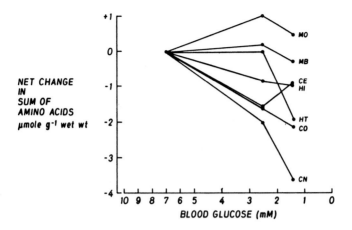

Fig. 6. Regional changes in sum of the amino acids (glutamate, glutamine, GABA and aspartate) in insulin hypoglycaemic. Legend as for Figure 2.

Previous studies in Siesjo's laboratory revealed that, during pronounced hypoglycaemia in which the EEG had been isoelectric for 15 min., cerebral cortex loses 10 μmole g^{-1} glutamate and 4 μmole g^{-1} glutamine and increased its aspartate concentration by 10 μmole g^{-1} (Siesjo 1978), ie: a net loss of 4 μmole g^{-1} amino acids. Results shown in Figure 6 suggest that a net loss of a similar magnitude is apparent in the metabolically more active regions of brain (cerebral cortex, caudate) early in hypoglycaemia. Interestingly, these more rostrally-situated brain regions in which early consumption of amino acids as alternative energy substrates appears to occur, are the regions of brain showing the greatest vulnerability to prolonged hypoglycaemic insult (Himwich 1951; Brierley et al., 1971).

Mobilization and utilisation of amino acids as alternative energy substrates clearly results in increased cerebral ammonia (reactions [1] and [4]) and several reports have suggested that increased concentrations of ammonia in brain may play a key role in the pathophysiology of hypoglycaemic encephalopathy. For example, cerebral ammonia levels in the range of 0.7 μmole g^{-1} are reportedly associated with disinhibition of pyramidal tract cells (Raabe 1981) and higher concentrations may block release of endogenous glutamate in hippocampal slices (Hamberger et al., 1979). During progression of hypoglycaemia, cerebral cortical ammonia levels rise from 0.2-0.3 µmole g^{-1} to 0.4 µmole g^{-1} at convulsive stages, progressing to levels in excess of 3 µmole g^{-1} during deep coma associated with isoelectric EEG's (Lewis et al., 1974). Thus, from this data, it would appear unlikely that increased cerebral cortical ammonia concentrations play a major role in early (preconvulsive) stages of insulin hypoglycaemia. Additional information on regional ammonia levels at various stages of hypoglycaemia will be required in order to more adequately resolve this question.

COMPARTMENTATION OF CEREBRAL AMINO ACID METABOLISM IN HYPO-GLYCAEMIA.

A simplified schematic representation of the steps involved in mobilisation of amino acids as alternative energy substrates according to reactions 1-4 is shown in Fig. 7.

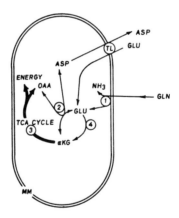

Fig. 7. Enzymes involved in amino acid oxidation in hypoglycaemia.

[1] glutaminase [2] aspartate aminotransferase [3] tricarboxylic acid cycle enzymes [4] glutamate dehydrogenase: TL: glutamate-aspartate translocase; MM: mitochondrial membrane.

Kinetic studies of the oxidation of labelled substrates indicate that the metabolism of glutamate and related compounds is compartmented in mammalian brain. Studies based on the fate of radiolabelled glucose have led for example, to the formulation of a model in which a 'large' glutamate compartment is assigned to neuronal structures and a 'small' glutamate compartment to astrocytes (Berl and Clarke 1969). Furthermore, there is evidence to suggest that astrocytes, by accumulation of neurotransmitter (glutamate and GABA) may be of major importance for the termination of its action. Since amino acid stores, as well as the enzymes necessary for their oxidation according to reactions 1-4 are localised to one (or more) cell types, it is possible that amino acids may be capable of fulfilling energy needs only in certain structures. For example, glutaminase activity is high in synaptosomes (of the order of 8 μmole min^{-1} g^{-1}, Bradford and Ward 1976); more than 4 times that found in astrocytes. Thus, if glutamine is to be used as an alternative energy substrate in nerve terminals, transport from astrocytes will be required. However, work from two laboratories in Canada has furnished results that, if confirmed, will raise serious questions concerning the ability of nerve terminals to utilise glutamate and glutamine as energy substrates. Firstly, a recent review article summarises evidence to suggest that glutamate and GABA in nerve terminals do not have access to a complete tricarboxylic acid cycle (Hertz 1979). This conclusion was based on findings from previous histochemical studies which showed that mitochondria in nerve endings were unable to metabolise α-ketoglutarate or succinate, suggesting a lack of α-ketoglutarate and succinate dehydrogenases (two enzymes necessary for energy production according to reaction [3]). Secondly, a study involving kainate degeneration of glutamate nerve terminals in rat striatum by McGeer and McGeer (1979) revealed no decrease in glutaminase activity leading to the conclusion that this enzyme may be absent from glutamate nerve terminals, at least in striatum. Use of glutamate and glutamine as alternative energy substrates therefore, during hypoglycaemia may be restricted to neuronal perikarya and astrocytes and glutamate/GABA nerve terminals may be particularly vulnerable to hypoglycaemia. Further studies will be required in order to evaluate such a possibility.

CONCLUSIONS

In insulin hypoglycaemia, as blood glucose falls below 2mM, there is evidence to suggest that the cerebral amino acids glutamate and glutamine are utilised as alternative energy substrates by reactions involving transamination and oxidative deamination. This utilisation of amino acids occurs first in the metabolically more active, rostrally-situated brain regions (cerebral cortex and caudate nucleus).

Since there is evidence to suggest that glutamate and glutamine are precursors of the releasable pools of GABA and glutamate respectively, their consumption as alternative energy substrates may lead to a disruption of the neuronal glial metabolic interrelationships leading to ultimate neuronal dysfunction. There is some evidence to suggest, however, that GABA and glutamate nerve terminals themselves may possess only a limited capacity to utilise these amino as energy substrates.

ACKNOWLEDGMENTS

Work described from the authors laboratory was accomplished with the skilled assistance of Dr Andrea Merkel-Drumheller and Ms France Landreville. The author thanks Ms Sylvie de Bellefeuille for assistance with the preparation of this manuscript and Dr Nico van Gelder for his invaluable critique and encouragement. Financial assistance for this work came from a grant from the Medical Research Council of Canada (MA 7889).

REFERENCES

Agardh CD, Kalimo H, Olsson Y, Siesjö BK (1980). Hypoglycaemic brain injury. Acta Neuropathol 50:31.

Agardh CD, Kalimo H, Olsson Y, Siesjö BK (1981). Hypoglycaemic brain injury. Metabolic and structural findings in rat cerebellar cortex during profound insulin induced hypoglycaemia and in the recovery period following glucose administration. J Cerebr Blood Flow and Metab 1:71.

Berl S, Clarke DD (1969). Compartmentation of amino acid metabolism. In Lajtha A (Ed)"Handbook of Neurochemistry vol 3, New York: Plenum, p.447.

Bradford HF, Ward HK (1976). On glutaminase activity in mammalian synaptosomes. Brain Res 110:115.

Brand MD, Chappell JB (1974). Glutamate and aspartate transport in rat brain mitochondria. Biochem J 140:205.

Brierley JB, Brown AW, Meldrum BS (1971). The nature and time course of the neuronal alterations resulting from oligaemia and hypoglycaemia in the brain of Macaca Mulatta. Brain Res 25:483.

Butterworth RF (1982). Prevention of hypoglycaemic convulsions by dilantin: role of amino acids. Trans Am Soc Neurochem 13:390.

Butterworth RF, Merkel AD, Landreville F (1982). Regional amino acid distribution in relation to function in insulin hypoglycaemia. J Neurochem 38:1483.

Chesler A, Himwich HE (1944). Effect of insulin hypoglycaemia on glycogen content of parts of the central nervous system of the dog. Arch Neurol Psych 52:114.

De Ropp RS, Snedeker EH (1961). Effects of drugs on amino acid levels in rat brain. J Neurochem 7:128.

Dolivo M (1974). Fedn Proc Fedn Am Soc Exp Biol 33:1043.

Ghajar JBG, Plum F, Duffy TE (1982). Cerebral oxidative metabolism and blood flow during acute hypoglycaemia and recovery in unanesthetized rats. J Neurochem 38:397.

Gibson GE, Blass JP (1967). Impaired synthesis of acetylcholine in brain accompanying mild hypoxia and hypoglycaemia. J Neurochem 27:37.

Gorell JM, Dolkart PH, Ferrendelli JA (1976). Regional levels of glucose, amino acids, high energy phosphates and cyclic nucleotides in the central nervous system during hypoglycaemic stupor and behavioural recovery. J Neurochem 27:1043.

Hamberger A, Hedquist B, Nyström B (1979). Ammonium ion inhibition of evoked release of endogenous glutamate from hippocampal slices. J Neurochem 33:1295.

Hertz L (1976). Functional interactions between neurons and astrocytes I. Turnover and metabolism of putative amino acid transmitters. Progr Neurobiol 13:277.

Hicks SP (1950). Brain metabolism in vivo. Arch Pathol 49:111.

Kvamme E, Olsen BE (1980). Substrate mediated regulation of phosphate-activated glutaminase in nervous tissue. Brain Res 181:228.

Lewis LD, Ljunggren B, Norberg K, Siesjö BK (1974). Changes in carbohydrate substrates, amino acids and ammonia in the brain during insulin-induced hypoglycaemia. J Neurochem 23:659.

McGeer EG, McGeer PL (1979). Localisation of glutaminase in the rat neostriatum. J Neurochem 32:1071.

Norberg K, Ljunggren, Siesjö BK (1975). Cerebral metabolism in relation to function in insulin-induced hypoglycaemia. In "Brain work", Alfred Benzon Symp VIII, Munksgaard, p.314.

Raabe WA (1981). Ammonia and disinhibition in cat motor cortex by ammonium acetate, monofluoroacetate and insulin-induced hypoglycaemia. Brain Res 210:311.

Ratcheson RA, Blank AC, Ferrendelli JA (1981). Regionally selective metabolic effects of hypoglycaemia in brain. J Neurochem 36:1952.

Saad SF (1972). Further observations on the role of γ-aminobutyric acid in insulin-induced hypoglycaemic convulsions. Eur J Pharmacol 17:152.

Siesjö BK (1978). Hypoglycaemia. In Siesjö BK (ed): "Brain Energy Metabolism", New York: John Wiley and Sons, p.380.

Tews JK, Carter SH, Stone WE (1965). Chemical changes in the brain during insulin hypoglycaemia and recovery. J Neurochem 12:679.

Van den Berg CJ (1970). Glutamate and glutamine. In Lajtha A (ed): "Handbook of Neurochemistry vol 3: Metabolic reactions in the nervous system", New York: Plenum, p.355.

Glutamine, Glutamate, and GABA
in the Central Nervous System, pages 609–618
© 1983 Alan R. Liss, Inc., 150 Fifth Avenue, New York, NY 10011

INVOLVEMENT OF GLUTAMATE DEHYDROGENASE IN DEGENERATIVE NEUROLOGICAL DISORDERS

Andreas Plaitakis, M.D. and Soll Berl, M.D.

Mount Sinai School of Medicine
New York, New York 10029

There is considerable evidence to suggest that acidic amino acids with putative neuroexcitatory function such as glutamate or aspartate can cause neurotoxic effects when present in excess in the nervous tissue.   Thus, Lucas and Newhouse (1957) observed degeneration of retinal neurons of pre-mature mice treated with systemic administration of monosodium glutamate (MSG). Olney et al. (1969, 1971) found hypothalamic lesions in similarly treated pre-mature mice and primates.   Furthermore, local injection of glutamate, and particularly its potent analogs kainic and ibotenic acids, into brain areas of experimental animals can produce selective destruction of regional neurons while sparing other structures such as glial cells, nerve terminals or axons passing through these areas (McGeer et al., 1978). Several lines of evidence suggest that the neurotoxicity of these substances may be directly related to their neuroexcitatory properties (excitotoxin theory). Olney et al. (1971) specifically proposed that substances with strong neuroexcitatory effects may cause neuronal degeneration by excessively depolarizing post–synaptic neurons.

Because the histologic and biochemical changes produced by the experimental use of potent excitotoxic compounds such as kainic acid, are similar to those found in patients wih degenerative disorders, e.g. Huntington's chorea (McGeer and McGeer, 1976), the possibility has been raised that abnormal accumulation of similar endogenous substances may occur in the brains of these patients and cause neuronal degeneration.   However, attempts to detect kainic acid-like compounds have not yet yielded positive results.   An alternative possibility is that neuronal degeneration in human disorders may be the result of altered metabolism of acidic amino acids normally present in the nervous system. Thus, a delicate balance may exist between the function of these substances as excitatory transmitters and their capacity to cause premature nerve cell death. In disease processes associated with abnormal neuroexcitatory mechanisms or faulty metabolism of acidic amino acids, this balance may be altered resulting in neurotoxic effects.

Data presented in this paper support this latter possibility by showing that faulty systemic metabolism of the major excitatory amino acid glutamate occurs in patients with recessive olivopontocerebellar atrophy (OPCA), a genetic neurological disorder associated with partial deficiency of glutamate dehydrogenase (GDH) (Plaitakis et al., 1980-1982). In addition, the nature of this enzymatic defect is further elucidated by data showing that an almost complete lack of a "heat-labile" GDH component is present in leukocytes of affected patients. These data support the possibility that a genetic alteration or absence of one GDH "isoenzyme" may be the primary defect of the disorder. Since GDH in the brain appears to play an important role in glutamate oxidation (Yu et al., 1982), the present results suggest that a genetically determined malfunction of this enzyme could lead to impaired glutamate catabolism within the nervous system with resultant neuronal degeneration.

METHODS

Subjects: Patients with adult-onset recessive OPCA were the subjects of this study. As previously described (Plaitakis et al., 1980-1983), these patients were affected by a progressive multi-system neurological disorder characterized by cerebellar ataxia, extrapyramidal features (Parkinsonism), bulbar nerve dysfunction, oculomotor disturbances and sometimes by muscle fasciculations and amyoatrophy. About half of these cases were familial and their genetic data suggested an autosomal recessive mode of inheritance. Two control groups were used for comparison: The 1st included normal adult individuals (healthy controls) and the 2nd, patients with various types of degenerative neurological disorders other than recessive OPCA (diseased controls).

Leukocyte preparations - enzyme assays: Leukocyte pellets were prepared from patients and controls as previously described (Plaitakis et al., 1980). The cells were disrupted by 3-4 cycles of freeze-thaw and homogenized by a motor driven (300 r.p.m.) glass homogenizer (0,004"-0.006" clearance) in 50 mm, pH 7.40, Tris HCL buffer. Whole homogenates (40-50 ul) were used for GDH assay, which was done fluorometrically, essentially as previously described (Plaitakis et al., 1980, 1981) but with the addition of 0.025% Triton

X-100 and 1 mM ADP, final concentrations, to the reaction mixture. Triton X-100 (0.16%) has been found to be inhibitory in the absence of ADP (Plaitakis et al., 1980).

Recent studies (Plaitakis et al., 1983) revealed that two GDH fractions can be prepared from human leukocytes and cultured skin fibroblasts: a "particulate" form found in the 100,000 xg pellet and a "soluble" form present in the 100,000 xg supernate prepared from whole leukocyte homogenates by differential centrifugation. Heat inactivation studies (Plaitakis et al., 1983) further suggested that these GDH forms may be "isoenzymes", since they were found to differ in heat stability. Thus, incubation at $47.5^{\circ}C$ largely inactivated the "particulate" fraction whereas the "soluble" enzyme remained stable under the same conditions. In view of this, a "heat-labile" and a "heat-stable" GDH component were determined by heat inactivation of leukocyte homogenates from patients and controls. Whole leukocyte homogenates (0.5-0.8 ml, about 7-10 mg protein/ml) were incubated at $47.5^{\circ}C$ in 10 x 7 mm capped Falcon tubes after measuring baseline GDH activity as described above. At exactly 60 minutes after starting incubation, aliquots of homogenates equal to those used for baseline measurements (40-60 µl) were removed and assayed with the addition of Triton X-100 (0.025%) and ADP (1 mM) to the reaction mixture. Activity found was considered "heat-stable" GDH; this was subtracted from the baseline activity in order to calculate the "heat-labile" GDH.

Determinaton of plasma amino acid, α-ketoglutarate, lactate and pyruvate levels: After overnight fasting, blood samples were obtained the following morning by venipuncture from patients and controls. The blood was transferred immediately to pre-chilled (0-$5^{\circ}C$) EDTA-containing tubes and the plasma was separated by centrifugation at 19,000 xg for 10 minutes. Protein was precipitated by perchloric acid (0.4N final concentration) and the final extract was obtained by another (19,000 xg 10 minutes) centrifugation. This was immediately stored at $-80^{\circ}C$ until just before analysis of each sample. An amino acid profile was measured with a Technicon TSM amino acid analyzer. Lactate, pyruvate, and α-ketoglutarate were measured enzymatically (Plaitakis et al., 1982).

Oral glutamate loading test: To perform glutamate loading test, fasted patients and controls received orally 60 mg/kg body weight of monosodium glutamate dissolved in 100-150 ml of water; blood samples were then drawn after 30, 60, 90 and 120 minutes for measurement of plasma substrates as above.

RESULTS

As shown in Figure 1 the "heat-labile" GDH fraction was markedly decreased (by about 90%, p $<$ 0.0005) in the patients with recessive OPCA as compared to healthy and diseased controls. In contrast, the "heat-stable" GDH was not different in the patients as compared to either control group.

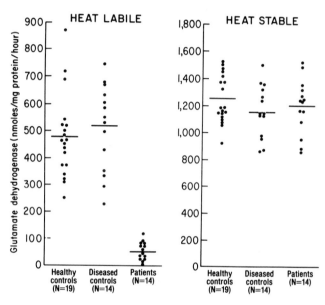

Figure 1.

Activities of glutamate dehydrogenase "heat-labile" and "heat-stable" components in leukocytes from patients and controls. Enzyme activities were determined by heat inactivation at 47.5°C in whole leukocyte homogenates as described in the Methods. Dots represent average activities for each individual and lines the mean value for each group.

Fasting plasma glutamate levels were significantly increased in the patients with GDH deficiency as compared to healthy and diseased controls (by 117-148%, p $<$ .0005) (Figure 2). In contrast, the fasting plasma levels of α-ketoglutarate were significantly decreased (by 21-26%; p $<$ 0.005) (Figure 2). Following oral intake of MSG, plasma glutamate and aspartate rose to significantly higher levels in the patients than in the controls (Figure 3). In contrast, there were no significant changes in plasma glutamine or alanine after MSG intake in the patients or controls. The lactate to pyruvate ratio increased significantly in the controls after 60 min of oral glutamate loading, but no such increase occurred in the patients with GDH deficiency; they showed a flat curve (Figure 3).

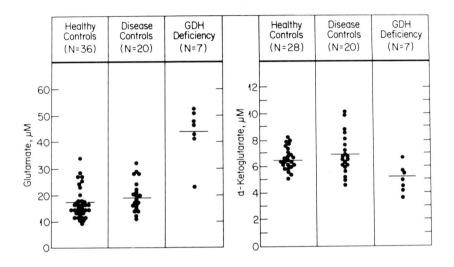

Figure 2.
    Fasting plasma glutamate and α-ketoglutarate levels in patients with GDH-deficient OPCA and controls. Dots represent average levels for each individual and lines the mean value for each group. Reprinted from Plaitakis et al., Science, 216: 193, 1982. By permission of the American Association for the Advancement of Science (Copyright (c) 1982).

DISCUSSION

    Under olivopontocerebellar atrophy (OPCA) are included several heterogenous neurological disorders which share some common neuropathological features such as degeneration of the olivocerebellar pathways, cerebellar cortex, pons and/or basal ganglia. Thus, the OPCAs are disorders with multiple system atrophy that link the spinocerebellar degenerations with the extrapyramidal diseases. Recent studies (Plaitakis et al., 1980–1982) showed that a late adult-onset form of OPCA, which is probably recessively inherited, is associated with partial deficiency of GDH.

    Although no isoenzymes for mammalian GDH are known to

date, recent studies in our laboratory revealed evidence for the presence of at least two forms of the enzyme in human tissues. (Plaitakis et al., 1983). One form is "particulate" and "heat-labile" and another "soluble" and "heat-stable". In the present study, the

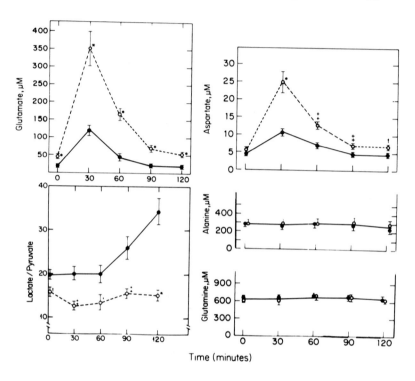

Figure 3.

Glutamate loading test. Patients (O) (N = 6) and controls (●) (N = 13) received orally 60 mg/kg body weight of MSG after overnight fasting. Blood samples were drawn at the time points indicated and processed as described in the Methods. Dots represent mean values and bars 1 standard error. *p < 0.001; †p < 0.01; ‡p < 0.05. Reprinted from Plaitakis et al., Science, 216:193, 1982. By permission of the American Association for the Advancement of Science (Copyright (c), 1982).

two GDH components were determined in leukocytes from OPCA patients (with partial deficiency of the total GDH activity) and controls by measurements before and after heat inactivation. Results revealed that the defect in GDH) was limited to its "heat labile" form. Furthermore, the decrease (by about 90%) in this GDH component is of the magnitude expected of a recessively inherited primary enzymatic defect. These data suggest that a genetically determined defect in of one GDH form, probably an "isoenzyme", is involved in the pathogenesis of this neurological disorder. Since the brain is the only organ involved in OPCA, these results raise the possibility for an important role for the "heat-labile" GDH in nervous tissue function. This remains to be explored by future studies.

The studies on the systemic metabolism of the substrates involved in the GDH-catalyzed reaction, showed evidence for impaired catabolism of glutamate in the GDH deficient patients. Thus, the fasting plasma levels of this amino acid were significantly elevated and those of α-ketoglutarate significantly decreased. Furthermore, an excessive elevation in plasma glutamate occurred in these patients after oral intake of MSG. The plasma lactate to pyruvate ratio increased significantly in the controls but not in the GDH–deficient patients following glutamate loading. Since GDH is thought to play a role in maintaining the NAD/NADH potentials (Miller et al., 1973), these data suggest that oxidation of the glutamate load by GDH in these individuals produced sufficient amounts of reduced NADH to increase the ratio of NADH to NAD as reflected in the increased plasma lactate to pyruvate ratio. The flat curve observed in the GDH–deficient patients, is consistent with a systemic defect in the oxidative deamination of glutamate in these individuals.

Because the present data suggest that a genetic mutation of one GDH "isoenzyme", a defect expressed in tissues outside the nervous system, may underly the disease, and because the systemic metabolic distortions found in this study are consistent with a defect in glutamate disposition, rather than in glutamate synthesis, it seems possible that the GDH "isoenzyme" involved may function specifically in glutamate oxidation in the various tissues. Impaired glutamate catabolism within the nervous tissue could result in excessive accumulation of this amino acid and neuronal degeneration according to the excitotoxin theory. The enzyme may be particularly associated with glutamatergic nerve terminals (Quastel, 1978) and/or glial cells (Berl, 1971). Its activity in neuronal cell bodies is relatively low (Kuhlman & Lowry, 1956). Cultured astrocytes have indeed been shown to oxidize glutamate in rather high rates via the GDH pathway (Yu, 1982). Faulty catabolism of glutamate at the nerve terminals or glial cells could result in the accumulation of increased amounts of the amino acid in the synaptic cleft during neurotransmission and this could cause degeneration of the post-synaptic neurons. Elderly patients may be particularly sensitive to glutamate neurotoxicity since the release of this amino acid from human brain tissue has been shown to increase significantly with aging (Smith et al., 1983).

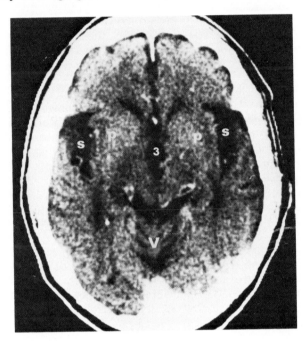

Figure 4.
    Head CT scan of a 75-year old patient with GDH deficient OPCA. A. Note the markedly dilated 3rd ventricle (3) and Sylvian fissures (S). The latter may to be the result of putamen (P) involvement. B. Atrophy of superior vermis (V) of the cerebellum is also visible.

Recent studies (Huang and Plaitakis, 1983), exploring the in vivo brain morphological changes of patients with GDH deficiency, as shown by a high resolution CT scans, revealed a topographic degeneration pattern that tends to support the "excitotoxin" pathogenesis of the disorder. Thus, the most striking abnormality found was dilatation of the anterior 3rd ventricle due to involvement of the hypothalamus and the adjacent part of the thalamus. Other morphological changes observed were atrophy of the cerebellum, brain stem and frontal cortex, as well as widening of the Sylvian fissures (Figure 4). Previous pathological studies have established that disappearance of the Purkinje cells may be the earliest histologic change occurring in the cerebellar cortex of OPCA patients. Since these cells receive direct glutamatergic innervation (parallel fibers), they may degenerate as a result of increased glutamate accumulation during neurotransmission. Involvement of the granule cells and the olivocerebellar fibers, also known to occur in OPCA, may be the result of a transneuronal degeneration process (Coyle, 1982). One important putative glutamatergic system in the brain is the corticostriate pathway, which in primates has been shown to project primarily to ipsilateral putamen (Jones et al., 1977). Atrophy of the putamen could lead to enlargement of the Sylvian fissures as found in the GDH-deficient patients. Finally, the markedly enlarged anterior 3rd ventricle, reflecting hypothalamic and thalamic involvement, is of particular interest since a selective destruction of hypothalamus (Olney, 1969, 1971) with resultant enlargement of 3rd ventricle (Bodnar et al., 1980) has been produced experimentally by systemic administration of MSG. These observations suggest that anatomical correlates of glutamate neurotoxicity may exist in a human neurological disorder. Should this contention be supported by future studies, including post-mortem verification, GDH deficient OPCA will be the first structural neurological disorder in which a specific genetically determined metabolic defect has been found responsible for its characteristic topography of brain lesions.

Supported by N.I.H. Grants NS-16871, NS--11631, The Clinical Center for Research in Parkinson's and Allied Diseases and RR-71, Division of Research Resources, General Clinical Research Center Branch. We are indebted to Professor P.Y. Huang for his invaluable help in the study of the CT scans, Natalya Khelemskaya for her excellent technical assistance and Minerva Feliciano for her skillful assistance in the preparation of this manuscript.

Berl S (1971) Cerebral amino acid metabolism in hepatic coma. Exp Biol Med 4:78.

Bodnar RJ, Abrams GM, Zimmerman EA, Krieger DT, Nicholson G and Kizer JS (1980) Neonatal monosodium glutamate. Neuroendocrinology 30:280.

Coyle JT (1982) Neurotoxic amino acids in human degenerative disorders. Trends Neurosci 5:287.

Huang YP and Plaitakis A (1983) Computerized tomography of OPCA. In Duvoisin RC and Plaitakis A (Eds) "The Olivopontocerebellar Atrophies", Adv Neurol, New York, Raven Press, in press.

Jones EG, Coulter JD, Burton H and Porter R (1977) Cells of origin and terminal distribution of corticostriatal fibers arising in the sensory-motor cortex of monkeys. J Comp Neurol 173:53.

Kuhlman RE, Lowry OH (1956) Quantitative histochemical changes during the development of the rat cerebral cortex. J. Neurochem 1:173.

Lucas DR and Newhouse JP (1957) The toxic effect of sodium L-glutamate on the inner layers of retina. AMA Arch Ophthalmol 58:193.

McGeer EG and McGeer PL (1976) Duplication of biochemical changes of Huntington's chorea by intrastriatal injections of glutamic and kainic acids. Nature (Lond.) 263:517.

McGeer EG, Olney JW and McGeer PL (1978) "Kainic Acid as a Tool in Neurobiology", New York, Academic Press.

Miller AL, Hawkins RA and Veech RL (1973) The mitochondrial redox state of rat brain. J Neurochem 20:1393.

Olney JW and Sharpe LG (1969) Brain lesions in an infant rhesus monkey treated with monosodium glutamate. Science 166:386.

Olney JW, Ho OL and Rhee V (1971) Cytotoxic effects of acidic and sulfur containing amino acids of the infant mouse central nervous system. Exp Brain Res 14:61.

Plaitakis A, Nicklas WJ and Desnick RJ (1980) Glutamate dehydrogenase deficiency in three patients with spinocerebellar syndrome. Ann Neurol 7:297.

Plaitakis A, Berl S, Nicklas WJ and Yahr MD (19801) Glutamate dehydrogenase deficiency in spinocerebellar degenerations: Correlation with adult-onset recessive ataxia. Trans Am Neurol Assoc 105:476.

laitakis A, Berl S and Yahr MD (1981) Amino acids as putative transmitters: the role of aspartate and glutamate in nervous system dysfunction and degeneration. Proceedings of the 12th World Congress of Neurology. Neurology 568:259.

Plaitakis A, Berl S and Yahr MD (1982) Abnormal glutamte metabolism in an adult-onset degenerative neurological disorder. Science 216:193.

Plaitakis A, Berl S, and Yahr, MD (1983) Neurological disorders associated with deficiency of glutamate dehydrogenase. Ann Neurol, in press.

Quastel JH (1978) Cerebral glutamate-glutamine interelations in vivo and in vitro. In Schoffeniels E, Franck G, Hertz L (eds), "Dynamic Properties of Glial Cells", Oxford, Pergamon Press, p. 153.

Smith CCT, Bowen DM, and Davison AN (1983) The evoked release of endogenous amino acids from tissue prisms of human neocortex. Brain Res 269:103.

Yu AC, Schousboe A and Hertz L (1982) Metabolic fate of ^{14}C-labeled glutamate in astrocytes. J Neurochem 39:954.

Glutamine, Glutamate, and GABA
in the Central Nervous System, pages 619–624
© 1983 Alan R. Liss, Inc., 150 Fifth Avenue, New York, NY 10011

GLUCOSE OXIDATION IN THE BRAIN DURING SEIZURES: EXPERIMENTS
WITH LABELED GLUCOSE AND DEOXYGLUCOSE

Cees J. Van den Berg and Roel Bruntink

Studygroup Inborn Errors and Brain
Department of Psychiatry, Faculty of Medicine
University of Groningen, Groningen
The Netherlands

It is generally accepted that there is a close relation
between the level of neuronal function and the rate of glucose oxidation; both decrease in anaesthesia and increase
during seizures. There is a fair amount of evidence that
a tight coupling between glucose oxidation and changes in
the activity pattern of brain exists, the most convincing
evidence coming from studies with anaesthetic agents.

Seizures are commonly accepted to be conditions of increased neuronal activity, and the increase of the rate of
glucose utilization during seizures has been used to argue
that increases of neuronal activity are accompanied by
increases in the rate of glucose oxidation, thus providing
further support for a tight coupling between the two.

But does the rate of glucose oxidation in the brain
really increase during seizures? There is a large body of
literature, some more than a century old, that such increases
do occur, but almost all the positive claims came from experiments in which anaesthetized and/or ventilated animals
were used. This procedure in itself results in a decreased
rate of glucose oxidation. Hence it is not surprising that
glucose oxidation increases in these situations when seizures
occur. The question is whether such an increase in glucose
oxidation can also be found when seizures are induced in
awake, free moving animals? We will show that there is no
such increase of the rate of glucose oxidation during seizures induced in awake animals; we will also show that increases of deoxyglucose phosphorylation do occur, indicating
that one should be extremely careful in interpretating data

obtained with deoxyglucose in terms of changes in rates of glucose oxidation. The seizures were induced by agents which affect glutamate or GABA systems and it is possible that such systems are involved in mediating the diverse effects on glucose metabolism.

Glucose and Deoxyglucose Metabolism during Seizures
Induced by Kainic Acid

A few min after the administration of kainic acid a complex pattern of behavioral changes develops with seizure discharges occurring in the brain, most notably in the hippocampus (Ben-Ari et al. 1980; Lothman, Collins 1981). Increases of some 200-300% in deoxyglucose uptake and phosphorylation were observed using the autoradiographic technique (Lothman, Collins 1981).

While the rate of deoxyglucose phosphorylation in the undisturbed state is almost certainly linearly related to the rate of glucose oxidation (Sokoloff et al. 1977), insufficient evidence is available to generalize this relationship to other states of the brain. We, therefore, measured both the rate of deoxyglucose phosphorylation and the rate of glucose incorporation into glutamate and related amino acids during kainic acid induced seizures. The rate of incorporation of labeled glucose into glutamate and related amino acids is directly related to the rate of glucose oxidation, as glutamate and aspartate are in an almost instantaneous equilibrium with α-ketoglutarate and oxaloacetate respectively (see Gaitonde 1965; Van den Berg et al. 1969; Van den Berg, Garfinkel 1971; Hawkins et al. 1974).

Table 1 contains the data obtained after intravenous injection of kainic acid. It can be seen that deoxyglucose phosphorylation was increased, while only a small increase of glucose incorporation was found. These data suggest that glucose oxidation was increased little or none during seizures and that changes in the rate of deoxyglucose phosphorylation may not necessarily indicate changes in the rate of glucose oxidation.

It should be noted that the level of, and the rate of, incorporation of labeled glucose into lactic acid was doubled (data not shown); these changes may be related to the increased rate of deoxyglucose phosphorylation observed.

Table 1: Effect of kainic acid on the metabolism of labeled glucose and deoxyglucose in the hippocampus of rat brain.

	Control	Kainic acid
Labeled glucose:		
Brain extract	334±112 (4)	360±26 (8)
Glutamate	121± 18	156± 22^x
Amino acid fraction	168± 14	205± 14^x
Labeled deoxyglucose:		
Total in brain	125± 60 (12)	437±108 (7)^x
Deoxyglucose	139± 45	152± 37
Deoxyglucose phosphate	119± 26	238± 67^x
Total in blood	207± 18	228± 31

Labeled glucose and deoxyglucose were injected in the tail vein, followed in 30 sec by kainic acid (12 mg/kg); controls received saline. At 15 min the animals were killed by micro wave fixation, hippocampi dissected and extracted. Amino acids and deoxyglucose phosphate were separated with AG 1-X4. Data are given in dpm/mg wet weight ± S.D. for an injected dose of 25 µC/200 gram body weight. Between brackets: number of animals; x: increase significant: $p < 0.05$, student t test.

Glucose and Deoxyglucose Metabolism during Seizures Induced by Bicuculline

The results obtained with kainic acid strongly suggest that an increased rate of deoxyglucose phosphorylation can be found in the absence of an increase in the rate of glucose oxidation. Since these results may be atypical, we extended our investigation to bicuculline induced seizures. Bicuculline induces a steady pattern of seizures, lasting for a long time; during those seizures in ventilated animals evidence for a marked increase in glucose and oxygen uptake has been presented (Meldrum, Nilsson 1976; Chapman et al. 1977).

The results, presented in Table 2, clearly show that deoxyglucose phosphorylation was markedly increased in the bicuculline-treated animals, while the rate of glucose incorporation into the combined amino acid fraction was unchanged. The level of glucose was decreased, and that of lactic acid increased (data not shown).

Table 2: Effect of bicuculline on the metabolism of labeled glucose and deoxyglucose in the cortex of rat brain.

	Control	Bicuculline
Labeled glucose:		
Brain extract	488±82 (9)	546± 81 (10)
Amino acid fraction	233±50	235± 53
Labeled deoxyglucose:		
Total in blood	324±22	309± 26
Total in brain	316±50	633±140^x
% in deoxyglucose phosphate	42± 5.3	68± 12.8^x

Bicuculline, 1.2 mg/kg, was injected i.v. 2 min after the labeled precursors; 5 min later the animals were killed by microwave fixation. Average ± S.D. of 9 or 10 animals. x: increase significant: $p < 0.05$, student t test.

DISCUSSION

During both the kainic acid and bicuculline induced seizures we observed increases of deoxyglucose phosphoryla- tion - as has been reported by others - but we did not ob- serve increases in the rate of glucose oxidation (derived from glucose incorporation data). The absence of an in- creased rate of glucose incorporation into brain amino acids during seizures induced by picrotoxin, cardiazol and fluro- thyl has been reported earlier (Yoshino, Elliott 1970; Reynolds, Gallagher 1973).

Taking these data together, we would suggest that during seizures induced in free moving animals there is no increase in the rate of glucose oxidation (or only a very small one): the rate of glucose oxidation proceeds during those seizures at its normal, high rate. There is an increased rate of lactic acid formation, delivering, however, not much extra useful energy. Evidently, the complex elect- rical patterns of the seizures do not require more energy than is normally converted.

Almost all the claims of an increased rate of glucose oxidation during seizures were derived from experiments with previously anaesthetized animals, as mentioned in the intro- duction. It is quite natural that, in those experimental situations, glucose oxidation will increase during the seizures. This has been found repeatedly. In most cases, the highest rate of glucose oxidation observed was not higher than found in the free moving animal but, in a few cases, suggestive evidence for a higher rate of glucose oxidation has been presented (Meldrum, Nilsson 1976; Chapman et al. 1977). These discrepancies require further clarification.

Nevertheless, we want to suggest that glucose oxidation is proceeding at its maximal rate - or very close to it - in the brain of awake animals, only decreases being possible. The brain is not a machine like the muscle with rest/activity cycles where the rate of glucose oxidation during activity is markedly increased, in correspondence with the increased amount of mechanical work performed. The brain is always producing "brain work" maximally. Changes in brain function and the "underlying" neuronal activities are not coupled to changes in energy transformation; they require, of course, a high rate of energy transformation to proceed continously.

The use of the muscle analogy to understand brain function may have had its use in the past; it certainly has its limits.

REFERENCES

Ben-Ari Y, Tremblay E, Riche D, Ghilini G, Naquet R (1980). Injection of kainic acid into the amygdaloid complex of rat: An electrographic, clinical and histological study in relation to the pathology of epilepsy. Neuroscience 5:515.

Chapman A, Meldrum BS, Siesjo BK (1977). Cerebral metabolic changes during prolonged epileptic seizures in rats. J Neurochem 28:1025.

Gaitonde MK (1965). Rate of utilization of glucose and compartmentation of α-oxoglutarate and glutamate in rat brain. Biochem J 95:803.

Hawkins RA, Miller AL, Cremer JE, Veech RL (1974). Measurement of the rate of glucose utilization by rat brain in vivo. J Neurochem 23:917.

Lothman R, Collins RC (1981). Kainic acid induced limbic seizures: Metabolic, behavioral, electroencephalographic and neuropathological correlates. Brain Res 218:299.

Meldrum BS, Nilsson B (1976). Cerebral blood flow and metabolic rate early and late in prolonged epileptic seizures induced in rats by bicuculline. Brain 99:523.

Reynolds AP, Gallagher BB (1973). The effect of hexafluoro-diethyl ether (fluothyl) on the metabolism of rat brain amino acids labelled by [U-^{14}C]glucose. Life Sci 13:87.

Van den Berg CJ, Garfinkel D (1971). A simulation study of brain compartments. Biochem J 123:211.

Van den Berg CJ, Krzalic LJ, Mela P, Waelsch H (1969). Compartmentation of glutamate metabolism in brain. Biochem J 113:281.

Yoshino Y, Elliott KAC (1970). Incorporation of carbon atoms from glucose into free amino acids in brain under normal and altered conditions. Can J Biochem 48:228.

Glutamine, Glutamate, and GABA
in the Central Nervous System, pages 625–641
© 1983 Alan R. Liss, Inc., 150 Fifth Avenue, New York, NY 10011

EXCITATORY AMINO ACIDS AND ANTICONVULSANT DRUG ACTION

Brian S. Meldrum and Astrid G. Chapman

Department of Neurology, Institute of Psychiatry,
De Crespigny Park, London SE5 8AF, UK;
Department of Neurology, Rayne Institute,
and King's College Hospital Medical School

Excitatory neurotransmitters play a key role in the spread of epileptic activity and may also contribute to its initiation (Meldrum 1984). The dicarboxylic amino acids (and their sulfinic or sulfonic analogs) are the most universal and potent excitatory neurotransmitters identified in the central nervous system (Curtis, Johnston 1974).

Previously it has been considered that the most appropriate strategy in seeking an antiepileptic drug effect is to enhance inhibitory mechanisms (Meldrum 1983). GABA-mediated inhibition in the cortex, hippocampus and elsewhere provides both feed-forward and feedback inhibition that, when enhanced, will suppress abnormal activity without altering physiological function, because it is activated by the abnormal activity (Meldrum 1981).

However, it is possible that some of the mechanisms for impairing excitatory transmission listed in Table 1 can operate selectively against the pathologically enhanced activity in epilepsy and leave normal function intact. The synthetic capacity for glutamate and aspartate is present in great excess; thus partial inhibition of the synthetic capacity could permit normal function yet restrict excessive activity. Effects on synaptic release can show selectivity, both for excitatory versus inhibitory amino acids and possibly also for specific excitatory transmitters. Antagonists acting post-synaptically have differential effects against different patterns of excitation and may indeed be capable of selectively antagonizing certain pathological patterns of activity. Data relating to these various possibilities will be discussed in detail below.

Table 1. Mechanisms for diminishing excitatory transmission

---

1. Decrease maximal rate of synthesis of glutamate,
   aspartate, cysteinesulfinic acid, etc.

2. Decrease synaptic release (selectively)
   a) Presynaptic receptors
        (i)   Autoreceptors for glutamate etc.
       (ii) $GABA_A$ or $GABA_B$ receptors.
      (iii)   Adenoside receptors.
   b) Action on Ca^{++} calmodulin-dependent protein kinase
      hydantoin, benzodiazepines (?).

3. Decrease post-synaptic action
   a) Selective antagonists
      N-methyl-D-aspartate antagonists
   b) Down-regulation of receptors (?).

INHIBITION OF SYNTHESIS

The metabolic pathways and the control mechanisms for
the synthesis of neurotransmitter glutamate and aspartate
are not adequately understood. Roles for glutaminase (Bradford, Ward 1976) and for asparaginase (Reubi et al. 1980)
have been proposed, but not proven. Immunocytochemical
evidence for enhanced glutaminase activity in some presumed
glutamatergic pathways (e.g. the hippocampal mossy fiber
path) but not in others (e.g. perforant path to granule and
pyramidal cell dendrites) has been presented by Wenthold
(this volume). Glutamate dehydrogenase and glutamate and
aspartate transaminases provide alternate routes of synthesis.

Control of the synthesis of cysteinesulfinic acid,
cysteic acid and homocysteic acid is also poorly understood.
Mapping of the selective neuronal localization of cysteine
deoxygenase and of cysteinesulfinate oxidase remains to be
accomplished.

Among anticonvulsant drugs used clinically, acetazola-
mide has been shown to inhibit phosphate-activated glutaminase (Beaton 1961). However the strongest evidence for an
action on the synthesis of excitatory amino acids concerns
sodium valproate (Chapman et al. 1982a). In acute

experiments in rodents, anticonvulsant doses of valproate decrease brain aspartate concentration, with a time course similar to that of the anticonvulsant action (Schechter et al. 1978). The decreases in brain aspartate have a wider regional distribution than do increases in brain GABA content (Chapman et al. 1982b; see also Fig. 1). Evaluation of anticonvulsant action and biochemical changes induced by various analogs of valproic acid shows a better correlation of anticonvulsant potencies with brain aspartate changes than with brain GABA changes (Chapman et al. 1983).

The mechanism by which valproate acts to reduce brain aspartate concentration is not known. One possibility is impaired CO_2 fixation leading to diminished oxaloacetate formation, brought about either by impaired pyruvate transport into mitochondria (Benavides et al. 1982) or by inhibition of pyruvate carboxylase activity (Turnbull et al. 1983).

Before any anticonvulsant action of valproate can be attributed to reduced aspartate synthesis, it will be necessary to demonstrate that the synaptic release of aspartate is decreased after valproate and/or that excitatory activity within an aspartergic pathway is decreased.

RELEASE OF EXCITATORY AMINO ACIDS

Synaptic release of neurotransmitters is regulated by receptors on the presynaptic terminal. These variously control the ionic permeability of the terminal membrane, the synthesis of the neurotransmitter and, more directly, the mechanism of release.

Receptors which respond to the neurotransmitter itself ('autoreceptors') are commonly pharmacologically slightly different from the corresponding post-synaptic receptors. Studies in hippocampal slices have provided evidence for functionally significant glutamate autoreceptors, sensitive to glutamate, cysteate and homocysteate, but not to kainate, N-methyl-D-aspartate or aspartate (McBean, Roberts 1981).

Rather diverse experiments suggest that GABA receptors can control excitatory amino acid release. Effects mediated by a bicuculline-sensitive, $GABA_A$ type receptor (Baba et al. 1983) and by a bicuculline insensitive, baclofen responsive, $GABA_B$ receptor have been described (Potashner 1979).

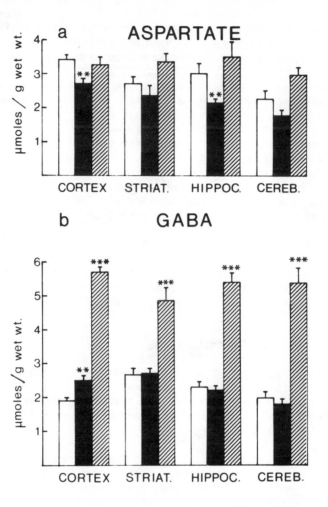

Fig. 1. Regional concentrations of aspartate and GABA in cortex, striatum, hippocampus and cerebellum from control rats (open bars) and rats given valproate, 400 mg/kg, i.p. (filled bars) or γ-vinyl-GABA, 1 g/kg, i.p. (hatched bars). Values are mean ± SEM, significance of differences from control **p < 0.01, ***p < 0.001. From Chapman et al. 1982.

In addition to baclofen, other central muscle relaxants decrease excitatory amino acid release. Tizanidine (DA 103-282) appears to have a highly selective action in the spinal cord, blocking polysynaptic excitation of the motoneuron (which depends on presumed aspartergic neurons, acting on N-methyl-D-aspartate sensitive receptors), but not monosynaptic excitation (which depends on primary afferents, possibly glutamatergic, acting on cis-2,3-piperidinedicarboxylic acid sensitive receptors (Davies, Watkins 1983). Thus the possibility of highly selective actions on neurotransmitter release merits consideration.

Reduction of excitatory neurotransmitter release is influenced by various endogenous compounds acting presynaptically, including proline and adenosine (Keller et al. 1981; Burnstock, Brown 1981). The effect of adenosine on presynaptic A-1 adenosine receptors is of physiological significance in the hippocampus (Dunwiddie 1980; Lee et al. 1983).

In in vitro studies using rat brain slices or 'mini-slices', several anticonvulsant drugs reduce the stimulated release of endogenous aspartate or of exogenous, isotopically-labelled compounds (^{3}H-D-aspartate, ^{3}H-glutamate or ^{14}C-cysteinesulfinic acid)(see Table 2).

Table 2. Reduction of K$^+$ stimulated excitatory amino acid release

	Conc. (μM)	Slice	Release of
Phenytoin (a)	25	Cortex (mini)	[^{3}H] D ASP
Phenobarbital (a)	100	Cortex (mini)	[^{3}H] D ASP
Pentobarbital (a)	1000	Cortex (mini)	[^{3}H] D ASP
Trimethadione (a)	100	Cortex (mini)	[^{3}H] D ASP
Diazepam (b)	10-100	Hippocamp.	[^{14}C] CSA
	10	Hippocamp.	[^{3}H] GLUT
Chlordiazepoxide (b)	100	Hippocamp.	[^{14}C] CSA
Chlordiazepoxide (c)	20	Olfactory Cortex	ASP

ASP = aspartate; CSA = cysteinesulfinic acid; GLUT - glutamate; (a) Skerrit, Johnston 1983; (b) Baba et al. 1983; (c) Collins 1981.

ANTAGONISTS OF POST-SYNAPTIC EXCITATORY RECEPTORS

Compounds that block excitation due to glutamate, aspartate and their analogs have been studied in vivo and in vitro (see Table 3).

Table 3. Test systems for excitatory amino acid antagonists

IN VITRO

Frog spinal cord - depolarization	Evans et al. 1982
Cultured mouse neurons - firing and membrane potential	MacDonald, Wojtowicz 1982
Brain slices - Na$^+$ release	Luini et al. 1981
Membrane potentials	Flatman et al. 1983

IN VIVO

Spinal cord motoneurons - firing	Peet et al. 1983
Caudate units - firing and membrane potentials	Herrling et al. 1983
Cerebral cortical units - firing	Perkins et al. 1981
	Birley et al. 1982

All test systems are broadly in accord that the receptors can be classified into three or four major types, according to their preferred agonist and the selective, or partially selective, actions of antagonists. Thus receptors preferentially activated by kainate, by quisqualate and by N-methyl-D-aspartate can be identified in all systems, and sometimes an additional 'glutamate preferring' receptor can be differentiated (Watkins, Evans 1981).

There is evidence not only that the receptor recognition sites differ in terms of agonist and antagonist effects, but also in terms of the associated ionophores. This difference is most decisive in the retina, where Type I and Type II bipolar cells receive presumably identical inputs (from the photoreceptors) but respond, respectively, with depolarization (due to opening of Na$^+$ channels) or hyperpolarization (due to closing of Na$^+$ channels). Glutamate may be the endogenous agonist; 2-amino-4-phosphonobutyric acid apparently acts as an agonist on the hyperpolarizing receptors (Slaughter, Miller 1981; Mitchell, Redburn 1982).

In spinal cord motoneurons, three patterns of action on membrane conductance, membrane potential and firing patterns have been described (Lambert et al. 1981). In this site, aspartate, glutamate and L-homocysteate all produce approximately the same response as quisqualate. N-Methyl-D-aspartate, ibotenate and D-homocysteate characteristically decrease membrane conductance (Engberg et al. 1983).

In caudate neurons in the cat, quisqualate and glutamate depolarize the membrane and increase firing rate, whereas N-methyl-D-aspartate and quinolinic acid induce, in two-thirds of the cells tested, a distinctive large plateau depolarization associated with a very rapid burst of firing (up to 100 Hz)(Herrling et al. 1983). The effect of aspartate is intermediate, sometimes resembling glutamate and sometimes reproducing the effect of N-methyl-D-aspartate. In cortical neurons in vitro, a similar pattern of depolarization and burst firing is induced by N-methyl-D-aspartate and aspartate and is shown to depend on an anomalous current-voltage relationship with a region of negative slope conductance (Flatman et al. 1983; MacDonald et al. 1982).

These specific effects of activation of the N-methyl-D-aspartate receptors are of immediate interest because they closely resemble the pattern of paroxysmal depolarization shift (in membrane potential) and burst firing that are characteristic of epileptic neurons in a focus and of normal units in hippocampus or cortex during a seizure discharge (Schwartzkroin, Wyler 1980).

Antagonists at the Post-synaptic Receptor

Table 4 presents some of the most potent of the antagonists currently available and indicates their selectivity in terms of receptor subtypes, evaluated in the spinal cord. Comparison of various studies suggests that there may be significant variation in the selectivity of antagonists according to the brain region studied, but systematic comparisons have not been reported.

It is evident that we have available potent and highly selective antagonists at the N-methyl-D-aspartate receptor (e.g. 2-amino-5-phosphonovaleric and 2-amino-7-phosphonoheptanoic acids). However, antagonists acting at the quisqualate or kainate receptors show less selectivity and potency.

Table 4. Antagonists of dicarboxylic amino acids:
potency against preferred agonists on the spinal cord

Antagonist	Potency against		
	N-Methyl-D aspartate	Kainate	Quisqualate
cis-2,3-piperidine-dicarboxylic acid	+++	+++	++
γ-D-glutamyl glycine	++++	+++	+
β-D-aspartyl-β-alanine	++++	+++	0
D-α-aminoadipate	+++	+	0
2-amino-4 phosphono-butyrate	0	++	0
2-amino-5-phosphono-valerate	++++	(+)	0
2-amino-7-phosphono-heptanoic acid	++++	(+)	0
Glutamic acid diethyl ester	0	0	++

From Peet et al. 1983; Watkins, Evans 1981.

ANTICONVULSANT ACTIONS OF EXCITATORY AMINO ACID ANTAGONISTS

Intracerebroventricular Injections in DBA/2 Mice

We have tested the anticonvulsant potency of a wide
range of antagonists by intracerebroventricular injection in
DBA/2 mice (Croucher et al. 1982). This inbred strain, at a
critical age range (18-23 days), responds to a loud sound
with a sequence of epileptic events (wild running, followed
by clonic jerking, tonic flexion and extension, and finally
respiratory arrest). It provides a convenient model for the
quantitative evaluation of drug effects on seizure threshold
(Chapman et al. 1984). Within the limitations provided by
water solubility and the volume of the injection (10 μl),
several antagonists were found to be inactive (e.g. glutamic
acid diethyl ester, D-α-aminoadipic acid, 2-amino-4-phosphon-
obutyric acid). However, all agents that are potent antagonists at the N-methyl-D-aspartate receptor produce significant anticonvulsant effects (see Table 5). Increasing the
dose of antagonist progressively decreases the incidence of

Table 5. Protection by intracerebroventricular injection of antagonists of excitation due to NMDA (and of diazepam and valproate) against the clonic seizure phase induced by sound stimulation in DBA/2 mice.

Antagonist	ED_{50} μmole
γ-D-glutamyl glycine	0.046
2-amino-5-phosphonopentanoic acid	0.022
2-amino-6-phosphonohexanoic acid	0.14
2-amino-7-phosphonoheptanoic acid	0.0018
cis-2,3-piperidinedicarboxylic acid	0.017
diazepam	0.011
valproate	6.00

From Croucher et al. 1982 and unpublished data; Chapman et al. 1984.

the later seizure phases until the response is totally abolished. By this route 2-amino-7-phosphonoheptanoic acid is as potent as the benzodiazepines, which are the most potent conventional anticonvulsants.

Anticonvulsant Actions by Systemic Administration

Intraperitoneal injection of the more potent antagonists (2-amino-7-phosphonoheptanoic acid, 2-amino-5-phosphonovaleric acid, and cis-2,3-piperidinedicarboxylic acid) also produces an anticonvulsant effect in DBA/2 mice (Meldrum et al. 1983a,b; and unpublished data), but the doses required are higher than for the anticonvulsant action of benzodiazepines.

2-Amino-7-phosphonoheptanoic acid administered intraperitoneally is also active against a variety of chemically-induced seizures (Cruczwar, Meldrum 1982)(see Table 6). Not surprisingly, it is active against seizures induced by N-methyl-D-aspartate, but not those induced by kainic acid.

There is anticonvulsant action against some agents generally considered to have a primary action on GABAergic transmission (e.g. 3-mercaptopropionic acid, thiosemicarbazide, picrotoxin and methyl 6,7-dimethoxy-4-ethyl-β-carboline carboxylate (DMCM). However, using in vitro preparations, these convulsants have been shown to enhance the stimulated

Table 6. Anticonvulsant action of 2-amino-7-phosphonoheptanoic acid (0.33 mmol/kg) against chemically-induced convulsions in Swiss S mice (from Czuczwar, Meldrum 1982)

| Convulsant | ED_{50} (mmol/kg, i.p.) for clonic convulsions | |
	Control	After 2 APH
N-Methyl-D,L-aspartate	1.38	2.32[++]
Kainic acid	0.38	0.35
3-Mercaptopropionic acid	0.33	0.48[+]
Thiosemicarbazide	0.11	0.28[++]
Bicuculline	0.012	0.013
Picrotoxin	0.0087	0.0156[++]
Methyl 6,7-dimethoxy-4-ethyl-β-carboline carboxylate	0.035	0.23[+++]

Significance of difference [+]$p<0.05$; [++]$p<0.01$; [+++]$p<0.001$.

release of endogenous or exogenous dicarboxylic acids (Kerwin, Meldrum 1983; Skerritt, Johnston 1983; Collins 1981). Thus release of excitatory amino acids acting on a 2-amino-7-phosphonoheptanoic acid sensitive receptor site appears to play a role in the development of seizures following administration of numerous agents acting on the GABA-benzodiazepine receptor complex.

Exposure to progressively increasing atmospheric pressure induces the 'high pressure neurological syndrome' characterized by tremors, myoclonus and convulsions (Halsey 1982). In rats, pretreatment with 2-amino-7-phosphonoheptanoic acid, or with cis-2,3-piperidinedicarboxylic acid, significantly delays the onset of tremor, myoclonus and convulsions (Meldrum et al. 1983a; Angel et al. 1983).

The animal model of epilepsy that corresponds most closely, in terms of neurophysiology and of responsiveness to anticonvulsant drugs, to syndromes of epilepsy in man is photically-induced epilepsy in the Senegalese baboon, Papio papio (Naquet, Meldrum 1972; Meldrum 1978). Given intravenously, 2-amino-7-phosphonoheptanoic acid (1 mmol/kg) completely abolishes myoclonic responses to photic stimulation for more than 5 h (Meldrum et al. 1983c). Cis-2,3-piperidinedicarboxylic acid and 2-amino-5-phosphonovaleric acid are somewhat less potent as anticonvulsants.

In summary, antagonists of excitation induced at the N-methyl-D-aspartate preferring receptor are potent anticonvulsants in a wide variety of animal test systems. Their activity by the systemic route of administration is not as great as would be predicted on the basis of their potency when administered intracerebroventricularly. This suggests that they suffer a pharmacokinetic disadvantage, most probably due to poor penetration of the blood-brain barrier.

ENTRY OF 2-AMINO-7-PHOSPHONOHEPTANOIC ACID INTO BRAIN

We have studied the entry of 2-amino-7-phosphonoheptanoic acid into mouse brain, following the intraperitoneal injection of 2-amino-7-phosphono[4,5-^{3}H]heptanoic acid (Chapman et al. 1983). Using HPLC analysis of dansylated brain extracts, the original labelled compound can be identified in the brain. The time course of its accumulation corresponds to the time course of its anticonvulsant action. The concentration in the brain is in the range 0.1-1.0 μM, which concentration is sufficient to antagonize excitatory effects of dicarboxylic amino acids in the in vitro frog spinal cord (Evans et al. 1982).

ACTIONS OF 2-AMINO-7-PHOSPHONOHEPTANOIC ACID ON REGIONAL BRAIN AMINO ACID CONTENT

We have studied the effect of a maximal anticonvulsant dose of 2-amino-7-phosphonoheptanoic acid (1 mmol/kg, i.p.) on regional brain amino acid content in rats and mice. Because hypoglycemia modifies brain glutamate and aspartate concentrations, we have studied fed and fasted animals and measured brain glucose content (Westerberg et al. 1983).

Glucose concentration falls by 25-30% in cortex and cerebellum of fasted mice and rats. Administration of 2-amino-7-phosphonoheptanoic acid does not change glucose in fed animals or alter the lowered content in fasted rats, but it restores glucose content to normal in fasted mice. Aspartate content tended to be increased in fasted animals.

In fed animals 2-amino-7-phosphonoheptanoic acid did not produce any changes in amino acid content that were consistent between species and brain regions (although there was a significant fall in aspartate content in mouse cortex).

In fasted animals a consistent pattern of changes was produced (see Fig. 2). Reductions in aspartate content were marked in the cerebellum, striatum and hippocampus. Proportionally smaller decreases in glutamate content occurred in the same regions. Glutamine content was increased, particularly in the striatum. GABA content tended to decrease. Taurine content showed no change.

These changes can be interpreted in terms of blockade of a post-synaptic receptor by 2-amino-7-phosphonoheptanoic acid and a compensatory increase in the synaptic release of the endogenous neurotransmitter (which would appear to be predominatly aspartate, with glutamate acting also as a transmitter in particular regions or under the special circumstances of postsynaptic blockade). In the presence of an inadequate precursor supply, this increased turnover leads to a fall in concentration of aspartate and glutamate. The increase in glutamine content is consistent with an increased turnover of glutamate, and the fall in GABA content could result from decreased glutamate levels. However, in the absence of direct evidence of the effects of 2-amino-7-phosphonoheptanoic acid on the relevant transaminases and decarboxylases, direct metabolic effects cannot be excluded.

SUMMARY

We have shown that antagonists of excitation due to dicarboxylic amino acids possess potent anticonvulsant activity in a wide range of animal models of epilepsy. This is most clearly seen with antagonists which act at sites preferentially responding to N-methyl-D-aspartate. The endogenous neurotransmitter acting at this site is not definitively known, but could be aspartate or a compound metabolically close to aspartate. Electrophysiological studies also suggest that this neurotransmitter receptor system may be particularly important in the abnormal discharges of epilepsy.

These findings emphasize the possible importance of changes in excitatory amino acid metabolism or transmitter action in the anticonvulsant action of known anticonvulsant drugs, and encourage the search for new anticonvulsant drugs in the direction of compounds that modify activity in these systems.

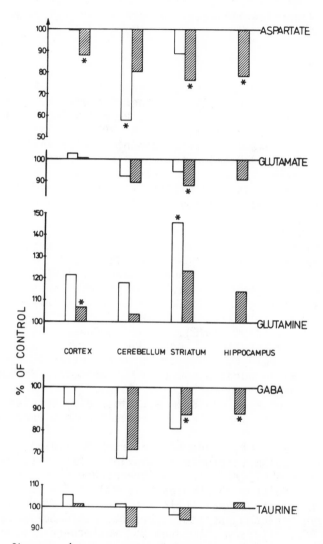

Fig. 2. Changes (as percent of fasted control) in regional aspartate, glutamate, glutamine, GABA and taurine concentrations 45 min after 2-amino-7-phosphonoheptanoic acid (1 mmol/kg) injected intraperitoneally in fasted mice (open bars) or rats (cross-hatched bars). (Mouse hippocampus not analyzed). *p<0.05 comparison with control (From Westerberg et al. 1983).

ACKNOWLEDGEMENT

We thank the Medical Research Council (U.K.) and the Wellcome Trust for financial support.

REFERENCES

Angel A, Halsey MJ, Little H, Meldrum BS, Ross JAS, Rostain J-C, Wardley-Smith B (1983). Specific effects of drugs at pressure: animal investigations. Proc Roy Soc B (in press).

Baba A, Okumura S, Mizuo H, Iwata H (1983). Inhibition by diazepam and γ-aminobutyric acid of depolarization-induced release of [^{14}C]cysteine sulfinate and [^{3}H]glutamate in rat hippocampus slices. J Neurochem 40:280.

Beaton T (1961). The inhibition by acetazoleamide of renal phosphate-activated glutaminase in rats. Can J Biochem Physiol 39:663.

Benavides J, Martin A, Ugarte M, Valdivieso F (1982). Inhibition by valproic acid of pyruvate uptake by brain mitochondria. Biochem Pharmacol 31:1633.

Birley S, Collins JF, Perkins MN, Stone TW (1982). The effects of cyclic dicarboxylic amino acids on spontaneous and amino acid-evoked activity of rat cortical neurones. Brit J Pharmacol 77:7.

Bradford HF, Ward HK (1976). On glutaminase activity in mammalian synaptosomes. Brain Res 110:115.

Burnstock G, Brown CM (1981). An introduction to purinergic receptors. In Burnstock G (ed): "Purinergic Receptors," London: Chapman and Hall Ltd, p 1.

Chapman AG, Keane PE, Meldrum BS, Simiand J, Vernieres JC (1982a). Mechanism of action of valproate. Prog Neurobiol 19:315.

Chapman AG, Riley K, Evans MC, Meldrum BS (1982b). Acute effects of sodium valproate and γ-vinyl GABA on regional amino acid metabolism in the rat brain. Neurochem Res 7:1089.

Chapman AG, Meldrum BS, Mendes E (1983). Acute anticonvulsant activity of structural analogs of valproic acid and changes in brain GABA and aspartate content. Life Sci 32:2023.

Chapman AG, Collins JF, Meldrum BS, Westerberg E (1983). Uptake of a novel anticonvulsant compound, 2-amino-7-phosphonoheptanoic [4,5-^{3}H] acid into mouse brain. Neurosci Lett 37:75.

Chapman AG, Croucher MJ, Meldrum BS (1984). Evaluation of anticonvulsant drugs in DBA/2 mice with sound-induced seizures. Arzneimit Forschung (in press).

Collins GGS (1981). The effects of chlordiazepoxide on synaptic transmission and amino acid neurotransmitter release in slices of rat olfactory cortex. Brain Res 224:389.

Croucher MJ, Collins JF, Meldrum BS (1982). Anticonvulsant action of excitatory amino acid antagonists. Science 216:899.

Curtis DR, Johnston GAR (1974). Amino acid transmitters in the mammalian central nervous system. Ergeb Physiol Biol Chem Exp Pharmacol 69:97.

Cruczwar SJ, Meldrum B (1982). Protection against chemically induced seizures by 2-amino-7-phosphonoheptanoic acid. Eur J Pharmacol 83:335.

Davies J, Watkins JC (1983). Role of excitatory amino acid receptors in mono- and polysynaptic excitation in the cat spinal cord. Exp Brain Res 49:280.

Dunwiddie TV (1980). Endogenously released adenosine regulates excitability in the in vitro hippocampus. Epilepsia 21:541.

Engberg I, Flatman JA, Lambert JDC, Lindsay A (1983). An analysis of bioelectrical phenomena evoked by microiontophoretically applied excitotoxic amino-acids in the feline spinal cord. In Fuxe K, Roberts PJ, Schwarcz R (eds): "Neurotoxic Effects of Excitatory Amino Acids," Pergammon Press.

Evans RH, Francis AA, Jones AW, Smith DAS, Watkins JC (1982) The effects of a series of ω-phosphonic α-carboxylic amino acids on electrically evoked and excitant amino acid-induced responses in isolated spinal cord preparations. Brit J Pharmacol 75:65.

Flatman JA, Schwindt PC, Crill WE, Stafstrom CE (1983). Multiple actions of N-methyl-D-aspartate on cat neocortical neurons in vitro. Brain Res 266:169.

Halsey MJ (1982). Effects of high pressure on the central nervous system. Phys Rev 62:1342.

Herrling PL, Morris R, Salt TE (1983). Effects of excitatory amino acids and their antagonists on membrane and action potentials of cat caudate neurones. J Physiol 339:207.

Keller E, Davis JL, Tachiki KH, Cummins JT, Baxter C (1981).. L-Proline inhibition of glutamate release. J Neurochem 37:1335.

Kerwin RW, Meldrum BS (1983). Effect on cerebral ^{3}H-D-aspartate release of 3-mercaptopropionic acid and methyl 6,7-dimethoxy-4-ethyl-β-carboline-3-carboxylate. Eur J Pharmacol 89:265.

Lambert JDC, Flatman JA, Engberg I (1981). Actions of

excitatory amino acids on membrane conductance and potential in motoneurones. In Di Chiara G, Gessa GL (eds): "Glutamate as a Neurotransmitter," N. Y.: Raven Press, p 205.

Lee KS, Schubert P, Reddington M, Kreutzberg GW (1983). Adenosine receptor density and the depression of evoked neuronal activity in the rat hippocampus in vitro. Neurosci Lett 37:81.

Luini A, Goldberg O, Teichberg VI (1981). Distinct pharmacological properties of excitatory amino acid receptors in the rat striatum: A study by a Na$^+$ efflux assay. Proc Natl Acad Sci 78:3250.

McBean GJ, Roberts PJ (1981). Glutamate-preferring receptors regulate the release of D-^{3}H-aspartate from rat hippocampal slices. Nature 291:593.

MacDonald JF, Wojtowicz JM (1982). The effects of L-glutamate and its analogue upon the membrane conductance of central murine neurones in culture. Can J Physiol Pharmacol 60:282.

MacDonald JF, Porietis AV, Wojtowicz JM (1982). L-Aspartic acid induces a region of negative slope conductance in the current-voltage relationship of cultured spinal cord neurons. Brain Res 237:248.

Meldrum BS (1978). Photosensitive epilepsy in Papio papio as a model for drug studies. In Cobb WA, Van Duijn H (eds): "Contemp Clin Neurophys," Suppl 34: "Electroenceph Clin Neurophysiol," Amsterdam: Elsevier Scientific Publishing Co., p 317.

Meldrum B (1981). Epilepsy. In Davison AN, Thompson RHS (eds): "The Molecular Basis of Neuropathology," London: Edward Arnold Ltd, p 265.

Meldrum BS (1983). Pharmacological considerations in the search for new anticonvulsant drugs. In Pedley TA, Meldrum BS (eds): "Recent Advances in Epilepsy," Vol. I. London: Churchill Livingstone.

Meldrum BS (1984). GABA and other amino acids. In Frey HH, Janz D (eds): "Handbook of Experimental Pharmacology. Antiepileptic Drugs," Berlin: (in press).

Meldrum B, Wardley-Smith B, Halsey H, Rostain J-C (1983a). 2-Amino-7-phosphonoheptanoic acid protects against the high pressure neurological syndrome. Eur J Pharmacol 87:501.

Meldrum BS, Croucher MJ, Czuczwar SJ, Collins JF, Curry K, Joseph M, Stone TW (1983b). A comparison of the anticonvulsant potency of (±) 2-amino-5-phosphonoheptanoic acid and (±) 2-amino-7-phosphonoheptanoic acid. Neuroscience (in press).

Meldrum BS, Croucher MJ, Badman G, Collins JF (1983c). Anti-epileptic action of excitatory amino acid antagonists in the photosensitive baboon, Papio papio. Neurosci Lett (in press).

Mitchell CK, Redburn DA (1982). 2-Amino-4-phosphonobutyric acid and N-methyl-D-aspartate differentiate between ^3H glutamate and ^3H aspartate binding sites in bovine retina. Neurosci Lett 28:241.

Naquet R, Meldrum BS (1972). Photogenic seizures in baboons In Purpura D, Penry JK, Tower DB, Woodbury DB, Walter RD (eds): "Experimental Models of Epilepsy," New York: Raven Press, p 373.

Peet MJ, Leah JD, Curtis D (1983). Antagonists of synaptic and amino acid excitation of neurones in the cat spinal cord. Brain Res 266:83.

Perkins MN, Stone TW, Collins JF, Curry K (1981). Phosphon-oate analogues of carboxylic acids as amino acid antagon-ists on rat cortical neurones. Neurosci Lett 23:333.

Potashner SJ (1979). Baclofen: Effects on amino acid release in slices of guinea pig cerebral cortex. J Neurochem 32:103.

Reubi JC, Toggenburger G, Cuenod M (1980). Asparagine as precursor for transmitter aspartate in corticostriatal fibres. J Neurochem 35:1015.

Schechter PJ, Tranier Y, Grove J (1978). Effect of n-dipro-pylacetate on amino acid concentrations in mouse brain: correlations with anticonvulsant activity. J Neurochem 31:1325.

Schwartzkroin PA, Wyler AR (1980). Mechanisms underlying epileptiform burst discharge. Ann Neurol 7:95.

Skerritt JH, Johnston GAR (1983). Modulation of excitant amino acid release by convulsant and anticonvulsant drugs. In Fariello RG (ed): "Neurotransmitters, Seizures and Epilepsy," II. New York: Raven Press.

Slaughter MM, Miller RF (1981). 2-Amino-4-phosphonobutyric acid: a new pharmacological tool for retina research. Science 211:182.

Turnbull DM, Bone AJ, Bartlett K, Koundakjian PP, Sherratt HSA (1983). The effects of valproate on intermediary metabolism in isolated rat hepatocytes and intact rats.

Watkins JC, Evans RH (1981). Excitatory amino acid trans-mitters. Ann Rev Pharmacol Toxicol 21:165.

Westerberg E, Chapman AG, Meldrum BS (1983). The effect of 2-amino-7-phosphonoheptanoic acid on regional brain amino acid levels in fed and fasted rodents. J Neurochem (in press).

**Glutamine, Glutamate, and GABA
in the Central Nervous System, pages 643–652
© 1983 Alan R. Liss, Inc., 150 Fifth Avenue, New York, NY 10011**

TRANSMITTER AMINO ACIDS AND THEIR ANTAGONISTS IN EPILEPSY

D.W. Peterson, J.F. Collins* and H.F. Bradford

Department of Biochemistry, Imperial College,
London SW7 2AZ, United Kingdom; *Department of
Chemistry, City of London Polytechnic, Jewry
Street, London EC1, United Kingdom.

Considerable interest continues to be attached to the
possible involvement of amino acid neurotransmitters in the
basic mechanisms of epilepsy. The principal compounds
concerned are glutamate, aspartate and GABA (Bradford, Dodd
1975; Van Gelder 1981). These three substances are present
in the brain at very high concentrations (2-10 mM) compared
with other neurotransmitters due to their involvement in
mainstream metabolism as well as in neurotransmission.

GABA is a major inhibitory transmitter and failure in
its synthesis, or the loss of inhibitory interneurons which
release GABA, would lead to an imbalance in favour of excitatory transmission. This is easily simulated by applying
agents which reduce the activity of glutamate decarboxylase,
the pyridoxal-phosphate-dependent enzyme synthesizing GABA
(Bradford, Dodd 1975). Thus, as might be expected, antipyri-
doxal agents (e.g. thiosemicarbazide, hydrazides) are potent
convulsant agents. Raising brain GABA levels (usually by
blocking its breakdown via the GABA transaminase pathway)
causes an imbalance in favour of inhibition, and drugs which
have this action tend to be anticonvulsants (e.g. sodium dipropylacetate; γ-vinyl-GABA). Glutamate and aspartate, on
the other hand, are excitatory neurotransmitters. Increased
release or contact between these compounds and their receptors will lead to lowered thresholds for hyperactivity. When
injected intracerebrally or systematically (Bradford, Dodd
1977) these agents cause convulsion. Equally, a reduced
ability of brain tissue to remove extracellular or synaptic
accumulations of these substances by the usual process of
high affinity transport could be expected to lead to hyper-

activity or convulsions (Bradford, Dodd 1975; Van Gelder 1981). In addition, excitatory pathways employing glutamate or aspartate might well be involved in the spread of epileptic hyperactivity from one brain region to another.

Studies of Glutamate Release

Our own group (Fig. 1) (Bradford, Dodd 1977) and others (Fig. 2) (Coutinho-Netto et al. 1981) have shown a close

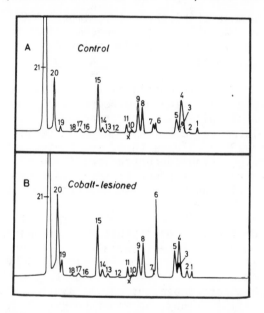

Fig. 1. Patterns of amino acid release. Representative chromatograms of samples from a control animal (A) and a cobalt-lesioned animal (B), both collected at the same post-operation time (day 4, midnight to 04.00 h BST) are shown. Amino acids: 1, methionine sulfoxide; 2, aspartate; 3, threonine; 4, glutamine; 5, serine; 6, glutamate; 7, citrulline;; 8, glycine; 9, alanine; 10, cysteine; X, unknown; 11, valine 12, methionine; 13, isoleucine; 14, leucine; 15, norleucine (added as internal standard); 16, tyrosine; 17, phenylalanine; 18, GABA; 19, histidine; 20, possibly some lysine, al-, though this peak occurs in the input solution (not used); 21 ammonia (most of which comes from the sample purifier). In this particular case, both animals were being superfused from the same supply of artificial CSF (from Dodd, Bradford 1976).

parallelism between an enhanced release of glutamate from various experimental epileptic foci and the onset of epileptic hyperactivity (Bradford, Dodd 1975,1977; Koyama 1972; Dodd et al. 1980). Decreases in tissue glutamate in excised epileptic focal tissue have also been demonstrated (Van Gelder 1981; Bradford, Dodd 1975). It does not seem likely that the observed glutamate release is due to tissue damage or degeneration, since equivalent lesions produced in cerebral cortex by nickel implants caused neither the equivalent levels of glutamate release, nor the epileptic conditions (Fig. 3) (Dodd et al. 1980). In fact cobalt is almost unique

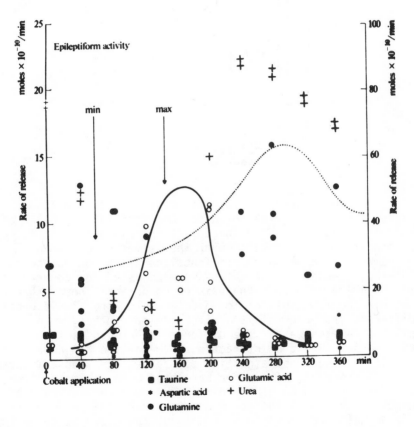

Fig. 2. Glutamate release from cobalt-focus in vivo ---- glutamate patterns; .... glutamine pattern (adapted from Koyama 1972).

among metals in causing this epileptic condition. In animals
with cobalt-implants that did not develop epilepsy, the lower
level of glutamate release was seen, similar in extent to
that in inactive nickel-implants (Fig. 3) (Dodd et al. 1980).

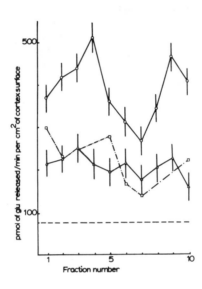

Fig. 3. Time-course of glutamate release from cobalt and
nickel foci. Both types of disc were used in each batch of
animals implanted. When the cobalt animals were active,
each animal was cannulated over the lesion site. Amino
acids were assayed in 20 min fractions using norleucine as
internal standard. The values were adjusted for covariance
with alanine release. Analysis of covariance showed that
overall the two types of lesioned animals were significantly
different from controls and also from each other, with
p<0.001 in each case. The differences between different
time periods and the interaction between time period and
animal type were not significant. Values are means of three
experiments each. The error bars have been estimated from
the calculated S.E. of the difference between each pair of
experimental means and are meant to serve as a guide only.
The animals were conscious throughout the superfusion period.
0, cobalt; Δ, nickel; --, average rate from unlesioned
tissue. Also shown (□) is a single experiment where an
inactive Co focus was superfused (from Dodd et al. 1980).

An exaggerated release of glutamate was also seen to parallel epileptiform activity in chronically denervated cerebral cortex produced by undercutting. Stimulation of the undercut cortex produces an epileptiform discharge which is accompanied by a 3-fold increase in glutamate release compared with the response of control intact cortex (Koyama, Jasper 1977).

Where there is a decrease in the tissue content of glutamate, aspartate and GABA in cobalt-induced epilepsy, there seems to be a close correlation between the extent of these changes and the severity of the epilepsy (Van Gelder, Coutois 1972). Such decreases have been detected in a wide range of experimental epilepsies (Bradford, Dodd 1975) and in spontaneous epilepsy in cats (Koyama 1978). Falls in aspartate and GABA levels could well be the result of loss of glutamate from the tissue.

Thus, a great deal of circumstantial and direct evidence exists for a release of glutamate from epileptogenic tissue which occurs in close parallelism with the onset of epileptic hyperactivity. However, whether these two events stand in a cause or effect relationship cannot easily be determined.

The Use of Amino Acid Receptor Antagonists

More recently, however, a causal connection between the release of excitatory amino acids and the onset of the hyperactivity has been indicated by the use of specific receptor antagonists of α-amino dicarboxylic amino acids (ω-substituted phosphono-derivatives of α-amino carboxylic acids, C_4 to C_7; Watkins, Evans 1981). Thus α-amino-4-phosphonobutyrate (APB) and α-amino-5-phosphonovalerate (APV), superfused in the concentration range 0.5 to 1.0 mM, effectively blocked contralateral forepaw myoclonic limb jerks and epileptiform EEG in cobalt-induced epilepsy in rats (Fig. 4) (Coutinho- Netto et al. 1981), whilst APV and α-amino-7-phosphonoheptanoate (APH) have been shown to block both audiogenic epilepsy and chemically induced seizures in mice (Croucher et al. 1982; Czuczwar, Meldrum 1982). Among the phosphono compounds tested so far in these various animals, the most potent agent is APH.

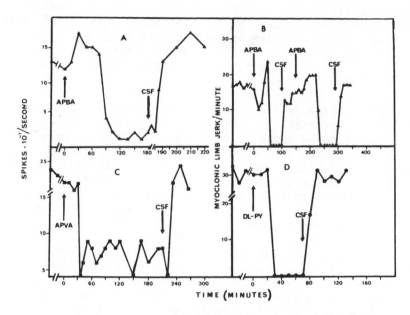

Fig. 4. Effect of glutamate antagonists on cobalt-induced epilepsy in the rat sensorimotor cortex. A.B: The effects of α-amino-4-phosphonobutyrate (APBA), 0.55 mM, administered directly onto epileptic focus via the superfusion cannula on the frequency of forelimb myoclonic jerks (B, Koyama 1978) and number of epileptic spikes (A) counted from the electro-corticograms. C: The action of α-amino-5-phosphonovalerate (APVA), 1.0 mM, on the frequency of epileptic spikes. D: The action of Dl-pyroglutamic acid (DL-PY), 0.775 mM, on the contralateral myoclonic limb-jerk frequency. Each point represents the mean value for at least 2 different animals. The total number of animals tested was as follows: APBA, 12; APVA, 3; DL-PY, 4 (from Coutinho-Netto et al. 1981).

The Kindling Model of Epilepsy

We have now tested these drugs on the "kindling-model" of epilepsy, the animals being rats with kindled amygdala (Peterson et al. 1983). In this case APH, APV and APB were superfused into the ipsilateral lateral ventricle of fully kindled rats. In these animals stimulation (250-350 μA) caused stage 5 seizures (full bilateral tonic-clonic seiz-

ures) and after-discharges of about 100 sec (Fig. 5). All
of these amino acid receptor blockers showed anticonvulsant
properties in this sequence of descending potency (ie. APH>
APV> APB; Table 1). Superfusion was for 45 min prior to
stimulation using 1 mM or 3 mM solutions of the drug as
appropriate. This could be shown to deliver a total dose of
0.5 or 1.5 µmole per animal. In the case of APH and APV,
the lower dose entirely prevented the seizures evoked by
electrical stimulation of the amygdala in some rats (Table
1). In these cases there were signs of hypoactivity and
incoordination in the rats. On the other hand, APB, which
reduced the after-discharge time, did not cause these
locomotor effects or prevent the onset of stage 5 seizures
at the concentrations tested (3 mM; dose 1.5 µmole per
animal).

Table 1. Antagonism of amygdaloid kindled seizures by
amino acid antagonists

Treatment µmoles total	Seizure stage 1 - 5*	After discharge % predrug	No.showing diminished response[+]	No. totally blocked
APB 0.5	4.7	95 ± 3	1/3	0/3
APB 1.5	5.0	74 ± 8**	2/3	0/3
APV 0.5	2.4**	42 ± 15**	6/7	3/7
APH 0.5	1.9**	28 ± 13**	6/7	3/7

For identification of receptor antagonists see text.
+ After discharge <75% of control.
* Racine scale (from Racine 1972).
** Student t-test $p<0.05$.
The afterdischarge was recorded in the amygdala. Values are
mean ± SEM for the numbers of animals shown (from
Peterson et al. 1983).

Thus, while both APB and APV effectively diminished
both myoclonic limb jerks and epileptiform EEG in the cobalt
model, APB did not prevent the kindled seizures in kindled
rats, but did reduce afterdischarge time recorded in the
amygdala and representing the hyperactive stage in this
brain region.

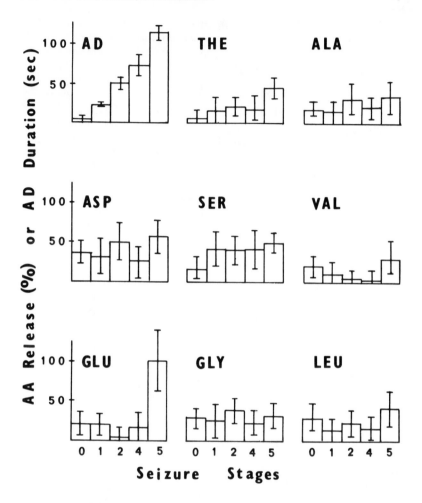

Fig. 5. Increased after-discharge duration (upper left) and release of amino acids into lateral ventricular perfusates with increasing stages of kindled amygdala seizures. The amino acid contents of samples collected during stimulation of the amygdala and in the 5 min after the stimulation were averaged and presented as the mean ± SEM percent increase above the levels in the sample preceding the stimulus. N=6. Most rats did not exhibit stage 3 seizures so no data are presented for this stage.

Abbreviations used: AD=afterdischarge; ASP=aspartate; GLU=glutamate; THE=threonine, SER=serine; GLY=glycine; ALA=alanine; VAL=valine; LEU=leucine (from Peterson et al. 1983)

Studies on the release of nine amino acids to the ventricular fluid on the ipsilateral side during the kindling process (Peterson et al. 1983) showed that only glutamate was significantly changed. In these experiments the lateral ventricles of rats were perfused with saline containing $CaCl_2$ and 5 min samples of perfusate collected. The amygdala was electrically stimulated and the after-discharge recorded on an EEG. When ventricular levels of glutamate at the pre-kindling stage (stage 0, before after-discharge duration was augmented) were compared with those found after a stage 5 seizure, the latter were found significantly increased by 79% (Fig. 5). Aspartate showed a 19% increase in level but this was not significant.

In summary, these results show a correlation which can be interpreted as indicating a causal role for excitatory dicarboxylic amino acids in the kindling process. Thus, glutamate shows a sharp increase in the amount released on stimulation as kindling progresses in severity from stage 4 to stage 5 and tonic-clonic convulsions appear. Aspartate, in contrast, shows lower but still elevated rates of release throughout (Fig. 5). At the same time, these specific blockers of dicarboxylic amino acid receptors (Watkins, Evans 1981) will prevent the seizures and either eliminate or reduce the associated increase in after-discharge duration.

Whether glutamate, aspartate or both are the excitatory agents cannot be unequivocally determined by these results. However, glutamate shows the most significantly enhanced release, both in these experiments on the kindling model of epilepsy, and in previous work on the cobalt-model (Bradford, Dodd 1975; Van Gelder 1981; Koyama 1972; Dodd, Bradford 1976; Dodd et al. 1980).

REFERENCES

Bradford HF, Dodd PR (1975). Biochemistry and Basic Mechanisms in Epilepsy. In Davison AN (ed): "Biochemistry and Neurological Disease", Oxford: Blackwells, Ch. 3.

Bradford HF, Dodd PR (1977). Convulsions and activation of epileptic foci induced by monosodium glutamate and related compounds. Biochem Pharmacol 26:253.

Coutinho-Netto JC, Abdul-Ghani AS, Collins JF, Bradford HF (1981). Is glutamate a trigger factor in epileptic hyperactivity? Epilepsia 22:289.

Croucher MJ, Collins JF, Meldrum BS (1982). Anticonvulsant action of excitatory amino acid antagonists. Science 216: 899.

Cruczwar SJ, Meldrum BS (1982). Protection against chemically-induced seizures by 2-amino-7-phosphonoheptanoic acid. Eur J Pharmacol 83:335.

Dodd PR, Bradford HF (1976). Release of amino acids from the maturing cobalt-induced epileptic focus. Brain Res 111:377.

Dodd PR, Bradford HF, Abdul-Ghani AS, Cox DWG, Coutinho-Netto J (1980). Release of amino acids from chronic epileptic and sub-epileptic foci in vivo. Brain Res 193:505.

Koyama I (1972). Amino acids in the cobalt-induced epileptogenic and non-epileptogenic cat's cortex. Can J Physiol Pharmacol 50:740.

Koyama I, Jasper H (1977). Amino acid content of chronic undercut cortex of the cat in relation to electrical afterdischarge: comparison with cobalt epileptogenic lesions. Can J Physiol Pharmacol 55:523.

Peterson DW, Collins JF, Bradford HF (1983). The kindled amygdala model of epilepsy: anticonvulsant action of amino acid antagonists. Brain Res (in press).

Racine R (1972). Modification of seizure activity by electrical stimulation. II Motor seizure. Electroenceph Clin Neurophysiol 32:281.

Van Gelder NM (1981). A role of taurine and glutamic acid in the epileptic process: a genetic predisposition. Rev Pure Appl Pharmacol Sci 2:293.

Van Gelder NM, Courtois A (1972). Close correlation between changing content of specific amino acids in epileptogenic cortex of cats and severity of epilepsy. Brain Res 43: 477.

Watkins JC, Evans RH (1981). Excitatory amino acid transmitter. Ann Rev Pharmacol Toxicol 21:165.

Glutamine, Glutamate, and GABA
in the Central Nervous System, pages 653–667
© 1983 Alan R. Liss, Inc., 150 Fifth Avenue, New York, NY 10011

THE EFFECTS OF ANESTHETIC AGENTS ON GABA METABOLISM IN RAT BRAIN SYNAPTOSOMES

Sze-Chuh Cheng and Edward A. Brunner

Department of Anesthesia
Northwestern University Medical School
Chicago, Illinois 60611

We have proposed a neurochemical mechanism for the action of anesthetic agents based on potentiation of GABA inhibition (Cheng, Brunner in press). The proposal is based primarily on: 1) an increased GABA content with a simultaneous reduced GABA synthesis and breakdown in rat brain slices; and 2) a decreased formation of CO_2 from exogenous GABA ("disposal") by rat brain synaptosomes (Cheng, Brunner 1981a, 1981b, 1981c). A correlation was proposed for ED_{50} and ID_{10} (disposal) in the latter work. This paper presents analyses of individual processes in GABA "disposal" which includes GABA uptake, GABA release, GABA-transaminase (GABA-T) and GABA binding. Since ID_{10} for disposal, the overall process, was equated to ED_{50}, all these processes were also evaluated with their respective ED_{10} or ID_{10} values. Those for midazolam were reported earlier.

Synaptosomes were prepared from rat (Sprague-Dawley) forebrain according to the sucrose density gradient centrifugation method; methods for protein assay, radioactivity determination, and the studying of synaptosomal GABA-T activity, GABA release and GABA uptake had been reported previously.

Several general anesthetic agents were studied as well as some other neurotropic agents which were included for comparison. They were shown in all tables and their sources were reported in the above citations. Usually 4-6 experiments were performed for each concentration of a drug followed by 2-tailed t-tests against their respective controls and regression line analyses. Both mean$\pm$S.E.M.

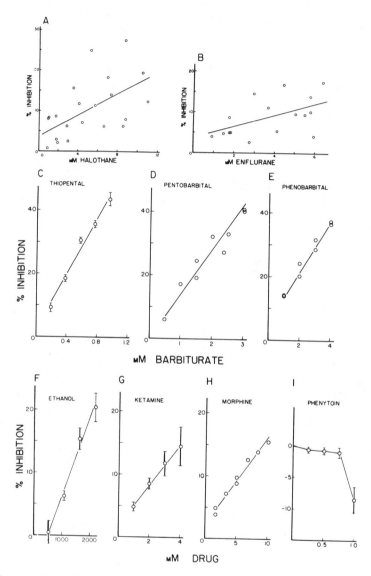

Figure 1. Effect of drugs on synaptosomal GABA-T activity. Synaptosomes were incubated at 30°C and pH 8.1 in 1 ml of TRIS 50mM, Triton-X-100 0.5%, dithiothreitol 1mM, pyridoxal phosphate 0.4mM, GABA 75mM, 2-oxoglutarate 5mM, aldehyde dehydrogenase 0.25 unit, NAD 8.3mM, NADH 17 μM and a drug (when required). Increases in A_{340nm} were observed and the difference between 10' and 40' values represented GABA-T activity and were converted to μmoles/hr.

TABLE 1. EFFECTS OF DRUGS ON GABA-T ACTIVITY

Drug	ED_{50}	ID_{10}	ID_{10}/ED_{50}	N;r
Halothane	1.0%	12%	12	22;0.58
Enflurane	1.7%	11%	6.5	16;0.54
Ether	3.2%	-	-	-
Thiopental	0.24mM	0.17mM	0.71	54;0.92
Pentobarbital	0.07mM	0.60mM	8.6	9;0.97
Phenobarbital	0.11mM	0.56mM	5.1	8;0.99
Paraldehyde	4.7mM	-	-	-
Ketamine	0.13mM	2.5mM	19	20;0.69
Ethanol	28mM	1310mM	47	26;0.88
Morphine	0.15mM	5.5mM	37	8;0.99
Phenytoin	0.085mM	-	-	12; -
Midazolam	0.008mM	0.62mM	78	21;0.92

with number of experiments (N) and correlation coefficients
(r) were reported whenever applicable. Concentrations were
given in mM or % v/v which referred to volume of gas in 100
volumes of solvent. ED_{50} for volatile anesthetics were
minimum alveolar concentration values.

Synaptosomal GABA-T was assayed at 340nm after Triton-
X100 solubilization and aldehyde dehydrogenase coupling
(Cheng, Brunner 1979). The control activity was 0.439 +
0.013 μmoles/hr/mg protein (N = 331) which agreed with
values in the literature (Buu, van Gelder 1974). The inhibitory effects of various anesthetic agents were shown in
Figure 1 and summarized in Table 1. Both ether and paralde-
hyde, not shown in Figure 1, caused increases at 340nm which
was used to measure the formation of NADH. Best estimates
showed that they both lacked effect on synaptosomal GABA-T
activity.

Thiopental (Cheng, Brunner 1979), phenobarbital (Sawaya
et al. 1975) and midazolam (Cheng, Brunner 1981c) inhibited
synaptosomal GABA-T activity while phenytoin stimulated it
at high concentration (Sawaya et al. 1975). These are all
consistent with our present findings. Pentobarbital showed
no inhibition (Sutton, Simmonds 1974) and the effects of
ethanol (Rawat 1974) and ketamine (Krishnan et al. 1981)
varied. Of the calculated ID_{10} (GABA-T) values, only
thiopental showed a value comparable to its ED_{50} and ID_{10}
(disposal) (Table 1). Therefore, only thiopental among

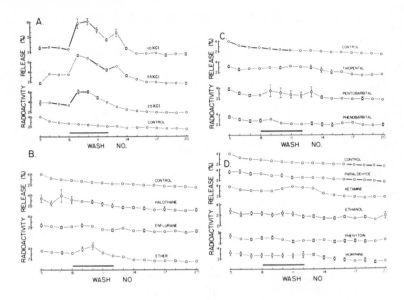

Figure 2. Resting release of preloaded 14C-GABA by synaptosomes and the effects of drugs. Synaptosomes (0.6 mg protein) were sedimented onto a piece of cloth, packed tight
with centrifugation, covered with another piece of cloth
and clamped in a silver frame for easy handling. After 5'
preloading of these beds in $[1-^{14}C]GABA$ (10 μM, 0.5 μCi/ml)
containing phosphate-Ringer's solution (20mM phosphate,
124mM NaCl, 5mM KCl, 2.6mM $CaCl_2$, 1.3mM $MgSO_4$, 10mM glucose,
pH 7.3), they were transferred serially through 20 washes
(each for 2.5') of phosphate-Ringer's solutions at 30°C.
Drugs were added to washes 9-12 (bar in figure) when required.
After washing, the beds were solubilized and both protein
and radioactivity were determined. Washes 9-12 were chosen
because the rate of radioactivity release usually reached a
steady value. Drugs were mostly near their maximal solubility in these experiments (Cheng, Brunner, 1981c).

---

these agents may exert its pharmacologic action via GABA-T
inhibition.

Resting release of preloaded $[1-^{14}C]GABA$ (Amersham/
Searle) in synaptosomes were studied using a method where a
clamped synaptosomal bed (0.6 mg protein) was transferred
serially through wash media (2 ml of Krebs-Ringer solution).
Most of the drugs studied were at their maximal concentra-

tion attainable in this system. They were added to some of
the wash media (washes 9-12) after the rate of radioactivity
washout achieved a steady value (Figure 2). After 20
washes, each 2.5 minutes, the remaining synaptosomes were
solubilized. Radioactivity in all the washes as well as
the synaptosomes after washes were monitored.

Water soluble drugs were added as a concentrated stock
solution and no precipitate could be observed in the final
solution. Volatile anesthetic agents were introduced as a
gas mixture (20% O_2 and the balance made up with N_2, H_2O
vapor and anesthetics). This mixture was continuously
flushed over the wash medium during 30 minutes preincubation as well as during its incubation. The concentration
of the anesthetic agent was monitored by gas chromatography.
With KCl, the solution became hypertonic since the KCl
added was not compensated by deleting NaCl accordingly.
Regardless, a clear K+-stimulation effect was observed
(Haycock et al. 1978; Osborne, Bradford 1975; Raiteri et
al. 1975).

Control radioactivity release (N=63) amounted to, in
% of total, 9.36+0.37 for washes 9-12 (when a drug might be
present), 23.55+0.86 for washes 9-20 and 63.45+1.46 in synaptosomal residue (Table 2). These figures were trans-
lated respectively to 0.154+0.016, 0.392+0.041 and 1.020+
0.078 in nmoles GABA/mg protein. The amount released per
minute per ml was just less than 1% and was in accordance
with other reports (Haycock et al. 1978; Osborne, Bradford
1975; Raiteri et al. 1975). This amount of GABA released
was insufficient to cause further GABA-stimulated release of
GABA nor was homoexchange possible under these conditions.
No attempt was made to distinguish whether the radioactivity
pertained solely to GABA, since the amount released was so
small. Also, no GABA-T inhibitor, such as AOAA, was added
to reduce metabolic breakdown of GABA.

Effects of elevated K+ concentration and drugs on resting GABA release, when compared to their corresponding controls, were illustrated in Figure 2 and summarized in Table
2. Increasing amounts of KCl elicited progressively more
release. A second peak of radioactivity release appeared
in the wash immediately after transferring the synaptosomes
out of the K+-rich medium. This may be an osmotic effect
since the K+-rich medium was increasingly hypertonic as
the K+ concentration increased. On the other hand, in

TABLE 2. RADIOACTIVITY RELEASE FROM SYNAPTOSOMES UNDER THE INFLUENCE OF VARIOUS DRUGS

Drug	Con'n	N	Sum of Washes 9-12	Sum of Washes 9-20	Synaptosomal Residue
Control		63	9.36+0.37	23.55+0.86	63.45+1.46
KCl	25mM	5	20.08+1.06*	35.91+1.31*	50.60+2.00
	55mM	5	23.53+0.55*	41.71+0.60*	43.69+0.78*
	110mM	5	25.97+0.84*	42.29+2.32*	46.59+3.24*
Halothane	8.5%	5	10.09+0.80	21.34+2.07	65.54+3.66
Enflurane	3.3%	6	7.73+1.14	18.74+2.92	72.32+4.34
Ether	7.4%	5	6.39+1.26	14.07+2.39	79.76+3.50
	14.1%	6	14.62+1.47*	30.69+1.69	55.84+2.37
Thiopental	0.8mM	5	12.25+0.69	28.18+2.67	60.43+3.49
Pentobarbital	10mM	5	11.85+3.56	28.22+4.12	60.88+5.11
Phenobarbital	25mM	5	9.81+0.51	26.46+1.68	61.41+3.20
Paraldehyde	38mM	5	10.56+1.17	26.03+1.50	60.38+2.68
Ketamine	2mM	5	5.99+1.76	13.88+3.19	78.22+5.17
	4mM	5	13.66+0.31*	29.67+0.28*	57.24+0.69
Ethanol	271mM	7	10.78+0.80	26.84+1.38	51.06+4.11
Morphine	10mM	5	10.98+2.19	25.94+3.79	62.46+5.76
Phenytoin	0.7mM	5	6.19+0.63	16.17+1.91	75.81+2.51
Midazolam	0.25mM	5	7.21+1.70	18.24+3.62	72.64+5.03
	0.50mM	5	14.85+3.83	40.65+7.59*	48.98+8.87*
	0.75mM	5	30.68+8.93*	63.63+6.98*	27.76+7.75*
	1.00mM	5	56.49+9.68*	84.92+4.37*	8.02+4.45*

Radioactivity (given in percentage of total) in treated samples when differed statistically ($p<0.05$) from their corresponding controls were indicated with a *.

---

the midazolam experiments (Cheng, Brunner 1981c), a strong tailing effect of radioactivity efflux was observed. Consequently, in Table 2, two columns on the sums of radioactivity were reported, sums of washes 9-12, when a drug might be present, and sums of washes 9-20. The last column recorded the residual radioactivity in the synaptosomes after all the washing. None of the drugs studied here potentiated resting release of GABA except high concentrations of ether and ketamine. Midazolam was reported previously to induce release (Table 2) at concentrations higher than ED_{50} (Cheng, Brunner 1981c). Therefore, these drugs do not appear to act pharmacologically through a potentiation of resting GABA release. The lack of effect by halothane was in agreement with previous findings (Berl

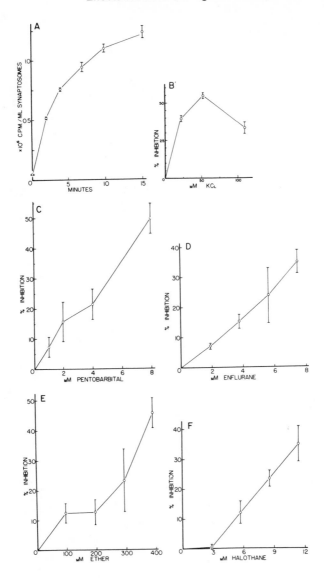

Figure 3-1

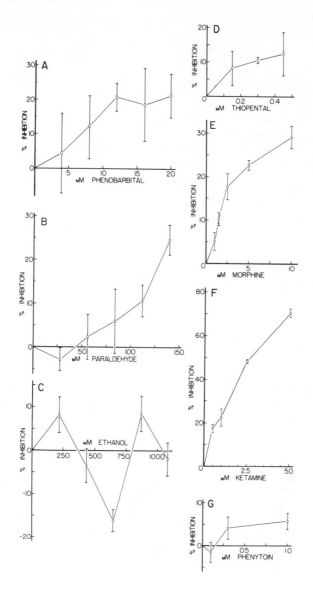

Figure 3-2

Figure 3. Synaptosomal uptake of 3H-GABA and the effects of drugs. Synaptosomes were incubated in a medium (0.5 ml) of one part synaptosomes (0.8 mg protein) in 0.32M sucrose and four parts of HEPES-Ringer's solution (20mM HEPES, 124mM NaCl, 5mM KCl, 2.6mM $CaCl_2$, 1.3mM $MgSO_4$, 10mM glucose, pH 7.3) containing [2,3-3H]GABA (25 nmoles, 1 μCi) and a drug (if required). Incubation was for 10' at 30°C. Samples were withdrawn after 0' and 10', diluted 10-times in ice-cold phosphate-Ringer containing 50mM GABA, and pelleted with a microfuge. After two superficial rinses and solubilization, the radioactivity in the pellets was determined. The difference in radioactivity between 0' and 10' represented uptake. Effects of drugs were compared with their respective controls. Figure 1A showed the time course of uptake in this assay system. The rest of the figures showed the effects of KCl and drugs (Cheng, Brunner, 1981c).

----

et al. 1979) but pentobarbital had been reported to inhibit resting release (Haycock et al. 1977). No ED_{10}/ED_{50} values can be derived from these results, they must be much larger than the corresponding ratios based on GABA disposal if any release could be induced at all.

Effect of drugs on the uptake of GABA was compared after 10-minute incubation of synaptosomes (with approximately 0.8 mg protein) in 3H-GABA containing Hepes-Ringer's solution between drug-treated synaptosomes and their corresponding controls. Samples of incubation mixture before and after 10 minute incubation were diluted in ice-cold 50-mM GABA-containing Ringer's solution, mixed immediately and followed by centrifugation in a microfuge. The pellets were rinsed twice superficially, solubilized and its radioactivity assessed. The difference between samples before and after incubation represented uptake.

The time course of uptake was shown in Figure 3-1A and the magnitude of uptake, as measured in this manner, was 96.6+4.0 (N = 71) pmoles/mg protein which was comparable to those previously reported (Levi, Raiteri 1973; Martin 1973; Ryan, Roskoski 1977). As in release experiments, the added KCl (Figure 3-1B) was not compensated by removing corresponding amounts of NaCl. Therefore, the lack of linear response to increasing K^+ concentration might have resulted from increased external osmotic concentration. Nevertheless, these results clearly confirmed the K^+ depolarization effect (Martin 1973; Ryan, Roskoski 1977).

TABLE 3. EFFECTS OF DRUGS ON SYNAPTOSOMAL GABA UPTAKE

Drug	ED_{50}	ID_{10}	ID_{10}/ED_{50}	N;r
Halothane	1.0%	15.7%	15.7	16;0.89
Enflurane	1.7%	16.7	9.8	21;0.69
Ether	3.2%	21.9%	6.9	25;0.56
Thiopental	0.24mM	0.28mM	1.45	15;0.18
Pentobarbital	0.07mM	1.46mM	21	20;0.83
Phenobarbital	0.11mM	6.83mM	62	15;0.35
Paraldehyde	4.7mM	92.0mM	19.6	30;0.63
Ketamine	0.13mM	0.12mM	0.92	14;0.93
Ethanol	28mM	-	-	35; -
Morphine	0.15mM	1.11mM	7.4	16;0.73
Phenytoin	0.085mM	1.56mM	18.4	15;0.45
Midazolam	0.008mM	0.013mM	1.63	29; -

Most of these drugs required a concentration higher than their respective ED_{50} to inhibit GABA uptake (Figure 3 and Table 3). Thiopental, which gave an ID_{10}/ED_{50} ratio of 1.45, should be considered to act via GABA uptake inhibition. However, owing to the erratic results (r=0.18) and the solubility limitation, so that its concentration in the assay system could not be increased to produce more consistent and meaningful inhibition, we chose not to emphasize this result. A similar ratio of 0.92 for ketamine confirmed a previous finding (Wood, Hertz 1980), so was the lack of effect by halothane and enflurane substantiated (Berl et al. 1979). Therefore, only ketamine may exert its pharmacological effects via a GABA uptake inhibition mechanism.

The binding of GABA to synaptic membrane was studied by binding 3H-GABA to membrane fragments prepared from either P_2B or P_2 fractions derived from rat forebrain (Willow, Johnston 1981). These fractions were lysed by water and washed extensively with phosphate and Tris-HCl buffers. A specific binding:non-specific binding ratio was usually between 5 and 6. Muscimol inhibited about 50% of specific binding at 50nM (Figure 4A). Both these parameters indicated that these membrane fragments could be used for binding studies. However, not all preparations could be used since not all of them exhibited a pentobarbital stimulation effect (Asano, Ogasawara 1982; Olsen, Snowman 1982; Whittle, Turner 1982; Willow, Johnston 1981).

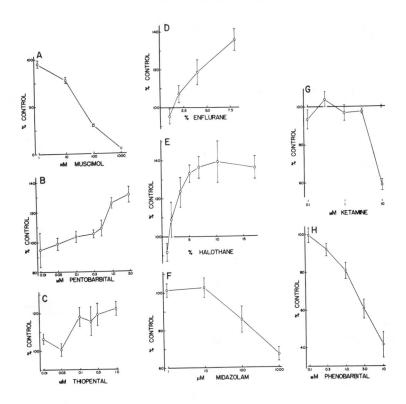

Figure 4. Effects of drugs on GABA binding by synaptosomal membrane. Synaptosomal membrane fragments (0.5 mg protein) were incubated at 0°C for 15' with [2,3-3H]GABA (5nM, 0.3 µCi/ml), TRIS-chloride (50mM, pH 7.4) and a drug or GABA (0.1mM) in a total volume of 0.5 ml. Those with halothane and enflurane were for 5' in a total volume of 1.3 ml. The membranes were subsequently sedimented in a microfuge and superficially rinsed twice. The pellet was solubilized and its radioactivity determined. Radioactivity from samples with 0.1mM GABA represented non-specific GABA binding. Effects of drugs were compared with corresponding controls.

Our data on pentobarbital stimulation (Figure 4) indicated that more than 1mM was required to obtain a significant increase in specific binding. Thiopental stimulation occurred at a lower concentration (0.1mM). Ketamine had no effect and midazolam inhibited. Two volatile anesthetic agents, halothane and enflurane, studied with only 5 minutes

incubation, showed a dose-related stimulation of specific
GABA binding but required concentrations higher than their
ED_{50} values. The significance of these data requires
further clarification. We are not ready to propose the
hypothesis, similar to that with pentobarbital (Willow,
Johnston 1981), that a prolonged opening of chloride channel
due to increased GABA binding to its receptor forms the
basis of the action of general anesthetics.

Since there was no good evidence to delineate the
underlying mechanism of GABA disposal inhibition by volatile anesthetic agents, attention was turned to the in-

TABLE 4. SUMMARIZED EFFECTS OF DRUGS ON SYNAPTOSOMAL GABA
DISPOSAL AND ITS INDIVIDUAL PROCESSES. VALUES
ARE ED_{10}/ED_{50}.

Drug	Disposal	GABA-T Inhibition	Induced GABA Release	GABA Uptake Inhibition	GABA Binding[2]
Halothane	0.55	12	large[1]	15.7	2.1
Enflurane	0.71	6.5	"	9.8	2.6
Ether	1.4	-	"	6.9	n.d.
Thiopental	1.1	0.71	"	1.45	0.38
Pentobarbital	6.4	8.6	"	21	0.50
Phenobarbital	30	5.1	"	62	-
Paraldehyde	3.6	-	"	21	n.d.
Ketamine	4.8	19	"	0.92	5.3
Ethanol	5.0	47	"	-	n.d.
Morphine	18	37	"	7.4	n.d.
Phenytoin	-	-	"	18.4	n.d.
Midazolam	1.6	78	"	1.63	-

1-"large" indicated concentrations tested were ineffective.
Either higher concentrations of a drug were required to
induce 10% more release or that the drug had no effect on
release. 2-Best estimation from curves in Figure 4.
"-" for inhibition and "n.d." for not determined.

tegrity of synaptosomal membrane. High concentrations of
anesthetics (Richter et al. 1978) did cause enzyme leakage
in beef heart mitochondria. In synaptosomes, an extra
synaptosomal membrane was also encountered if any enzyme
should leak out. Halothane induced GABA-T leakage in a
dose-related manner (Cheng, Brunner in press). A reduced

leakage was found with succinic semialdehyde dehydrogenase and essentially no effect was observed on glutamate decarboxylase, lactate dehydrogenase, malate dehydrogenase and creatine phosphokinase. Unfortunately, a 5% halothane was required to give a 10% effect. And this was five times the ED_{50} value. But the specificity toward GABA-T leakage is intriguing.

In summary, after advancing a correlation of ED_{50} and ID_{50} for GABA disposal in our pursuit of the mode of anesthetic action, we tried to define the exact mechanism for this correlation. We found that (Table 4) correlation could be established for thiopental to GABA-T inhibition and both midazolam and ketamine to GABA uptake. The mechanism for volatile anesthetics could reside in potentiation of GABA binding, but this suggestion requires further verification. In addition, altered membrane integrity should not be overlooked because of a possible specific leakage of GABA-T in vivo.

ACKNOWLEDGEMENT

The authors deeply appreciate the highly competent technical help of Mrs. Irena Minieka and the assistance of Mrs. Peggy Collins in preparing this manuscript. We also wish to thank the following publishers in granting permission to reproduce some of the data published in their publications: American Society of Anesthesiologists, ANKHO International Inc., Plenum Publishing Company, and Raven Press.

REFERENCES

Asano T, Ogasawara N (1982). Stimulation of GABA receptor binding by barbiturates. Eur J Pharmacol 77:355.

Azzaro AJ, Smith DJ (1977). The inhibitory action of ketamine HCl on [3H]5-hydroxytryptamine accumulation by rat brain synaptosomal-rich fractions: Comparison with [3H]-catecholamine and [3H]γ-aminobutyric acid uptake. Neuropharmacol 16:349.

Berl S, Getzow JJ, Nicklas WJ, Mahendran C (1979). Effect of halogenated hydrocarbons on synaptosomal uptake and release of neurotransmitters. Prog Clin Biol Res 27:135.

Buu NT, van Gelder NM (1974). Differences in biochemical properties of γ-aminobutyric acid aminotransferase from synaptosome-enriched and cytoplasmic mitochondria-enriched subcellular fractions of mouse brain. Can J Physiol Pharmacol 52:674.

Cheng S-C, Brunner EA (1979). Thiopental inhibition of γ-aminobutyrate transaminase in rat brain synaptosomes. Biochem Pharmacol 28:105.

Cheng S-C, Brunner EA (1981a). Inhibition of GABA metabolism in rat brain slices by halothane. Anesthesiology 55:26.

Cheng S-C, Brunner EA (1981b). Effects of anesthetic agents on synaptosomal GABA disposal. Anesthesiology 55:34.

Cheng S-C, Brunner EA (1981c). Inhibition of GABA metabolism in rat brain synaptosomes by midazolam (RO-21-3981). Anesthesiology 55:41.

Cheng S-C, Brunner EA (in press). A proposed GABA mechanism for anesthesia. In Paolatti R, Tiengo M (eds.): "Pharmacological Basis of Anaesthesiology," New York: Raven Press.

Haycock JW, Levy WB, Cotman CW (1977). Pentobarbital depression of stimulus-secretion coupling in brain - Selective inhibition of depolarization-induced calcium-dependent release. Biochem Pharmacol 26:159.

Haycock JW, Levy WB, Denner LA, Cotman CW (1978). Effects of elevated $[K^+]_o$ on the release of neurotransmitters from cortical synaptosomes: Efflux or secretion? J Neurochem 30:1113.

Krishnan H, Baquer NZ, Singh R (1981). Changes in γ-aminobutyric acid-shunt enzymes in regions of rat brain with ketamine anaesthesia. Neuropharmacol 20:567.

Levi G, Raiteri M (1973). GABA and glutamate uptake by subcellular fractions enriched in synaptosomes: Critical evaluation of some methodological aspects. Brain Res 57:165.

Martin DL (1973). Kinetics of the sodium-dependent transport of gamma-aminobutyric acid by synaptosomes. J Neurochem 21:345.

Olsen RW, Snowman AM (1982). Chloride-dependent enhancement by barbiturates of γ-aminobutyric acid receptor binding. J Neurosci 2:1812.

Osborne RH, Bradford HF (1975). The influence of sodium, potassium and lanthanum on amino acid release from spinal-medullary synaptosomes. J Neurochem 25:35.

Raiteri M, Federico R, Coletti A, Levi G (1975). Release and exchange studies relating to the synaptosomal uptake of GABA. J Neurochem 24:1243.

Rawat AK (1974). Brain levels and turnover rates of presumptive neurotransmitters as influenced by administration and withdrawal of ethanol in mice. J Neurochem 22: 915.

Richter JJ, Sunderland E, Juhl U, Kornguth S (1978). Extraction of mitochondrial proteins by volatile anesthetics. Biochim Biophys Acta 543:106.

Ryan LD, Roskoski R, Jr. (1977). Net uptake of γ-aminobutyric acid by a high affinity synaptosomal transport system. J Pharmacol Exp Ther 200:285.

Sawaya MCB, Horton RW, Meldrum BS (1975). Effects of anticonvulsant drugs on the cerebral enzymes metabolizing GABA. Epilepsia 16:649.

Sutton I, Simmonds MA (1974). Effects of acute and chronic pentobarbitone on the γ-aminobutyric acid system in rat brain. Biochem Pharmacol 23:1801.

Whittle SR, Turner AJ (1982). Differential effects of sedative and anticonvulsant barbiturates on specific [3H]GABA binding to membrane preparations from rat brain cortex. Biochem Pharmacol 31:2891.

Willow M, Johnston GAR (1981). Enhancement by anesthetic and convulsant barbiturates of GABA binding to rat brain synaptosomal membranes. J Neurosci 1:364.

Wood JD, Hertz L (1980). Ketamine-induced changes in the GABA system of mouse brain. Neuropharmacol 19:805.

Glutamine, Glutamate, and GABA
in the Central Nervous System, pages 669–673
© 1983 Alan R. Liss, Inc., 150 Fifth Avenue, New York, NY 10011

EFFECTS OF ETHANOL TREATMENT ON GLUTAMINERGIC
NEUROTRANSMISSION

J.T. Cummins, E. Keller and M. Frolich

Addiction Research Laboratory, V.A. Medical Center,
Sepulveda, CA 91343 and Dept. Psychiatry and Human
Behavior, UCLA

Although ethanol is classified as a sedative/hypnotic,
excitatory activity is observed in both acute and chronic
stages of ethanol treatment (Pohorecky, 1976). The nature
of these excitatory effects is not known, but they are
likely to involve either direct or indirect influences of
ethanol on excitatory neurotransmitters. Even though glutamate is a prime candidate for involvement in some of the
observed excitations, there are surprisingly few studies on
the effects of ethanol on glutaminergic neurotransmission.
Glutamate binding studies do show changes in glutamate
binding parameters due to both in vivo and in vitro ethanol
treatments (Michaelis, Michaelis and Freed, 1980). This
paper demonstrates that there are also effects of chronic
ethanol treatment on presynaptic glutaminergic neurotransmission and suggests regional differences among postsynaptic
effects.

METHODS

Male Sprague-Dawley rats with a starting weight of 250 g
were addicted to ethanol by supplying 6% ethanol in a liquid
diet as the sole food source for 21-25 days (Lieber and
DeCarli, 1973). After sacrifice, the striatum and hippocampus were removed and either sliced on a Sorvall TC-2 tissue
chopper set at 0.22 mm or frozen on dry ice. The tissue
slices were maintained in standard Krebs-Ringer bicarbonate
at $37 \pm 2^{\circ}$ and gassed with 95% O_2/5% CO_2.

^{3}H-Glutamate uptake was measured by incubating the slices for 25 min. in the isotope and stopping the uptake by centrifugation (1000 RPM, 2 min., 0°C). Aliquots of the solubilized tissue were taken for protein determination and liquid scintillation counting.

For studies on K^+ depolarized endogenous glutamate release, the chopped tissue was bedded out under a slight vacuum on filter paper in 13 mm Swinnex chambers and Krebs-Ringer bicarbonate was pumped through the tissue bed for 25 min. to stabilize the baseline. The tissue was depolarized with 45mM K^+. Glutamate in the efflux collected before and after depolarization was determined by enzymatic procedures (Graham and Aprison, 1966).

^{22}Na efflux activity was measured by the method of Teichburg (1982). Procedures described by Lehman and Scatton (1982) to measure glutamate-stimulated acetylcholine release were followed.

RESULTS AND DISCUSSION

Table 1 summarizes the effects of ethanol treatment on three presynaptic and one postsynaptic glutamate activity in the striatum. Glutamate levels are significantly elevated 36 hours after the withdrawal of ethanol, but there is no change in glutamate level in rats chronically treated with ethanol. ^{3}H-glutamate uptake in striatal slices at normal K^+ is significantly elevated both in the ethanol addicted and withdrawn rat. However, there is no significant effect of ethanol treatment on endogenous glutamate release following depolarization with elevated K^+, nor is there an effect on glutamate stimulated ^{3}H-acetylcholine release.

The effect of chronic ethanol treatment on some hippocampal glutamate activities are presented in Table 2. In the hippocampus, ethanol withdrawal raises both glutamate levels and K^+-stimulated endogenous glutamate release. ^{3}H-glutamate uptake activity is increased in the ethanol addicted state and returns to control values following withdrawal. There appears to be no effect of chronic ethanol treatment on glutamate stimulated ^{22}Na-efflux activity in the hippocampus.

TABLE 1: Effects of Ethanol Treatment on Rat Striatal Glutamate

	Control	Addicted	Withdrawn
Glu Levels nmoles/mg prot	26±2.0 (7)	30±1.3 (4)	*38±1.6 (5)
Glu Uptake CPM/mg prot	23,000 (4)	*36,000 (4)	*39,000 (4)
Glu Release nmoles/mg prot	6.5±0.7 (6)	8.4±0.7 (7)	7.2±0.7 (8)
3H-Acetylcholine Release (o)	1.5±0.1 (7)	1.6±0.2 (5)	1.6±0.2 (6)

* Significantly different from control values, P(t)<0.05.
o Rate before stimulation/Rate after stimulation

TABLE 2: Effects of Ethanol Treatment on Rat Hippocampal Glutamate

	Control	Addicted	Withdrawn
Glu Levels nmoles/mg prot	26±1.9 (8)	32±1.7 (8)	*43±2.2 (8)
Glu Uptake CPM/mg prot	28,000 (4)	*41,000 (4)	29,000 (4)
Glu Release nmoles/mg prot	4.7±0.6 (8)	3.6±0.2 (7)	*6.0±0.6 (8)
22Na-Efflux Δo, min^{-1}	0.16±.02 (4)	0.15±.02 (4)	0.15±.02 (3)

* Significantly different from control, P(t)<0.05.
o The difference between the average specific efflux rate two min. before stimulation and two min. after stimulation.

In general, it would be expected that ethanol-induced changes in glutamate release will result in changes in sensitivity of postsynaptic receptors. Thus, the observation that ethanol treatment does not change glutamate-induced striatal ^{3}H-acetylcholine release may be seen as the expected effect due to the negative effect of ethanol on glutamate release in this brain area. This mechanism cannot be evoked to explain the lack of change in glutamate-induced ^{22}Na-efflux in hippocampal slices from the withdrawn rat because in that tissue glutamate release is elevated. The effect(s) on receptor sensitivity of changes in glutamate uptake are not clear and require further investigation.

Regional patterns of changes in binding activity are indicated by the ethanol independence of glutamate binding in these two brain areas and the demonstration that total binding activity increases with addiction (Michaelis, Michaelis and Freed, 1980).

The results presented here and those published for the cortex (Keller, Cummins and von Hungen, 1983) demonstrate that ethanol-induced changes in these brain regions differ as to the type of glutamate activity affected and to the time and direction of effect. The observation of these regional differences is in accord with a recent trend in alcoholism research, based on genetic and behavioral data, which indicates multiple expressions of ethanol action (Tabakoff, 1983). That there are a number of neurochemical actions of ethanol on the CNS is compatible with theories postulating that the primary action of ethanol is to "fluidize" membrane systems (Chin and Goldstein, 1976), implying that there are no specific receptors involved in the actions of ethanol and that numerous homeostatic changes follow this "fluidity" effect. This seems to be the case here where large changes related to glutaminergic neurotransmission are observed and which no doubt affect excitatory behavior.

REFERENCES

1. Chin JH, Goldstein DB (1976). Drug tolerance in biomembranes: A spin label study of the effects of ethanol. Science 196:684.

2. Graham LT, Aprison MH (1966). Fluorometric determination of aspartate, glutamate and gamma-aminobutyric acid in nerve tissue using enzymatic methods. Anal Biochem 15:487.
3. Keller E, Cummins JT, von Hungen K (1983). Regional effects of ethanol on glutamate levels, uptake and release in slice and synaptosome preparations from rat brain. Subst Alc Actions/Misuse: In Press.
4. Lieber CS, DeCarli LM (1973). Ethanol dependence and tolerance: A nutritionally controlled experimental model in the rat. Res Comm Chem Path Pharmacol 6:983.
5. Lehman J, Scatton B (1982). Characterization of the excitatory amino acid receptor-mediated release of [^{3}H] acetylcholine from rat striatal slices. Brain Res 252: 77.
6. Michaelis EK, Michaelis ML, Freed WJ (1980). Chronic ethanol intake and synaptosomal glutamate binding activity. Adv Exp Med Biol 126:43.
8. Pohorecky LA (1976). Biphasic action of ethanol. Biobehav Rev 1:231.
9. Tabakoff B (1983). Current trends in biologic research on alcoholism. Drug Alc Depend 11:33.
10. Teichberg VL, Goldberg O, Luini A (1982). The stimulation of ion fluxes in brain slices by glutamate and other excitatory amino acids. Cell Biochem 39:281.

Glutamine, Glutamate, and GABA
in the Central Nervous System, pages 675–688
© 1983 Alan R. Liss, Inc., 150 Fifth Avenue, New York, NY 10011

PHARMACOLOGY OF GABA METABOLISM AT THE SUBCELLULAR LEVEL

J. D. Wood and J. W. Geddes,

Department of Biochemistry,
University of Saskatchewan,
Saskatoon, Saskatchewan,
Canada. S7N 0W0

INTRODUCTION

The importance of amino acids as neurotransmitter
substances in the central nervous system (CNS) is becoming
increasingly apparent. While γ-aminobutyric acid (GABA) and
glycine have been well established as inhibitory transmitters for several years (Krnjevic 1974), glutamate and
aspartate are only now gaining like-status as excitatory
transmitters (Roberts, Storm-Mathisen, Johnston 1981).
However, the specific contribution of the individual amino
acid transmitter systems towards the establishment of the
state of excitability of the CNS remains uncertain. Complicating the interpretation of data obtained in this area
of research are two factors: (1) the compartmentation of
the amino acids into pools with various cellular and subcellular locations (Berl, Lajtha, Waelsch 1961; Bradford
1982), and (ii) the close metabolic relationships between
aspartate, glutamate and GABA (Shank, Graham 1978). Adding
to the complexity of the situation is the very major role
played by aspartate and glutamate in the "general" metabolism of the cell.

Various researchers have investigated the possibility
that changes in the functioning of an amino acid transmitter
system bring about changes in the excitable state of the
brain. These studies focussed primarily on the GABA system,
and, although some limited correlations were obtained, it
became clear that no simple relationship existed between
whole brain GABA levels and the excitable state of the brain
(Wood 1975). One possible reason for this lack of correla-

tion is the afore-mentioned compartmentation of GABA. The
critical concentration of GABA with respect to its neurotransmitter function is that at the post-synaptic receptor
site (i.e. in the synaptic cleft), and changes in this GABA
concentration are not necessarily reflected in like-changes
in whole brain levels of the amino acid. Unfortunately,
determination of the GABA concentration in the synaptic
cleft is beyond the capability of current methodologies,
but, in view of the critical role played by nerve endings in
controlling neurotransmitter function, changes in the GABA
content of nerve endings might reflect more accurately
concurrent changes in the concentration of the amino acid at
its receptor site. Accordingly, we directed our research
towards an evaluation of the changes in nerve ending GABA
content induced by selected convulsant and anticonvulsant
drugs, and a comparison of these changes with the excitable
state of the brain. Since previous work (Wood 1981)
indicated that changes in amino acid levels in synaptosomes
prepared from brain tissue were likely to reflect accurately
the drug-induced changes in the "parent" nerve endings, the
synaptosomal model was used in these studies. In view of
the close metabolic relationship among GABA, glutamate and
aspartate as well as with glutamine, the effect of the
convulsant and anticonvulsant drugs on the synaptosomal
levels of all these amino acids was monitored. A review of
the resulting data and our interpretation of the findings
constitute the major thrust in this presentation.

METHODS

Male Swiss mice weighing 25-30 g were used in the
experiments. Convulsant and anticonvulsant drugs were
dissolved in 0.9% (w/v) NaCl and injected intramuscularly
into the animals. Synaptosomes were prepared from brain
tissue by differential and Ficoll-sucrose density gradient
centrifugation as described by Cotman (1974) with the
modification described previously (Wood, Russell, Kurylo,
Newstead 1979). Analysis of GABA was carried out in the
initial studies by the enzymatic-fluorometric procedure of
Graham and Aprison (1966) as modified by Balcom, Lennox and
Meyerhoff (1975). This procedure was subsequently replaced
by an HPLC technique which allowed the simultaneous analyses
of all the amino acids under study. The HPLC method was
essentially that of Lenda and Svenneby (1980) with the modifications described previously (Geddes, Wood 1983).

TABLE 1. GABA LEVELS IN MOUSE BRAIN AT ONSET OF SEIZURES.

Convulsant agent (mmol/kg body wt)	Time to Onset of seizures (min)	GABA Whole brain (umol/g)	GABA Synaptosomes (nmol/mg protein)	Δ GABA syn (%)
None		2.08 ± 0.03	31.6 ± 1.6	
Hydrazine (4.0)	28	2.46 ± 0.09	22.2 ± 1.8	-30
INH (2.2)	29	1.71 ± 0.06	23.6 ± 1.5	-25
AOAA (3.6)	8	2.03 ± 0.07	22.3 ± 0.1	-29

Values are mean ± SEM for 4 - 6 samples.
Data from Wood, Russell, Kurylo, Newstead (1979).

RESULTS AND DISCUSSION

Effect of Convulsant and Anticonvulsant Drugs on GABA Levels

Aminooxyacetic acid (AOAA), isonicotinic acid hydrazide (INH) and hydrazine all alter GABA metabolism in brain and induce seizures in animals. If there is a cause and effect relationship between the two parameters, it might be expected that the changes in GABA levels at the onset of seizures would be the same for all three convulsant agents. This is clearly not the case with whole brain GABA levels, an increase, a decrease and no significant change being observed in mice at the onset of seizures induced by hydrazine, INH and AOAA respectively (Table 1). In contrast, the synaptosomal GABA levels were decreased by similar amounts at the onset of seizures induced by all three convulsant agents. These results clearly illustrate the compartmentation of GABA between nerve endings and other cellular structures, and highlight the importance of the GABA content of the nerve terminals with respect to the functioning of the CNS.

AOAA (at low dosage levels), gabaculine, ethyl nipecotate and dipropylacetate (DPA) all possess anticonvulsant properties (Simler, Ciesielski, Maitre, Randrianarisoa, Mandel 1973; Matsui, Deguchi 1977; Frey, Popp, Loscher 1979; Horton, Collins, Anlezark, Meldrum 1979; Kuriyama, Roberts, Rubinstein 1966), but their action on the GABA system varies considerably. AOAA and gabaculine are potent inhibitors of 4-aminobutyrate-2-oxoglutarate aminotransferase (GABA-T), and their injection into mice causes large increases in GABA levels in both nerve endings (synaptosomes) and whole brain, the latter increase (expressed as a percentage of control values) being much greater than that in the synaptosomes (Fig. 1). This finding raises the question as to whether the increase in synaptosomal GABA content arises from exogenous sources (i.e. the very high GABA levels extant in structures other than nerve endings), or whether it arises from endogenous sources (e.g. other amino acids in the nerve terminals). In contrast to the results with the potent GABA-T inhibitors, the administration of DPA which is a weak inhibitor of GABA-T activity, causes only moderate increases in both synaptosomal and whole brain GABA levels, and in this case the synaptosomal GABA increase is the greater of the two (Fig. 1). In addition, the effects of DPA are

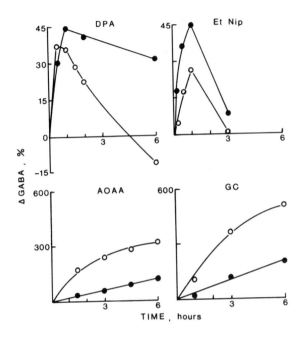

Fig. 1. Changes in GABA levels after administration of
various drugs to mice. ● —— ● , synaptosomes; o —— o ,
whole brain; DPA, dipropylacetate (2.82 mmol/kg); Et nip,
ethyl nipecotate (0.22 mmol/kg); AOAA, aminooxyacetic acid
(0.23 mmol/kg); GC, gabaculine (0.58 mmol/kg). Data from
Wood, Kurylo, Tsui 1981; Wood, Russell, Kurylo 1980; Wood,
Schousboe, Krogsgaard-Larsen 1980.

shorter-lasting than are those of AOAA or gabaculine. The
administration of ethyl nipecotate also induces moderate,
short term increases in the levels of GABA, and here too
the elevation in synaptosomal GABA content was greater than
that in the whole brain (Fig. 1). The increase in GABA level
within the nerve endings is rather surprising given the
properties of nipecotic acid as a GABA uptake inhibitor.
The most plausible explanation for this phenomenon is that
the GABA uptake by neuronal perikarya or nearby glial cells
is inhibited to a greater extent than is the reuptake by
nerve endings, resulting in an increase in extracellular
GABA concentration which more than compensates for the
impairment in the uptake system of the nerve terminals.

TABLE 2. INTERREFFECTS OF A CONVULSANT AGENT (ISONICOTINIC ACID HYDRAZIDE) AND ANTICONVULSANT AGENTS ON SYNAPTOSOMAL GABA LEVELS.

Anticonvulsant drug (mmol/kg)	Time* (h)	GABA (nmol/mg protein)		Δ GABA (%)
		At injection of convulsant	At onset of seizures	
None		29.9 ± 1.3	22.1 ± 1.9	−26
AOAA (0.23)	6	63.1 ± 3.7	46.0 ± 2.0	−27
AOAA (0.23)	15	46.1 ± 1.7	34.0 ± 0.6	−26
L-cycloserine (0.25)	3	43.3 ± 1.6	30.7 ± 1.0	−29
L-cycloserine (0.5)	3	59.5 ± 1.0	39.4 ± 1.1	−33
L-cycloserine (1.0)	3	69.9 ± 1.0	51.0 ± 1.2	−27

Values are mean ± SEM for 4 – 9 samples.
*Time between injection of anticonvulsant drugs and INH.
Data from Wood, Russell, Kurylo (1980).

Relationship Between Synaptosomal GABA Content and the
Excitable State of the Brain

The relationship between seizure activity and the magnitude of the decrease in synaptosomal GABA levels induced
by the convulsant agents has been illustrated above. In
contrast, the relationship between the two parameters becomes more complex when the treatments combine both convulsant and anticonvulsant agents. For example, although the
prior administration of potent GABA-T inhibitors such as
AOAA or L-cycloserine delayed the onset of drug-induced
seizures, the delay being directly proportional to the
elevation in synaptosomal GABA level at the time of injection of the convulsant agent (Fig. 2), the seizures still
occurred and at synaptosomal GABA levels which were above
those in control mice (Table 2). Interestingly, the per-

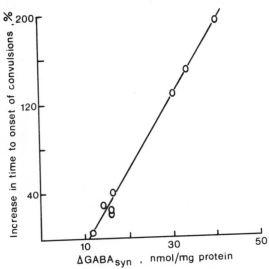

Fig. 2. Correlation between the increase in synaptosomal
GABA levels and the delay in the onset of seizures
$\Delta GABA_{syn}$ indicates the increase in GABA level due to drug
pretreatment at the time of injection of the convulsant
agent. Convulsant agents used were isonicotinic acid
hydrazide, unsymmetrical dimethylhydrazine and amino-
oxyacetic acid. Anticonvulsant agents were L-cycloserine,
aminooxyacetic acid and dipropylacetate. Data from Wood,
Kurylo, Tsui 1981; Wood, Russell, Kurylo 1980.

centage decrease in synaptosomal GABA level from the time of injection of the convulsant agent to the onset of seizures was similar (28 ± 1) regardless of whether the initial GABA content was normal or elevated by pretreatment with the GABA-T inhibitors. These results strongly suggest the presence in nerve endings of a transmitter pool of GABA which is critically important for the functioning of the GABA transmitter system, and of one or more non-transmitter pools of GABA which render impossible a simple relationship between synaptosomal GABA content and seizure activity. Nevertheless, the data suggest some connection between the transmitter and non-transmitter pools, otherwise the constancy of the percentage decrease in GABA level mentioned above would be unlikely to occur.

We conclude from the above studies that the elevation in synaptosomal GABA levels does play a role in the anticonvulsant activity of the potent GABA-T inhibitors. In contrast, the anticonvulsant activity of DPA (Wood, Kurylo, Tsui 1981) does not correlate with the DPA-induced elevation in synaptosomal GABA levels (Fig. 1). Moreover, the maximum increase in the latter parameter is 11 nmol/mg protein, an elevation in GABA level which brings about a negligible delay in the time to onset of seizures (Fig. 2). We therefore conclude that changes in synaptosomal GABA content are not responsible for the anticonvulsant action of DPA. Similarly, the small increases in synaptosomal GABA level induced by ethyl nipecotate are unlikely to be involved in the anticonvulsant action of the drug. A more likely explanation is that an ethyl nipecotate-induced elevation in extracellular GABA concentration was responsible for the anticonvulsant effects.

Relationship Between Drug-induced Changes in Synaptosomal Levels of GABA, Glutamate, Glutamine and Aspartate.

The convulsant drugs used in our studies not only lowered synaptosomal GABA levels, but also increased the glutamate content of the nerve endings, both changes occurring prior to seizure activity (Fig. 3). Unlike Matsuda, Hoshino and Sakurai (1978) who reported that the injection of pyridoxine along with toxopyrimidine prevented the onset of toxopyrimidine-induced seizures and changes in glutamate levels, but not the changes in GABA content, we found that the simultaneous administration of pyridoxine

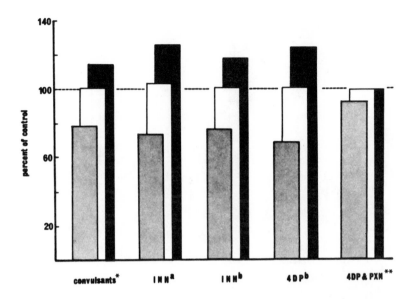

Fig. 3. Effect of convulsant agents on synaptosomal GABA and glutamate levels. Black histograms represent glutamate levels; grey histograms represent GABA levels; white histograms represent combined GABA + glutamate levels; *, at the onset of seizures induced by five convulsant agents; INH[a], immediately prior to isonicotinic acid hydrazide induced seizures; INH[b], onset of INH-induced seizures; 4DP[b], onset of 4-deoxypyridoxine induced seizures; 4DP + PXN**, non-convulsed animals treated simultaneously with 4DP and pyridoxine and sampled at a time equivalent to onset of seizures with 4DP alone. Data from Geddes, Wood (1983).

and 4-deoxypyridoxine prevented all three phenomena due to the latter drug (Fig. 3). The results presented in Fig. 3 are in accord with what might be expected of drugs which inhibit the synthesis of GABA from glutamate (glutamate decarboxylase). Although the more uniform decreases in GABA levels suggest that this is the primary factor in the seizure mechanism, the possibility cannot be ignored that the elevated glutamate levels play a role in the onset of the seizures.

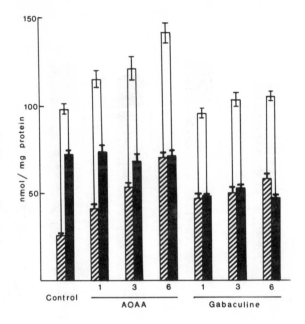

Fig. 4. Effect of AOAA (0.91 mmol/kg) and gabaculine (0.5 mmol/kg) on amino acid levels in synaptosomes. Hashed columns, GABA; solid columns, glutamate + glutamine + aspartate; open columns, GABA + glutamate + glutamine + aspartate; 1, 3 and 6 represent the time in hours after injection of the drugs; C, control. Data from Geddes, Wood (1983).

Although AOAA and gabaculine are potent GABA-T inhibitors, their effects on the amino acid contents of nerve endings differ dramatically (Fig. 4). The administration of gabaculine to mice induced not only an increase in synaptosomal GABA levels, but also decreases in the levels of aspartate, glutamate and glutamine such that the total content of the four amino acids in the nerve endings remains unchanged. A possible scenario for these related changes is as follows: The gabaculine-induced inhibition of GABA-T activity causes an increase in the concentration of substrate (GABA) and a decrease in the concentration of product (glutamate). The latter change, in turn, modulates positively the activity of glutaminase (Kvamme 1979) causing a decrease in glutamine level. In addition, the low (substrate) glutamate levels will reduce the activity of aspartate aminotransferase resulting in a decreased concentration of the product (aspartate). The constancy of the "four amino acid pool" after treatment of the mice with gabaculine suggests that the increased GABA content of nerve endings occurs at the expense of the related amino acids in the terminals, and is not due to exogenous GABA; thus answering the question raised earlier.

TABLE 3. EFFECT OF GABACULINE AND AOAA ON ENZYME ACTIVITIES IN MOUSE BRAIN

	Inhibition (%)	
ENZYME	Gabaculine	AOAA
Glutamate decarboxylase	2	41
GABA aminotransferase	62	100
Aspartate aminotransferase	3	35
Glutaminase	(-6)	1

Enzyme activities were measured in brain homogenates prepared from animals three hours after administration of gabaculine (0.5 mmol/kg) or AOAA (0.91 mmol/kg). Data from Geddes and Wood (1983).

In contrast to the situation with gabaculine, the administration of AOAA to mice causes increases in synaptosomal glutamate levels, decreases in aspartate levels and no change in glutamine levels, such that the total content of the three amino acids remains constant (Fig. 4). In view of the concomitant increases in the GABA levels, the total content of the four amino acids in the nerve endings rises dramatically with time after administration of AOAA. A probable explanation for these inter-related changes is the lack of specificity of AOAA with respect to enzyme inhibition (Table 3). AOAA inhibits both glutamate decarboxylase and GABA-T activities resulting in an increase in glutamate level due to the former inhibition, and a decrease in glutamate concentration due to the latter enzyme inhibition. The resulting overall change is a small increase in glutamate level which would appear insufficient to alter glutaminase activity and thus glutamine levels.

The AOAA-induced decrease in synaptosomal aspartate level would seem to be due to a direct inhibition of GABA-T activity (Table 3) and not to any lack of substrate as was the case with gabaculine.

SUMMARY AND CONCLUSIONS

The series of investigations described in this presentation clearly indicate the important role which the GABA content of the nerve endings plays in the functioning of the GABA inhibitory transmitter systems, and hence in controlling the excitable state of the brain. In addition they draw attention to the various factors which hinder a complete understanding of the situation, such as (i) the possible role of the excitatory amino acid transmitter substances in determining the excitable state of the brain; (ii) the compartmentation of GABA in the nerve endings and its implication with respect to the functioning of the GABA system; and (iii) the complex metabolic inter-relationships among the amino acids which also act as neurotransmitters. Clearly, much further study is required before a full understanding is possible.

ACKNOWLEDGEMENT

The authors thank the Medical Research Council of Canada (Grant No. MT 3301) for their financial support of the projects.

REFERENCES

Balcom GJ, Lennox TH, Meyerhoff JL (1975). Regional γ-amino buryric acid levels in rat brain determined after microwave fixation. J. Neurochem 24:609.

Berl S, Lajtha A, Walsch H (1961). Amino acid and protein metabolism. VI Cerebral compartments of glutamic acid metabolism. J. Neurochem 7:186.

Bradford HF (1982). "Neurotransmitter Interaction and Compartmentation" New York: Plenum Press, pp 1-839.

Cotman CW (1974). Isolation of synaptosomal and synaptic plasma fractions. In Fleischer S, Packer L (eds): "Methods in Enzymology, Vol 31", New York: Academic Press, p 445.

Frey H-H, Popp C, Loscher W (1979). Influence of inhibitors of the high affinity GABA uptake on seizure thresholds in mice. Neuropharmacol. 18:581.

Geddes JW, Wood JD (1983). Changes in the amino acid content of nerve endings (synaptosomes) induced by drugs which alter the metabolism of glutamate and GABA. J Neurochem (in press).

Graham LT, Aprison MH (1966). Fluorometric determination of aspartate, glutamate and γ-aminobutyrate in nerve tissue using enzymic methods. Anal Biochem 15:487.

Horton RW, Collins JF, Anlezark GM, Meldrum BS (1979). Convulsant and anticonvulsant actions in DBA/2 mice of compounds blocking the reuptake of GABA. Eur J Pharmacol 59:75.

Kuriyama K, Roberts E, Rubinstein MK (1966). Elevation of γ-aminobutyric acid in brain with aminooxyacetic acid and susceptibility to convulsive seizures in mice. A quantitative re-evaluation. Biochem Pharmacol 15:221.

Kvamme E (1979). Regulation of glutaminase and its possible implication for GABA metabolism. In Mandel P, DeFeudis FV (eds): "GABA Biochemistry and CNS Function", New York: Plenum Press, p 111.

Lenda K. Svenneby G (1980). Rapid high performance liquid chromatographic determination of amino acids in synaptosomal extracts. J Chromatog 198:516.

Matsuda M, Hoshino M, Sakurai T (1978). Synaptosomal γ-aminobutyric acid and glutamic acid contents and its relationships to convulsions. Jikeikai Med J 25:

Matsui Y, Deguchi T (1977). Effects of gabaculine, a potent new inhibitor of gamma-aminobutyrate transaminase, on the brain gamma-aminobutyrate content and convulsions in mice. Life Sci 20:1291.

Roberts PJ, Storm-Mathisen J, Johnston GAR (1981). "Glutamate: Transmitter in the Central Nervous System". New York: John Wiley and Sons Ltd, pp 1-226.

Shank RP, Graham LT (1978). The multiple roles of glutamate and aspartate in neural tissues. In Agranoff BW, Aprison MH (eds): "Advances in Neurochemistry, Vol 3", New York: Plenum Press, p 165.

Simler S, Ciesielski L, Maitre M, Randrianarisoa H, Mandel P (1973). Effect of sodium n-dipropylacetate on audiogenic seizures and brain γ-aminobutyric acid level. Biochem Pharmacol 22:1701.

Wood JD (1975). The role of γ-aminobutyric acid in the mechanism of seizures. Prog Neurobiol 5:77.

Wood JD (1981). Evaluation of a synaptosomal model for
    monitoring in vivo changes in the GABA and glutamate
    content of nerve endings. Int J Biochem 13:543.
Wood JD, Kurylo E, Tsui S-K (1981). Interactions of di-n-
    propylacetate, gabaculine and aminooxyacetic acid:
    anticonvulsant activity and the γ-aminobutyrate system.
    J Neurochem 37:1440.
Wood JD, Russell MP, Kurylo E, Newstead JD (1979). Stability
    of GABA levels and their use in determining the in vivo
    effects of drugs: convulsant agents. J Neurochem 33:61.
Wood JD, Russell MP, Kurylo E (1980). The γ-aminobutyrate
    content of nerve endings (synaptosomes) in mice after
    the intramuscular injection of γ-aminobutyrate-elevating
    agents: a possible role in anticonvulsant activity.
    J Neurochem 35:125.
Wood JD, Schousboe A, Krogsgaard-Larsen P (1980). In vivo
    changes in the GABA content of nerve endings (synap-
    tosomes) induced by inhibitors of GABA uptake.
    Neuropharmacol 19:1149.

Index